Microbial Approaches to Personalized Nutrition

Neethu Asokan
https://orcid.org/0000-0003-0742-3594
Sri Sathya Sai University for Human Excellence, India

Abdel Rahman Mohammad Said Al-Tawaha
Department of Biological Sciences, Al Hussein bin Talal University, Jordan

Santosh Kumar Singh
Sri Sathya Sai University for Human Excellence, India

Rajeshwari Ullagaddi
Sri Sathya Sai University for Human Excellence, India

IGI Global Scientific Publishing
Publishing Tomorrow's Research Today

Vice President of Editorial Melissa Wagner
Director of Acquisitions Mikaela Felty
Director of Book Development Jocelynn Hessler
Production Manager Mike Brehm
Cover Design Jose Rosado

Published in the United States of America by
IGI Global Scientific Publishing
701 East Chocolate Avenue
Hershey, PA, 17033, USA
Tel: 717-533-8845 | Fax: 717-533-7115
Website: https://www.igi-global.com E-mail: cust@igi-global.com

Library of Congress Cataloging-in-Publication Data

LCCN: 2025950948 (CIP Data Pending)
ISBN13: 9798337343822
Isbn13Softcover: 9798337343839
EISBN13: 9798337343846
British Cataloguing in Publication Data
A Cataloguing in Publication record for this book is available from the British Library.

"The end of education is character." — Bhagwan Sri Sathya Sai Baba

This book is humbly dedicated with reverence and gratitude to Almighty and whose eternal teachings help to light the way to knowledge, caring, and selfless services. We do dedicate this work with a lot of love to our students, scholars, and researchers whose quest to learn keeps the flame of inquiry burning. We offer our heartfelt tribute to our late Prof. Al-Tawaha *that through his wisdom, scholarship and guidance we still find ourselves being influenced by his genius even after his demise. It is dedicated to our families whose unwavering support, sacrifices and never-ending faith enabled us to have this scholastic pilgrimage.*

Table of Contents

Detailed Table of Contents

The human microbiome is a large group of microbes which plays a key role in nutrition and health. These microbes aid in digestion of food, production of vitamins and breakdown of dietary fibers. Microbial community also assist in regulating immune system and how one's body uses nutrients. An imbalanced microbiome (dysbiosis) can make us sick and develop obesity, diabetes and inflammation. The microbiome is influenced by birth method, breastfeeding and mother's diet in early life and can affect health. Researchers now have new tools; metagenomics, metabolomics which help understand how these microbes work and interact with body. The trend of using microbiome data for personalized nutrition is thinking to optimize health with respect to specific diets, probiotics, prebiotics. This chapter reviews how microbiome and nutrition interact and the roles that key functions play in impacting health and to put this knowledge into use in nutrition and medicine. This connection will enable us to develop better ways of dealing with diet-related diseases and to help prevent future health problems.

The synergy of microbiome analysis and metagenomics has transformed diet-microbe-host relationships, and this chapter delves into how bioinformatics tools and high-throughput sequence technologies are utilized to decipher gut microbiome structure and function and its pivotal role in human nutrition. Investigating microbial diversity, metabolic capacity, and relations between hosts and microbiomes reveals personalized dietary response and pathways underlying nutrient processing, energy homeostasis, and risk factors of chronic disease. This chapter outlines methodological strategies such as sequence analysis of the 16S rRNA gene, shotgun metagenomics, and integration of metabolomics and uses of these in personalized nutrition, biomarker development, and dietary intervention. Obstacles, implications, and future views of microbiome-guided nutrition are presented. This chapter offers an in-depth overview to inform investigators, clinicians, and nutrition experts working to apply microbiome information to precision health and optimal dietary regimes.

Nutritional sciences have been profoundly affected by the shift from malnourishment to overnutrition in various regions owing to factors including cultural diversity, lifestyle choices, environmental instability and food sustainability. By customizing dietary therapies to meet the unique needs of each person, personalized nutrition reimagines the role of probiotics, prebiotics, postbiotics, and synbiotics in healthy eating, with a focus on gastrointestinal illnesses and other condition-specific issues. With the advancement in technologies in-depth characterization of gut microbiota, revealing its composition, functional dynamics, and extensive microbial diversity have been enabled. Considering all aspects, in this chapter, we discussed how societal influence and advancements in functional biotics foods are driving individualized nutrition strategies for therapeutic and preventive healthcare. The main focus on gut biotics is at the forefront of innovations in human health, propelled by collaborative efforts paving the way for a new era of personalised and targeted healthcare.

The convergence of epigenomic and microbiome research marks a transformative step in precision medicine. The human microbiome, a diverse ecosystem shaping digestion, immunity, and metabolism, interacts with epigenetic mechanisms such as DNA methylation, histone modifications, and non-coding RNAs influenced by diet and microbial metabolites. Compounds like short-chain fatty acids, folate, and bile acid derivatives regulate key epigenetic enzymes (DNMTs, HATs, HDACs), modulating chromatin accessibility and gene expression tied to metabolic and immune functions. Epigenetic biomarkers, being reversible and environmentally responsive, offer dynamic insight into nutritional status and disease trajectories. Integrating metagenomic and epigenomic data enables stratification of microbiota-dependent epigenetic phenotypes, supporting personalized nutrition strategies. This chapter discusses mechanistic, clinical, and methodological advances shaping microbiome-driven precision nutrition.

The gut microbiome plays a pivotal role in shaping human metabolic health through complex interactions with diet. Dietary components influence microbial composition and activity, which in turn regulate nutrient metabolism and the production of microbial metabolites such as short-chain fatty acids, bile acid derivatives, and indoles. These metabolites act as signaling molecules affecting insulin sensitivity, inflammation, energy balance, and gut integrity. Inter-individual differences in gut microbiota partly explain variable responses to identical diets, highlighting the limitations of generalized dietary recommendations. This has led to the emergence of personalized and precision nutrition approaches that integrate microbiome profiles with dietary patterns to optimize metabolic outcomes. By linking diet–microbe interactions to

Food allergy is known to result due to a highly intricate interplay between food antigens, host immunity, and intestinal microbe composition. Imbalances in these factors could result in hypersensitivity. Pathways in food allergy include alterations in epithelial cell/tissue regeneration, along with improper immunity against food antigens, which leads to a boosted T-helper cell type 2 (Th2) response. Intestinal epithelial cells, which include stem cells, Paneth cells, mucus secreting goblet cells, and tuft cells, have been analyzed in terms of epithelial integrity. Inclusion of intestinal microbe composition also discovers gut microbe roles in epithelial cell/pathophysiology, which underlines short-chain fatty acid-mediated functions, microbial lactate, which points to other microbe metabolites. Inclusion of gut microbe composition on gut epithelial cell/pathophysiology also underlines microbe functions in maintaining epithelial cell/pathophysiology, clues of which include microbe-mediated secure functioning of tight junction proteins.

Microbial dysbiosis, defined as an imbalance in the composition and functional activity of microbial communities, has emerged as a major factor influencing host metabolic health. The human microbiota, which is mostly located in the Gut, Oral Cavity, Skin, and Vagina, is essential for nutrition metabolism, homeostasis, and immune system control. Changes in microbial abundance and diversity are linked to metabolic illnesses such as type 2 Diabetes, Obesity, Non-Alcoholic Fatty Liver Disorder, and even Metabolic Syndrome. These changes can be attributed to either an increase in opportunistic (e.g., Escherichia coli, Staphylococcus aureus, Prevotella) or decreased beneficial pathogens. The breakdown of intestinal barrier function, systemic inflammation, endotoxemia, changes in the production of Short-Chain Fatty Acids (SCFA), and distortion of the metabolism of glucose and fats are among the processes of dysbiosis. Additionally, microbial compounds such as Trimethylamine-N-Oxide (TMAO) promote insulin resistance with cardiovascular risk.

The gut microbiota is a critical component in the complex interplay of processes underlying cancer formation, progression, and treatment, which is now receiving recognition due to the abundance of microbes, numbering in the trillions, within the human gut. Advancements in microbiota-targeted approaches, including faecal microbiota transplantation (FMT), probiotic therapy, and dietary modification, hold significant potential for restoring microbial homeostasis, enhancing immune-mediated anti-tumour responses, mitigating treatment side effects, and addressing existing challenges such as protocol uniformity in microbiota manipulation, safety, long-term efficacy, and the complexity of microbial relationships. This review synthesises the cumulative insights into the dual role of gut microbiota as both an ally and an adversary in understanding cancer biology and treatment, serving as a salient biomarker and therapeutic target, and highlights research gaps that could be exploited to incorporate microbiome technology into personalised cancer management, aiming to maximise effectiveness.

Sumira Malik, Amity University, Ranchi, India
Rupjyoti Bharali, Biswanath College, India
Humayun Samir Ahmed Barbhuyan, St. John College, India
Jutishna Bora, Amity University, Ranchi, India
Smita Lata, Amity University, Ranchi, India
Ayush Madan, People's University, India

Microorganisms residing in the host gut collectively known as gut microbiota, plays a crucial role in the health of the host. The gut microbiota influences the immune system, cognitive abilty and other functions in an individual contributing towards the well-being of the individual. These gut colonizers eventually change throughout the life of an individual that are specific in nature. However, there is a set of conserved gut microbiota which is present in every individual. Longevity has been related to healthy aging referring to disease-free health in individuals which is further related to composition of gut microbiota. Life-style and dietary habits have been linked directly to impact the composition of these gut colonizers. An inclusive understanding of impact of gut microbiota interactions in longevity and on human body, are discussed in this chapter.

Saloua Mabsor-Zgandaoui, Biology and Health Laboratory, Department of Biology, Faculty of Sciences, Ibn Tofail University, Morocco

Ionizing radiation, whether environmental, diagnostic, or therapeutic, profoundly alters the gut microbiota, a key regulator of metabolism, nutrient absorption, and immunity. Radiation exposure disrupts microbial diversity, reduces beneficial taxa, and favors opportunistic species, impairing functions such as short-chain fatty acid production, vitamin synthesis, and bile acid metabolism. These disturbances weaken intestinal integrity and trigger systemic inflammation. In radiotherapy, especially for abdominal or pelvic cancers, dysbiosis is linked to gastrointestinal toxicity,

The microbiome-based nutrition is a revolutionary change in nutritional science since it identifies the gut microbiome as the key node between diet and human health. The conventional dietary advice has been mostly based on the population-wide guidelines, but there is increasing evidence to show that how individuals respond to food is highly dependent on the composition and the capacity of the gut microbial communities. Human gut microbiome, which contains trillions of microorganisms, is a dynamic and metabolic and immunological organ that regulates nutrient usage, energy, inflammatory response, and host physiology by generating bioactive metabolites, including short-chain fatty acid, vitamins, and signaling molecules. Recent developments in the high-throughput sequencing, multi-omics technologies, bioinformatics and artificial intelligence have sped up the comprehension of diet-microbiome-host interactions and made the possibility of precision and personalized nutrition strategies possible.

Preface

The recent developments in the microbiome science field have radically changed the knowledge of human nutrition, health, and disease. There is growing evidence to support that the gut microbiota is one of the most important factors involved in the digestion of nutrients, the regulation of metabolism, the regulation of the immune system, the neural signalling, and the maintenance of physiological homeostasis. The interactive processes of nutrients and microbial communities affect nutrient bioavailability and energy balance as well as predisposition to chronic diseases like obesity, diabetes, inflammatory diseases, cancer and neurological conditions. The findings have triggered the rise of personalized nutrition shifting away from generalized dietary advice to individualized nutritional plans by the constitution of microbiomes and metabolic reactions.

Personalized nutrition is becoming increasingly popular in the modern global setting as the healthcare frameworks are transformed into precision medicine and preventive health models. Conventional generalized dietary prescriptions are not usually capable of considering inter-individual variation caused by genetics, way of living, setting and diversity of microbes. The recent developments in the high-throughput sequencing, metagenomics, metabolomics, artificial intelligence and digital health technologies have rendered it more possible to profile individual microbiomes and design specific nutritional interventions. Microbial nutrition practices are an essential scientific area within this dynamic landscape that has proactive consequences on the overall health of the population, the nursing profession and wellness management.

Microbial Approaches to Personalized Nutrition is a compilation of interdisciplinary research on the nexus of microbiology and nutrition science and biotechnology and digital health. It discusses the role of gut microorganisms in the metabolism of nutrients, energy, immune system, disease susceptibility, and therapeutic effects. The amount of information to be found in the volume combines basic biological knowledge with translational and applied ones, providing understanding of microbial metabolites, probiotics and prebiotics, fermented foods, dysbiosis-related disorders, microbiome-based precision nutrition, and integration of new technologies, including metagenomics, artificial intelligence, and wearable health monitoring systems.

The targeted audience of this edited volume will be researchers, clinicians, nutritionists, biotechnologists, healthcare professionals, policy planners, graduate and post-graduate students. The book facilitates both theoretical research and the practical application with the integration of theoretical underpinnings and application-focused discourse. It is especially applicable to a person who is interested in learning how microbial science can be used to design personalized nutritional plans to promote health, prevent diseases, and optimize treatment.

INTRODUCTION TO CHAPTER CONTRIBUTIONS

Introduction to the Microbiome and Nutrition.

The chapter gives a background review of human microbiome and its connection to nutrition. It presents the major microbial communities, their formation and how they are useful during digestion and metabolism, which forms the conceptual framework that sequences the next chapters.

Metagenomics and Microbiome Analysis to get Nutritional Insights.

Giving a technological view, this chapter includes metagenomic tools and analytical methods to study the microbial communities, with the focus on the application of these methods in the nutritional studies and individual health assessment.

Custom sustenance through gut biotics, a promising way for gut well-being through a personalised manner

Nutritional sciences have been profoundly affected by the shift from malnourishment to overnutrition in various regions owing to factors including cultural diversity, lifestyle choices, environmental instability and food sustainability. By customizing dietary therapies to meet the unique needs of each person, personalized nutrition reimagines the role of probiotics, prebiotics, postbiotics, and synbiotics in healthy eating, with a focus on gastrointestinal illnesses and other condition-specific issues. With the advancement in technologies in-depth characterization of gut microbiota, revealing its composition, functional dynamics, and extensive microbial diversity have been enabled. Considering all aspects, in this chapter, we discussed how societal influence and advancements in functional biotics foods are driving individualized nutrition strategies for therapeutic and preventive healthcare. The main focus on gut biotics is at the forefront of innovations in human health, propelled by collaborative efforts paving the way for a new era of personalised and targeted healthcare.

Epigenetic Biomarkers In Microbiome-Driven Nutrition Therapy

The convergence of epigenomic and microbiome research marks a transformative step in precision medicine. The human microbiome, a diverse ecosystem shaping digestion, immunity, and metabolism, interacts with epigenetic mechanisms such as DNA methylation, histone modifications, and non-coding RNAs influenced by diet and microbial metabolites. Compounds like short-chain fatty acids, folate, and bile acid derivatives regulate key epigenetic enzymes (DNMTs, HATs, HDACs), modulating chromatin accessibility and gene expression tied to metabolic and immune functions. Epigenetic biomarkers, being reversible and environmentally responsive, offer dynamic insight into nutritional status and disease trajectories. Integrating metagenomic and epigenomic data enables stratification of microbiota-dependent epigenetic phenotypes, supporting personalized nutrition strategies. This chapter discusses mechanistic, clinical, and methodological advances shaping microbiome-driven precision nutrition.

Feeding Your Microbes Why What You Eat Matters

The gut microbiome plays a pivotal role in shaping human metabolic health through complex interactions with diet. Dietary components influence microbial composition and activity, which in turn regulate nutrient metabolism and the production of microbial metabolites such as short-chain fatty acids, bile acid derivatives, and indoles. These metabolites act as signaling molecules affecting insulin sensitivity, inflammation, energy balance, and gut integrity. Inter-individual differences in gut microbiota partly explain variable responses to identical diets, highlighting the limitations of generalized dietary recommendations. This has led to the emergence of personalized and precision nutrition approaches that integrate microbiome profiles with dietary patterns to optimize metabolic outcomes. By linking diet–microbe interactions to metabolic health, nutrition science is shifting toward targeted, microbiome-informed strategies for disease prevention and health promotion.

Microbial Metabolites and their role in human health.

This chapter dwells upon the systemic effects of microbial-derived metabolites including short-chain fatty acids, bile acid derivatives and neurotransmitter precursors that thrive in one-on-one nutrition programs, as they are particularly relevant in personalized nutrition.

Microbiota in Food Sensitivities and Allergies.

In this chapter, the authors examine the role of gut microbiota in food sensitivities and allergic reactions, the mechanisms of microbes, diagnostic, and nutritional interventions.

Dysbiosis in microbes and Metabolic Disorders.

The emphasis of this chapter is placed on microbial imbalance, which is related to metabolic imbalances, including obese, diabetes, and inflammatory diseases. It raises the issue of diagnostic signals and nutrition plans to restore the stability of microbes.

The Microbiota of the gut and cancer.

The chapter dwells upon the contribution of gut microbiota to cancer development, progression, and treatment response as the potential of personalized cancer treatment through nutrition and microbial strategies.

The Microbiota of the Gut and Longevity.

This chapter focuses on aging and lifespan; it talks on the impact of gut microbial composition on longevity, healthy aging, and age-associated metabolic and inflammatory alterations.

Intestinal Microbiota and the brain.

Dwelling upon the gut-brain axis, the chapter discusses the impact of microbes on neurological functions, mental health and behaviour, with the dietary modulation as a treatment approach.

Wearable and Digital health technologies in microbiome monitoring.

The chapter has been dedicated to the consideration of digital innovation, and it is based on wearable devices and digital platforms that facilitate real-time health tracking, dietary monitoring, and nutritional decisions based on microbiome information.

Nutritional Health AI-Based Microbiome Bio-markers.

In this chapter, the authors talk about the combination of artificial intelligence and machine learning to detect microbiome-based biomarkers. It emphasizes predictive modelling and information-based techniques of precision nutrition and health tracking.

Future View and Ethical Standpoints of Microbiome-Based Nutrition.

The final chapter is concerned with the new tendencies, ethical issues, data privacy, and regulatory aspects related to microbiome-based personalized nutrition.

Collectively, the chapters of this volume show a detailed and progressive view of microbial techniques on individual nutrition. This book helps in the development of the growing areas of precision nutrition and preventive medicine by combining the basics of science with technological advances and practice. It focus on research about the role of the microbiome in human health and offers future studies, clinical applications, and policy-making an opportunity. As individualized nutrition is becoming an inseparable part of the healthcare system, this book can be used as a key reference when formulating the research questions and enhancing patient health results with the help of microbiome-based dietary recommendations.

Acknowledgement

The editors wish to express their profound gratitude to all the contributing authors in their professional effort, intellectuality, and excellent endeavours to ensure the completion of this volume. Their professional skills, cooperation, and involvement into the peer-review and revision process have played a key role in creating an interdisciplinary and extensive resource on microbial responses to personalized nutrition.

We are very grateful to Sadguru Sri Madhusudan Sai, Chancellor, whose foresight, consistent encouragement, and unswerving emphasis on academic excellence and research-based programs have been very helpful. We also take this opportunity to express our gratitude and recognition of the directions and support of the Administrator, the Vice Chancellor Dr Srikanta Murthy and Registrar Dr Hanumanth Rao Naidu, who has developed the environment of study, cooperation and knowledge sharing in her administrative leadership and dedication to scholarly development.

The editors appreciate the great contributions of the reviewers to the quality, clarity and the level of scientific rigor of the chapters, as well as to the overall quality of the paper. The editorial and production staff of IGI Global is also given a special credit of the professional guidance and the support it offered and the careful coordination throughout the publication process.

The editors also note the support given by their respective universities and research facilities that have been supportive and institutional in encouraging interdisciplinary collaboration and innovation. Finally, we would like to thank the colleagues, mentors, and students whose intellectual discussions, enthusiasm and curiosity are continued to inspire research at the nexus of microbiology and nutrition science.

Introduction

A holistic appreciation of human microbiome is needed in understanding the ways humans participate and use nutrients. Conventional nutritional advice is conventionally based on the average values of the population, and it does not consider the individual differences in metabolism, genetics, lifestyle, and microflora. Personalized nutrition offers a solution to this shortcoming by customizing dietary plans to meet the profiles of the microbiome and other metabolic reactions in the individual.

Microbiological investigations have demonstrated that gut microbes are the centre stage in the digestion, macronutrient absorption, vitamin production, immunological regulation and even in the mental state. Whereas some microbial communities increase nutrient bioavailability and energy efficiency, microbial imbalances (dysbiosis) are becoming increasingly linked to obesity, diabetes, inflammatory diseases and cancer, as well as neurodegenerative conditions.

The viewpoints of microbiology, biotechnology, nutrition science, and digital health are combined in this book to offer a holistic overview of microbiome-based personalized nutrition. Some of the modern areas are microbial metabolites, functional foods, fermented foods, epigenetic and AI-based biomarkers, microbiome sequencing technologies, and wearable technologies that allow monitoring real-time health. The book is directed to the researchers, medical workers, nutritionists, and students, and it demonstrates the potential of microbial solutions to revise the approach to dietary interventions and play a role in the future of preventive and precision healthcare.

Chapter 1

Introduction to Microbiome and Nutrition

Aliza Falak
Quaid-i-Azam University, Islamabad, Pakistan

Banzeer Ahsan Abbasi
https://orcid.org/0000-0003-3036-4481
Rawalpindi Women University, Pakistan

Sameel Hassan
https://orcid.org/0009-0001-7559-5550
University of Tuscia, Italy

Tabassum Yaseen
Bacha Khan University, Charsadda, Pakistan

Muhammad Anas
https://orcid.org/0000-0001-5127-8043
Selçuk University, Turkey

Madiha Imtiaz
Bacha Khan University, Charsadda, Pakistan

Javed Iqbal
https://orcid.org/0000-0002-9032-2622
Bacha Khan University, Charsadda, Pakistan

ABSTRACT

The human microbiome is a large group of microbes which plays a key role in nutrition and health. These microbes aid in digestion of food, production of vitamins and breakdown of dietary fibers. Microbial community also assist in regulating immune system and how one's body uses nutrients. An imbalanced microbiome (dysbiosis) can make us sick and develop obesity, diabetes and inflammation. The microbiome is influenced by birth method, breastfeeding and mother's diet in early life and can affect health. Researchers now have new tools; metagenomics, metabolomics which help understand how these microbes work and interact with body. The trend of using microbiome data for personalized nutrition is thinking to optimize health with respect to specific diets, probiotics, prebiotics. This chapter reviews how microbiome and

DOI: 10.4018/979-8-3373-4382-2.ch001

nutrition interact and the roles that key functions play in impacting health and to put this knowledge into use in nutrition and medicine. This connection will enable us to develop better ways of dealing with diet-related diseases and to help prevent future health problems.

TABLE OF CONTENTS

INTRODUCTION

The human body is host to a vast and dynamic population of microorganisms collectively known as the microbiome *(*Gilbert et al., 2018*)*. Several types of microbes including bacteria, archaea, viruses and fungi live in our bodies specially in the gut where they form the largest studied community. Gut contains trillions of microbes arranged in a close relationship with us that affect many parts of human health *(*Rahman et al., 2023*)*. The microbial community participating inside our bodies takes active part in multiple nutrition and metabolism processes. Scientists have changed their understanding of biology by showing that the complex link between body systems and the different microbes matters in how the human body operates *(*Fan & Pedersen, 2021*)*.

Nutritional science previously studied macronutrients and micronutrients only now studies the essential role gut bacteria play in digestion and metabolism. Through fermentation the gut microbiota helps break down complex polysaccharides and produces SCFAs like acetate and butyrate when manufacturing vitamins B12 K and folate. The human body requires these vital functions since its genome lists few enzymes to break down specific food components. The digestive system in microbiota operates as a separate organ set to help the body digest nutrients beyond its basic capacity and boost its dietary intake (Rowland et al., 2018). The gut microbiota helps protect the host immune system and keeps the intestines intact by managing inflammation. The metabolism and immune systems of the microbiome work together through metabolism products that send signals that control energy balance eating habits and fat processing. A mismatch between community structures or diversity in gut microbiota triggers metabolic conditions which lead to obesity type 2 diabetes heart diseases and insulin resistance. Nutritional wellness depends on the presence of the microbiome both as a factor that shapes health and a mediator of its outcomes (Kim, 2018).

The makeup of gut microbiota changes constantly under influence of environmental and personal factors. Eating more fruits and plants adds diverse microbes to the gut while choosing many saturated fats and sugars leads to fewer healthy bacteria in the intestine. Individual gut bacteria patterns respond to various influences like age evolution, hereditary traits, stress levels, physical movement levels, antibiotic treatments and contact with external environments. Our bodies' adaptive responses to dietary changes drive new strategies that customize eating plans by analyzing what microbes are present and how they work in each person (Kolodziejczyk et al., 2019). Our microbiome develops its basic features and abilities during early childhood that shape our body's health through adulthood. Initial development of gut microbes starts in a newborn subject to various delivery methods and factors like breast milk feeding and feeding choices. Early life disruptions affect how our metabolism and immune system grow which may raise our risk to develop lifelong health problems. Research into how the microbiome develops between infancy and adulthood will help create strategies that preserve good health throughout life (Dogra et al., 2021).

New sequencing technologies and analytical tools help doctors understand both how many types and what types of microbes live inside us through microbe research studies. Research methods like Metagenomics and Meta-transcriptomics plus Metabolomics and Proteomics help scientists better understand how bacteria affect health and disease which leads to microbiome-based medical treatments. Doctors now treat digestive conditions with live beneficial microbes and non-digestible food ingredients along with their combinations. These approaches offer potential ways to improve nutrition status and help the gut system better process food while returning to a healthy balance (Hadrich, 2018). People in the nutrition field increasingly want to bring microbiome knowledge into public health programs. Successful treatment depends on joining many fields of research plus testing solid effects and following ethical rules about changing body bacteria. By combining microbiome research with nutrition experts can use tailored diets to benefit health at the individual level while protecting against diseases (Wilkinson et al., 2021).

THE HUMAN MICROBIOME: COMPOSITION AND FUNCTIONS

The human microbiome includes many microorganisms living in different body parts such as the skin, mouth, lungs, urogenital system, and especially the gut. The gut microbiome represents the most complex and active microbial community by hosting approximately 100 trillion microorganisms which exceed human cell counts by factor of 1.3:1. The primary bacterial phylum groups found in human guts are Firmicutes along with Bacteroidetes and Actinobacteria and Proteobacteria. The microbiome shows major differences between individuals because different genetic and environmental and lifestyle elements shape each person's unique microbiome picture (Scepanovic et al., 2019).

The intestinal environment demonstrates irregular distribution patterns regarding microbial populations. The stomach together with the small intestine contain reduced microbial counts because of acidic conditions and rapid food movement but the colon functions as the main space for microbial fermentation and nourishment and microbial cell expansion. Host bacteria establish positive microbial relationships which help the host acquire nutrients while defending the body from infectious agents and manage immune responses while preserving health in the mucosal lining (Cao et al., 2022).

The digestion along with fermentation of complex dietary polysaccharides exists as a vital function of the microbiome. The gastrointestinal tract uses carbohydrate-active enzymes (CAZymes) from microbes to decompose complex plant fibers into small-chain fatty acids that include mainly acetate propionate and butyrate. Butyrate and other SCFAs serve two functions within the colon first as cellular energy sources for colonocytes whereas secondly, they function as signaling molecules which affect both lipid metabolism and glucose regulation and neurological functions through the gut-brain axis (Myhrstad et al., 2020).

Nutrients necessary for human health are produced by the microbiome in conjunction with its SCFA production capability. Gut bacteria possess the ability to create B-group vitamins including folate together with biotin and thiamine and riboflavin and vitamin K. The biosynthetic pathways augment the nutritional needs of the host organism and substantially support total micronutrient balance levels. The gut flora enables the transformation and deconjugation of bile acids through its enzymes which result in changes to both lipid digestion and cholesterol metabolic processes (Ramírez-Pérez et al., 2018).

The immune system of the host undergoes developmental training by the gut microbiota starting from childhood. The gut-associated lymphoid tissue (GALT) develops through this mechanism while the balance between pro-inflammatory and anti-inflammatory immune responses regulates, and mucosal barrier integrity improves because the microbiota promotes production of mucus and antimicrobial peptides. Commensal microbes maintain healthy resistance against pathogens by creating space through colonization resistance that stops harmful species from growing (Dogra et al., 2021).

Health professionals regard both diversity and resilience of microbiomes as crucial markers in assessing overall health status. The composition of microbiota affects both the adaptability of organisms and their range of metabolic functions in positive ways. Medical research has shown that reduced microbial diversity leads to various health problems including inflammatory bowel disease yet also produces metabolic syndrome alongside neurodevelopmental complications and certain types of cancer. For humans to function at their optimal best it is necessary to hold bacteria at equilibrium (Bello et al., 2018).

The human microbiome serves as an essential biological component that runs the body like a system with digestive capabilities and immunity defense alongside nutrient synthesis and metabolic control functions. The microbiome demonstrates flexible composition and operations to adjust to environmental changes but its ability to thrive becomes a risk factor during encounters with poor diet or infections and antibiotic overuse events. The fundamental knowledge about microbiome baseline characteristics and core functions creates a base for investigating its relationship with nutrition which follows in later sections (Kim, 2018).

Table 1. Key features of the gut microbiome, including its dominant phyla, density, anatomical distribution, and core functions such as SCFA production. The table summarizes foundational aspects of microbial composition and activity, highlighting their role in digestion, nutrient processing, and gut health.

Feature/Aspect	Description	Key Microbial Players/ Mechanisms	Citation
Dominant Phyla	Major bacterial groups in the gut	Firmicutes, Bacteroidetes, Actinobacteria, Proteobacteria	(Alam et al., 2020)
Microbial Density	Microbial cell numbers in the gastrointestinal tract	~100 trillion microbial cells in the gut	(Flint, 2020)
Anatomical Distribution	Distribution varies across gastrointestinal sections	Low in stomach; high in colon	(Collins et al., 2024)
SCFA Production	Fermentation of dietary fibers to produce energy-rich short-chain fatty acids	Acetate, propionate, butyrate	(Quagebeur et al., 2023)
Vitamin Biosynthesis	Microbial synthesis of essential vitamins	B1, B2, B6, B12, folate, biotin, vitamin K	(Yuan et al., 2020)
Carbohydrate Degradation	Breakdown of complex polysaccharides	Carbohydrate-active enzymes (CAZymes)	(Wardman et al., 2022)

continued on following page

Table 1. Continued

Feature/Aspect	Description	Key Microbial Players/ Mechanisms	Citation
Bile Acid Metabolism	Microbial transformation and deconjugation of bile acids	Involves bile salt hydrolases (BSH)	(Foley et al., 2019)
Immune System Modulation	Education and regulation of host immune responses	Development of GALT, regulation of cytokines, Treg induction	(Delgobo et al., 2019)
Barrier Integrity Support	Maintenance of intestinal epithelial barrier	Stimulates mucus, antimicrobial peptides	(Okumura & Takeda, 2018)
Colonization Resistance	Protection against pathogens through competition	Competitive exclusion, niche occupation	(Quinn et al., 2022)
Neuroactive Compound Production	Synthesis of molecules influencing brain function	GABA, serotonin, dopamine precursors	(Wall et al., 2014)
Metabolic Regulation	Influence on host lipid, glucose, and energy metabolism	SCFA-mediated signaling pathways	(Shimizu et al., 2019)
Inflammation Control	Modulation of pro- and anti-inflammatory responses	IL-10 induction, NF-κB pathway modulation	(Preshaw, 2018)
Microbial Diversity	Richness and evenness of microbial species	Marker of resilience and health	(Philippot et al., 2021)
Dysbiosis	Disruption in microbiota composition	Associated with diseases like obesity, IBD, diabetes	(Gao et al., 2018)
Inter-Individual Variability	Differences in microbiome composition between individuals	Influenced by genetics, diet, environment, lifestyle	(Chen et al., 2022)
Influence of Antibiotics	Alteration of microbial communities	Reduces diversity may cause opportunistic infections	(Huang et al., 2022)
Role in Nutrient Absorption	Microbes facilitate uptake of minerals and nutrients	Increases bioavailability of calcium, iron, magnesium	(Sardans et al., 2023)
Maturation of Immune Tissues	Helps develop immune architecture in early life	Gut-associated lymphoid tissue (GALT)	(Bemark et al., 2024)
Developmental Programming	Early-life microbiome shapes long-term health	Influences metabolic and immune trajectories	(Zhou et al., 2019)

GUT MICROBIOTA AND NUTRIENT METABOLISM

The gut microbiota plays a central role in modulating nutrient metabolism, extending far beyond passive interaction with dietary intake. This community is metabolically versatile and, by direct biochemical transformations that supplement the host enzymatic limitations, directly contributes to the host's energy balance and nutrient acquisition (Rowland et al., 2018). Dietary fibres that are not digestible by human enzymes can be fermented by the gut microbiota into short chain fatty acids (SCFAs) which is one of the most studied metabolic functions of the gut microbiota. Acetate, propionate, and butyrate (the metabolites) are key energy sources for colonocytes and exert systemic effects, by modulating glucose homeostasis, appetite regulation and lipid metabolism. Butyrate is necessary to maintain intestinal epithelial integrity, and possesses anti-inflammatory effects (Barone et al., 2022). The microbiota also improves the absorption of micronutrients. In such a case, microbial metabolism may alter non absorbable dietary forms of iron to more bioavailable states or synthesize vitamins e.g. folate, biotin, riboflavin that contribute to the host's vitamin pool. The role of vitamin K2 (mainly produced by bacterial species Bacteroides, Eubacterium, etc.) in blood coagulation, deciduous bone metabolism is very important. Some Lactobacillus and Bifidobacterium strains produce B group vitamins and as such, some of the microbiota's contribution to micronutrient sufficiency can be considered comparable (Das et al., 2019).

Vanillin is synthesized in protein metabolism by microbial deamination and decarboxylation processes, the products of which are also bioactive amines and branched chain fatty acids. Some of these compounds are positive for gut health, but others, like ammonia, phenols and hydrogen sulfide, can be bad if produced to excess, particularly under high protein, low fiber dietary patterns (Brown et al., 2023). As a result, the balance between good and bad metabolites derives from the diet and depends on the existing microbial composition. The microbiome also influences lipid metabolism through the modulation of the bile acid profile. Microbial enzymes convert primary bile acids synthesized in the liver into secondary bile acids that are important for lipid digestion, cholesterol reabsorption, and deter lipid and glucose homeostasis through farnesoid X receptor (FXR) and G protein coupled bile acid receptor 1 (TGR5) as signaling molecules (Kolodziejczyk et al., 2019).

Another crucial territory where gut microbiota works is the polyphenol metabolism. Due to their antioxidant properties, this plant derived compounds are extensively metabolized by gut microbes into smaller more absorbable and more bioactive molecules. The polyphenol interindividual bioavailability variability is primarily dependent on the composition and enzymatic capacity of the gut microbiota, and the association between microbial diversity and individual responses to certain food components is established (Bešlo et al., 2023; Yao et al., 2024).

In addition, microbiomes play a key role in microbial metabolism of amino acids such as the synthesis of essential amino acids, such as tryptophan, which is a precursor for serotonin, kynurenine and indole derivatives (Ma & Ma, 2019). The concentrations of these metabolites also affect the gut and influence several neurological and immunological axes, leading to direct links between nutritional metabolism and systemic health through the gut immune and brain axes (Hou et al.,

2023). Collectively, these functions establish the microbiota as a tissue critical for a functionally integrated, metabolic organ that can aid in nutrient breakdown and synthesis as well as signal host physiology via a complex metabolic dialogue. The type of metabolic products that can be used by the host is mediated by a balanced diet that provides optimal microbiota-mediated nutrient metabolism (Lee et al., 2022).

INFLUENCE OF DIET ON MICROBIAL COMPOSITION

Diet stands as one of the most potent and modifiable factors influencing the composition, diversity, and function of the gut microbiota. The composition and nutrients found in what people eat determine precisely how their gut bacteria will grow. Our daily eating habits lead to microbial changes that happen fast, yet our regular food choices create lasting microbial patterns. Through its response to external events the microbiome connects the inside of the body to the outside world (Rinninella et al., 2019). A plant-rich diet with plenty of fiber helps Bifidobacterium and Lactobacillus bacteria grow to ferment complex sugars into SCFAs. Butyrate and other SCFAs produced by gut microbes enhance living tissue in the intestine and act as an anti-inflammatory agent with metabolic control functions. Having a diet that includes real grains, beans, fruits, and vegetables leads to more types of gut bacteria in our system which defines its ability to stay healthy and operate effectively (Oliver et al., 2021).

Western eating habits make the gut environment more suitable for Alistipes and Bilophila bacteria while lowering total friendly gut bacteria. Eating habits that promote proteolytic fermentation in the digestive system produce dangerous metabolic waste products that break down gut walls and increase body-wide inflammation. Protein source also matters. Different dietary fats support various microbes in our gut since polyunsaturated and monounsaturated acids foster anti-inflammatory patterns yet saturated fats foster species that initiate endotoxemia and insulin resistance. Fermented foods including yogurt and sauerkraut supply live microorganisms with bioactive components that improve the diversity of gut microorganisms. Eating healthy foods rich in polyphenols changes gut bacteria and creates a positive loop that helps gut and body health (Christ et al., 2019).

Consuming foods with non-digestible fibers benefits microbiota through their use specifically by beneficial gut microorganisms. Inulin and other natural fiber compounds help good bacteria named Bifidobacteria and Lactobacilli grow while reducing harmful bacteria populations by boosting SCFA production (Mukherjee et al., 2024). Research shows that artificial sweeteners saccharin and sucralose cause changes to the gut microbiome which harm glucose metabolism and make gut conditions unhealthy. Our gut bacteria need both new types of food plus various food items to reach their full number. When diets have limited variety, they help less microbes grow which weakens our resistance to stress and protects us against infection. The eating patterns of today's cities affect how people mostly eat as they consume many processed foods with low fiber content (Cantu-Jungles & Hamaker, 2020).

MICROBIOME-DRIVEN NUTRITIONAL DISORDERS

Alterations in the gut microbiota, commonly referred to as dysbiosis, have been increasingly recognized as both contributors to and indicators of various nutritional and metabolic disorders. The irregular microbial mix creates problems with metabolism and nutrient processing while starting inflammation throughout the body. Research now shows that microbiome imbalances play a main role in developing chronic diseases, especially nutritional disorders (Singh et al., 2021).

Research has thoroughly examined how obesity relates to gut microbiota balance issues. People who have obesity tend to show a decrease in their species variety and a shift in bacterium types especially between Firmicutes and Bacteroidetes, but results differ among studies. The gut microorganisms in obese bodies enhance food breakdowns particularly through boosting carbohydrate fermentation into easy-to-absorb short-chain fatty acids. The inflammatory response in the body from gram-negative bacteria lipopolysaccharides (LPS) spreads through the intestinal walls to create low-grade body wide infection which affects insulin sensitivity and damages fat cells (Vallianou et al., 2019).

The signatures of decreased SCFA-producers and more harmful bacteria seen in microbiome samples of T2D patients also appear in samples from insulin-resistant people. The reduced number of butyrate-producers weakens gut protection which lets microbial components enter the system and trigger inflammation problems while breaking down glucose control and insulin response. Pathological processes driving metabolic endotoxemia start with LPS produced by microbiome bacteria as its main initiator (Scheithauer et al., 2020).

Microbes contribute significantly to the development of heart diseases known as CVDs. Gut bacteria process choline and L-carnitine nutrients from red meat and eggs to form TMA which the liver converts into TMAO. Microbial metabolism produces TMAO which strongly increases cardiovascular disease risk and damages blood vessels demonstrating how gut bacteria impact remote body parts. Undernutrition together with micronutrient deficiency creates damage to microbial health. Studies show that severe malnourished children have poor gut microbiota that fails to produce enough energy and helps proper immune development. Lack of certain vitamins in the diet makes the gut microbiota unhealthy while microbiota problems worsen mineral absorption into the system. These two processes feed off each other in harmful loops (Zhen et al., 2023).

People with inflammatory bowel diseases Crohn's and ulcerative colitis present a clear gut bacterial imbalance of disease when they show less helpful *Faecalibacterium prausnitzii* and more harmful *Enterobacteriaceae* bacteria. These transformations boost intestinal inflammation and damage the intestinal barrier while changing how the body soaks up nutrients. The inflammatory bowel diseases show how microbe problems directly affect proper nutrient absorption (Kundra et al., 2021).

Celiac disease shows special ways through which the microbiome affects the health of gluten-sensitive patients. Research shows that microbiome imbalances occur equally in celiac patients who have not started treatment and in patients receiving treatment. Some scientists believe that specific microbial signatures trigger gluten intolerance when combined with immune reactions. The damaged intestine from villous atrophy stops absorbing nutrients and causes iron, calcium, folate, fat-soluble vitamin, and other nutrient shortfalls (Valitutti et al., 2019).

Microbiota's interaction with our digestive system helps our body break down milk sugar at those who have lactose intolerance. After consuming dairy foods people without enough lactase support their digestion when microbiota contains *Lactobacillus* or *Bifidobacterium* bacteria which transform lactose in the colon to ease digestive symptoms (JanssenDuijghuijsen et al., 2024).

These results prove that natural microbe changes affect our diet and wellness by various body system impacts. Research on how microbes affect nutritional diseases reveals new treatment options best achieved by balancing gut microorganisms using food choices and medical procedures. Our health objective is to restore gut bacteria balance to aid proper nutrient breakdown and fight illness advancement (Abdulsalam et al., 2024).

Figure 1. Microbiome-driven nutritional disorders and associated health impacts. Dysbiosis alters gut microbial composition, contributing to various metabolic, immune, and gastrointestinal conditions including obesity, type 2 diabetes, cardiovascular diseases, undernutrition, inflammatory bowel diseases, celiac disease, and lactose intolerance.

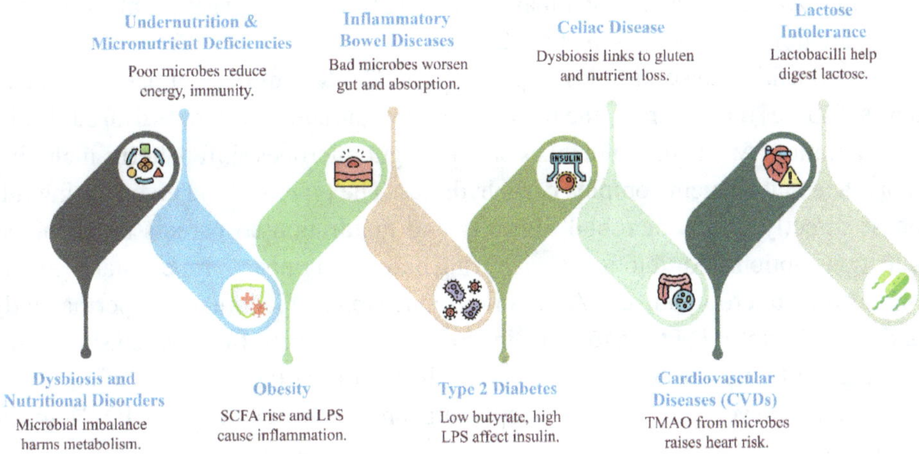

EARLY-LIFE MICROBIOTA AND LONG-TERM HEALTH

The establishment of the gut microbiota begins at birth and undergoes rapid changes during the first three years of life, a critical window during which foundational microbial communities are shaped. At a young age microbe colonization sets up biological processes that affect metabolic health as well as protect against disease and determine brain function. When the gut microbiota development gets disrupted, it leads someone more likely to develop health problems like allergic reactions, weight problems, autoimmune conditions, and metabolic issues (Walker, 2017).

The baby receives most of the early microbial exposure through the birth process. Newborns delivered through the vagina obtain their first microbial passengers mainly from their mother's vaginal and intestinal system which contains *Lactobacillus*, *Prevotella*, and *Bifidobacterium* microorganisms. Children born through cesarean delivery receive more skin-related bacteria because their exposure to hospital germs combines with Staphylococcus, Corynebacterium, and Propionibacterium species. Studies show cesarean delivery raises a child's chances of developing asthma problems with their skin and becoming obese over time (Korpela, 2021).

The microorganisms living inside a nursing infant strongly depend on whether a mother breastfeeds or not. Human breast milk contains vital nutrients and bioactive compounds such as HMOs that specially support the growth of *Bifidobacterium longum* subsp. *infantis*. Formula-fed infants tend to develop a more diverse but less beneficial microbial profile, often with a greater abundance of *Clostridium* and *Enterobacteriaceae*, which may contribute to increased risk of infections and Inflammation (Van den Elsen et al., 2019).

The transition to solid foods, typically around 4 to 6 months of age, introduces new substrates that diversify the microbiome and initiate a shift toward an adult-like configuration. As the new diet takes effect the gut microbes shift patterns including more taxa that ferment complex carbohydrates. The types of food given during this phase directly affect microbial diversity and maturation so parents must choose nutritious options. Antibiotics taken during babyhood impact proper establishment of intestinal microorganisms. Antibiotics reduce many good microbes permanently and allow harmful bacteria to grow inappropriately. Scientific research shows that starting antibiotics early in life raises the chance of getting obese, allergic, type 1 diabetic, and developing neurodevelopmental problems including ADHD (Nogacka et al., 2018).

Immunity develops through each stage of early life that depends on the presence of gut microbiome. Gut microbes help develop regulatory T cells while strengthening immune defenses in the body's surfaces plus producing immunoglobulin A. When the gut bacteria maintain a proper balance, it helps the body to tolerate normal substances while lowering the chances of developing immune and allergic conditions. Poor immune education results when microbiota is not properly balanced or developed leading to increased risk of chronic inflammation and immune system disorders (Jain, 2020).

Scientists now believe that the first microbiome influences brain growth through its connection to the gut and the nervous system. Metabolic activity of gut bacteria produces SCFAs and indole derivatives alongside neurotransmitter precursors which affect how the brain responds to stress and controls behavior. Studies indicate that different gut microbiota patterns at birth lead to variations in infant temperament and cognitive abilities, but scientists need to explore the direct links (Cong et al., 2015).

The types of bacteria that exist during infancy drive our future health outcomes. The path of microbial growth depends on how babies enter the world plus what they eat while newborn and how much time they spend exposed to antibiotics plus their daily living environment. The health of the early microbiome depends on supporting practices like vaginal delivery first, extended breast milk feeding, late antibiotics usage and adding fiber in solid foods. Future research will test methods to improve a mother's microbial profile before birth to strengthen her infant's natural microbial development (Martinez, 2014).

PERSONALIZED NUTRITION AND MICROBIOME PROFILING

The concept of personalized nutrition represents a significant advancement in dietary science, recognizing that individual responses to foods are not uniform and are heavily influenced by the gut microbiome. Microbial communities are very different in all individuals and have direct influences on how we process, absorb and use nutrients. As a tool, microbiome profiling of the composition and functional potential of an individual's gut microbiota has become foundational in the process of deciding precisely which nutrients to recommend helping individuals best achieve desired health outcomes (Li, 2023).

Normal dietary guidelines are population adapted, with broad intentions of applicability. Although, increasing evidence shows that two people having the same meals may have very diverse glycemic responses, lipid profiles, or metabolite outputs. Part of these differences are explained by different microbial taxa and enzymatic and metabolite production. For instance, some bacteria may be better at fermenting complex carbohydrates forming SCFAs, others to increase amino acid or polyphenol bioavailability, etc. The variability of (healthy) microbes behind this principle that "one size does not fit all when it comes to nutrition" for supporting optimal metabolic health (van Zanten, 2023).

Personalized nutrition utilizing microbiome data consists of sequencing microbial DNA from stool samples using technologies such as 16S rRNA gene sequencing or whole metagenome shotgun sequencing. These impose not only the microbial taxa but also their genes for functional, pathways from a metabolic point of view and how they may interact with dietary components. Microbiome profiles coupled with metabolic, phenotypic and lifestyle data can inform the development of dietary plans to promote beneficial microbes and suppress harmful ones (Zmora, 2019).

Microbiome guided nutrition is one of the practical ways to manage postprandial glycemic control. In second scenario, people were presented with personalized diets that would mitigate glycemic spikes according to their microbiota composition, dietary behaviour and blood markers. The results showed that the intervention outperformed standard dietary advice, supporting microbiome data as an indicator for the prediction of how personalized nutrition strategies will impact future health (Rouskas et al., 2025).

An area of use is also weight management. Certain microbial signatures have been linked to increased abilities to store energy, inflammation and fat. Personalized interventions may modulate the abundance of such microbes through specific prebiotics, probiotics, or dietary patterns for bettering metabolic flexibility and weight loss. In addition, personalized nutrition also pertains to micronutrient optimization. For instance, such individuals can consider dietary modifications or supplementation since they have low abundance of vitamin B12 producing microbes. In a parallel, diets rich in polyphenols may be more advantageous in individuals with microbes that can metabolize such polyphenols to bioactive forms (Eslami et al., 2025).

Artificial intelligence and machine learning can be combined with microbiome research, which greatly improves the potential of personalized nutrition. And predictive algorithms can look through millions of datasets for patterns and fill an algorithm where the food item could be matched with an individual's specific microbiota profile and health goals. As more data is available, these models are refined and the models become more and more precise at personalizing (Verma et al., 2018).

Despite its promise, challenges remain. The composition of the microbiome is dynamic, thereby susceptible to changes as short as the duration and timing of diet, and use of medications, circadian rhythms and psycho-social stress. Thus, to be suitable for temporal variability and applicable over time, personalized nutrition models are needed. Ethical considerations, data privacy, and the need for robust clinical validation also warrant attention before widespread clinical application (Verma et al., 2018).

In brief, the profile of personal microbiome reveals a new way to individualize dietary intervention instead of conventional generalized intervention. It is possible to design diets that maximize health, prevent disease and support overall well being by taking advantage of each person's own unique metabolic capabilities, those of their gut microbiota. The significance of this paradigm shift is that it heralds in a new era of nutritional science that is data driven, microbiome informed and highly personalized (Bhuiyan & Nahid, 2025).

PROBIOTICS, PREBIOTICS, AND DIETARY INTERVENTIONS

Modulating the gut microbiome through diet offers a promising strategy to enhance health and prevent or manage disease. Dietary tools known as probiotics and prebiotics with their combination synbiotics represent the most studied and effective dietary instruments to support this purpose. These treatments work to preserve the microbial equilibrium while boosting beneficial bacteria and inhibiting dangerous microorganisms and growing health-promoting substances made by the microbes *(Bandyopadhyay & Mandal, 2014)*.

The definition of probiotics entails living microorganisms that produce health benefits to their human recipients when consumed in recommended dosages. The most frequently used probiotic microorganisms within the gut microbiome belong to Lactobacillus, Bifidobacterium, Saccharomyces and specific Bacillus species. These healthy bacteria effectively maintain gut membrane health while adjusting immune reactions and treat irritable bowel syndrome (IBS) symptoms and help the microbiota recover after antibiotic treatments. Through their actions probiotics execute three functions: they claim colonization sites from pathogens and produce antimicrobial agents and adjust cytokine production in the host. Strains of these organisms can provide two vital functions by generating vitamins B12 and folate as well as enhancing lactose tolerance and absorption (Maldonado Galdeano et al., 2015).

Prebiotics represent non-digestible compounds in dietary substances that trigger beneficial microbial development and improved function of helpful microorganisms in the body. The prebiotic compounds primarily include fibers together with oligosaccharides which include inulin and fructo-oligosaccharides (FOS) and galacto-oligosaccharides (GOS). Since prebiotics function as food sources within the digestive system for beneficial bacteria they generate short-chain fatty acids (SCFAs) that both influence pH levels and block harmful microbes and promote healthy epithelial tissue. Studies show prebiotics used routinely improve intestinal calcium absorption rates as well as immune system responses and lipid profile health and create greater feelings of satiety in users (Valero-Cases et al., 2020).

Synbiotics unite prebiotics with probiotics to improve probiotic survival in the gut along with stimulating beneficial bacteria naturally present in the human body. Studies using clinical subjects demonstrate that synbiotics produce better metabolic disorder results and decreased inflammation levels while improving nutrient absorption better than when using probiotics or prebiotics separately *(Bandyopadhyay & Mandal, 2014)*.

Wider changes in food consumption prove to have substantial long-term impacts on how the microbiome develops. Consuming foods containing multiple types of fiber from whole grains and legumes and fruits and vegetables supports saccharolytic bacteria that generate health-essential butyric acid and other short-chain fatty acids. Multiple research studies show how polyphenol-rich foods enhance *Akkermansia muciniphila* and Bifidobacterium together with Lactobacillus species while positively affecting the microbiome. These foods include berries, tea, cocoa and extra virgin olive oil. Food fermentation creates products like kefir, yogurt, kimchi, sauerkraut and miso which bring beneficial microorganisms plus natural compounds that rebuild gut biodiversity and strengthen mucosal defenses and generate a healthy gut environment. Consistent intake of such foods produces parallel reductions in inflammatory markers along with gastrointestinal improvements (Whitman et al., 2024).

The consumption of high-fat together with sugary diet along with ultra-processed foods results in decreased microbiome diversity while creating a pro-inflammatory environment that allows bile-tolerant bacteria. The dysbiosis changes affect how the body absorbs nutrients while simultaneously producing metabolic endotoxemia that leads to long-term diseases. The long-term dietary preferences shape the gut microbiota more strongly compared to short-period usage of probiotics or prebiotics. The emergence of precision prebiotics targets selected microbial pathways while postbiotics refers to non-viable cells and metabolites produced from microorganisms that deliver health advantages. Scientifically developed products from new research areas show promise as therapeutic agents despite their inability to preserve viability and shelf life of live microorganisms (Zinöcker & Lindseth, 2018).

The three strategies of probiotics prebiotics along with dietary measures create a complete system which advances microbiome health by improving nutrient management and immune control alongside gastrointestinal intactness. A variety of elements such as specific bacterial strain types, exact dosage amounts, food consumed, and the makeup of the host microbial community determine how effective these microbiome interventions will be. Food-based fiber-rich diets along with minimal nutrient-processing present the foundation for supporting both microbial health and overall nutritional well-being (Fang et al., 2025).

TECHNOLOGICAL ADVANCES IN MICROBIOME RESEARCH

Recent technological breakthroughs have revolutionized our understanding of the human microbiome, transforming it from a mysterious "black box" into a highly accessible and quantifiable component of human biology. These advances have allowed scientists to move beyond taxonomic composition of microbial communities to their functional roles, interactions, and contributions to health and disease, with a focus on nutrition as a crucial factor (Utreja, 2023). Next generation sequencing (NGS), particularly 16S rRNA gene sequencing, is one of the most transformative tools, which allows identification of bacterial taxa on the basis of conserved genetic markers. It gives a detailed overview of the composition of the microbial community, and it's possible to compare individuals, populations and dietary interventions. While 16S sequencing can only provide taxonomic resolution it is still widely used because it is cost effective and highly scalable (Almonacid et al., 2017).

Whole-metagenome shotgun sequencing (WMGS) is a technique that sequences all genomic content within a sample for deeper insights into microbial functionality. Our approach reveals functional genes and metabolic pathways and reveals strain level changes that yield a much greater understanding of how microbiota affects nutrient metabolism, drug interactions and immune response (Joseph & Pe'er, 2021). Using constraints from these studies, paired with the gene model established by assembly of the genome, WMGS was instrumental in mapping microbial capabilities including ability to synthesize vitamins, ferment fiber, transform bile acids and metabolize amino acids. Unlike metagenomics, meta-transcriptomics shows which microbial genes are active under certain diets or conditions. It is critical to achieve this level of temporal resolution to understand the dynamic impact of dietary changes or interventions on microbial activity beyond stating they are present (Zhang et al., 2021).

Genomic approaches are complemented by metabolomics that identify the metabolites produced by microbiota at the small molecule level. Consequently, many of the SCFAs, amino acid derivatives, bile acids and neurotransmitter precursors directly mediate host physiology. Metabolomic profiling is commonly used on platforms of mass spectrometry and nuclear magnetic resonance (NMR) spectroscopy, and these aids in linking microbial activity to the metabolic outputs and nutritional status. In addition to genomics, proteomics offers functional insights into microbial proteins such as enzymes that breakdown nutrients and produce metabolites. Researchers can correlate specific proteins with metabolic pathways to understand the mechanistic underpinnings of microbiome-host interactions (Saak et al., 2023; Tang, 2011).

These multi-omics systems are integrated into the systems biology to provide a holistic view of the microbiome's role in human nutrition. Vast datasets are processed and interpreted with advanced bioinformatics pipelines and machine learning algorithms, and biomarkers are identified while complex diet, microbiota, and host health interactions are modeled. These serve as tools in developing predictive models for personal nutrition as well as therapeutic interventions (Son et al., 2020). Recently, cultivation culturomics using a MALDI-TOF mass spectrometry platform has recently revived interest in the isolation and characterization of novel 'unculturable' microbes. This method increases diversity of known microbiomes and allows testing function of isolated strain in controlled environment, which experimentally confirms sequencing findings (Lagier et al., 2015). At the same time, gnotobiotic animal models (especially germ-free mice colonized with defined microbial communities) have become essential tools in the study of mechanisms. These models allow researchers to observe connections between specific microbes or microbial consortia and nutrient metabolism, immune responses and behavioral outcomes without changes in the composition of the gastrointestinal or oral flora (Tedeschi, 2019).

Table 2. Overview of key technological tools advancing microbiome research, highlighting their functions in understanding microbial composition, activity, and contributions to nutrient metabolism.

Technology/Tool	Key Function	Citation
16S rRNA Sequencing	Identifies microbial taxa; cost-effective and scalable	(Watts et al., 2017)
WMGS	Reveals genes, pathways, and strain-level variations	(Walsh et al., 2023)
Meta-transcriptomics	Shows active genes under diet-specific conditions	(Shi et al., 2018)
Metabolomics	Detects SCFAs, bile acids, neurotransmitter precursors	(Zhong et al., 2023)
Proteomics	Links microbial proteins to nutrient metabolism	(Melin, 2004)

continued on following page

Table 2. Continued

Technology/Tool	Key Function	Citation
Culturomics	Isolates and tests unculturable microbes	(Lagier et al., 2016)
Gnotobiotic Models	Links microbes to metabolism and host responses	(Kubelkova et al., 2016)

Moreover, open access microbiome data repositories including the Human Microbiome Project (HMP), MetaHIT and American Gut Project have been used to compare and generate hypotheses. These databases are essential to defining microbial "signatures" associated with health states, disease phenotypes, and dietary patterns. Despite these advances, challenges remain (Abusleme et al., 2021). Carefully interpreting microbiome data is needed; not only is this dependent on host genetics, environment and the medication that has been taken, it is also dependent on our circadian rhythms. Additionally, numerous microbial functions are context dependent and are affected by complex interactions between host and microbe and between the various microbes, which are not adequately captured by the current tools (Shanahan et al., 2021).

Yet progress in developing high throughput omics technologies and computational biology has advanced the frontiers of microbiome science. These tools further the understanding of the microbiome–nutrition axis, complementing the repertoire for devising novel diagnostics, targeted therapies and precision dietary recommendation grounded on microbial ecology (Vijay et al., 2025).

FUTURE PERSPECTIVES & CHALLENGES

The future of microbiome-nutrition research is moving toward precision health strategies that utilize individual microbial profiles to design tailored dietary interventions. Next generation sequencing, metabolomics, and artificial intelligence have opened the door for personalized diets, specific probiotics, engineered prebiotics to 'fine tune' the microbiome with high specificity. CRISPR and synthetic biology may enable microbiome editing to fine tune functions of microbes for nutrient metabolism and preventing disease. Also, real time monitoring tools and microbiome biomarkers will serve as adaptive nutritional therapies, so that clinical nutrition could become a dynamically responsive discipline.

However, several challenges remain. Standardization is complicated by the inherent variability of microbiomes amongst genetics, geography and lifestyle. Data is most often obtained from Western populations and therefore is not globally applicable. In addition, given the sensitivity of the microbiome to daily influences like dietary choice, medication, and circadian rhythms, a longitudinal approach is warranted. Stem cells, microbiome manipulation, data privacy and commercial use are all serious subjects to consider in ethical terms. To bridge this gap, robust, reproducible trials and interdisciplinary collaboration, to support safe, effective and equitable use in research settings is required.

CONCLUSION

Human nutrition and metabolism with immunity function depend fundamentally on the gut microbiome. The metabolic system uses the gut to break down complex carbohydrates in addition to producing essential vital nutrients and maintaining inflammatory and metabolic processes. The imbalance of this microbially dominated ecosystem leads to different nutritional conditions that result in both obesity along with diabetes and inflammatory bowel diseases and malnutrition. Dietary changes together with the use of probiotics and lifestyle adjustments create a strong method to restore microbiome equilibrium thus enhancing health results.

The quick development of microbiome science now forces nutrition experts to transition from broad population recommendations toward specific individual strategies that use microbial data to guide their decisions. The new approach selects the preservation of diversified microbial communities achieved by consuming plant-based foods abundant in fibers together with established early-life microbiota protective actions as its fundamental principles. Future developments in microbiome understanding together with better tools will enable authorities to transform public health strategies through scientific insights about microbiomes thus promoting both individual health sustainability and community-wide wellness gains.

REFERENCES

Abdulsalam, M., Hamisu, A. A., Ahmad, A. M., Wakili, F. B., Annu, F. S., & Garba, M. M. (2024). Microbiome dynamics and strategic management strategies: Exploring synergies between integrative medicine modalities and microbial balance. *Biological Sciences*, *4*(3), 725–735. DOI: 10.55006/biolsciences.2024.4307

Abusleme, L., Hoare, A., Hong, B.-Y., & Diaz, P. I. (2021). Microbial signatures of health, gingivitis, and periodontitis. *Periodontology 2000*, *86*(1), 57–78. DOI: 10.1111/prd.12362 PMID: 33690899

Alam, M. T., Amos, G. C. A., Murphy, A. R. J., Murch, S., Wellington, E. M. H., & Arasaradnam, R. P. (2020). Microbial imbalance in inflammatory bowel disease patients at different taxonomic levels. *Gut Pathogens*, *12*(1), 1. DOI: 10.1186/s13099-019-0341-6 PMID: 31911822

Almonacid, D. E., Kraal, L., Ossandon, F. J., Budovskaya, Y. V., Cardenas, J. P., Bik, E. M., Goddard, A. D., Richman, J., & Apte, Z. S. (2017). 16S rRNA gene sequencing and healthy reference ranges for 28 clinically relevant microbial taxa from the human gut microbiome. *PLoS One*, *12*(5), e0176555. DOI: 10.1371/journal.pone.0176555 PMID: 28467461

Bandyopadhyay, B., & Mandal, N. C. (2014). Probiotics, prebiotics and synbiotics-in health improvement by modulating gut microbiota: The concept revisited. *International Journal of Current Microbiology and Applied Sciences*, *3*(3), 410–420.

Barone, M., D'Amico, F., Brigidi, P., & Turroni, S. (2022). Gut microbiome–micronutrient interaction: The key to controlling the bioavailability of minerals and vitamins? *BioFactors (Oxford, England)*, *48*(2), 307–314. DOI: 10.1002/biof.1835 PMID: 35294077

Bello, M. G. D., et al. (2018). Preserving microbial diversity. *science, 362*(6410), 33-34.

Bemark, M., Pitcher, M. J., Dionisi, C., & Spencer, J. (2024). Gut-associated lymphoid tissue: A microbiota-driven hub of B cell immunity. *Trends in Immunology*, *45*(3), 211–223. DOI: 10.1016/j.it.2024.01.006 PMID: 38402045

Bešlo, D., Golubić, N., Rastija, V., Agić, D., Karnaš, M., Šubarić, D., & Lučić, B. (2023). Antioxidant activity, metabolism, and bioavailability of polyphenols in the diet of animals. *Antioxidants*, *12*(6), 1141. DOI: 10.3390/antiox12061141 PMID: 37371871

Bhuiyan, M. N. I., & Nahid, M. (2025). Smart nutrition: AI and 3D printing for personalized diets. *Food and Nutrition*, *1*(2), 100032. DOI: 10.1016/j.fnutr.2025.100032

Brown, E. M., Clardy, J., & Xavier, R. J. (2023). Gut microbiome lipid metabolism and its impact on host physiology. *Cell Host & Microbe*, *31*(2), 173–186. DOI: 10.1016/j.chom.2023.01.009 PMID: 36758518

Cantu-Jungles, T., & Hamaker, B. (2020). New view on dietary fiber selection for predictable shifts in gut microbiota. *mBio*, *11*(1), 02179–02119. DOI: 10.1128/mBio.02179-19 PMID: 32071263

Cao, X., Dong, A., Kang, G., Wang, X., Duan, L., Hou, H., Zhao, T., Wu, S., Liu, X., Huang, H., & Wu, R. (2022). Modeling spatial interaction networks of the gut microbiota. *Gut Microbes*, *14*(1), 2106103. DOI: 10.1080/19490976.2022.2106103 PMID: 35921525

Chen, L., Zhernakova, D. V., Kurilshikov, A., Andreu-Sánchez, S., Wang, D., Augustijn, H. E., Vich Vila, A., Weersma, R. K., Medema, M. H., Netea, M. G., Kuipers, F., Wijmenga, C., Zhernakova, A., & Fu, J. (2022). Influence of the microbiome, diet and genetics on inter-individual variation in the human plasma metabolome. *Nature Medicine*, *28*(11), 2333–2343. DOI: 10.1038/s41591-022-02014-8 PMID: 36216932

Christ, A., Lauterbach, M., & Latz, E. (2019). Western diet and the immune system: An inflammatory connection. *Immunity*, *51*(5), 794–811. DOI: 10.1016/j.immuni.2019.09.020 PMID: 31747581

Collins, J. T.. (2024). Anatomy, abdomen and pelvis, small intestine. In *StatPearls* [Internet]. StatPearls Publishing.

Cong, X., Henderson, W. A., Graf, J., & McGrath, J. M. (2015). Early life experience and gut microbiome: The brain–gut–microbiota signaling system. *Advances in Neonatal Care*, *15*(5), 314–323. DOI: 10.1097/ANC.0000000000000191 PMID: 26240939

Das, P., Babaei, P., & Nielsen, J. (2019). Metagenomic analysis of microbe-mediated vitamin metabolism in the human gut microbiome. *BMC Genomics*, *20*(1), 208. DOI: 10.1186/s12864-019-5591-7 PMID: 30866812

Delgobo, M., Paludo, K. S., Fernandes, D., Oliveira, J. G., Ortolan, G. L., & Favero, G. M. (2019). Gut: Key element on immune system regulation. *Brazilian Archives of Biology and Technology*, *62*, e19180654. DOI: 10.1590/1678-4324-2019180654

Dogra, S. K., Chung, C., Wang, D., Sakwinska, O., Colombo Mottaz, S., & Sprenger, N. (2021). Nurturing the early life gut microbiome and immune maturation for long term health. *Microorganisms*, *9*(10), 2110. DOI: 10.3390/microorganisms9102110 PMID: 34683431

Eslami, M., Naderian, R., Bahar, A., Babaeizad, A., Rezanavaz Gheshlagh, S., Oksenych, V., & Tahmasebi, H. (2025). Microbiota as diagnostic biomarkers: Advancing early cancer detection and personalized therapeutic approaches through microbiome profiling. *Frontiers in Immunology*, *16*, 1559480. DOI: 10.3389/fimmu.2025.1559480 PMID: 40406094

Fan, Y., & Pedersen, O. (2021). Gut microbiota in human metabolic health and disease. *Nature Reviews. Microbiology*, *19*(1), 55–71. DOI: 10.1038/s41579-020-0433-9 PMID: 32887946

Fang, X., et al. (2025). Precision microbiome: A new era of targeted therapy with core probiotics. *Research, 8*, 0658.

Flint, H. J. (2020). *Why gut microbes matter*. Springer. DOI: 10.1007/978-3-030-43246-1

Foley, M. H., O'Flaherty, S., Barrangou, R., & Theriot, C. M. (2019). Bile salt hydrolases: Gatekeepers of bile acid metabolism and host-microbiome crosstalk in the gastrointestinal tract. *PLoS Pathogens*, *15*(3), e1007581. DOI: 10.1371/journal.ppat.1007581 PMID: 30845232

Gao, R., Zhu, C., Li, H., Yin, M., Pan, C., Huang, L., Kong, C., Wang, X., Zhang, Y., Qu, S., & Qin, H. (2018). Dysbiosis signatures of gut microbiota along the sequence from healthy, young patients to those with overweight and obesity. *Obesity (Silver Spring, Md.)*, *26*(2), 351–361. DOI: 10.1002/oby.22088 PMID: 29280312

Gilbert, J. A., Blaser, M. J., Caporaso, J. G., Jansson, J. K., Lynch, S. V., & Knight, R. (2018). Current understanding of the human microbiome. *Nature Medicine*, *24*(4), 392–400. DOI: 10.1038/nm.4517 PMID: 29634682

Hadrich, D. (2018). Microbiome research is becoming the key to better understanding health and nutrition. *Frontiers in Genetics*, *9*, 212. DOI: 10.3389/fgene.2018.00212 PMID: 29951086

Hou, Y., Li, J., & Ying, S. (2023). Tryptophan metabolism and gut microbiota: A novel regulatory axis integrating the microbiome, immunity, and cancer. *Metabolites*, *13*(11), 1166. DOI: 10.3390/metabo13111166 PMID: 37999261

Huang, C., Feng, S., Huo, F., & Liu, H. (2022). Effects of four antibiotics on the diversity of the intestinal microbiota. *Microbiology Spectrum, 10*(2), e01904–e01921. DOI: 10.1128/spectrum.01904-21 PMID: 35311555

Jain, N. (2020). The early life education of the immune system: Moms, microbes and (missed) opportunities. *Gut Microbes, 12*(1), 1824564. DOI: 10.1080/19490976.2020.1824564 PMID: 33043833

JanssenDuijghuijsen, L., Looijesteijn, E., van den Belt, M., Gerhard, B., Ziegler, M., Ariens, R., Tjoelker, R., & Geurts, J.JanssenDuijghuijsen. (2024). Changes in gut microbiota and lactose intolerance symptoms before and after daily lactose supplementation in individuals with the lactase nonpersistent genotype. *The American Journal of Clinical Nutrition, 119*(3), 702–710. DOI: 10.1016/j.ajcnut.2023.12.016 PMID: 38159728

Joseph, T. A., & Pe'er, I. (2021). An introduction to whole-metagenome shotgun sequencing studies. *Deep sequencing data analysis*, 107-122.

Kim, C. H. (2018). Immune regulation by microbiome metabolites. *Immunology, 154*(2), 220–229. DOI: 10.1111/imm.12930 PMID: 29569377

Kolodziejczyk, A. A., Zheng, D., & Elinav, E. (2019). Diet–microbiota interactions and personalized nutrition. *Nature Reviews. Microbiology, 17*(12), 742–753. DOI: 10.1038/s41579-019-0256-8 PMID: 31541197

Korpela, K. (2021). Impact of delivery mode on infant gut microbiota. *Annals of Nutrition & Metabolism, 77*(Suppl. 3), 11–19. DOI: 10.1159/000518498 PMID: 34515049

Kubelkova, K., Benuchova, M., Kozakova, H., Sinkora, M., Krocova, Z., Pejchal, J., & Macela, A. (2016). Gnotobiotic mouse model's contribution to understanding host–pathogen interactions. *Cellular and Molecular Life Sciences : CMLS, 73*(20), 3961–3969. DOI: 10.1007/s00018-016-2341-8 PMID: 27544211

Kundra, P., Rachmühl, C., Lacroix, C., & Geirnaert, A. (2021). Role of dietary micronutrients on gut microbial dysbiosis and modulation in inflammatory bowel disease. *Molecular Nutrition & Food Research, 65*(5), 1901271. DOI: 10.1002/mnfr.201901271

Lagier, J.-C., Hugon, P., Khelaifia, S., Fournier, P.-E., La Scola, B., & Raoult, D. (2015). The rebirth of culture in microbiology through the example of culturomics to study human gut microbiota. *Clinical Microbiology Reviews, 28*(1), 237–264. DOI: 10.1128/CMR.00014-14 PMID: 25567229

Lagier, J.-C., Khelaifia, S., Alou, M. T., Ndongo, S., Dione, N., Hugon, P., Caputo, A., Cadoret, F., Traore, S. I., Seck, E. H., Dubourg, G., Durand, G., Mourembou, G., Guilhot, E., Togo, A., Bellali, S., Bachar, D., Cassir, N., Bittar, F., & Raoult, D. (2016). Culture of previously uncultured members of the human gut microbiota by culturomics. *Nature Microbiology*, *1*(12), 16203. DOI: 10.1038/nmicrobiol.2016.203 PMID: 27819657

Lee, J.-Y., et al. (2022). The microbiome and gut homeostasis. *science, 377*(6601), eabp9960.

Li, C. (2023). Understanding interactions among diet, host and gut microbiota for personalized nutrition. *Life Sciences*, *312*, 121265. DOI: 10.1016/j.lfs.2022.121265 PMID: 36473543

Ma, N., & Ma, X. (2019). Dietary amino acids and the gut-microbiome-immune axis: Physiological metabolism and therapeutic prospects. *Comprehensive Reviews in Food Science and Food Safety*, *18*(1), 221–242. DOI: 10.1111/1541-4337.12401 PMID: 33337014

Maldonado Galdeano, C., et al. (2015). Role of probiotics and functional foods in health: gut immune stimulation by two probiotic strains and a potential probiotic yoghurt. *Endocrine, Metabolic & Immune Disorders-Drug Targets (Formerly Current Drug Targets-Immune, Endocrine & Metabolic Disorders), 15*(1), 37-45.

Martinez, F. D. (2014). The human microbiome. Early life determinant of health outcomes. *Annals of the American Thoracic Society*, *11*(Supplement 1), S7–S12. DOI: 10.1513/AnnalsATS.201306-186MG PMID: 24437411

Melin, P. (2004). Proteomics as a tool to study microbial interactions. *Current Proteomics*, *1*(1), 27–34. DOI: 10.2174/1570164043488261

Mukherjee, A., Breselge, S., Dimidi, E., Marco, M. L., & Cotter, P. D. (2024). Fermented foods and gastrointestinal health: Underlying mechanisms. *Nature Reviews. Gastroenterology & Hepatology*, *21*(4), 248–266. DOI: 10.1038/s41575-023-00869-x PMID: 38081933

Myhrstad, M. C., Tunsjø, H., Charnock, C., & Telle-Hansen, V. H. (2020). Dietary fiber, gut microbiota, and metabolic regulation—Current status in human randomized trials. *Nutrients*, *12*(3), 859. DOI: 10.3390/nu12030859 PMID: 32210176

Nogacka, A. M., Salazar, N., Arboleya, S., Suárez, M., Fernández, N., Solís, G., de los Reyes-Gavilán, C. G., & Gueimonde, M. (2018). Early microbiota, antibiotics and health. *Cellular and Molecular Life Sciences : CMLS*, *75*(1), 83–91. DOI: 10.1007/s00018-017-2670-2 PMID: 28988290

Okumura, R., & Takeda, K. (2018). Maintenance of intestinal homeostasis by mucosal barriers. *Inflammation and Regeneration*, *38*(1), 5. DOI: 10.1186/s41232-018-0063-z PMID: 29619131

Oliver, A., Chase, A. B., Weihe, C., Orchanian, S. B., Riedel, S. F., Hendrickson, C. L., Lay, M., Sewall, J. M., Martiny, J. B. H., & Whiteson, K. (2021). High-fiber, whole-food dietary intervention alters the human gut microbiome but not fecal short-chain fatty acids. *mSystems*, *6*(2), 00115–00121. DOI: 10.1128/msystems.00115-21 PMID: 33727392

Philippot, L., Griffiths, B. S., & Langenheder, S. (2021). Microbial community resilience across ecosystems and multiple disturbances. *Microbiology and Molecular Biology Reviews : MMBR*, *85*(2), 00026–00020. DOI: 10.1128/MMBR.00026-20 PMID: 33789927

Preshaw, P. M. (2018). Host modulation therapy with anti-inflammatory agents. *Periodontology 2000*, *76*(1), 131–149. DOI: 10.1111/prd.12148 PMID: 29193331

Quagebeur, R., Dalile, B., Raes, J., Van Oudenhove, L., Verbeke, K., & Vrieze, E. (2023). The role of short-chain fatty acids (SCFAs) in regulating stress responses, eating behavior, and nutritional state in anorexia nervosa: Protocol for a randomized controlled trial. *Journal of Eating Disorders*, *11*(1), 191. DOI: 10.1186/s40337-023-00917-6 PMID: 37884972

Quinn, A. M., Bottery, M. J., Thompson, H., & Friman, V.-P. (2022). Resistance evolution can disrupt antibiotic exposure protection through competitive exclusion of the protective species. *The ISME Journal*, *16*(10), 2433–2447. DOI: 10.1038/s41396-022-01285-w PMID: 35859161

Rahman, S.. (2023). Gut microbial metabolites and its impact on human health. *Annals of Gastroenterology*, *36*(4), 360. DOI: 10.20524/aog.2023.0809 PMID: 37396009

Ramírez-Pérez, O.. (2018). The role of the gut microbiota in bile acid metabolism. *Annals of Hepatology*, *16*(1), 21–26.

Rinninella, E., Cintoni, M., Raoul, P., Lopetuso, L. R., Scaldaferri, F., Pulcini, G., Miggiano, G. A. D., Gasbarrini, A., & Mele, M. C. (2019). Food components and dietary habits: Keys for a healthy gut microbiota composition. *Nutrients*, *11*(10), 2393. DOI: 10.3390/nu11102393 PMID: 31591348

Rouskas, K., Guela, M., Pantoura, M., Pagkalos, I., Hassapidou, M., Lalama, E., Pfeiffer, A. F. H., Decorte, E., Cornelissen, V., Wilson-Barnes, S., Hart, K., Mantovani, E., Dias, S. B., Hadjileontiadis, L., Gymnopoulos, L. P., Dimitropoulos, K., & Argiriou, A. (2025). The Influence of an AI-Driven Personalized Nutrition Program on the Human Gut Microbiome and Its Health Implications. *Nutrients*, *17*(7), 1260. DOI: 10.3390/nu17071260 PMID: 40219016

Rowland, I., Gibson, G., Heinken, A., Scott, K., Swann, J., Thiele, I., & Tuohy, K. (2018). Gut microbiota functions: Metabolism of nutrients and other food components. *European Journal of Nutrition*, *57*(1), 1–24. DOI: 10.1007/s00394-017-1445-8 PMID: 28393285

Saak, C. C., Pierce, E. C., Dinh, C. B., Portik, D., Hall, R., Ashby, M., & Dutton, R. J. (2023). Longitudinal, multi-platform metagenomics yields a high-quality genomic catalog and guides an in vitro model for cheese communities. *mSystems*, *8*(1), e00701–e00722. DOI: 10.1128/msystems.00701-22 PMID: 36622155

Sardans, J., Lambers, H., Preece, C., Alrefaei, A. F., & Penuelas, J. (2023). Role of mycorrhizas and root exudates in plant uptake of soil nutrients (calcium, iron, magnesium, and potassium): Has the puzzle been completely solved? *The Plant Journal*, *114*(6), 1227–1242. DOI: 10.1111/tpj.16184 PMID: 36917083

Scepanovic, P., Hodel, F., Mondot, S., Partula, V., Byrd, A., Hammer, C., Alanio, C., Bergstedt, J., Patin, E., Touvier, M., Lantz, O., Albert, M. L., Duffy, D., Quintana-Murci, L., & Fellay, J. (2019). A comprehensive assessment of demographic, environmental, and host genetic associations with gut microbiome diversity in healthy individuals. *Microbiome*, *7*(1), 130. DOI: 10.1186/s40168-019-0747-x PMID: 31519223

Scheithauer, T. P., Rampanelli, E., Nieuwdorp, M., Vallance, B. A., Verchere, C. B., van Raalte, D. H., & Herrema, H. (2020). Gut microbiota as a trigger for metabolic inflammation in obesity and type 2 diabetes. *Frontiers in Immunology*, *11*, 571731. DOI: 10.3389/fimmu.2020.571731 PMID: 33178196

Shanahan, E. R., McMaster, J. J., & Staudacher, H. M. (2021). Conducting research on diet–microbiome interactions: A review of current challenges, essential methodological principles, and recommendations for best practice in study design. *Journal of Human Nutrition and Dietetics*, *34*(4), 631–644. DOI: 10.1111/jhn.12868 PMID: 33639033

Shi, M., Zhang, Y.-Z., & Holmes, E. C. (2018). Meta-transcriptomics and the evolutionary biology of RNA viruses. *Virus Research*, *243*, 83–90. DOI: 10.1016/j.virusres.2017.10.016 PMID: 29111455

Shimizu, H.. (2019). Regulation of host energy metabolism by gut microbiota-derived short-chain fatty acids. *Glycative Stress Research, 6*(3), 181–191.

Singh, R., Zogg, H., Wei, L., Bartlett, A., Ghoshal, U. C., Rajender, S., & Ro, S. (2021). Gut microbial dysbiosis in the pathogenesis of gastrointestinal dysmotility and metabolic disorders. *Journal of Neurogastroenterology and Motility, 27*(1), 19–34. DOI: 10.5056/jnm20149 PMID: 33166939

Son, J. W., Shoaie, S., & Lee, S. (2020). Systems biology: A multi-omics integration approach to metabolism and the microbiome. *Endocrinology and Metabolism (Seoul, Korea), 35*(3), 507–514. DOI: 10.3803/EnM.2020.303 PMID: 32981293

Tang, J. (2011). Microbial metabolomics. *Current Genomics, 12*(6), 391–403. DOI: 10.2174/138920211797248619 PMID: 22379393

Tedeschi, L. O. (2019). ASN-ASAS SYMPOSIUM: FUTURE OF DATA ANALYTICS IN NUTRITION: Mathematical modeling in ruminant nutrition: approaches and paradigms, extant models, and thoughts for upcoming predictive analytics. *Journal of Animal Science, 97*(5), 1921–1944. DOI: 10.1093/jas/skz092 PMID: 30882142

Utreja, S. (2023). *Unlocking the Power of Next Generation Sequencing for Microbiome Analysis.* State University of New York at Buffalo.

Valero-Cases, E., Cerdá-Bernad, D., Pastor, J.-J., & Frutos, M.-J. (2020). Non-dairy fermented beverages as potential carriers to ensure probiotics, prebiotics, and bioactive compounds arrival to the gut and their health benefits. *Nutrients, 12*(6), 1666. DOI: 10.3390/nu12061666 PMID: 32503276

Valitutti, F., Cucchiara, S., & Fasano, A. (2019). Celiac disease and the microbiome. *Nutrients, 11*(10), 2403. DOI: 10.3390/nu11102403 PMID: 31597349

Vallianou, N., Stratigou, T., Christodoulatos, G. S., & Dalamaga, M. (2019). Understanding the role of the gut microbiome and microbial metabolites in obesity and obesity-associated metabolic disorders: Current evidence and perspectives. *Current Obesity Reports, 8*(3), 317–332. DOI: 10.1007/s13679-019-00352-2 PMID: 31175629

Van den Elsen, L. W., Garssen, J., Burcelin, R., & Verhasselt, V. (2019). Shaping the gut microbiota by breastfeeding: The gateway to allergy prevention? *Frontiers in Pediatrics, 7*, 47. DOI: 10.3389/fped.2019.00047 PMID: 30873394

van Zanten, A. R. (2023). Personalized nutrition therapy in critical illness and convalescence: Moving beyond one-size-fits-all to phenotyping and endotyping. *Current Opinion in Critical Care, 29*(4), 281–285. DOI: 10.1097/MCC.0000000000001060 PMID: 37431268

Verma, M., ... (2018). Challenges in personalized nutrition and health. In (Vol. 5, pp. 117): Frontiers Media SA. DOI: 10.3389/fnut.2018.00117

Vijay, J., ... (2025). Precision Nutrition Through Nutritional Informatics: Futuristic Technologies for Health Advancement. In *Exploration of Transformative Technologies in Healthcare 6.0* (pp. 329-360). IGI Global Scientific Publishing.

Walker, W. A. (2017). The importance of appropriate initial bacterial colonization of the intestine in newborn, child, and adult health. *Pediatric Research, 82*(3), 387–395. DOI: 10.1038/pr.2017.111 PMID: 28426649

Wall, R., et al. (2014). Bacterial neuroactive compounds produced by psychobiotics. *Microbial endocrinology: The microbiota-gut-brain axis in health and disease*, 221-239.

Walsh, L. H., Coakley, M., Walsh, A. M., O'Toole, P. W., & Cotter, P. D. (2023). Bioinformatic approaches for studying the microbiome of fermented food. *Critical Reviews in Microbiology, 49*(6), 693–725. DOI: 10.1080/1040841X.2022.2132850 PMID: 36287644

Wardman, J. F., Bains, R. K., Rahfeld, P., & Withers, S. G. (2022). Carbohydrate-active enzymes (CAZymes) in the gut microbiome. *Nature Reviews. Microbiology, 20*(9), 542–556. DOI: 10.1038/s41579-022-00712-1 PMID: 35347288

Watts, G., Youens-Clark, K., Slepian, M. J., Wolk, D. M., Oshiro, M. M., Metzger, G. S., Dhingra, D., Cranmer, L. D., & Hurwitz, B. L. (2017). 16S rRNA gene sequencing on a benchtop sequencer: Accuracy for identification of clinically important bacteria. *Journal of Applied Microbiology, 123*(6), 1584–1596. DOI: 10.1111/jam.13590 PMID: 28940494

Whitman, J. A., Doherty, L. A., Pantoja-Feliciano de Goodfellow, I. G., Racicot, K., Anderson, D. J., Kensil, K., Karl, J. P., Gibson, G. R., & Soares, J. W. (2024). In vitro fermentation shows polyphenol and fiber blends have an additive beneficial effect on gut microbiota states. *Nutrients, 16*(8), 1159. DOI: 10.3390/nu16081159 PMID: 38674850

Wilkinson, J. E., Franzosa, E. A., Everett, C., Li, C., Bae, S., Berzansky, I., Bhosle, A., Bjørnevik, K., Brennan, C. A., Cao, Y. G., Chun, E., Clay, S. L., Fenn, K., Hall, A. B., Lennon, D., Lobel, L., Ma, S., Ma, W., Maharjan, S., & Huttenhower, C. (2021). A framework for microbiome science in public health. *Nature Medicine, 27*(5), 766–774. DOI: 10.1038/s41591-021-01258-0 PMID: 33820996

Yao, S., Zhou, C., Li, S., Li, Y., Shen, C., Tao, Y., & Li, X. (2024). Microbial diversity across tea varieties and ecological niches: Correlating tea polyphenol contents with stress resistance. *Frontiers in Microbiology, 15*, 1439630. DOI: 10.3389/fmicb.2024.1439630 PMID: 39252833

Yuan, P.. (2020). Microbial production of vitamins. In *Systems and synthetic biotechnology for production of nutraceuticals* (pp. 159–187). Springer.

Zhang, Y., Thompson, K. N., Branck, T., Yan Yan, , Nguyen, L. H., Franzosa, E. A., & Huttenhower, C. (2021). Metatranscriptomics for the human microbiome and microbial community functional profiling. *Annual Review of Biomedical Data Science, 4*(1), 279–311. DOI: 10.1146/annurev-biodatasci-031121-103035 PMID: 34465175

Zhen, J., Zhou, Z., He, M., Han, H.-X., Lv, E.-H., Wen, P.-B., Liu, X., Wang, Y.-T., Cai, X.-C., Tian, J.-Q., Zhang, M.-Y., Xiao, L., & Kang, X.-X. (2023). The gut microbial metabolite trimethylamine N-oxide and cardiovascular diseases. *Frontiers in Endocrinology, 14*, 1085041. DOI: 10.3389/fendo.2023.1085041 PMID: 36824355

Zhong, J.-G., Lan, W.-T., Feng, Y.-Q., Li, Y.-H., Shen, Y.-Y., Gong, J.-H., Zou, Z., & Hou, X. (2023). Associations between dysbiosis gut microbiota and changes of neurotransmitters and short-chain fatty acids in valproic acid model rats. *Frontiers in Physiology, 14*, 1077821. DOI: 10.3389/fphys.2023.1077821 PMID: 37035670

Zhou, X., et al. (2019). Early-life food nutrition, microbiota maturation and immune development shape life-long health. *Critical reviews in food science and nutrition, 59*(sup1), S30-S38.

Zinöcker, M. K., & Lindseth, I. A. (2018). The western diet–microbiome-host interaction and its role in metabolic disease. *Nutrients, 10*(3), 365. DOI: 10.3390/nu10030365 PMID: 29562591

Zmora, N. (2019). *Microbiome-based personalized interventions.* The Weizmann Institute of Science.

Chapter 2
Metagenomics and Microbiome Analysis for Nutritional Insights:
Decoding Microbial Signatures for Precision Nutrition

Renu Agarwal
https://orcid.org/0000-0002-5366-5773
Shrimathi Devkunvar Nanalal Bhatt Vaishnav College for Women, University of Madras, Chennai, India

R. Vijaya Vahini
https://orcid.org/0000-0002-8482-8037
Shrimathi Devkunvar Nanalal Bhatt Vaishnav College for Women, University of Madras, Chennai, India

V. Subasshini
https://orcid.org/0000-0002-5880-869X
Shrimathi Devkunvar Nanalal Bhatt Vaishnav College for Women, University of Madras, Chennai, India

R. Subaratinam
Shrimathi Devkunvar Nanalal Bhatt Vaishnav College for Women, University of Madras, Chennai, India

ABSTRACT

The synergy of microbiome analysis and metagenomics has transformed diet-microbe-host relationships, and this chapter delves into how bioinformatics tools and high-throughput sequence technologies are utilized to decipher gut microbiome

DOI: 10.4018/979-8-3373-4382-2.ch002

structure and function and its pivotal role in human nutrition. Investigating microbial diversity, metabolic capacity, and relations between hosts and microbiomes reveals personalized dietary response and pathways underlying nutrient processing, energy homeostasis, and risk factors of chronic disease. This chapter outlines methodological strategies such as sequence analysis of the 16S rRNA gene, shotgun metagenomics, and integration of metabolomics and uses of these in personalized nutrition, biomarker development, and dietary intervention. Obstacles, implications, and future views of microbiome-guided nutrition are presented. This chapter offers an in-depth overview to inform investigators, clinicians, and nutrition experts working to apply microbiome information to precision health and optimal dietary regimes.

OVERVIEW OF MICROBIOME AND NUTRITION

The gut microbiome of humans hosts trillions of microbes with an aggregate genome several orders of magnitude larger than that of the host(mortal Microbiome Project Consortium, 2012). It is responsible for nutrient metabolism, vulnerable function, and homeostasis (Valdes et al., 2018). Diet too is a significant adjustable determinant of function and composition of microbiome with goods of fibre, fat, proteins, and micronutrients on particular microbial communities(Zhang et al., 2022). Metagenomics has enhanced understanding of these intricate relations through the eventuality of culture-independent description of microbial communities along with their functional capacity(Quince et al., 2017).

The microbiome participates in digestion by degrading complex polysaccharides, generating short- chain adipose acids(SCFAs), vitamin product, and corrosiveness acid metabolism modulation(Ríos- Covián et al., 2016). In addition to this, dysbiosis or microbial imbalance has been associated with metabolic conditions like rotundity, diabetes, and cardiovascular complaint (Kim & Shin, 2018). This places high significance on the operation of microbiome- targeted salutary interventions in maintaining health.

HISTORICAL CONTEXT

Before the genomics period, microbiome exploration was grounded substantially on civilization, which did not reflect the enormous population of gut microbes that were n't cultivable(Eckburg et al., 2005). 16S rRNA gene sequencing has made it possible to now taxonomically classify bacterial communities on a high-outurn scale(Janda & Abbott, 2007). Shotgun metagenomics has lately allowed for detailed perceptivity into microbial gene content and apparent function(Qin et al., 2010).

These technological advances gave the drive for systems similar to the mortal Microbiome Project, which set the healthy mortal microbiome and complaint-concentrated reference norms(Turnbaugh et al., 2007). Functional reflection and pathway analysis are now made possible with metagenomic approaches, connecting microbial diversity to biochemical functions applicable to nutrition and complaint(-Franzosa et al., 2015).

THE RELATION BETWEEN GUT-MICROBIOME AND NUTRITIONAL PHYSIOLOGY

According to previous study, bacterial phyla include Bacteroidetes, Firmicutes, Actinobacteria, and Proteobacteria are present in the human gut (Eckburg et al., 2005). Their relative cornucopia impacts nutrient processing and host metabolism

- Firmicutes include rubrics similar as Clostridium and Faecalibacterium, complete in fiber declination and SCFA product, particularly butyrate, which contributes to gut hedge health (Louis & Flint, 2017).
- Bacteroidetes are effective at catabolizing polysaccharides and proteins; they help prize energy from salutary filaments unapproachable to the host (Flint et al., 2012).
- Actinobacteria, particularly Bifidobacterium spp., are important for stirring oligosaccharides and synthesizing essential vitamins (Pompei et al., 2007).
- Proteobacteria generally have low cornucopia in the healthy gut but bloom during inflammation and dysbiosis (Shin, Whon, & Bae, 2015).

MICROBIAL DONATION TO NUTRIENT METABOLISM

Gut microbes raise inedible carbohydrates producing SCFAs like acetate, propionate, and butyrate, which contribute to colonic energy sources and systemic metabolic regulation(Koh et al., 2016). Microbes also synthesize vitamins including K and B12 and influence corrosiveness acid metamorphosis impacting fat solubilization and cholesterol metabolism(Ridlon, Kang, & Hylemon, 2006).

Differences in microbiota composition modulate nutrient immersion effectiveness, impacting host energy balance. This is apparent in studies showing shifts in FirmicutesBacteroidetes rate relating with rotundity and insulin resistance(Turnbaugh et al., 2009). Likewise, microbial metabolites act as signaling motes that regulate appetite, glucose homeostasis, and vulnerable function(Goulet, 2015).

Figure 1. Metagenomic Methods Workflow

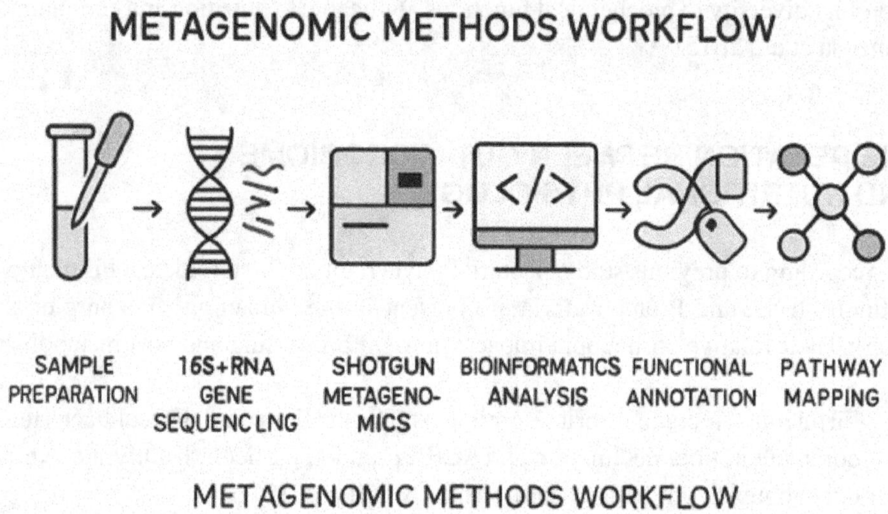

Source: Original infographic based on workflow steps described by Franzosa et al. (2018), Quince et al. (2017), and Janda & Abbott (2007).

METAGENOMIC STYLES IN MICROBIOME STUDIES

Sequencing of the 16S rRNA Gene

This system targets conserved regions of the 16S ribosomal RNA gene unique to bacteria, enabling taxonomic bracket and community profiling(Janda & Abbott, 2007). It's extensively used due to affordability and fairly simple analysis but limited in its functional sapience since it focuses solely on bacterial taxonomy.

Shotgun Metagenomics

Shotgun metagenomics sequences the total microbial DNA allowing analysis of bacterial, archaeal, viral, and eukaryotic genomes simultaneously(Qin et al., 2010).

It provides deep insight into the genes present, allowing pathway reconstruction and functional implicit estimation(Franzosa et al., 2015). This approach enables discovery of new genes and microbial relations critical to nutrition.

Functional Reflection and Pathway Analysis

Bioinformatics tools analogous as HUMAnN2, KEGG, and MetaCyc annotate microbial genes to metabolic pathways, relating gene cornucopia with physiological functions(Franzosa et al., 2018). Metagenomic datasets combined with metabolomic lives enable linking microbial gene content with metabolic labors applicable to salutary factors and host health(Zierer et al., 2018).

MICROBIOME- DIET RELATIONS

Microbial Response to Dietary Components

Salutary input profoundly influences gut microbiome composition and functional capacity. Specific nutrients act as modulating microbial diversity, substrates, and metabolic affairs(Valdes et al., 2018).

Salutary fibers, especially answerable bones like inulin and resistant brio, stimulate the growth of salutary microbial taxa analogous as Bifidobacterium and Faecalibacterium prausnitzii, performing in increased product of short- chain adipose acids(SCFAs) that support mucosal health(Koh, De Vadder, Kovatcheva- Datchary, & Bäckhed, 2016). Again, high- fat or high- protein diets have been associated with increases in cattiness-- seditious taxa analogous as Bilophila and Alistipes(David et al., 2014).

Figure 2. Microbiome–Diet Relations

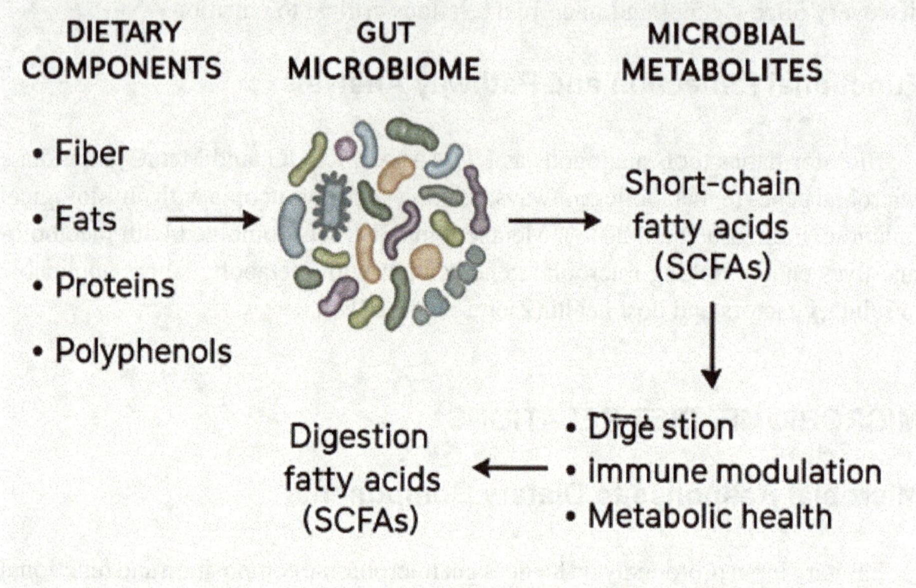

Source: Original figure created for this chapter using concepts from Valdes et al. (2018), Koh et al. (2016), and Cardona et al. (2013).

Food complements, polyphenols, and micronutrients further modify microbial ecology. Polyphenols have antimicrobial and prebiotic- suchlike goods, perfecting taxa associated withanti- seditious and antioxidative parcels(Cardona, Andrés-Lacueva, Tulipani, Tinahones, & Queipo- Ortuño, 2013). These nutrient- microbe relations accentuate the severity and rigidity of the microbial ecosystem in response to salutary variation.

Positive effects on Digestion, absorption, and Metabolism

Microbial transformation of salutary factors enhances nutrient bioavailability and influences host metabolism. Fermentation of indigestible carbohydrates by gut microbes results in SCFAs product — acetate, propionate, and butyrate which serve as energy substrates for colonocytes, modulate glucose and lipid metabolism, and regulate appetite via gut- brain axis signaling (Koh et al., 2016).

Microbial enzymes contribute to mineral immersion (e.g., calcium, magnesium) and conflation of vitamins (B group and K vitamins) essential for mortal physiology (Hill, 2012). Dysbiosis alters these metabolic processes, frequently leading to disabled nutrient immersion, increased gut permeability, and systemic inflammation, which have counteraccusations in metabolic conditions including rotundity and type 2 diabetes (Ley, Turnbaugh, Klein, & Gordon, 2006).

OPERATIONS IN PERSONALIZED NUTRITION

Microbiome- Grounded Salutary Recommendations

Arising substantiation supports acclimatizing diets grounded on individual microbiota biographies to enhance metabolic health issues (Zmora, Zeevi, Korem, Segal, & Elinav, 2019). Individualized nutrition platforms influence metagenomic data to recommend foods that widely promote salutary taxa or modulate microbial metabolites relating to better glycemic control and lipid biographies (Ghaisas, Maher, & Kanthasamy, 2016).

Clinical trials demonstrate that microbiome- guided salutary interventions can outperform generalized guidelines in managing weight, insulin perceptivity, and seditious countries. For illustration, Zeevi et al.(2015) showed that personalized postprandial glucose prognostications grounded on microbiome composition achieved superior glycemic control in prediabetic subjects.

Prophetic Models and Case Studies

Machine literacy algorithms integrating microbiome and clinical data ameliorate vaticination of diet response and personalization of interventions (Tremaroli & Bäckhed, 2012). These models use microbial taxa cornucopia, gene content, and metabolite biographies to stratify cases and prognosticate efficacity of specific salutary factors.

Case studies in rotundity operation have stressed the role of microbiome diversity and specific SCFA directors as predictors of response to high- fiber diets(Cotillard et al., 2013). Likewise, interventions targeting microbiota composition have demonstrated defensive goods against cardiovascular threat factors through corrosiveness acid metabolism modulation(Joyce & Gahan, 2016).

Figure 3. Microbial Biomarkers of Nutritional Status

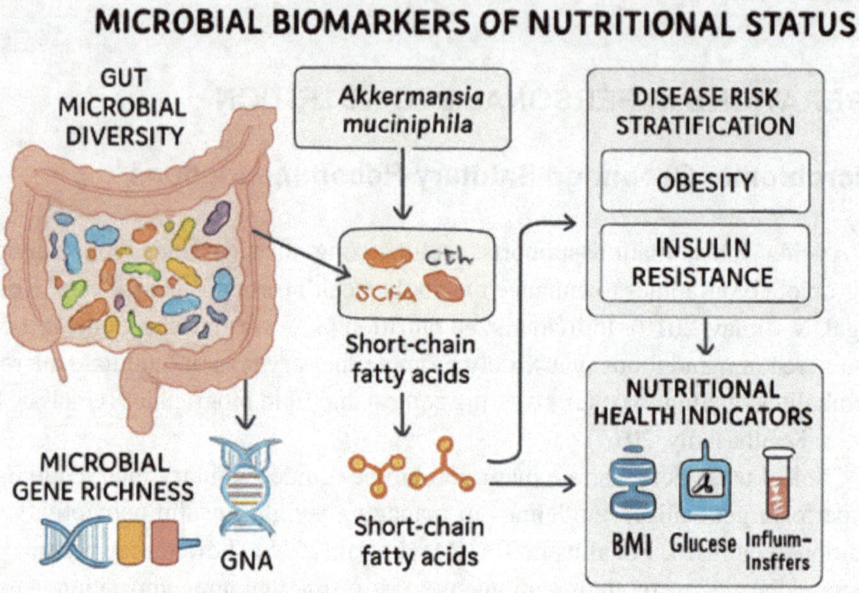

Sources: Le Chatelier et al., 2013, Everard et al., 2013, Franzosa et al., 2018, Cotillard et al., 2013

Identification of Microbial Autographs

Microbial community indicators, including nascence diversity and gene uproariousness, serve as labels for nutritive health status and complaint vulnerability(Le Chatelier et al., 2013). Specific taxa similar as Akkermansia muciniphila have been linked as salutary microbes linked to leanness and bettered glucose metabolism(Everard et al., 2013).

Metagenomic functional profiling reveals microbial pathways involved in inflammation, energy crop, and xenobiotic metabolism that relate with nutritive biomarkers and clinical phenotypes(Franzosa et al., 2018).

Disease Risk Stratification

Assessment of microbial gene content and metabolite product facilitates threat position for metabolic and seditious conditions. Low microbial gene uproariousness and functional redundancy have been associated with rotundity and insulin resistance, guiding remedial decision- making and covering responses(Cotillard et al., 2013).

similar microbial biomarkers are decreasingly incorporated into clinical trials and epidemiological studies.

INTEGRATION WITH OTHER OMICS

Metabolomics, Proteomics and Transcriptomics

The integration of metagenomics with metabolomics, proteomics, and transcriptomics provides a comprehensive view of microbial and host physiology relations(Li et al., 2020). Metabolomics measures the pool of small molecules produced by microbes and host cells, linking heritable eventuality to active biochemical processes.

Proteomic studies yield insight into microbial protein expression and enzymatic exertion, while transcriptomics lives gene expression dynamics under different salutary conditions(Franzosa et al., 2015). Thismulti-omics approach helps interpret unproductive connections and nonsupervisory networks bolstering nutritional responses.

Systems Biology Approaches

Systems biology leverages computational models to integratemulti- omic datasets and prognosticate microbial community behavior and host responses(Altay et al., 2019).

LIMITATIONS AND CHALLENGES

Technical and Analytical Barriers

Despite significant advances, technical challenges limit the reproducibility and community of microbiome disquisition. Variations in sample collection, sequencing protocols, and bioinformatics channels introduce impulses (Pollock, Glendinning, Wisedchanwet, & Watson, 2018). Standardization of methodologies and data sharing remain priorities for the field.

Individual Variation

Naturally high interpersonal variability in microbiome composition, told by genetics, terrain, and life, complicates the development of universal salutary recommendations(Zhernakova et al., 2016). Longitudinal and large cohort studies are necessary to decrypt stable microbial traits and responses.

Ethical and sequestration Issues

The generation and use of large substantiated microbiome datasets raise ethical enterprises regarding sequestration, concurrence, and implicit abuse of particular health data(Kumar, 2019). Regulatory fabrics must balance invention with patient rights and data security.

UNBORN DIRECTIONS AND TRANSLATIONAL IMPLICIT

Microbiome- Targeted rectifiers

Unborn curatives include developer probiotics, prebiotics, postbiotics, and fecal microbiota transplantation aimed at reshaping gut microbiota to optimize nutritive health(Suez, Zmora, Zilberman- Schapira, Mor, & Elinav, 2019). Engineered microbial colleges and substantiated microbial supplements open avenues for perfection nutrition interventions.

Their part in Global Public Health and Nutrition

Microbiome- informed nutrition strategies remain implicit for public health by enabling early identification of at- threat populations and substantiated salutary guidelines at scale(Smits et al., 2019). Integrating microbiome data into nutrition policy and education could alleviate habitual complaint burdens encyclopedically.

CONCLUSION

Metagenomics and microbiome analysis have readdressed understanding of diet- host- microbe functional networks, enabling slice- edge substantiated nutrition. Comprehensive multi-omics and systems biology tools unlock complex relations that govern digestion, metabolism, and complaint threat. Despite challenges, advancing microbiome- targeted interventions and ethical fabrics can revise public health nutrition and perfection drug.

REFERENCES

Altay, O.. (2019). Systems biology perspective for studying the gut microbiota interactions. *Frontiers in Physiology*, *10*, 1177. DOI: 10.3389/fphys.2019.01177

Cardona, F., Andrés-Lacueva, C., Tulipani, S., Tinahones, F. J., & Queipo-Ortuño, M. I. (2013). Benefits of polyphenols on gut microbiota and implications in human health. *The Journal of Nutritional Biochemistry*, *24*(8), 1415–1422. DOI: 10.1016/j.jnutbio.2013.05.001 PMID: 23849454

Cotillard, A., Kennedy, S. P., Kong, L. C., Prifti, E., Pons, N., Le Chatelier, E., Almeida, M., Quinquis, B., Levenez, F., Galleron, N., Gougis, S., Rizkalla, S., Batto, J.-M., Renault, P., Doré, J., Zucker, J.-D., Clément, K., Ehrlich, S. D., Blottière, H., & Layec, S. (2013). Dietary intervention impact on gut microbial gene richness. *Nature*, *500*(7464), 585–588. DOI: 10.1038/nature12480 PMID: 23985875

David, L. A., Maurice, C. F., Carmody, R. N., Gootenberg, D. B., Button, J. E., Wolfe, B. E., Ling, A. V., Devlin, A. S., Varma, Y., Fischbach, M. A., Biddinger, S. B., Dutton, R. J., & Turnbaugh, P. J. (2014). Diet rapidly and reproducibly alters the human gut microbiome. *Nature*, *505*(7484), 559–563. DOI: 10.1038/nature12820 PMID: 24336217

Eckburg, P. B., Bik, E. M., Bernstein, C. N., Purdom, E., Dethlefsen, L., Sargent, M., Gill, S. R., Nelson, K. E., & Relman, D. A. (2005). Diversity of the human intestinal microbial flora. *Science*, *308*(5728), 1635–1638. DOI: 10.1126/science.1110591 PMID: 15831718

Everard, A., Belzer, C., Geurts, L., Ouwerkerk, J. P., Druart, C., Bindels, L. B., Guiot, Y., Derrien, M., Muccioli, G. G., Delzenne, N. M., de Vos, W. M., & Cani, P. D. (2013). Cross-talk between Akkermansia muciniphila and intestinal epithelium controls diet-induced obesity. *Proceedings of the National Academy of Sciences of the United States of America*, *110*(22), 9066–9071. DOI: 10.1073/pnas.1219451110 PMID: 23671105

Flint, H. J., Scott, K. P., Duncan, S. H., Louis, P., & Forano, E. (2012). Microbial degradation of complex carbohydrates in the gut. *Gut Microbes*, *3*(4), 289–306. DOI: 10.4161/gmic.19897 PMID: 22572875

Franzosa, E. A., Huang, K., Meadow, J. F., Gevers, D., Lemon, K. P., Bohannan, B. J. M., & Huttenhower, C. (2015). Identifying personal microbiomes using metagenomic codes. *Proceedings of the National Academy of Sciences of the United States of America*, *112*(22), E2930–E2938. DOI: 10.1073/pnas.1423854112 PMID: 25964341

Franzosa, E. A., McIver, L. J., Rahnavard, G., Thompson, L. R., Schirmer, M., Weingart, G., Lipson, K. S., Knight, R., Caporaso, J. G., Segata, N., & Huttenhower, C. (2015). Species-level functional profiling of metagenomes and metatranscriptomes. *Nature Methods*, *15*(11), 962–968. DOI: 10.1038/s41592-018-0176-y PMID: 30377376

Franzosa, E. A., McIver, L. J., Rahnavard, G., Thompson, L. R., Schirmer, M., Weingart, G., Lipson, K. S., Knight, R., Caporaso, J. G., Segata, N., & Huttenhower, C. (2018). Species-level functional profiling of metagenomes and metatranscriptomes. *Nature Methods*, *15*(11), 962–968. DOI: 10.1038/s41592-018-0176-y PMID: 30377376

Ghaisas, S., Maher, J., & Kanthasamy, A. (2016). Gut microbiome in health and disease: Linking the microbiome-gut-brain axis and environmental factors in the pathogenesis of systemic and neurodegenerative diseases. *Pharmacology & Therapeutics*, *158*, 52–62. DOI: 10.1016/j.pharmthera.2015.11.012 PMID: 26627987

Hill, M. J. (2012). Microbial vitamin K and cardiovascular disease. *Microbial Biotechnology*, *5*(1), 98–107. DOI: 10.1111/j.1751-7915.2011.00228.x PMID: 21958386

Janda, J. M., & Abbott, S. L. (2007). 16S rRNA gene sequencing for bacterial identification in the diagnostic laboratory: Pluses, perils, and pitfalls. *Journal of Clinical Microbiology*, *45*(9), 2761–2764. DOI: 10.1128/JCM.01228-07 PMID: 17626177

Kim, S. A., & Shin, J. (2018). Role of the gut microbiome in obesity and metabolic syndrome. *Experimental & Molecular Medicine*, *50*(11), 1–9. DOI: 10.1038/s12276-018-0178-y PMID: 30429461

Koh, A., De Vadder, F., Kovatcheva-Datchary, P., & Bäckhed, F. (2016). From dietary fiber to host physiology: Short-chain fatty acids as key bacterial metabolites. *Cell*, *165*(6), 1332–1345. DOI: 10.1016/j.cell.2016.05.041 PMID: 27259147

Koh, A., De Vadder, F., Kovatcheva-Datchary, P., & Bäckhed, F. (2016). From dietary fiber to host physiology: Short-chain fatty acids as key bacterial metabolites. *Cell*, *165*(6), 1332–1345. DOI: 10.1016/j.cell.2016.05.041 PMID: 27259147

Kumar, A. (2019). Ethical considerations in microbiome research. *Frontiers in Microbiology*, *10*, 1801. DOI: 10.3389/fmicb.2019.01801

Le Chatelier, E., Nielsen, T., Qin, J., Prifti, E., Hildebrand, F., Falony, G., Almeida, M., Arumugam, M., Batto, J.-M., Kennedy, S., Leonard, P., Li, J., Burgdorf, K., Grarup, N., Jørgensen, T., Brandslund, I., Nielsen, H. B., Juncker, A. S., Bertalan, M., & Pedersen, O. (2013). Richness of human gut microbiome correlates with metabolic markers. *Nature*, *500*(7464), 541–546. DOI: 10.1038/nature12506 PMID: 23985870

Ley, R. E., Turnbaugh, P. J., Klein, S., & Gordon, J. I. (2006). Microbial ecology: Human gut microbes associated with obesity. *Nature*, *444*(7122), 1022–1023. DOI: 10.1038/4441022a PMID: 17183309

Louis, P., & Flint, H. J. (2017). Formation of propionate and butyrate by the human colonic microbiota. *Environmental Microbiology*, *19*(1), 29–41. DOI: 10.1111/1462-2920.13589 PMID: 27928878

Pollock, J., Glendinning, L., Wisedchanwet, T., & Watson, M. (2018). The madness of microbiome: Attempting to find consensus "best practice" for 16S microbiome studies. *Applied and Environmental Microbiology*, *84*(7), e02627–e17. DOI: 10.1128/AEM.02627-17 PMID: 29427429

Pompei, A.. (2007). Genome sequence and characterization of Bifidobacterium breve strain UCC2003. *Journal of Bacteriology*, *189*(19), 6878–6884. DOI: 10.1128/JB.00719-07

Qin, J., Li, R., Raes, J., Arumugam, M., Burgdorf, K. S., Manichanh, C., Nielsen, T., Pons, N., Levenez, F., Yamada, T., Mende, D. R., Li, J., Xu, J., Li, S., Li, D., Cao, J., Wang, B., Liang, H., Zheng, H., & Wang, J. (2010). A human gut microbial gene catalogue established by metagenomic sequencing. *Nature*, *464*(7285), 59–65. DOI: 10.1038/nature08821 PMID: 20203603

Quince, C., Walker, A. W., Simpson, J. T., Loman, N. J., & Segata, N. (2017). Shotgun metagenomics, from sampling to analysis. *Nature Biotechnology*, *35*(9), 833–844. DOI: 10.1038/nbt.3935 PMID: 28898207

Ridlon, J. M., Kang, D. J., & Hylemon, P. B. (2006). Bile salt biotransformations by human intestinal bacteria. *Journal of Lipid Research*, *47*(2), 241–259. DOI: 10.1194/jlr.R500013-JLR200 PMID: 16299351

Ríos-Covián, D., Ruas-Madiedo, P., Margolles, A., Gueimonde, M., de los Reyes-Gavilán, C. G., & Salazar, N. (2016). Intestinal short chain fatty acids and their link with diet and human health. *Frontiers in Microbiology*, *7*, 185. DOI: 10.3389/fmicb.2016.00185 PMID: 26925050

Smits, S. A.. (2019). Public health interventions targeting the microbiome: A new frontier in disease prevention. *Nature Reviews. Microbiology*, *17*(9), 654–668. DOI: 10.1038/s41579-019-0236-9

Suez, J., Zmora, N., Zilberman-Schapira, G., Mor, U., & Elinav, E. (2019). Personalized microbiome-based approaches to prophylaxis against food allergy and other non-communicable diseases. *Trends in Immunology*, *40*(8), 682–700. DOI: 10.1016/j.it.2019.06.008

Tremaroli, V., & Bäckhed, F. (2012). Functional interactions between the gut microbiota and host metabolism. *Nature*, *489*(7415), 242–249. DOI: 10.1038/nature11552 PMID: 22972297

Turnbaugh, P. J., Hamady, M., Yatsunenko, T., Cantarel, B. L., Duncan, A., Ley, R. E., Sogin, M. L., Jones, W. J., Roe, B. A., Affourtit, J. P., Egholm, M., Henrissat, B., Heath, A. C., Knight, R., & Gordon, J. I. (2009). A core gut microbiome in obese and lean twins. *Nature*, *457*(7228), 480–484. DOI: 10.1038/nature07540 PMID: 19043404

Turnbaugh, P. J., Ley, R. E., Hamady, M., Fraser-Liggett, C. M., Knight, R., & Gordon, J. I. (2007). The human microbiome project. *Nature*, *449*(7164), 804–810. DOI: 10.1038/nature06244 PMID: 17943116

Valdes, A. M., Walter, J., Segal, E., & Spector, T. D. (2018). Role of the gut microbiota in nutrition and health. *BMJ (Clinical Research Ed.)*, *361*, k2179. DOI: 10.1136/bmj.k2179 PMID: 29899036

Zeevi, D., Korem, T., Zmora, N., Israeli, D., Rothschild, D., Weinberger, A., Ben-Yacov, O., Lador, D., Avnit-Sagi, T., Lotan-Pompan, M., Suez, J., Mahdi, J. A., Matot, E., Malka, G., Kosower, N., Rein, M., Zilberman-Schapira, G., Dohnalová, L., Pevsner-Fischer, M., & Segal, E. (2015). Personalized nutrition by prediction of glycemic responses. *Cell*, *163*(5), 1079–1094. DOI: 10.1016/j.cell.2015.11.001 PMID: 26590418

Zhang, P.. (2022). Influence of foods and nutrition on the gut microbiome and implications for intestinal health. *Frontiers in Nutrition*, *9*, 833968. DOI: 10.3389/fnut.2022.833968 PMID: 36076980

Zhernakova, A., Kurilshikov, A., Bonder, M. J., Tigchelaar, E. F., Schirmer, M., Vatanen, T., Mujagic, Z., Vila, A. V., Falony, G., Vieira-Silva, S., Wang, J., Imhann, F., Brandsma, E., Jankipersadsing, S. A., Joossens, M., Cenit, M. C., Deelen, P., Swertz, M. A., Weersma, R. K., & Fu, J. (2016). Population-based metagenomics analysis reveals markers for gut microbiome composition and diversity. *Science*, *352*(6285), 565–569. DOI: 10.1126/science.aad3369 PMID: 27126040

Zmora, N., Zeevi, D., Korem, T., Segal, E., & Elinav, E. (2019). Personalized gut mucosal colonization resistance to empiric probiotics is associated with unique host and microbiome features. *Cell*, *174*(6), 1388–1405.e21. DOI: 10.1016/j.cell.2018.08.041 PMID: 30193112

Chapter 3
Custom Sustenance Through Gut Biotics:
A Promising Way for Gut Well-Being Through a Personalised Manner

Debdut Manna
https://orcid.org/0009-0001-7923-5173
Indian Agricultural Research Institute, India

Rosalin Laishram
Indian Agricultural Research Institute, India

Debjyoti Das
Bidhan Chandra Krishi Viswavidyalaya, India

Anil Dahuja
Indian Agricultural Research Institute, India

ABSTRACT

Nutritional sciences have been profoundly affected by the shift from malnourishment to overnutrition in various regions owing to factors including cultural diversity, lifestyle choices, environmental instability and food sustainability. By customizing dietary therapies to meet the unique needs of each person, personalized nutrition reimagines the role of probiotics, prebiotics, postbiotics, and synbiotics in healthy eating, with a focus on gastrointestinal illnesses and other condition-specific issues. With the advancement in technologies in-depth characterization of gut microbiota, revealing its composition, functional dynamics, and extensive microbial diversity have been enabled. Considering all aspects, in this chapter, we discussed how societal

DOI: 10.4018/979-8-3373-4382-2.ch003

influence and advancements in functional biotics foods are driving individualized nutrition strategies for therapeutic and preventive healthcare. The main focus on gut biotics is at the forefront of innovations in human health, propelled by collaborative efforts paving the way for a new era of personalised and targeted healthcare.

1. INTRODUCTION

Personalised nutrition is a relatively new trend in the health and wellness industry that seeks to address people's unique nutritional needs by taking into account their unique genetic makeup, phenotypic, microbiota, and personal preferences. The growing concern over physical and mental health. These conditions are diagnosed through abnormalities in one's cognitive abilities or through therapeutic screening markers that do not have the typical pathophysiologic symptoms (Luo et al., 2019). So, one of the most important things about modern nutrition and healthcare is coming up with effective intervention techniques and novel approaches that take into account the specific gut microbiota of each individual and how it may be used to improve health (Wilmanski et al., 2021). Modifying host–microbiota interactions by personalised nutrition represents a novel therapeutic approach for illness management and prevention. The composition and function of gut microbiota are established throughout infancy, as individuals are colonised by bacteria from carers and their surroundings, significantly impacting the microbiota's makeup in maturity (Gomez de Agüero et al., 2016). Recent research investigating the effects of functional foods, particularly probiotics, prebiotics and postbiotics on human health have emerged in response to the expanding understanding of the role of gut microbiota in maintaining overall health. In order to provide specific health benefits beyond their fundamental nutritional value, functional foods are prepared or augmented with biologically active substances, such as vitamins, minerals, herbs, or other beneficial nutrients.

The scientific core of personalized nutrition is combined with genetics and epigenetics. Nutrigenetics involves the study of the interactions between genetic differences and the effects of nutrients. Thereby it describes why some people might be affected by some foods, including lactose intolerance or the way a body metabolizes folate. Nutrigenomics tells us about the influences that nutrients and bioactive substances have on gene expression and metabolic pathways and emphasizes the interactive nature in which diet and the genome interact to maintain health and prevent diseases (Lagoumintzis & Patrinos, 2023). Epigenetics has further taken a step in observing the reversible modifications of the gene activity which include variations involving DNA methylation or modification of histone that are affected by dietary constituents and even extend to successive generations. Future convergence of these disciplines opens the possibility to shift the current paradigm of generalized dietary guidelines to the highly specific, individualized nutrition design focused on disease prevention, maximum metabolic health, and overall well-being via gene-diet interactions.

Microbial diversity can only be partially characterized using conventional culture-based methods. Other methods that have made a greater impact in taxonomic and functional profiling by providing high-resolution data with the culture-independent approach include 16S rRNA gene sequencing, whole metagenome sequencing and shotgun metagenomics. In addition to DNA-based techniques, meta-transcriptomics, meta-proteomics, and meta-metabolomics enable the study of microbial activity, protein expression, and metabolite interactions in an integrated manner of host-microbe dynamics. These technologies not only add insight to our developing science on microbial ecology, but they can also contribute to translational applications to precision nutrition, diagnostics and therapy (Hemmati et al., 2024).

Within this framework, the term gut biotics includes prebiotics, probiotics, metabolites derived from probiotics called postbiotics and also species that combine probiotics and prebiotics known as synbiotics. Probiotics have therefore a massive therapeutic potential for maintaining epithelial homeostasis and modulating systemic health. Probiotics are live microorganisms, e.g., Lactobacillus and Bifidobacterium spp., that confer health benefits through competitive inhibition of pathogen microorganisms, synthesis of beneficial metabolic substances and modulation of immune responses. Prebiotics, such as inulin, galacto-oligosaccharides (GOS) and fructo-oligosaccharides (FOS) preferentially stimulate the growth of these beneficial gut bacteria and the resulting short-chain fatty acids (SCFAs) decrease colonic pH, improve intestinal barrier integrity and modulate lipid and glucose metabolism. To avoid the issue of viability, which is justified for live probiotics, postbiotics are thermal inactivated microbial cells and their metabolic products with antioxidant, anti-microbial and immunomodulatory activity (Kandari et al. 2024). As synbiotics are the combination of probiotics with complementary prebiotics, it has a synergistic effect that increases the microbial resistance, the absorption of nutrients and the host immunity (Smolińska et al., 2025).

They have been shown efficacy for controlling different syndromes of inflammatory bowel diseases like colitis, intestinal infections, irritable bowel syndrome and colon cancer. In addition to classical GI effects, growing evidence suggests that selective regulation of the intestinal microbiota can have a beneficial effect on the evolution of COVID-19 (Xavier-Santos et al., 2022). In this regard, Akour (2020) stated administration of probiotics or prebiotics as an adjuvant therapy may help to reduce the risk of developing the secondary infections by repopulating the dysregulated microbiota in the infected patients. Furthermore, clinical trials are ongoing that suggest synbiotic supplementation can reduce diarrhoea duration, increase stool consistency and reduce inflammation associated with dysbiosis, further demonstrating the potential of gut biotics for preventive as well as restorative healthcare.

Despite many advancements, clinical translation of gut biotics continues to be difficult. This may be because of individual variations in gut microbiota composition, the lack of appropriate standardization of dosages, the paucity of long-term randomised controlled trials (RCTs), and stability issues, especially for probiotics. New regulatory environment, i.e. strain-specific characterisation and clinical evidence of health claims are required in Europe by the European Food Safety Authority (EFSA), while in the US probiotics are used as dietary supplements and in general undergo only a limited pre-market review by the US Food and Drug Administration (US FDA). Furthermore, new types of products such as psychobiotics for mental health and next generation designed mixed microbial consortiums create new complexity in safety assessment and ethical considerations. (Zommiti et al., 2020; Alagiakrishnan & Halverson, 2021).

Taken together, these developments exemplify the potential of gut biotics for targeted and preventative nutrition. Apart from these strategies for alleviating gastrointestinal disease manifestations, they also have a beneficial potential in modulating extra-intestinal diseases, such as obesity, type 2 diabetes, inflammatory bowel disease, and neuroimmune disorders. The subsequent sections of this chapter will provide mechanistic insights, summarise clinical evidence, explore technological innovations, and discuss regulatory challenges shaping the future of gut biotics in precision health.

2. PERSONALIZED NUTRITION IN TERMS OF GENETICS AND EPIGENETICS

In personalised nutrition, people have different dietary needs and responses because of their unique genetic and epigenetic make-up. Therefore, the establishment of dietary interventions depending upon the genetic and epigenetic features can be viewed as an evidence-based approach to health improvement and reduction of disease development. The key to this approach is nutrigenetics and nutrigenomics. Nutrigenetics focuses on the effect of variation in the genetic makeup through alteration of nutrient intake, metabolism, and absorption (Bouchard & Ordovas, 2012). On the other hand, nutrigenomics is the study of how nutrients can exert this regulatory effect on gene expression, most prominently as a nuclear transcription factor. Nutritional elements can also indirectly influence gene expression by modulating gene regulatory factors such as epigenetic markers, which include DNA methylation and miRNA (Holzapfel et al., 2022). Nutrigenetics can have an extremely significant impact on both nutrigenomic and epigenetic outcomes. The effects, in turn, regulate personal status and disease prone-ness.

2.1 Nutrigenetics and Nutrigenomics

Nutrigenomics, as an emerging discipline that was developed by the Human Genome Project and the post-genomic age, employs the use of high through-put omics platforms to describe the effect of dietary inputs on gene expression (Lagoumintzis & Patrinos, 2024). Whereas, nutrigenetics tends to focus on single nucleotide polymorphisms (SNPs) and the flanking haplotypes as the main objects of the analysis using Genome-wide association studies (GWAS) (Marcum, 2020).

The most visible example is CYP1A2 gene, coding a liver-specific enzyme, demethylating caffeine. Certain variants are capable of promoting the process of demethylation faster than other ones (Chaudhary et al., 2025). Polymorphism in PNPLA3 consists of three different genotypic variants, all of which predispose the occurrence of non-alcoholic fatty liver disease (NAFLD). The result of carrying the G allele in both adults and paediatrics leads to isoleucine-methionine conversion, which heightens the lipogenesis, triggers the triglyceride production and stores in hepatocytes. Various factors such as glucose and insulin also regulate PNPLA3 gene in human hepatocytes and this regulation is quite sensitive to changes in nutritional status (Oh et al., 2023). Moreover, fasting and re-feeding states modulate the level of PNPLA3 mRNAs expression as the mRNA levels are also higher in obese insulin-dependent mice (Huang et al., 2010). Obesity itself represents a leading risk factor to a variety of numerous diseases, particularly diabetes type 2, cardiovascular disease and some cancers. Fat mass and obesity-associated (FTO) gene is one of the genetic determinants of adiposity. FTO gene not only enhances repair of DNA and RNA, but also increases metabolism specific to various pathways, especially that of proteins controlling hunger and satiety. In the brain, higher FTO expression is associated with greater obesity, and carriers of certain FTO polymorphisms have increased body mass, increased food consumption, reduced satiety, and increased circulating levels of leptin-a hormone involved in appetite regulation (Górczyńska-Kosiorz et al., 2024; St Germain et al., 2025). Empirical evidence suggests that this gene has a very strong effect on the development of paediatric obesity, and there is a need to explain the role of this gene in interaction with dietary patterns when seeking innovative treatment opportunities in obesity. Cardiovascular disease is controlled by Apolipoprotein E (APOE) by maintaining cholesterol homeostasis. They have three functional APOE alleles, including APOE2, APOE3 and APOE4, which have significant effects towards cardiovascular disease susceptibility and Alzheimer disease (AD). APOE allelic status, and thereby risk of disease, is a joint product of two SNPs. Individuals who possess two APOE4 alleles are subjected to significant increased risk of Alzheimer, whereas people possessing a combination of APOE4 and APOE3 allele are highly susceptible to AD as well as coronary artery disease. The susceptibility is lowered in approximately 50 per cent of general population, through the APOE3/APOE3 and APOE2/APOE2 genotypes (Abondio et al., 2019; Mullins et al., 2020). Lifestyle changes, which predominantly comprise dietary modification and habitual exercise have been found to moderate cardiovascular morbidity and are most effective in both groups that bear APOE4 alleles. In case of folate metabolism, MTHFR gene provides the coding target of the methylenetetrahydrofolate reductase enzyme that changes the 5,10-methyleneTHF to 5-methylTHF, the bioactive folate acknowledged as vital in haematopoiesis and transformation of homocysteine to methionine. The muter-exchange effect common on the MTHFR gene significantly reduces enzyme activity, especially on people with t/t genotype (Kassem et al., 2023). The reduced circulating folate and elevated circulating homocysteine is attributed to this genotype. Increased homocysteine is an increased risk of many medical diseases.

In a nutshell, nutrigenetics and nutrigenomics complement one another through reciprocal interactions, allowing them specialty to provide a comprehensive picture of an individual's integrated metabolism in order to construct a personalized diet to avoid illness and potential health risks, as well as promote health and longevity.

2.2 Nutritional Influences on Epigenetics

Epigenetics refers to heritable changes in gene expression that are not caused by changes in the DNA sequence but include DNA methylation, histone modifications (acetylation and methylation), and the regulatory activities of non-coding RNAs (miRNAs and lncRNAs). The epigenetic marks are a dynamic network of modifications that incorporates extrinsic signalling, including dietary inputs. Methyl group donors of S-adenosylmethionine (SAM) include one-carbon metabolism molecules like folate, vitamin B12, vitamin B6, choline, methionine etc. When these cofactors are deficient in the diet, it leads to defective patterns of methylation. DNA hypomethylation and Colorectal cancer risk as well as predisposition to other cancers has been linked to clinical folate deficiency (Tiffon, 2018; Wang et al., 2022). On the other hand, excessive consumption of these micronutrients has a significant effect on epigenetic cell programming.

There are also direct regulatory effects of dietary components on the enzymes that add and remove epigenetic marks. Substances such as polyphenols and other phytochemicals that occur in fruits and vegetables block DNA methyltransferases (DNMTs) and thus make tumor-suppressor genes prone to demethylation. There is empirical evidence that green tea catechins, curcumin in turmeric, and genistein in soy inhibit DNMT in vitro and reactivate silenced genes (Carlos-Reyes et al., 2019).

Epigenome-wide association studies (EWASs) have found a number of DNA methylation markers linked to a variety of disorders, and new research is investigating the function of DNA methylation in influencing the response to food and lifestyle changes. A systematic review combined the evidence pointing to maternal dieting habits during pregnancy and placental and offspring epigenetic modifications. Other studies demonstrated the impact of dietary micronutrients on gene expression and health in early life, later life health and disease. Large-scale DNA methylation analysis identified associated CpG sites with folate and vitamin B12 intake in adults, while habitual diet quality reported a link to differential leukocyte DNA methylation levels (Holzapfel et al., 2022).

2.3 Gut Microbiota in Relationship with Nutrigenetics, Nutrigenomics and Epigenetics

Intestinal microbiota is a critical gut-host interface between genetics, epigenetics and diet. Diet includes bioactive molecules produced by microorganisms of the gastrointestinal tract through the metabolism of dietary components and have an effect on the networks of host genes. Gut microbiota ferments dietary fibers in colon and synthesizes short-chain fatty acids (SCFAs), especially butyrate, which acts as a HDAC inhibitor and also express protective genes (Tiffon, 2018). Similarly, gut bacteria produce vitamins (folate, biotin, vitamin K and some B vitamins) that make up the host one-carbon pool and hence affect DNA methylation (Lagoumintzis & Patrinos, 2023). The bacterial metabolism of dietary polyphenols and amino acids generates urolithins and tryptamine, which can bind host receptors, as well as initiate epigenetically-induced effects, although these mechanisms have not been yet fully described.

On the other hand, microbial ecosystem is also conditioned by host genotypic and epigenetic influences. Each gene responsible in immune recognition and mucosal physiology predetermines the ability of microbes to inhabit the intestine. Nutrigenetic individuality results in quantitatively and qualitatively different microbial communities; these microbial populations, in turn, adjust the host metabolic and epigenome state. Modern-day research highlights a triangular relationship in which a personalized nutrition paradigm is conceptualized not just in terms of the host genome and its diet, but also the metagenome, which is the sum of the microbial genomes (Lagoumintzis & Patrinos, 2023; Kussmann & van Bladeren, 2011). According to recent studies in vitamin D and folate metabolism, the microbiome differentiation is highly related to the VDR or MTHFR genotype, thus, indicating a two-way association between host and microbe (Meral et al., 2024).

Nutrigenetics, nutrigenomics and epigenomics form a combined system on which personalized nutrition is based. Gut microbiota acts as a primary intermediate impacting the availability of nutrients and producing signaling molecules that trigger modulatory effects on the host genome and epigenome. The overall objective is to conceptualize nutrition to create dietary patterns, materialized to be in agreement with the genetic makeup, epigenetic status as well as microbiome of an individual, thus improving health outcomes in an entirely personalized sense.

3. INTERFERENCE OF PROBIOTICS AS PERSONALIZED NUTRITION

The significance of adequate nutrition for health is universally recognized, which is why it is integrated into public health efforts to promote optimal well-being in all facets of life. Despite the significant challenges, it is important to incorporate the individual functionalities of different foods in terms of their health benefits for developing personalized nutrition concepts. The market for functional products is dominated by foods that include probiotics, making them one of the most ubiquitous substances in this category. The term "probiotics" refers to supplemental living organisms that have the ability to change the microbiota of the host intestine through colonization and implantation and have positive benefits at optimal doses (Gasbarrini et al., 2016). What began in 1907 with the pioneering research of Russian researcher Elie Metchnikoff on phagocytosis as an endogenous immunological process in fighting infection, has evolved into the present-day era of probiotics. Thus, Metchnikoff came up with the concept of intestinal auto-intoxication which he believed is responsible for the degeneration of healthy tissues and the premature aging (Casado, 2017). Parker first introduced the word probiotic as the name for a category of micro-organisms that help to restore the healthy microbial environment to the human gut. Lactic acid bacteria (LAB) are the most common type of probiotic microorganisms and are categorised as "Generally Recognized as Safe (GRAS)". LAB belongs to the family *Lactobacillales*, the phylum *Firmicutes*, and the class *Bacilli*. They are grouped based on utilization of various sugar sources, fermentation of glucose by themselves, optimum temperature for growth and their cell's size and shape (Huynh et al., 2023). *Lactobacillus* and *Bifidobacterium* are the most prevalent genera for probiotic microbes. Other, less common species may belong to genera including *Streptococcus, Lactococcus, Enterococcus, and Bacillus* (Sniffen et al., 2018). Further, in light of increasing knowledge on the human-associated microbiota followed by discovery of methodologies, new potential probiotics such as *Roseburia intestinalis, Faecalibacterium prausnitzii, Eubacterium spp., Bacteroides spp., Clostridium butyricum*, and *Akkermansia muciniphila* have emerged as new generation probiotics (O'Toole et al., 2017).

A good way to choose probiotics is important to make sure they are good for your health. Additionally, for probiotics to be effective, the microorganisms used to make them must meet certain criteria, such as being safe for humans to consume, having the capacity to survive in the digestive tract, adhering to the intestinal epithelium, colonizing the gastrointestinal tract, producing antimicrobial substances, and remaining viable and stable throughout processing and storage (Yoha et al., 2022). To ensure safety and efficacy in effective targeted delivery, contemporary protective technologies and methodologies such as edible coating formulation, bio-encapsulation, high/low temperature drying, electrospray coating and 3D printing techniques have been adopted and refined by the scientific community (Zhang et al., 2024). Viability of live microorganisms (7 log CFU/mL) is required throughout production, storage and throughout the shelf life of the product for survival through the gastrointestinal tract (Korčok et al., 2018).

When consumed in adequate amounts, probiotics show beneficial effects on human health and physiology. Promising potential in health regulation and health promotion can be linked with values like survival, activity, quorum sensing, unique structural components, metabolites, as well as mechanisms of action. (Sadeghi et al., 2023). They are reported to be health-promoting, including the ability to maintain epithelial barrier functions, reduce the risk of type 2 diabetes development, prevent inflammatory bowel disease, improve intestinal health, digestion, and absorption, regulate immune system, alleviate allergies, combat cancer and lower serum cholesterol (Das et al., 2022). Probiotics are taken to supplement exact dose and type of advantageous microorganisms to the gastrointestinal tract (GIT) system. A healthy gut microbiome, which can be facilitated by nutritional and lifestyle changes, such as the intake and use of a wide range of probiotics, can help the gut to avoid living with neurological illnesses, digestive illnesses, gastric ulcers, atopic diseases, and lactose intolerance (Dhopatkar et al., 2023; Yeşilyurt et al., 2021).

There has been much discussion about personalizing probiotics for quite some time. The current global marketing of probiotic products is based on the premise that all people can benefit from these proven health benefits. The health condition, dietary habits, and predominant GI microbiota of an individual determine the effectiveness of a probiotic (Kashyap et al., 2017). The identification of specific microbiome types and their characteristics that can be utilized to predict the beginning, progression and effectiveness of disease is a major goal of microbiome research. Such results underscore the necessity for more authentic strategies in modifying host microbiota, with probiotics emerging as a potentially transformative intervention that could positively affect health (Veiga et al., 2020; Liu et al., 2018). Hence, there is a critical need for the development of personalized probiotics to allow concerns relevant populations of the probiotic effects.

4. INTERFERENCE OF PREBIOTICS IN PERSONALIZED NUTRITION

In the current era of precision medicine, growing recognition of the gut microbiome community's influence on human biology is expanding. The recognition of substantial inter-personal variation in microbiome composition-function and the manipulation of these microbial communities through personalised nutrition strategies has become a promising frontier. The human gut microbiome, often described as an essential organ, contributes to host physiology through nutrient metabolism, immune modulation and even neuro-behavioral regulation. Among the most powerful dietary modulators of the gut microbiome community configuration are Microbiota-Directed Foods (MDFs), particularly prebiotics. The concept of prebiotic arises with the discovery of the beneficial gut bacteria which promotes human health (György *et al.*, 1954) up to the selective fermentation of the carbohydrates (Yazawa, 1978). The term prebiotic was first formally introduced by Gibson and Roberfroid in their seminal paper, 1995. The current consensus definition promulgated by the International Scientific Association for Probiotics and Prebiotics (ISAPP), supported by the International Probiotics Association (IPA) in 2022, defines prebiotics as "substrates that are selectively utilized by host microorganisms conferring a health benefit." Prebiotics comprise diverse oligosaccharides (inulin, FOS, GOS, XOS, IMO) and synthetic compounds (lactulose, polydextrose, lactitol, protein hydrolysates) that nourish gut microbiota (Refer Table 1). These non-digestible compounds resist enzymatic hydrolysis in the upper gastrointestinal tract and reach the colon intact, where they serve as fermentable substrates for beneficial bacteria such as *Bifidobacterium, Lactobacillus*. Their substrate selectivity also extends to other beneficial taxa, including *Akkermansia muciniphila, Faecalibacterium prausnitzii, and Roseburia* (Li *et al.*, 2019; You *et al.*, 2022). Depending on structural properties, for example, the degree of polymerization and the structure of a monosaccharide they ferment to produce SCFAs such as acetate, propionate, and butyrate. (Davani-Davari *et al.*, 2019).

Prebiotics that have gained popularity as a functional ingredient in the food industry and are added in multiple food matrixes, such as dairy products, dairy alternative drinks, gluten free foods to encourage gut health. Several prebiotics, including inulin, FOS and GOS can serve as a carrier for probiotic enhancing their viability in the gut, improving sensory properties and add value addition to the final products. Furthermore, the SCFAs produced during prebiotic fermentation link gut microbiota activity to both food sensory properties and human health by activating umami taste receptors (TAS1R1 and TAS1R3) in enteroendocrine cells through G protein–coupled receptor pathways, thereby enhancing the perception of savoury flavours. This improves taste perception and overall palatability in prebiotic-enriched fermented foods like cheeses, yoghurts, and fermented beverages. Concurrently, SCFAs contribute to physiological benefits, including antimicrobial effects, gut barrier strengthening, and immune modulation, exemplifying their significance in microbiome-targeted functional foods. In drinks they enhance mouthfeel, add functional fibre content and help in sensory enhancement. The prebiotics help in maintaining moisture in bakery items, increase elastin, and the products act as fat and sugar substitutes hence increases the nutritional content without compromising taste. The Prebiotic enrichment converts normal foods to specific functional foods intended to stimulate microbiome modulation and enhanced host physiology. (Jackson et al., 2022; Verma et al., 2023).

Emerging prebiotics through enzyme-based bio-conversion, microbial sources or underutilized plant-sources include agro-residues, ciceritol found in legumes, legumes by-products are under consideration as an alternative inexpensive source of prebiotics. These will expand more healthier food products options in existing functional food markets which also promotes sustainability. Recent analysis of patent fillings in prebiotic research and their application across various food products are gaining innovation. The number of patents in prebiotic has steadily increase since 2013 which include gut-friendly food applications, drug delivery systems and synbiotic food development (Zang et al. 2024). Among food companies, Nestec SA is leading in the number of patents filed. Alongside, the technological applications extend to improving food characteristics and developing novel delivery methods (Dixit et al., 2016). The expanding patent landscape reflects the growing market interest and potential of prebiotics in varied dominant market sectors.

Table 1. Different sources of prebiotics and their functional roles in Human health.

Source	Prebiotic Type(s)	Functional Properties	Applications	Benefits	References
Chicory root, Jerusalem artichoke, onion	Inulin: Long-chain β-(2→1) linked fructans, DP >10	Soluble dietary fiber regulates satiety and gut motility	Functional foods, beverages, snacks	↑ Sustained SCFA production; ↑ gut barrier integrity; modulates lipid and glucose metabolism	Qin et al.,2023; Mudannayake et al., 2022
Various plants (legumes, beans, grains)	Raffinose Family Oligosaccharides (RFOs): α-galactosyl derivatives of sucrose (raffinose, stachyose)	Oligosaccharides resistant to digestion	Functional foods, supplements	↑ Selective fermentation by probiotics; ↑ SCFA; immune modulation; flatulence side effect	Clemente, A., & Olias, R.,2017.
Milk lactose (via enzymatic process)	Galactooligosaccharides (GOS): β-1,4 and β-1,6 galactose-linked oligomers	Potent bifidogenic oligosaccharides	Infant formulas, supplements	↑ Immune development; ↑ calcium absorption; stimulates *bifidobacteria*	Ambrogi et al., 2023
Plant xylans (corncobs, sugarcane bagasse)	Xylooligosaccharides (XOS): β-(1→4) xylose oligomers	Derived from hemicellulose	Fibre supplements, functional foods	↑ Selective microbiota stimulation; ↓ pathogen growth	Nascimento et al., 2022 ; Marim & Gabardo,, 2021.
Grains, unripe bananas, legumes	Resistant Starch: α-1,4 glucan polysaccharides resistant to mammalian digestion	Slowly fermentable polysaccharide	Bakery, cereals	↑ Butyrate production; ↑ bowel motility; improves glycemic control	Ghare et al., 2024
Cereals (oats, barley), mushrooms	Beta-glucans: Soluble β-1,3/1,6 glucans	Cholesterol-lowering soluble fiber	Cereals, functional beverages	↑ Immune modulation; ↓ LDL cholesterol	Ames et al.,2018; Lante et al., 2023
Food-processed starch (synthetic)	Polydextrose: Synthetic glucose polymer	Low-calorie bulking agent; soluble fiber	Food additives, fibre supplements	↑ Gut microbiota balance; ↑ laxation	do Carmo et al.,2016
Starch fermentation products	Isomalto-oligosaccharides (IMO): α-1,6 linked glucooligosaccharides	Fermentation derivatives from starch	Synbiotics, fiber-enriched foods	↑ Supports *bifidobacteria* and *lactobacilli* growth	Tiangpook et al.,2023
Fruit peels (apple, citrus)	Pectin: Complex galacturonic acid heteropolysaccharide	Soluble fiber	Fibre supplements, beverages	↑ Enhances microbial diversity; regulates lipid metabolism; and immune modulation, cancer prevention	Emran et al., 2022
Soybean residue (Okara)	Insoluble and soluble fibers; raffinose, stachyose; proteins; isoflavones	Nutrient-dense byproduct	Nutraceuticals, synbiotics, functional foods	↑ Prebiotic substrate for *Lactobacillus*, *Bifidobacterium*; ↑ SCFA production; immunomodulation; gut barrier support	Swallah et al., 2021
Microalgae (*Spirulina*, *Chlorella*)	Sulfated and branched polysaccharides	Bioactive dietary fiber and antioxidants	Nutraceuticals, functional foods	↑ Antioxidant, antiviral, immunomodulatory; ↑ prebiotic effects	Feng et al.,2023

continued on following page

Table 1. Continued

Source	Prebiotic Type(s)	Functional Properties	Applications	Benefits	References
Polygonatum sibiricum (medicinal plant)	Glucofructan polysaccharides	Medicinal plant polysaccharides	Nutraceuticals	↑ Antioxidant activity; modulates gut microbiota diversity	Liu et al.,2024
Poria cocos (medicinal mushroom)	Mushroom-derived heteropolysaccharides	Traditional medicinal polysaccharides	Nutraceuticals, medicinal foods	↑ Anti-inflammatory; modulates obesity-related gut dysbiosis	Liu et al.,2025
Brewer's spent grain (BSG) (agro-industrial byproduct)	Arabinoxylan-oligosaccharides (XOS); cellulose; hemicellulose	Rich in fiber and protein; soluble arabinoxylan	Functional foods, animal feed; synbiotic formulations	↑ Bifidogenicity; ↑ SCFA (acetate, propionate); antioxidant capacity	Kaur et al.,2025;Falade et al., 2025
Grape pomace (fruit processing byproduct)	Pectin, cellulose, hemicellulose; polyphenols (flavonoids, resveratrol)	Soluble and insoluble fibers; antioxidants	Nutraceuticals, functional foods	↑ Gut microbial diversity; ↓ intestinal inflammation; ↑ SCFA production	Sinrod et al.,2023
Lactose (synthetic)	Lactulose: Synthetic disaccharide of galactose-fructose	Pharmaceutical prebiotic	Food supplements	↑ Bifidobacteria growth; ↑ bowel motility; ↓ ammonia toxicity	Ruszkowski et al.,2019.
Agricultural by-products (wheat/rice/corn bran, sugarcane bagasse), Legumes (e.g., chickpeas), Microbial synthesis	Xylooligosaccharides (XOS), arabinoxylan-oligosaccharides; ciceritol (galactosyl cyclitol); β-1,2-Galactooligosaccharides synthesized by microbes	Sustainable production; highly selective substrates for beneficial gut bacteria	Functional foods, supplements, precision nutrition formulations	↑ Targeted stimulation of bifidobacteria and lactobacilli; ↑ SCFA production; ↑ pathogen resistance; sustainable sourcing	Valladares-Diestra et al.,2024;de Mattos et al., 2024

5. INTERFERENCE OF POSTBIOTICS AS PERSONALIZED NUTRITION

Postbiotics, also referred as metabiotic, are defined as metabolites/cell-free supernatants (CFS) and soluble factors like peptides, vitamins, organic acids, and enzymes secreted by probiotics. In 1993 researchers begin exploring the potential health benefits of microbial fermentation products. While in 2004 the term "post-biotics" to describe about beneficial compounds produced by probiotic microorganisms. In order to govern the different biological impacts of these substances, different research teams have utilized terminology such as para-probiotics, ghost biotics, metabiotics, tantalized probiotics, and para-psychobiotics in past (Islam et al., 2024). In 2021, ISAPP defined postbiotics as "a product derived from inanimate microorganisms and/or their components, offering a beneficial effect on the host's well-being" (ISAPP 2022). The problem of dose standardization and unpredictability is well known to affect live bacteria called probiotics, but similar problems do not affect postbiotics. Because they don't include virulence factors or antibiotic resistance genes, are simpler to handle and store, have a longer shelf life, better quality control, and faster production times (Żółkiewicz et al., 2020).

Postbiotics are soluble molecules comprising cell remnants, cellular components, cell-wall fractions, secretions, and metabolites derived from probiotic cells, which, when ingested in adequate amounts, confer health benefits to the host (Cicenia et al., 2016). These molecules have been found in bodily fluids in different forms like peptidoglycan-derived muropeptides, exopolysaccharides (EPS), teichoic acids, peptides, protein chains, lactic acid, acetic acid, vitamins, cofactors, cell-free supernatant and antimicrobial peptides (Thorakkattu et al., 2022; Aghebati-Maleki et al., 2021). It is also important to note that postbiotics like prebiotics develop probiotics in each individual's digestive tract instead of adding new strains to the gut microbiota. To conquer this problem and bring postbiotics closer to the end user in a personalized nutrition setting, there is a need for safety evaluation, optimization of the different methods for extraction and identification of their chemical content, and their function in biological systems (Abbasi et al. 2022). There is a potential for using postbiotics with medicinal and health promotion applications which could be exploited for personalized nutrition. By better understanding the impact of these metabolites on these systems, and advancing the use of these metabolites, we hope to unlock alternate therapeutic treatments for metabolic disease, immunity, and improve gut health.

A number of technological protocols can be used for the production of postbiotics from inactivated probiotics. While considering postbiotics, it is always important to keep in mind that their inactivation process must preserve all of the beneficial properties of their live counterparts. These include heat treatment, pressurization, irradiation, radiation, chemical treatment, enzymatic processing and drying, ultrasonication and pH fluctuations among many others (de Almada et al., 2016). These techniques have an impact on DNA, nucleic acids, cell membranes, denaturation of proteins, chemical modifications, enzyme inactivation, and protein coagulation. To increase the economy of manufacturing and storage of such substances, some process steps such as centrifugation, freeze drying, dialysis and extraction are used for extracting the desired compound from the plant extract. Subsequently, several qualitative and quantitative analyses, including GC-MS, LC-MS, TLC, spectroscopy, NMR, MALDI-TOF, and FTIR, have been employed to check the volume of postbiotics and their chemical compositions associated with positive effects (Moradi et al., 2021).

Postbiotics have gained in popularity in the scientific and industrial field for their proven benefits of improving human gut health, extending the shelf life and sensory characteristics of fermented foods, and improving their nutritional content. This further provides greater choices for personalized nutrition to customers (Vera-Santander et al, 2023). Their reported benefits (Table 2) include supporting lactose intolerance, reduce cancer risk, improving heart health, modulating immune and inflammatory responses, lowering cholesterol, reducing cancer risk, alleviating acute diarrhea, mitigating food allergies, improving nutrient bioavailability, protecting oral health, reducing signs of ageing, and supporting respiratory health (Bourebaba et al., 2022; de Almada et al., 2016).

Table 2. Overview of postbiotic components, their microbial sources, and documented health benefits.

Postbiotics	Sources	Health benefits	References
SCFAs	*Butyricicoccus pullicaecorum* LMG 24109 T	Management of IBD, defence against immune illnesses, reduction of inflammation and control of obesity	Geirnaert et al., 2017
Bacteriocin	*Pediococcus acidilactici* LAC5-17	Exhibits anti-microbial activity against *Listeria monocytogenes* through the depolarisation of cell membranes and changes their shape and ultrastructure	Xia et al., 2023
EPS	*Lactobacillus plantarum* L-14	Suppressed adipogenesis via TLR2 and AMPK signalling pathways, resulting in decreased levels of PPARγ, p-ACC, SREBP-1c, and increased levels of adiponectin, AKT.	Lee et al., 2021
Peptidoglycan	*L.rhamnosus* CRL1505	Influencing the immune system (Th1/ Th2-led responses during humoral or cellular immunological responses) and reducing inflammation.	Salva et al., 2021
Heat-inactivated bacteria	*Lactobacillus brevis* KU15176	Anti-proliferative impact on human gastric cancer cell lines by controlling the expression of Bax, Caspase-3, and Caspase-9.	Hwang et al., 2022
GABA	*Lactobacillus plantarum* 90sk & *Bifidobacterium adolescentis* 150	Mediating the relationship between gut flora and mental health, including a variety of disorders such as autism spectrum disorder, anxiety, depression, stress, seizures, and epilepsy	Yunes et al., 2020
Cell-free supernatant	*Bifidobacterium bifidum* DS0908 and *Bifidobacterium longum* DS0950	Anti-obesity, improving insulin sensitivity and glucose metabolism	Rahman et al., 2022
Teichoic acid	*Bifidobacterium animalis* subsp. lactis BPL1	Lipid regulator, inhibits fat oxidation (IGF-1) and reduces synthesis of pro-inflammatory cytokines (IL-6, TNF, and IL-1).	Balaguer et al., 2022
Enzymes	*Lactobacillus casei* BL23	Regulating various reactive oxygen and nitrogen species	Wang et al., 2017

continued on following page

Table 2. Continued

Postbiotics	Sources	Health benefits	References
Enterocins	*Enterococcus casselifavus* MI001	Pore development and suppression of protein production provide antimicrobial action against *Pseudomonas aeruginosa.*	Indira et al., 2018
Organic acids	Lactic acid Bacteria	Prevent food from deteriorating by eliminating harmful bacteria and other organisms, making them a good natural preservative.	Sharafi et al., 2024
Vitamins	*Lacticaseibacillus rhamnosus* GG	Synthesize folate and acts as a regulator in one-carbon metabolism, DNA replication, nucleotide synthesis and epigenetic changes.	Cucick et al., 2024
Extracellular vesicles	*Lactobacillus rhamnosus* GG	Activity against colorectal cancer by reducing the growth of HT-29 and SW-480 cells	Keyhani et al., 2022
Cell surface proteins	*Pediococcus pentosaceus*	Suppressing the occurrence of colorectal cancer by triggering a halt in cell proliferation in DLD-1 cells by reducing CDK1/Cyclin B1 expression.	An et al., 2023

6. IMPACT OF PERSONALISED NUTRITION ON GUT MICROBIOTA AND HUMAN HEALTH

In Personalised Nutrition, the dietary intervention is a critical step in the real-world implementation, as it evaluates each individual to oversee the pattern of intake and supports adherence to individual meal plans. These help to customises diet based on an individual's gut microbiome composition, genetic makeup and metabolic profile, providing effective inflection of the microbial ecosystem thereby improved microbiome-related health benefits (Abeltino et al., 2024) (Figure 1).

Figure 1. Role of gut biotics in the modulation of gut microbiota and prevention of various health conditions

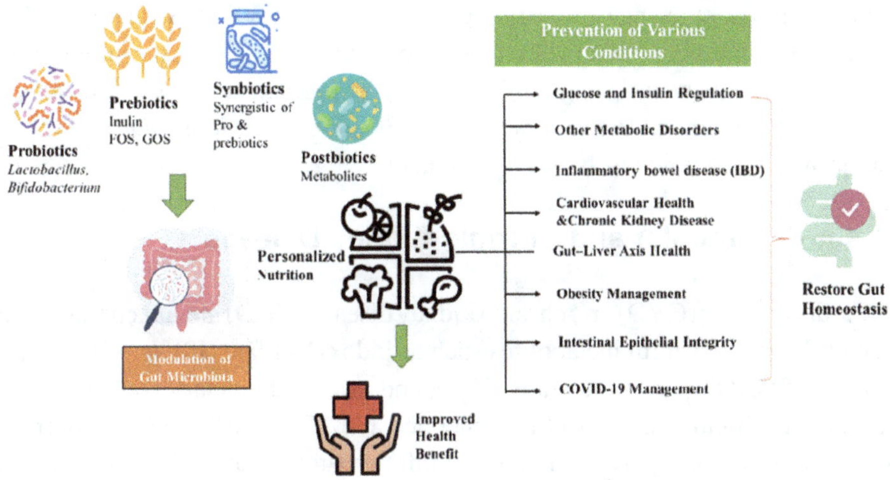

6.1 Regulation of Insulin and Glucose Metabolism

Gut microbiome composition is fundamental for glucose homeostasis and insulin sensitivity. Dysbiosis marked by reduced beneficial bacterial population over pathogenic bacteria in gut leads to impair insulin sensitivity and glucose metabolism. This gives rise to various metabolic disorders such as obesity, type 2 diabetes (T2D). Clinical studies reported that ingestion of strain specific probiotic mitigates metabolic disorders. For example, the reduction of serum cholesterol and HbA1c in patients with T2DM by modulating *Bacteroidetes* and *Bifidobacterium* was achieved with *Lactobacillus reuteri* strains ADR-1 and ADR-3. Among these strains, ADR-3 contribute to other benefits reducing blood pressure and changes in the abundance of *Firmicutes*. Similarly, the daily consumption of Bifidobacterium *lactis* BB-12 and *Lactobacillus acidophilus* La-5 (10^9 CFU) fermented milk over six weeks improved serum fructosamine, HbA1c and anti-inflammatory cytokine (IL-10).

In addition, it has been shown that, over sixteen weeks, fermented milk prepared with *Lactobacillus casei* Shirota can help inhibit gut microbe translocation into the blood, favoring the increase of desirable fecal microbes like *Clostridium coccoides*, *Clostridium lepultum*, and *Lactobacillus*. SCFAs enhance insulin signalling, inflammatory metabolism as well as glucose metabolism. For instance, incorporation of *Coix lacryma-jobi* into probiotic yogurt improved weight management and fasting blood glucose levels (Tiderencel et al., 2020; Ayesha et al., 2023). However, other studies indicate that synbiotics may offer limited benefits on diabetic biomarkers, and some interventions showed improvements in HbA1c, BMI, and microalbuminuria without significant changes in fasting glucose (Li et al., 2021). Such personalized dietary interventions include fibrous and specific prebiotic dietary supplements, which enhance the beneficial gut microbes, e.g., *Bifidobacterium adolescentis*, *Bifidobacterium longum*, *Anaerostipes hadrus*, *Bacteroides xylanisiolvens* and result in improved glycaemic levels and metabolism.

6.2 Cardiovascular and Chronic Kidney Disease

Cardiovascular (CVD) and chronic kidney disease (CKD) are linked through the accumulation of harmful metabolites such as indoxyl sulfate (IS), trimethylamine-N-oxide (TMAO), p-cresyl sulfate (PCS), and uric acid. Dietary sources choline, phosphatidylcholine, and carnitine generates TMAO by *Acinetobacter* promotes macrophage foam cell formation, arterial inflammation, platelet hyperactivity, and progression of atherosclerosis. The disruption in renal clearance occur in CKD build up TMAO and other uremic toxins incidence CVD risk. Gut biotics improve the balance of beneficial bacteria, reduce TMA producing bacteria, increased SCFA level. Dietary interventions with synbiotics containing prebiotic fibres and encapsulated combinations of *B. bifidum*, *L. delbrueckii*, and *S. thermophilus* shown lower uric acid and reduce IS and PCS accumulation levels. Furthermore, Probiotics such as *Lactobacillus DM9218* reduce serum uric acid, while *L. gasseri* PA-3 yoghurt uric acid lowering effect in CKD patients. (Luo *et al.*, 2018; Ramezani, A., & Raj, D. S., 2014).

6.3 Obesity Management

Obesity is closely associated with alteration in gut microbiome composition. The consumption of strain specific *Lactobacillus pentosus GSSK2*, *Lactobacillus plantarum GS26A*, and *Lactobacillus casei IMVB-7280*, exhibit anti-obesity effects, with efficacy influenced by bacterial viability. Although Live multi-strain combination of *Acetobacter, Bifidobacterium, Lactobacillus, and Propionibacterium* demonstrated improve anti-obesity effects, insulin resistance and adiponectin levels than lyophilised or single-strain probiotics. The intake of Prebiotics such as polyphenols and resistant starch, also aid advantages in increasing SCFA production with strengthen anti-obesity effects. Similarly in case of Synbiotics formulation for instance, *Bifidobacterium lactis, Lactobacillus rhamnosus* combination with oligofructose-enriched inulin synergistically enhance intestinal microenvironment regulation. In terms of Post biotics where it includes microbial metabolites and secreted proteins, also contribute to anti-obesity effects. Thus, gut biotics altogether has an amplifying effect of anti-obesity and can be effectively employs in personalised effective weight management. (Li et al., 2021).

6.4 Inflammatory bowel disease (IBD)

Adequate administration of single or multi-strain specific probiotic formulations induce remission in patients with ulcerative colitis (UC) and Crohn's disease (CD) reducing stool frequency, enhance gut barrier function, and improve endoscopy. Synbiotic formulation effectively reduce disease activity scores, CRP levels, and TNF-α, increases beneficial gut microbial ratio. While Postbiotics has gained attention as a safe and stable therapeutic methods for the prevention and management of IBD. Postbiotics derived from *Lacticaseibacillus rhamnosus* and *Lactobacillus delbrueckii* CIDCA 133 demonstrated strong anti-inflammatory effects in IBD models by reducing levels of pro-inflammatory cytokines, IL-6 and TNF-α. (Yassine et al., 2025; Roy, S., & Dhaneshwar, S.,2023).

6.5 Gut–Liver Axis

Impairment of intestinal barrier integrity encourages bacterial translocation and endotoxemia, leading to hepatocyte injury, portal hypertension, and cancer-promoting inflammation. Translocated microbial cell parts and products stimulate the signalling of the toll-like receptors, leading to hepatic inflammation, fibrosis, and genotoxicity. influencing the development and progression of hepatocellular carcinoma (HCC), non-alcoholic fatty liver disease (NAFLD), and metabolic disorders such as type 2 diabetes. The Gut-liver axis is the route of administration of gut biotics aiming at restoring the microbial balance (Cho et al., 2018). Other Clinical studies also support that perioperative pro-/synbiotics significantly reduce infection rates after liver surgery, though their effects on liver function are variable (Kahn et al., 2020).

6.6 Gut Intestinal Integrity

Prebiotics protect intestinal epithelial cells against heat- or hypoxia-induced damage by maintaining trans-epithelial electrical resistance, decrease paracellular permeability and preserving tight junction proteins ZO-1 and claudin-3. Prebiotic ingestion of FOS improved tight junction assembly in T84 cells via the CaMKKβ-AMPK pathway. While Inulin-type fructans (ITFs) also prevent epithelial barrier disruption induced by calcium ionophore A23187 and reduce IL-8 production. (Daguet et al., 2016) Probiotics *Lactobacillus*, *Bifidobacterium*, and *Clostridium butyricum*, regains colonic mucosa by promoting epithelial proliferation through the production of SCFAs, which will serve as energy for enterocytes. These microbes reduce intestinal permeability highly depend on strain, dosage, and treatment duration. Other proteins that mediate gut barrier function in postbiotics are secreted proteins (p40, p75, HM0539), SCFAs, bacteriocins (nisin, pediocin PA-1), organic acids, pili/fimbriae and surface layer (S-layer) proteins. They stimulate epithelial growth, induce mucin (MUC2) and IgA synthesis, have antioxidant effects and pathogen inhibitory effects, blocking epithelial apoptosis. Therefore, gut biotics act through complementary mechanisms structural reinforcement, antimicrobial activity, immune modulation, and microbial ecosystem optimisation, to preserve epithelial integrity, and improve gastrointestinal health. (Kandari et al., 2024; Smolińska et al.,2025).

6.7 COVID-19 Management

The supplementation of specific probiotic strain as an adjunctive treatment for COVID-19 demonstrated multiple protective effects. Probiotics can able to regulate cytokine level, stimulate IgA secretion, activate phagocytosis, induce dendritic cell maturation, strengthen mucosal barriers, and limit viral entry. These altogether may facilitate viral clearance by reducing the risk of bacterial co-infections associated with COVID-19. Few probiotic strains produce bioactive peptides with angiotensin-converting enzyme (ACE) inhibitory activity, which block SARS-CoV-2 entry into host cells. These peptides regulate blood pressure by inhibiting the conversion of angiotensin-I to angiotensin-II Moreover, the administration of Prebiotics also support these effects by promoting probiotic growth and inhibit ACE production. Peptidoglycan, lipoteichoic acid, and phospho-polysaccharides can bring gut immune homeostasis with postbiotics. Gut microbiota modulate immunity and improve lung infections by regulating oxidative stress. (Xavier-Santos et al., 2022; Allali et al., 2021).

7. INVOLVEMENT OF CUTTING-EDGE TECHNOLOGIES FOR EXPLORING MICROBIOTA COMPOSITION

Host metabolism, immunity and health are closely linked to the human gut microbiota. Its characterization holds paramount importance in further development of an individualized nutrition approach. In the past decade, omics technologies have made tremendous advances and shifted microbiome research from the phenotypic interrogation i.e., community profiling, to the functional and genome-resolved interrogation (Hemmati et al. 2024). It is now possible to characterize both microbial composition and activity in detail using approaches that include 16S rRNA sequencing, shotgun sequencing, and other multi-omics technologies. Such tools grant unparalleled chances in correlating microbiome dynamics with personal dietary responses, and such a prospect can lead to the introduction of precision nutrition interventions based on the microbial make-up of an individual (Pedroza Matute & Iyavoo, 2023). Although data measured by bulk sequencing and meta-omics methods have offered unprecedented understanding of gut microbial ecology, these methods tend to obscure the contributions of rare or uncultured organisms as well as disregard functional diversity within communities. To overcome these shortcomings, several recent developments including single-cell genomics, reverse genomics, Raman-activated cell sorting, live-fluorescence in situ hybridization, iChip etc. have been introduced as innovative tools that can supplement existing multi-omic tools and allow direct access to microbial diversity to strain and cellular levels (Figure 2).

Figure 2. Overview of multi-omics approaches and specialized tools used to analyze and characterize microbial communities

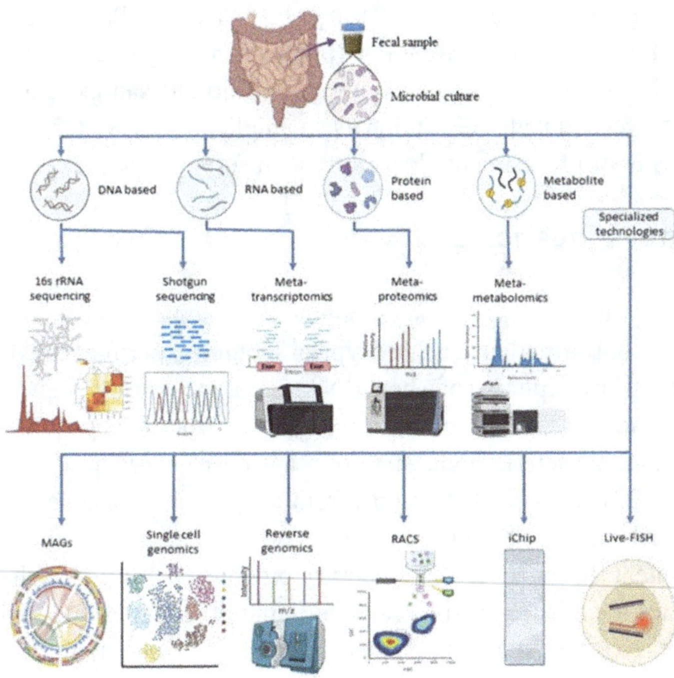

7.1 16s rRNA sequencing

High-throughput omics have transformed the way the human gut microbiota can be described. As an example, sequencing of 16s rRNA genes has remained as the conventional means of bacterial community composition profiling. In this method conserved areas of the small-subunit rRNA gene are PCR-amplified and sequenced to provide a fast taxonomic overview of the bacteria in the gut (Church et al., 2020). 16S rRNA gene amplicon sequencing is the commonly used technique to study microbiota using the next-generation sequencing technologies (Kameoka et al., 2021). This approach allows detection of the dominant bacterial phyla and genera found in stool or biopsies by targeting one or more hypervariable regions (e.g. V3-V4, V4, V1-V2) of the ~1.5 kb 16S gene. It has the benefit of being easy and more affordable and therefore is applied in large human cohorts. Nevertheless, several limitations are associated with 16S-based profiling. Generally, the reads are not enough long, which makes the resolution to genus level, and abundance measurements are subject to PCR and primer bias that may tilt the results (Johnson et al., 2019). It too gives only taxonomic (phylogenetic) data rather than functional data. Recent third-generation sequencing, e.g., PacBio and Nanopore, allows reading of full-length 16S and better resolution as an amplicon survey at the species/strain level, but 16S is still fundamentally an amplicon survey of who is present.

7.2 Shotgun sequencing

In contrast, whole-metagenome (shotgun) sequencing amplifies all DNA in a sample, and not only a marker gene. In a typical shotgun experiment total community DNA, following any depletion of a host DNA, is fragmented and sequenced in bulk. This generates reads that are sampled throughout all microbial genomes within the intestines including bacteria, archaea, viruses and even eukaryotes (Sharpton, 2014; Portik et al., 2022). Since reads can come from any position in a genome, like coding genes, marker loci, etc., shotgun sequencing offers an unbiased census of species and gene content. In practice, contemporary pipelines are utilizing those reads to predict species abundances and to catalogue microbial genes and pathways. The major advantage is that shotgun data instantaneously capture both, who is present and what can be done. As an example, antibiotic-resistance genes or metabolic mechanisms might be identified in gut microbiomes using 16S, and otherwise not. The approach of shotgun metagenomics has been frequently applied in the studies of human gut, e.g., Human Microbiome Project, with the aims to obtain finer taxonomic resolution and functions profiling (Vogtmann et al., 2016). Shotgun datasets are simplistic, large and extensive to compute and always need assembly and binning algorithms. This can be used to gain information about community biodiversity and function by recovering reads of taxonomic markers and coding genes (Sharpton, 2014). Overall, whole-genome metagenomics is a potent culture-free method of identifying the genetic space of the intestinal microbiome.

7.3 Meta-transcriptomics

In addition to DNA, multi-omics techniques also record the community activity in the gut. Meta transcriptomics sequences RNA in a community, typically after depletion of abundant rRNA, as a method of gene expression profiling. Sequencing all the cDNA, created by converting total RNA of the microbes in the gut, gives the investigator a picture of all the genes being expressed by the microbes at the time of sampling. This demonstrates which pathways of metabolism are being realistically utilized under given diets or conditions. Indicatively, recent work established that the human gut transcriptional signature harbored a core set of genes expressed in all individuals and a variable set of genes that was distinct and person specific (Pereira-Marques et al., 2024). Meta-transcriptome of the gut is usually more distinct than the metagenomic gene pool, implying that gut microbes will adjust their behaviors according to host factors (Tanca et al., 2024). This technique in practice has been employed to observe microbiota changes in response to nutrients or treatment, e.g., upregulation of carbohydrate-degrading enzyme or inflammatory genes. The limitation is that RNA is fragile and any processing must be done with care. But, with improved technologies, meta-transcriptomics is playing a significant layer in the planned hierarchical omics.

7.4 Meta-proteomics

Meta-proteomics takes this one unit further to identify the proteins of microorganisms contained in a gut sample, typically via mass spectrometry identification. In this method, extraction and subsequent digestion of all proteins are followed by liquid chromatography- tandem mass spectrometry (LC-MS/MS). The identified spectra of peptides are compared with the repositories containing the information about the microbes, and what enzymes and structural proteins can be contained there and in what concentration (Chignell et al., 2018; Peters et al., 2019). This gives first-hand testimony of in situ microbial activity. Gut metaproteomics, can support direct insights into functional activity of microbial activities in the colonic environment (Tanca et al., 2024). Meta-transcriptomics indicates a gene is transcribed, whereas checking by metaproteomics will reveal whether this is an actual protein product or not. These experiments have guided to the identification of stable core metabolic functions, e.g. glycolysis enzymes, butyrate synthesis enzymes etc., that were common to healthy guts and dynamic proteins implicated in environmental sensing and stress responses. Accordingly, metaproteomics connects taxonomy with the functionality by demonstrating which taxa provide what proteins. Within the personalized nutrition, it would be possible to trace the microbial enzyme abundance and adapt diet based on the level.

7.5 Meta-metabolomics

This technique also gives a side vision by quantifying the end products of the microbiota as well as the host. Usually, samples containing stool, urine or serum are tested using high-resolution mass spectrometry or NMR to determine and measure metabolites. The short-chain fatty acids, bile acids, amino acids, and myriad signaling compounds products of diet-microbe interactions are a few examples of metabolites. This strategy is an effective method of capturing the output of the microbiome which can be correlated against host physiology. Gut-metabolomics is a novel method of gathering the complicated metabolic exchanges between the host and its peculiar microbial partners (Vernocchi et al., 2016). This technique may be used to identify small molecules/products synthesized by intestinal microbes and establish biochemical metabolites pathways. As an example, products of microbial fermentation, like acetate, propionate, butyrate, may be measured and related to diet and health. Metabolomics is commonly applied to identify disease biomarkers, e.g., metabolites that are higher in obesity or IBD, and so can be applied to precision nutrition (Peters et al., 2019). Metabolomics complements DNA/RNA/protein analysis by matching gut community composition with real-time metabolism and fills the incomplete picture.

7.6 Metagenome-assembled genomes (MAGs)

Finally, the contemporary sequencing analysis frequently generates MAGs. Rather than considering shotgun reads as anonymous fragments, the bioinformaticians assemble reads into draft genomes. Each MAG is a nearly complete genome of the microbial species in the gut sample. The first step in reconstructing a genome is to divide contigs into groups based on the amount of sequence composition and coverage, and it requires advanced algorithms to perform this task. WMS, as advanced algorithms, is well suited to the task of reconstruction. The outcome of this technique is a genome-resolved microbiota. We can retrieve genomes of bacteria that live in the intestine but can never be cultured in the laboratory. This reference microbial catalog has expanded to the enormity of genome-resolved metagenomics rapidly. Over the last decade, alone thousands of MAGs have been accumulated on the research on human gut (Kim et al., 2024). The MAGs contain complete genetic blueprints of a strain providing a detailed metabolic and niche specialization. This method is currently being deployed to find novel species and can be used to examine population genetics of the microorganism. In personalized nutrition, MAGs enable functional genes of interest within certain taxa to be tracked, such as the presence of antibiotic-resistance or certain enzyme genes in the gut flora (Heinken et al., 2021).

7.7 Single-cell genomics

It is a methodology involving the isolation of individual microbial cells belonging to large complex communities, amplifying their genomes, and sequencing them individually. This method is an improvement over metagenomics where mixed species data is assembled and does not reveal low abundance species. Studying the genomic content of single cells enables investigators to determine previously undescribed lineages, metabolic capabilities and strain-level diversity without a prior cultivation requirement (Xu & Zhao, 2018). It also gives functional annotation to biomolecules hard to culture, alongside correlating genes to likely functional contributions at an unprecedented level of detail.

7.8 Reverse genomics

This technology has provided an additional approach of using genomic information to develop specific culturing methods to isolate previously uncultured organisms. Rather than randomly growing cultures, reverse genomics applies selective probes or antibodies made to surface proteins or predicted functional genes encoded on the microbial genome and use this specification to capture live cells of interest. It is a viable method of isolating the unique microbes in the human gut with a genomic signature alone and increased the culturable diversity of the microbiota (Cross et al. 2019). To the personalized nutritional area, these targeted isolations yield living strains that can be characterized in vitro, or as advanced probiotics with specified functional characteristics.

7.9 Raman-mediated cell sorting (RACS)

RACS is a novel technology fusing single-cell Raman spectroscopy and microfluidics to characterize and isolate single microbial cells based on their biochemical composition. Raman spectra present a non-destructive molecular fingerprint of cellular metabolites lipids, nucleic acids or short-chain fatty acids, without requiring tagging. Integrating Raman detection with optical tweezers or microfluidic droplet sorting, RACS can be used to isolate high-throughput phenotype-based isolation of a functional subset of microbes within complex gut communities. Such as Lee et al. (2019), who used RACS to specifically enrich bacteria that produce butyrate in fecal samples, and showed that they have a functional relationship to dietary fiber metabolism. This functionality driven targeting of microbes is direct evidence of metabolic members of a heterogeneous community.

7.10 Live-FISH (fluorescence in situ hybridization of viable cells)

It is a method of nucleic acid hybridization facilitated with the preservation of viability sample preparation strategy of microbial cell identification and sorting against species-specific probes. In contrast to the conventional FISH, where fixation is usually performed and kills the cells, it is possible to use live- FISH to perform downstream cultivation and functional studies of the labeled microbes. Live-FISH was shown to allow the selective separation of live microbes in the gastrointestinal tract to culture or genome sequence individual organisms (Su *et al.*, 2017), filling the gap between the identifications based on phylogeny and their functional characterization. The given technology is highly applicable in the connection between taxonomic identity and ecological role in the existence of living things, a central pillar in personalized dietary interventions.

7.11 Isolation chip (iChip)

This facility is a breakthrough toward cultivating previously unculturable microbes. iChip is a diffusion chamber, in which single cells of microorganisms are entrapped in separate micro-wells isolated with semi-permeable membranes, then incubated under natural conditions. This enables microbes to grow in native nutrient and signaling conditions, but keep physically separated in order to form colonies. The actual progress of iChip led to the finding of of *Eleftheria terrae* and its new anti-bacterial molecule teixobactin (Ling et al., 2015). Since that time iChip-based approaches have been used to study the gut and soil microbiota to uncover new taxa that do not readily grow in the laboratory.

In combination, these leading-edge techniques provide a multi-dimensional perspective of the human gut microbiome. The multi-omics integrative approach has unprecedented resolution of the gut ecosystem. As another example, we may find bacterial species via 16S or WGS, further prove that it produces important enzymes via transcriptomics/proteomics, and finally monitor its metabolic products via metabolomics, a complete evidence chain. Microbiome-informed personalized nutrition is based on such complex profiling. These technologies can provide the means of highly specific dietary intervention in a certain detail by disclosing which microbes are there and active in a particular person and how they change with the change of diet. Meta-transcriptomics, meta-proteomics, metabolomics, and MAG analysis, in conjunction with high-throughput 16S and shotgun sequencing, are revolutionizing gut microbiota studies as well as precision nutrition. Beside this, the other novel technologies allow the researcher to resolve the hidden majority of uncultured or rare communities and directly correlate microbial identity to phenotype. Such innovations are not only expanding the microbial reference databases, but also providing living strains applicable to mechanistic studies, that would help in better translation of microbiome science to practical personalized nutrition approaches.

8. REGULATORY ASPECTS AND MARKET APPROACHES FOR PERSONALIZED NUTRITION

Reliance on personalized nutrition, including probiotics, prebiotics and postbiotics, is inevitable due to factors such as poor lifestyles and inadequate exercise, which contribute to its prevalence. Despite the growing global popularity of functional foods, many countries are facing challenges in ensuring the safety of these products. This highlights the critical need for functional food-specific legislation. In 2018, after the initial meeting for establishing a common understanding about probiotics and their related compounds, the ISAPP (International Society for the Science of Probiotics and Prebiotics) signed a white paper stating the minimum requirements for a standardized regulatory approach in food and dietary supplements (Chieffi et al., 2022). Globally, consumers' food safety concerns have driven the food industry to implement many food safety standards, including ISO 22000:2005, HACCP, IFS, and the British Retail Consortium (Kotsanopoulo and Arvanitoyannis., 2017). There is a lack of worldwide harmony even at the most fundamental levels of classification and regulation of probiotics and rest biotics, despite widespread recognition of the necessity to authenticate commodities and additives. Many regional and international bodies are responsible for overseeing the regulation. These include the European Food Safety Authority (EFSA) in the EU, the Association of Southeast Asian Nations (ASEAN) in SE Asia, the National Medical Products Administration (NMPA) in China, the Food for Specified Health Use (FOSHU) in Japan, the Food and Drug Administration (FDA) in the US, and the Food Safety and Standard Authority of India (FSSAI) in India (Arora and Baldi., 2017; Bhupathiraju *et al.*, 2019). These Regulatory agencies provide specific standards for microbiological identification, evaluation, labelling, health statements, dossiers, and lists in addition to limits on food safety, sanitation, and hygiene throughout the food production process.

In terms of global food safety and quality, the FAO and the WHO are among the most important organizations. They work together in administering the Codex Alimentarius Commission's Food Standards Programme. On the international level, organizations such as UNIDO, GATT, ISO, OCU, ICMSF, and IDF appear to be of a supporting role as regards food safety (Anyanwu and Jukes, 1990). The functional foods must be manufactured according to Good Manufacturing Practices (GMP) to guarantee they are safe for consumption. There should be comprehensive processes in place to make sure that various biotic substances in functional foods and those released by the manufacturer are safe, high-quality, identifiable, pure, and potent (Owusu-Apenten and Vieira, 2023; FDA, 2007). Implementing GMPs would yield quantifiable advantages assessable through critical metrics such as microbiological indicators, pre- and post-implementation costs, and the PDCA cycle, which encompasses four stages: planning, doing, checking, and acting (Lockis et al., 2011).

Considerable advances have been made in understanding the health effects and potential uses of some strains and their metabolites. Some prominent loopholes like overstated beneficial effects, label inaccuracy, and mismanagement of nutritional compositions still persist in the market. These uncertainties have led the WHO to recommend implementing both mandatory and voluntary nutrition labelling programs to reduce the prevalence of unhealthy dietary behaviors (Jackson et al., 2019). A certain proportion of healthy options should be labelled on all foods, with government procurement standards setting annual targets for the purchase and sale of nutritious foods. Additionally, food assistance programs should offer incentives to encourage the purchase of healthy meals (Griffith et al., 2017). Research with quantifiable outcomes shows significant evidence that, with appropriate food labelling strategies in place, it is possible to boost sales of healthy options and reduce sales of unhealthy ones (Roberto et al., 2021).

To ensure the safe, high-quality, and stability of probiotic-based functional foods requires strict compliance with product and site licensing regulations, product and site licensing must be strictly followed. To avoid contaminants in probiotics, it's important to sanitize regularly its source along with verifying the stock, checking viability, cell growth dilemma, harvesting procedures, purification, and other procedures for maintaining the integrity of functional foods by which people can take it for their personalized purposes.

Many people are increasingly demanding food products which are tailored to meet personal tastes and preferences, life habits, and certain health requirements. Consumer awareness creation via common education forums and open labelling is extremely crucial in increasing the level of consumer acceptance of functional foods. Moreover, marketing surveys are effective to introduce valuable information that assists professionals to obtain a better idea of how individuals actually perceive functional foods. The main way to boost the intake of the functional food and particularly the consumption of fresh and minimally processed food involves the use of consumer surveys. As having a healthy gut microbiota isn’t a minor health advantage, it should be motivation in itself to make consumers be able to find the corresponding products without any difficulties. Because of that, the process of encouraging the health benefits of these foods by providing future communications and educational programs may need to be delivered in an easy and convincing way. Focusing on their safety, natural ingredients, and sustainability will go the extra miles in alleviating the fear held by consumers, breed confidence and foster greater acceptance. (Topolska et al., 2021).

9. CHALLENGES AND FUTURE PROSPECT

Personalized nutrition utilising gutbiotics concepts faces several significant challenges that limit its broad commercial application. Primary challenges is the high inter-individual variability in gut microbial composition shaped by genetics, diet and several environmental cue. This heterogeneity makes it difficult to develop universally effective dietary interventions with individuals will exhibit different responses to the same dietary pattern. The field lacks standardized biomarkers to reliably assess the predictability of personalized nutrition approaches and shortage of long-term randomized controlled trials (RCTs) that can confirm the sustainability and safety of these interventions over extended periods. The integration of multi-omics, metagenomics, metabolomics, and nutrigenomics for effective and precise profiling, remains costly and limits its accessibility for large-scale public health use. Different regulatory frameworks leading microbiome-based dietary interventions are still developing, with inconsistencies in strain authentication, safety assessments, and health claim validation.

Future research and innovation should focus on developing precision synbiotics designed to target specific microbial profiles, integrates artificial intelligence and machine learning to create predictive well structure personalised dietary plans. The integration of personalized nutrition with mental and immune health will provide new therapeutic avenues, while reducing the cost of microbiome testing and expanding access through digital globalised health platforms.

10. CONCLUSION

Personalized nutrition using gut biotics positively influences potential health issues by improving gut microbial composition and benefiting the overall wellbeing of the system. Advancement in different multiomics approaches have been explores to dietary strategies which strengthen immune function, modulate inflammatory pathways, and reduce the risk of chronic diseases such as obesity, type 2 diabetes, and colorectal cancer. Despite these, the field continues to face limited barriers such as high costs associated with advanced profiling techniques, insufficiently validated biomarkers, and fragmented regulatory policies that delay widespread clinical translation and mass global adoptions. In order to achieved long-term adherence remains a behavioural and cultural challenge that consider socioeconomic disparities and individual preferences. The future of personalized nutrition will be driven by multidisciplinary collaboration between researchers, healthcare professionals, regulatory authorities, and industry partners, ensuring the development of cost-effective, scientifically validated, and ethically guided interventions. Incorporation of AI-driven predictive models, precision synbiotics, and microbiome-editing tools like CRISPR-Cas and phage therapies, customised dietary intervention and precision-based healthcare is within reach. Personalized nutrition is poised to become a basis of both preventive and therapeutic reshaping global health models.

REFERENCES

Abbasi, A., Rad, A. H., Ghasempour, Z., Sabahi, S., Kafil, H. S., Hasannezhad, P., Rahbar Saadat, Y., & Shahbazi, N. (2022). The biological activities of postbiotics in gastrointestinal disorders. *Critical Reviews in Food Science and Nutrition*, *62*(22), 5983–6004. DOI: 10.1080/10408398.2021.1895061

Abeltino, A., Hatem, D., Serantoni, C., Riente, A., De Giulio, M. M., De Spirito, M., De Maio, F., & Maulucci, G. (2024). Unraveling the Gut Microbiota: Implications for Precision Nutrition and Personalized Medicine. *Nutrients*, *16*(22), 3806. DOI: 10.3390/nu16223806

Abondio, P., Sazzini, M., Garagnani, P., Boattini, A., Monti, D., Franceschi, C., Luiselli, D., & Giuliani, C. (2019). The Genetic Variability of APOE in Different Human Populations and Its Implications for Longevity. *Genes*, *10*(3), 222. DOI: 10.3390/genes10030222

Aghebati-Maleki, L., Hasannezhad, P., Abbasi, A., & Khani, N. (2021). Antibacterial, antiviral, antioxidant, and anticancer activities of postbiotics: A review of mechanisms and therapeutic perspectives. *Biointerface Research in Applied Chemistry*, *12*(2), 2629–2645. DOI: 10.33263/BRIAC122.26292645

Akour, A. (2020). Probiotics and COVID-19: Is there any link? *Letters in Applied Microbiology*, *71*(3), 229–234. DOI: 10.1111/lam.13334

Alagiakrishnan, K., & Halverson, T. (2021). Microbial therapeutics in neurocognitive and psychiatric disorders. *Journal of Clinical Medicine Research*, *13*(9), 439–459. DOI: 10.14740/jocmr4575

Allali, I., Bakri, Y., Amzazi, S., & Ghazal, H. (2021). Gut-Lung axis in COVID-19. *Interdisciplinary Perspectives on Infectious Diseases*, *2021*(1), 6655380. DOI: 10.1155/2021/6655380

Ambrogi, V., Bottacini, F., Cao, L., Kuipers, B., Schoterman, M., & van Sinderen, D. (2023). Galacto-oligosaccharides as infant prebiotics: Production, application, bioactive activities and future perspectives. *Critical Reviews in Food Science and Nutrition*, *63*(6), 753–766. DOI: 10.1080/10408398.2021.1953437

Ames, N., Storsley, J., & Thandapilly, S. J. (2018). In Beta, T., & Camire, M. E. (Eds.), *Functionality of beta-glucan from oat and barley and its relation with human health. Cereal Grain-based Functional Foods: Carbohydrate and Phytochemical Components* (pp. 147–166). The Royal Society of Chemistry., DOI: 10.1039/9781788012799-00147

An, B. C., Ahn, J. Y., Kwon, D., Kwak, S. H., Heo, J. Y., Kim, S., Ryu, Y., & Chung, M. J. (2023). Anti-cancer roles of probiotic-derived P8 protein in colorectal cancer cell line DLD-1. *International Journal of Molecular Sciences*, *24*(12), 9857. DOI: 10.3390/ijms24129857

Anyanwu, R. C., & Jukes, D. J. (1990). Food safety control systems for developing countries. *Food Control*, *1*(1), 17–26. DOI: 10.1016/0956-7135(90)90116-T

Arora, M., & Baldi, A. (2017). Comparative study of regulatory framework for probiotics: Current status and future recommendations. *Applied Clinical Research, Clinical Trials and Regulatory Affairs*, *4*(2), 140–156. DOI: 10.2174/2213476X04666170620100145

Ayesha, I. E., Monson, N. R., Klair, N., Patel, U., Saxena, A., Patel, D., & Ayesha, I. E. (2023). Probiotics and their role in the management of type 2 diabetes mellitus (Short-term versus long-term effect): A systematic review and meta-analysis. *Cureus*, *15*(10). Advance online publication. DOI: 10.7759/cureus.46741

Balaguer, F., Enrique, M., Llopis, S., Barrena, M., Navarro, V., Álvarez, B., Chenoll, E., Ramón, D., Tortajada, M., & Martorell, P. (2022). Lipoteichoic acid from Bifidobacterium animalis subsp. lactis BPL1: A novel postbiotic that reduces fat deposition via IGF-1 pathway. *Microbial Biotechnology*, *15*(3), 805–816. DOI: 10.1111/1751-7915.13769

Bouchard, C., & Ordovas, J. M. (2012). Fundamentals of nutrigenetics and nutrigenomics. *Progress in Molecular Biology and Translational Science*, *108*, 1–15. DOI: 10.1016/B978-0-12-398397-8.00001-0

Bourebaba, Y., Marycz, K., Mularczyk, M., & Bourebaba, L. (2022). Postbiotics as potential new therapeutic agents for metabolic disorders management. *Biomedicine and Pharmacotherapy*, *153*, 113138. DOI: 10.1016/j.biopha.2022.113138

Carlos-Reyes, Á., López-González, J. S., Meneses-Flores, M., Gallardo-Rincón, D., Ruíz-García, E., Marchat, L. A., Astudillo-de la Vega, H., Hernández de la Cruz, O. N., & López-Camarillo, C. (2019). Dietary Compounds as Epigenetic Modulating Agents in Cancer. *Frontiers in Genetics*, *10*, 79. DOI: 10.3389/fgene.2019.00079

Casado, J. M. R. (2017). Centenario de Elie Metchnikoff (1845-1916). *Educación Médica*, *18*(2), 136–143. DOI: 10.1016/j.edumed.2016.11.009

Chaudhary, D., Guleria, D., Aggarwal, H., Mishra, V., Chauhan, A., Dufossé, L., & Joshi, N. C. (2025). Nutrigenomics and Personalized Diets-Tailoring Nutrition for Optimal Health. *Applied Food Research*, *100980*(1), 100980. Advance online publication. DOI: 10.1016/j.afres.2025.100980

Chieffi, D., Fanelli, F., & Fusco, V. (2022). Legislation of probiotic foods and supplements. In *Probiotics for human nutrition in health and disease* (pp. 25–44). Academic Press., DOI: 10.1016/B978-0-323-89908-6.00013-3

Chignell, J. F., De Long, S. K., & Reardon, K. F. (2018). Meta-proteomic analysis of protein expression distinctive to electricity-generating biofilm communities in air-cathode microbial fuel cells. *Biotechnology for Biofuels*, *11*(1), 121. DOI: 10.1186/s13068-018-1111-2

Cho, M. S., Kim, S. Y., Suk, K. T., & Kim, B. Y. (2018). Modulation of gut microbiome in nonalcoholic fatty liver disease: Pro-, pre-, syn-, and antibiotics. *Journal of Microbiology (Seoul, Korea)*, *56*(12), 855–867. DOI: 10.1007/s12275-018-8346-2

Church, D. L., Cerutti, L., Gürtler, A., Griener, T., Zelazny, A., & Emler, S. (2020). Performance and application of 16S rRNA gene cycle sequencing for routine identification of bacteria in the clinical microbiology laboratory. *Clinical Microbiology Reviews*, *33*(4), 10–1128. DOI: 10.1128/CMR.00053-19

Cicenia, A., Santangelo, F., Gambardella, L., Pallotta, L., Iebba, V., Scirocco, A., Marignani, M., Tellan, G., Carabotti, M., Corazziari, E. S., Schippa, S., & Severi, C. (2016). Protective role of postbiotic mediators secreted by Lactobacillus rhamnosus GG versus lipopolysaccharide-induced damage in human colonic smooth muscle cells. *Journal of Clinical Gastroenterology*, *50*(Supplement 2), S140–S144. DOI: 10.1097/MCG.0000000000000681

Clemente, A., & Olias, R. (2017). Beneficial effects of legumes in gut health. *Current Opinion in Food Science*, *14*, 32–36. DOI: 10.1016/j.cofs.2017.01.005

Cross, K. L., Campbell, J. H., Balachandran, M., Campbell, A. G., Cooper, C. J., Griffen, A., Heaton, M., Joshi, S., Klingeman, D., Leys, E., Yang, Z., Parks, J. M., & Podar, M. (2019). Targeted isolation and cultivation of uncultivated bacteria by reverse genomics. *Nature Biotechnology*, *37*(11), 1314–1321. DOI: 10.1038/s41587-019-0260-6

Cucick, A. C. C., Bedani, R., Ribeiro, L. S., Franco, B. D. G. D. M., & Saad, S. M. I. (2024). Effect of fruit by-products and orange pectin on folate (vitamin B9) production by selected starter and probiotic strains. *International Journal of Food Science & Technology*, *59*(6), 3929–3938. DOI: 10.1111/ijfs.17141

Daguet, D., Pinheiro, I., Verhelst, A., Possemiers, S., & Marzorati, M. (2016). Arabinogalactan and fructooligosaccharides improve the gut barrier function in distinct areas of the colon in the Simulator of the Human Intestinal Microbial Ecosystem. *Journal of Functional Foods*, *20*, 369–379. DOI: 10.1016/j.jff.2015.11.005

Das, T. K., Pradhan, S., Chakrabarti, S., Mondal, K. C., & Ghosh, K. (2022). Current status of probiotic and related health benefits. *Applied Food Research*, *2*(2), 100185. DOI: 10.1016/j.afres.2022.100185

de Almada, C. N., Almada, C. N., Martinez, R. C., & Sant'Ana, A. S. (2016). Paraprobiotics: Evidences on their ability to modify biological responses, inactivation methods and perspectives on their application in foods. *Trends in Food Science & Technology*, *58*, 96–114. DOI: 10.1016/j.tifs.2016.09.011

de Mattos, P. B. G., de Souza Vandenberghe, L. P., Valladares-Diestra, K. K., Neyra, L. C. R., Vieira, S., Letti, L. A. J., & Soccol, C. R. (2024). Recent developments in xylooligosaccharides: Sustainable production, characterization, beneficial properties and applications. *Food Research International*, *197*, 115206. DOI: 10.1016/j.foodres.2024.115206

Dhopatkar, N., Keeler, J. L., Mutwalli, H., Whelan, K., Treasure, J., & Himmerich, H. (2023). Gastrointestinal symptoms, gut microbiome, probiotics and prebiotics in anorexia nervosa: A review of mechanistic rationale and clinical evidence. *Psychoneuroendocrinology*, *147*, 105959. DOI: 10.1016/j.psyneuen.2022.105959

Dixit, Y., Wagle, A., & Vakil, B. (2016). Patents in the field of probiotics, prebiotics, synbiotics: A review. *J Food Microbiol Saf Hyg*, *1*(02), 1–13. DOI: 10.4172/2476-2059.1000111

do Carmo, M. M., Walker, J. C., Novello, D., Caselato, V. M., Sgarbieri, V. C., Ouwehand, A. C., Andreollo, N. A., Hiane, P. A., & Dos Santos, E. F. (2016). Polydextrose: Physiological Function, and Effects on Health. *Nutrients*, *8*(9), 553. DOI: 10.3390/nu8090553

Emran, T. B., Islam, F., Mitra, S., Paul, S., Nath, N., Khan, Z., Das, R., Chandran, D., Sharma, R., Lima, C. M. G., Awadh, A. A. A., Almazni, I. A., Alhasaniah, A. H., & Guiné, R. P. F. (2022). Pectin: A Bioactive Food Polysaccharide with Cancer Preventive Potential. *Molecules (Basel, Switzerland)*, *27*(21), 7405. DOI: 10.3390/molecules27217405

. Falade, E. O., Kouamé, K. J. E., Zhu, Y., Zheng, Y., & Ye, X. (2025). A review: Examining the effects of modern extraction techniques on functional and structural properties of cellulose and hemicellulose in Brewer's Spent Grain dietary fiber. *Carbohydrate polymers, 348*(Pt A), 122883. https://doi.org/DOI: 10.1016/j.carbpol.2024.122883

Feng, Y., Wassie, T., Gan, R., & Wu, X. (2023). Structural characteristics and immunomodulatory effects of sulfated polysaccharides derived from marine algae. *Critical Reviews in Food Science and Nutrition, 63*(24), 7180–7196. DOI: 10.1080/10408398.2022.2043823

Food and Drug Administration, HHS. (2007). Current good manufacturing practice in manufacturing, packaging, labeling, or holding operations for dietary supplements. Final rule. *Federal Register, 72*(121), 34751–34958.

Gasbarrini, G., Bonvicini, F., & Gramenzi, A. (2016). Probiotics history. *Journal of Clinical Gastroenterology, 50*(Supplement 2), S116–S119. DOI: 10.1097/MCG.0000000000000697

Geirnaert, A., Calatayud, M., Grootaert, C., Laukens, D., Devriese, S., Smagghe, G., De Vos, M., Boon, N., & Van de Wiele, T. (2017). Butyrate-producing bacteria supplemented in vitro to Crohn's disease patient microbiota increased butyrate production and enhanced intestinal epithelial barrier integrity. *Scientific Reports, 7*(1), 11450. DOI: 10.1038/s41598-017-11734-8

Ghare, M., Vishwakarma, K., Tripathi, S., Dixit, G. P., & Soren, K. R. (2024). Unveiling the benefits of resistant starch in legumes: Overview of current and future prospective. *Stärke, 76*(7-8), 2300212. DOI: 10.1002/star.202300212

Gomez de Agüero, M., Ganal-Vonarburg, S. C., Fuhrer, T., Rupp, S., Uchimura, Y., Li, H., Steinert, A., Heikenwalder, M., Hapfelmeier, S., Sauer, U., McCoy, K. D., & Macpherson, A. J. (2016). The maternal microbiota drives early postnatal innate immune development. *Science, 351*(6279), 1296–1302. DOI: 10.1126/science.aad2571

Górczyńska-Kosiorz, S., Lejawa, M., Goławski, M., Tomaszewska, A., Fronczek, M., Maksym, B., Banach, M., & Osadnik, T. (2024). The Impact of Haplotypes of the FTO Gene, Lifestyle, and Dietary Patterns on BMI and Metabolic Syndrome in Polish Young Adult Men. *Nutrients, 16*(11), 1615. DOI: 10.3390/nu16111615

Griffith, R., O'Connell, M., & Smith, K. (2017). The importance of product reformulation versus consumer choice in improving diet quality. *Economica, 84*(333), 34–53. DOI: 10.1111/ecca.12192

Heinken, A., Basile, A., Hertel, J., Thinnes, C., & Thiele, I. (2021). Genome-scale metabolic modeling of the human microbiome in the era of personalized medicine. *Annual Review of Microbiology, 75*(1), 199–222. DOI: 10.1146/annurev-micro-060221-012134

Hemmati, M. A., Monemi, M., Asli, S., Mohammadi, S., Foroozanmehr, B., Haghmorad, D., Oksenych, V., & Eslami, M. (2024). Using new technologies to analyze gut microbiota and predict cancer risk. *Cells*, *13*(23), 1987. DOI: 10.3390/cells13231987

Holzapfel, C., Waldenberger, M., Lorkowski, S., & Daniel, H. (2022). Genetics and epigenetics in personalized nutrition: Evidence, expectations, and experiences. *Molecular Nutrition & Food Research*, *66*(17), 2200077. DOI: 10.1002/mnfr.202200077

Huang, Y., He, S., Li, J. Z., Seo, Y. K., Osborne, T. F., Cohen, J. C., & Hobbs, H. H. (2010). A feed-forward loop amplifies nutritional regulation of PNPLA3. *Proceedings of the National Academy of Sciences of the United States of America*, *107*(17), 7892–7897. DOI: 10.1073/pnas.1003585107

Huynh, U., & Zastrow, M. L. (2023). Metallobiology of Lactobacillaceae in the gut microbiome. *Journal of Inorganic Biochemistry*, *238*, 112023. DOI: 10.1016/j.jinorgbio.2022.112023

Hwang, C. H., Lee, N. K., & Paik, H. D. (2022). The anti-cancer potential of heat-killed Lactobacillus brevis KU15176 upon AGS cell lines through intrinsic apoptosis pathway. *International Journal of Molecular Sciences*, *23*(8), 4073. DOI: 10.3390/ijms23084073

Indira, M., Venkateswarulu, T. C., Prabhakar, K. V., Peele, K. A., & Krupanidhi, S. (2018). Isolation and characterization of bacteriocin producing Enterococcus casseliflavus and its antagonistic effect on Pseudomonas aeruginosa. *Karbala International Journal of Modern Science*, *4*(4), 361–368. DOI: 10.1016/j.kijoms.2018.09.002

ISAPP. (2022). Definition of postbiotics: A panel debate in Amsterdam. International Scientific Association for Probiotics and Prebiotics (ISAPP). Available at: https://isappscience.org/definition-of-postbiotics-a-panel-debate-in-amsterdam/ (Accessed 27 July 2025).

Islam, F., Azmat, F., Imran, A., Zippi, M., Hong, W., Tariq, F., Shehzadi, U., Fatima, A., Safdar, M., Ahmed, H., Ijaz, M., Zeeshan, F., Ali, R., Asif Shah, M., & Suleria, H. A. (2024). Role of postbiotics in food and health: A comprehensive review. *CYTA: Journal of Food*, *22*(1), 2386412. DOI: 10.1080/19476337.2024.2386412

Jackson, P. P. J., Wijeyesekera, A., & Rastall, R. A. (2022). Inulin-type fructans and short-chain fructooligosaccharides-their role within the food industry as fat and sugar replacers and texture modifiers-what needs to be considered! *Food Science & Nutrition*, *11*(1), 17–38. DOI: 10.1002/fsn3.3040

Jackson, S. A., Schoeni, J. L., Vegge, C., Pane, M., Stahl, B., Bradley, M., & Sanders, M. E. (2019). Improving end-user trust in the quality of commercial probiotic products. *Frontiers in Microbiology*, *10*, 739. DOI: 10.3389/fmicb.2019.00739

Johnson, J. S., Spakowicz, D. J., Hong, B. Y., Petersen, L. M., Demkowicz, P., Chen, L., Leopold, S. R., Hanson, B. M., Agresta, H. O., Gerstein, M., Sodergren, E., & Weinstock, G. M. (2019). Evaluation of 16S rRNA gene sequencing for species and strain-level microbiome analysis. *Nature Communications*, *10*(1), 5029. DOI: 10.1038/s41467-019-13036-1

Kahn, J., Pregartner, G., & Schemmer, P. (2020). Effects of both Pro- and Synbiotics in Liver Surgery and Transplantation with Special Focus on the Gut-Liver Axis-A Systematic Review and Meta-Analysis. *Nutrients*, *12*(8), 2461. DOI: 10.3390/nu12082461

Kameoka, S., Motooka, D., Watanabe, S., Kubo, R., Jung, N., Midorikawa, Y., Shinozaki, N. O., Sawai, Y., Takeda, A. K., & Nakamura, S. (2021). Benchmark of 16S rRNA gene amplicon sequencing using Japanese gut microbiome data from the V1–V2 and V3–V4 primer sets. *BMC Genomics*, *22*(1), 527. DOI: 10.1186/s12864-021-07746-4

Kandari, A., Odat, M. A., Alzaid, F., & Scott, K. P. (2024). Biotics and bacterial function: Impact on gut and host health. *The ISME Journal*, *18*(1), wrae226. Advance online publication. DOI: 10.1093/ismejo/wrae226

Kashyap, P. C., Chia, N., Nelson, H., Segal, E., & Elinav, E. (2017, December). Microbiome at the frontier of personalized medicine. In Mayo Clinic Proceedings (Vol. 92, No. 12, pp. 1855-1864). *Elsevier*. https://doi.org/DOI: 10.1016/j.mayocp.2017.10.004

Kassem, N. M., Abdelmegid, Y. A., El-Sayed, M. K., Sayed, R. S., Abdel-Aalla, M. H., & Kassem, H. A. (2023). Nutrigenomics and microbiome shaping the future of personalized medicine: A review article. *Journal of Genetic Engineering and Biotechnology*, *21*(1), 134. DOI: 10.1186/s43141-023-00599-2

Kaur, N., Pandey, S., & Bhushan, K. (2025). Recent Developments in Extraction, Molecular Characterization, Bioactivity, and Application of Brewers Spent Grain Arabinoxylans. *Journal of Food Science*, *90*(5), e70239. DOI: 10.1111/1750-3841.70239

Keyhani, G., Hosseini, H. M., & Salimi, A. (2022). Effect of extracellular vesicles of Lactobacillus rhamnosus GG on the expression of CEA gene and protein released by colorectal cancer cells. *Iranian Journal of Microbiology*, *14*(1), 90. DOI: 10.18502/ijm.v14i1.8809

Kim, N., Ma, J., Kim, W., Kim, J., Belenky, P., & Lee, I. (2024). Genome-resolved metagenomics: A game changer for microbiome medicine. *Experimental & Molecular Medicine*, *56*(7), 1501–1512. DOI: 10.1038/s12276-024-01262-7

Korčok, D. J., Tršić-Milanović, N. A., Ivanović, N. D., & Đorđević, B. I. (2018). Development of probiotic formulation for the treatment of iron deficiency anemia. *Chemical & Pharmaceutical Bulletin*, *66*(4), 347–352. DOI: 10.1248/cpb.c17-00634

Kussmann, M., & van Bladeren, P. J. (2011). The extended nutrigenomics – understanding the interplay between the genomes of food, gut microbes, and human host. *Frontiers in Genetics*, *2*, 21. DOI: 10.3389/fgene.2011.00021

Lagoumintzis, G., & Patrinos, G. P. (2023). Triangulating nutrigenomics, metabolomics and microbiomics toward personalized nutrition and healthy living. *Human Genomics*, *17*(1), 109. DOI: 10.1186/s40246-023-00561-w

Lagoumintzis, G., & Patrinos, G. P. (2024). Nutrigenomics and personalized nutrition: Advancing basic, clinical, and translational research. *Frontiers in Nutrition*, *11*, 1435475. DOI: 10.3389/fnut.2024.1435475

Lante, A., Canazza, E., & Tessari, P. (2023). Beta-glucans of cereals: Functional and technological properties. *Nutrients*, *15*(9), 2124. DOI: 10.3390/nu15092124

Lee, J., Park, S., Oh, N., Park, J., Kwon, M., Seo, J., & Roh, S. (2021). Oral intake of Lactobacillus plantarum L-14 extract alleviates TLR2-and AMPK-mediated obesity-associated disorders in high-fat-diet-induced obese C57BL/6J mice. *Cell Proliferation*, *54*(6), e13039. DOI: 10.1111/cpr.13039

Lee, K. S., Palatinszky, M., Pereira, F. C., Nguyen, J., Fernandez, V. I., Mueller, A. J., Menolascina, F., Daims, H., Berry, D., Wagner, M., & Stocker, R. (2019). An automated Raman-based platform for the sorting of live cells by functional properties. *Nature Microbiology*, *4*(6), 1035–1048. DOI: 10.1038/s41564-019-0394-9

Li, H. Y., Zhou, D. D., Gan, R. Y., Huang, S. Y., Zhao, C. N., Shang, A., Xu, X. Y., & Li, H. B. (2021). Effects and Mechanisms of Probiotics, Prebiotics, Synbiotics, and Postbiotics on Metabolic Diseases Targeting Gut Microbiota: A Narrative Review. *Nutrients*, *13*(9), 3211. DOI: 10.3390/nu13093211

Ling, L. L., Schneider, T., Peoples, A. J., Spoering, A. L., Engels, I., Conlon, B. P., Mueller, A., Schäberle, T. F., Hughes, D. E., Epstein, S., Jones, M., Lazarides, L., Steadman, V. A., Cohen, D. R., Felix, C. R., Fetterman, K. A., Millett, W. P., Nitti, A. G., Zullo, A. M., & Lewis, K. (2015). A new antibiotic kills pathogens without detectable resistance. *Nature*, *517*(7535), 455–459. DOI: 10.1038/nature14098

Liu, R., Zhang, X., Cai, Y., Xu, S., Xu, Q., Ling, C., Li, X., Li, W., Liu, P., & Liu, W. (2024). Research progress on medicinal components and pharmacological activities of polygonatum sibiricum. *Journal of Ethnopharmacology*, *328*, 118024. DOI: 10.1016/j.jep.2024.118024

Liu, W., Yu, L., Chen, Q., Zhang, C., Wang, L., Yu, N., Peng, D., Ou, J., Chen, W., Zhang, Y., & Wang, Y. (2025). Poria cocos polysaccharides alleviate obesity-related adipose tissue insulin resistance via gut microbiota-derived short-chain fatty acids activation of FGF21/PI3K/AKT signaling. *Food Research International*, *215*, 116671. DOI: 10.1016/j.foodres.2025.116671

Liu, Y., Tran, D. Q., & Rhoads, J. M. (2018). Probiotics in disease prevention and treatment. *Journal of Clinical Pharmacology*, *58*(S10), S164–S179. DOI: 10.1002/jcph.1121

Lockis, V. R., Cruz, A. G., Walter, E. H., Faria, J. A., Granato, D., & Sant'Ana, A. S. (2011). Prerequisite programs at schools: Diagnosis and economic evaluation. *Foodborne Pathogens and Disease*, *8*(2), 213–220. DOI: 10.1089/fpd.2010.0645

Luo, C., Xu, X., Wei, X., Feng, W., Huang, H., Liu, H., Xu, R., Lin, J., Han, L., & Zhang, D. (2019). Natural medicines for the treatment of fatigue: Bioactive components, pharmacology, and mechanisms. *Pharmacological Research*, *148*, 104409. DOI: 10.1016/j.phrs.2019.104409

Marcum, J. A. (2020). Nutrigenetics/nutrigenomics, personalized nutrition, and precision healthcare. *Current Nutrition Reports*, *9*(4), 338–345. DOI: 10.1007/s13668-020-00327-z

Marim, A. V. C., & Gabardo, S. (2021). Xylooligosaccharides: Prebiotic potential from agro-industrial residue, production strategies and prospects. *Biocatalysis and Agricultural Biotechnology*, *37*, 102190. DOI: 10.1016/j.bcab.2021.102190

Meral, G., Aslan, E. S., Tunaligil, V., Burkay, N., Alper Acar, E. G., & Alp, M. Y. (2024). The importance of nutrigenetics and microbiota in personalized medicine: From phenotype to genotype. *Cureus*, *16*(5), 61256. DOI: 10.7759/cureus.61256

Moradi, M., Molaei, R., & Guimarães, J. T. (2021). A review on preparation and chemical analysis of postbiotics from lactic acid bacteria. *Enzyme and Microbial Technology*, *143*, 109722. DOI: 10.1016/j.enzmictec.2020.109722

Mudannayake, D. C., Jayasena, D. D., Wimalasiri, K. M., Ranadheera, C. S., & Ajlouni, S. (2022). Inulin fructans–food applications and alternative plant sources: A review. *International Journal of Food Science & Technology*, *57*(9), 5764–5780. DOI: 10.1111/ijfs.15947

Mullins, V. A., Bresette, W., Johnstone, L., Hallmark, B., & Chilton, F. H. (2020). Genomics in Personalized Nutrition: Can You "Eat for Your Genes"? *Nutrients*, *12*(10), 3118. DOI: 10.3390/nu12103118

Nascimento, C. E. O., Simões, L. C. O., Pereira, J. C., da Silva, R. R., de Lima, E. A., de Almeida, G. C., Penna, A. L. B., Boscolo, M., Gomes, E., & da Silva, R. (2022). Application of a recombinant GH10 endoxylanase from Thermoascus aurantiacus for xylooligosaccharide production from sugarcane bagasse and probiotic bacterial growth. *Journal of Biotechnology*, *347*, 1–8. DOI: 10.1016/j.jbiotec.2022.02.003

O'Toole, P. W., Marchesi, J. R., & Hill, C. (2017). Next-generation probiotics: The spectrum from probiotics to live biotherapeutics. *Nature Microbiology*, *2*(5), 1–6. DOI: 10.1038/nmicrobiol.2017.57

Oh, S., Lee, J., Chun, S., Choi, J. E., Kim, M. N., Chon, Y. E., Ha, Y., Hwang, S. G., Choi, S. W., & Hong, K. W. (2023). Interaction between the PNPLA3 Gene and Nutritional Factors on NAFLD Development: The Korean Genome and Epidemiology Study. *Nutrients*, *15*(1), 152. DOI: 10.3390/nu15010152

Owusu-Apenten, R. K., & Vieira, E. R. (2023). *Elementary food science (No. 303022)*. Springer., DOI: 10.1007/978-3-030-65433-7

Pedroza Matute, S., & Iyavoo, S. (2023). Exploring the gut microbiota: Lifestyle choices, disease associations, and personal genomics. *Frontiers in Nutrition*, *10*, 1225120. DOI: 10.3389/fnut.2023.1225120

Pereira-Marques, J., Ferreira, R. M., & Figueiredo, C. (2024). A metatranscriptomics strategy for efficient characterization of the microbiome in human tissues with low microbial biomass. *Gut Microbes*, *16*(1), 2323235. DOI: 10.1080/19490976.2024.2323235

Peters, D. L., Wang, W., Zhang, X., Ning, Z., Mayne, J., & Figeys, D. (2019). Metaproteomic and metabolomic approaches for characterizing the gut microbiome. *Proteomics*, *19*(16), 1800363. DOI: 10.1002/pmic.201800363

Portik, D. M., Brown, C. T., & Pierce-Ward, N. T. (2022). Evaluation of taxonomic classification and profiling methods for long-read shotgun metagenomic sequencing datasets. *BMC Bioinformatics*, *23*(1), 541. DOI: 10.1186/s12859-022-05103-0

Qin, Y. Q., Wang, L. Y., Yang, X. Y., Xu, Y. J., Fan, G., Fan, Y. G., Ren, J. N., An, Q., & Li, X. (2023). Inulin: Properties and health benefits. *Food & Function*, *14*(7), 2948–2968. DOI: 10.1039/D2FO01096H

Rahman, M. S., Lee, Y., Park, D. S., & Kim, Y. S. (2022). Bifidobacterium bifidum DS0908 and Bifidobacterium longum DS0950 culture-supernatants ameliorate obesity-related characteristics in mice with high-fat diet-induced obesity. *Journal of Microbiology and Biotechnology, 33*(1), 96–105. DOI: 10.4014/jmb.2210.10046

Ramezani, A., & Raj, D. S. (2014). The gut microbiome, kidney disease, and targeted interventions. *Journal of the American Society of Nephrology, 25*(4), 657–670. DOI: 10.1681/ASN.2013080905

Roberto, C. A., Ng, S. W., Ganderats-Fuentes, M., Hammond, D., Barquera, S., Jauregui, A., & Taillie, L. S. (2021). The influence of front-of-package nutrition labeling on consumer behavior and product reformulation. *Annual Review of Nutrition, 41*(1), 529–550. DOI: 10.1146/annurev-nutr-111120-094932

Roy, S., & Dhaneshwar, S. (2023). Role of prebiotics, probiotics, and synbiotics in management of inflammatory bowel disease: Current perspectives. *World Journal of Gastroenterology, 29*(14), 2078–2100. DOI: 10.3748/wjg.v29.i14.2078

Ruszkowski, J., & Witkowski, J. M. (2019). Lactulose: Patient- and dose-dependent prebiotic properties in humans. *Anaerobe, 59*, 100–106. DOI: 10.1016/j.anaerobe.2019.06.002

Sadeghi, A., Ebrahimi, M., Kharazmi, M. S., & Jafari, S. M. (2023). Effects of microbial-derived biotics (meta/pharma/post-biotics) on the modulation of gut microbiome and metabolome; general aspects and emerging trends. *Food Chemistry, 411*, 135478. DOI: 10.1016/j.foodchem.2023.135478

Salva, S., Kolling, Y., Ivir, M., Gutiérrez, F., & Alvarez, S. (2021). The role of immunobiotics and postbiotics in the recovery of immune cell populations from respiratory mucosa of malnourished hosts: Effect on the resistance against respiratory infections. *Frontiers in Nutrition, 8*, 704868. DOI: 10.3389/fnut.2021.704868

Sharafi, H., Divsalar, E., Rezaei, Z., Liu, S. Q., & Moradi, M. (2024). The potential of postbiotics as a novel approach in food packaging and biopreservation: A systematic review of the latest developments. *Critical Reviews in Food Science and Nutrition, 64*(33), 12524–12554. DOI: 10.1080/10408398.2023.2253909

Sharpton, T. J. (2014). An introduction to the analysis of shotgun metagenomic data. *Frontiers in Plant Science, 5*, 209. DOI: 10.3389/fpls.2014.00209

Sinrod, A. J. G., Shah, I. M., Surek, E., & Barile, D. (2023). Uncovering the promising role of grape pomace as a modulator of the gut microbiome: An in-depth review. *Heliyon, 9*(10), e20499. DOI: 10.1016/j.heliyon.2023.e20499

Smolinska, S., Popescu, F. D., & Zemelka-Wiacek, M. (2025). A Review of the Influence of Prebiotics, Probiotics, Synbiotics, and Postbiotics on the Human Gut Microbiome and Intestinal Integrity. *Journal of Clinical Medicine*, *14*(11), 3673. DOI: 10.3390/jcm14113673
Smolinska, S., Popescu, F. D., & Zemelka-Wiacek, M. (2025). A Review of the Influence of Prebiotics, Probiotics, Synbiotics, and Postbiotics on the Human Gut Microbiome and Intestinal Integrity. *Journal of Clinical Medicine*, *14*(11), 3673. DOI: 10.3390/jcm14113673
Sniffen, J. C., McFarland, L. V., Evans, C. T., & Goldstein, E. J. (2018). Choosing an appropriate probiotic product for your patient: An evidence-based practical guide. *PLoS One*, *13*(12), e0209205. DOI: 10.1371/journal.pone.0209205

St Germain, M. M., Mortazavi, A., & Bakovic, M. (2025). Advancing Personalized Nutrition Through Genetic Nutritional Insights. *Nutrients*, *17*(13), 2166. DOI: 10.3390/nu17132166

Sturm, G., Mojarrad, M., & Kaster, A. K. (2023). Targeted cell labeling and sorting of prokaryotes for cultivation and omics approaches. *Microbial Physiology*, *33*(1), 63–84. DOI: 10.1159/000532088

Swallah, M. S., Fan, H., Wang, S., Yu, H., & Piao, C. (2021). Prebiotic Impacts of Soybean Residue (Okara) on Eubiosis/Dysbiosis Condition of the Gut and the Possible Effects on Liver and Kidney Functions. *Molecules (Basel, Switzerland)*, *26*(2), 326. DOI: 10.3390/molecules26020326

. Tanca, A., Palomba, A., Fiorito, G., Abbondio, M., Pagnozzi, D., & Uzzau, S. (2024). Metaproteomic portrait of the healthy human gut microbiota. *npj Biofilms and Microbiomes*, 10, 54. https://doi.org/DOI: 10.1038/s41522-024-00526-4

Thorakkattu, P., Khanashyam, A. C., Shah, K., Babu, K. S., Mundanat, A. S., Deliephan, A., Deokar, G. S., Santivarangkna, C., & Nirmal, N. P. (2022). Postbiotics: Current trends in food and pharmaceutical industry. *Foods*, *11*(19), 3094. DOI: 10.3390/foods11193094

Tiangpook, S., Nhim, S., Prangthip, P., Pason, P., Tachaapaikoon, C., Ratanakhanokchai, K., & Waeonukul, R. (2023). Production of a Series of Long-Chain Isomaltooligosaccharides from Maltose by *Bacillus subtilis* AP-1 and Associated Prebiotic Properties. *Foods*, *12*(7), 1499. DOI: 10.3390/foods12071499

Tiderencel, K. A., Hutcheon, D. A., & Ziegler, J. (2020). Probiotics for the treatment of type 2 diabetes: A review of randomized controlled trials. *Diabetes/Metabolism Research and Reviews*, *36*(1), e3213. DOI: 10.1002/dmrr.3213

Tiffon, C. (2018). The impact of nutrition and environmental epigenetics on human health and disease. *International Journal of Molecular Sciences*, *19*(11), 3425. DOI: 10.3390/ijms19113425

Topolska, K., Florkiewicz, A., & Filipiak-Florkiewicz, A. (2021). Functional food—Consumer motivations and expectations. *International Journal of Environmental Research and Public Health*, *18*(10), 5327. DOI: 10.3390/ijerph18105327

Valladares-Diestra, K. K., de Souza Vandenberghe, L. P., Vieira, S., Goyzueta-Mamani, L. D., de Mattos, P. B. G., Manzoki, M. C., Soccol, V. T., & Soccol, C. R. (2023). The Potential of Xylooligosaccharides as Prebiotics and Their Sustainable Production from Agro-Industrial by-Products. *Foods*, *12*(14), 2681. DOI: 10.3390/foods12142681

Veiga, P., Suez, J., Derrien, M., & Elinav, E. (2020). Moving from probiotics to precision probiotics. *Nature Microbiology*, *5*(7), 878–880. DOI: 10.1038/s41564-020-0721-1

Vera-Santander, V. E., Hernández-Figueroa, R. H., Jiménez-Munguía, M. T., Mani-López, E., & López-Malo, A. (2023). Health benefits of consuming foods with bacterial probiotics, postbiotics, and their metabolites: A review. *Molecules (Basel, Switzerland)*, *28*(3), 1230. DOI: 10.3390/molecules28031230

. Verma, S., Gupta, N., Reshi, M., Chib, A., & Kumari, A. (2023). APPLICATIONS OF PROBIOTICS AND PREBIOTICS IN THE FOOD INDUSTRY: A REVIEW. *Plant Archives (09725210)*, *23*(2). https://doi.org/DOI: 10.51470/PLANTARCHIVES.2023.v23.no2.075

Vernocchi, P., Del Chierico, F., & Putignani, L. (2016). Gut microbiota profiling: Metabolomics based approach to unravel compounds affecting human health. *Frontiers in Microbiology*, *7*, 1144. DOI: 10.3389/fmicb.2016.01144

Vogtmann, E., Hua, X., Zeller, G., Sunagawa, S., Voigt, A. Y., Hercog, R., Goedert, J. J., Shi, J., Bork, P., & Sinha, R. (2016). Colorectal cancer and the human gut microbiome: Reproducibility with whole-genome shotgun sequencing. *PLoS One*, *11*(5), e0155362. DOI: 10.1371/journal.pone.0155362

Wang, X., Zeng, H., Li, L., Fang, Z., Xu, L., Shi, W., Li, J., Qian, J., Tan, X., Li, J., Qian, Y., & Xie, L. (2022). Personalized nutrition intervention improves nutritional status and quality of life of colorectal cancer survivors in the community: A randomized controlled trial. *Nutrition (Burbank, Los Angeles County, Calif.)*, *103-104*, 11. DOI: 10.1016/j.nut.2022.111835

Wang, Y., Wu, Y., Wang, Y., Xu, H., Mei, X., Yu, D., & Li, W. (2017). Antioxidant properties of probiotic bacteria. *Nutrients*, *9*(5), 521. DOI: 10.3390/nu9050521

Wilmanski, T., Rappaport, N., Diener, C., Gibbons, S. M., & Price, N. D. (2021). From taxonomy to metabolic output: What factors define gut microbiome health? *Gut Microbes*, *13*(1), 1907270. DOI: 10.1080/19490976.2021.1907270

Xavier-Santos, D., Padilha, M., Fabiano, G. A., Vinderola, G., Gomes Cruz, A., Sivieri, K., & Costa Antunes, A. E. (2022). Evidences and perspectives of the use of probiotics, prebiotics, synbiotics, and postbiotics as adjuvants for prevention and treatment of COVID-19: A bibliometric analysis and systematic review. *Trends in Food Science & Technology*, *120*, 174–192. DOI: 10.1016/j.tifs.2021.12.033

Xia, T., Teng, K., Liu, Y., Guo, Y., Huang, F., Tahir, M., Wang, T., & Zhong, J. (2023). A novel two-component bacteriocin, acidicin P, and its key residues for inhibiting Listeria monocytogenes by targeting the cell membrane. *Microbiology Spectrum*, *11*(4), e05210–e05222. DOI: 10.1128/spectrum.05210-22

Xu, J., & Zhao, F. (2018). Single-cell metagenomics: Challenges and applications. *Protein & Cell*, *9*(5), 501–510. DOI: 10.1007/s13238-018-0544-5

Yassine, F., Najm, A., & Bilen, M. (2025). The role of probiotics, prebiotics, and synbiotics in the treatment of inflammatory bowel diseases: An overview of recent clinical trials. *Frontiers in Systems Biology*, *5*, 1561047. DOI: 10.3389/fsysb.2025.1561047

Yeşilyurt, N., Yılmaz, B., Ağagündüz, D., & Capasso, R. (2021). Involvement of probiotics and postbiotics in the immune system modulation. *Biologics (Basel, Switzerland)*, *1*(2), 89–110. DOI: 10.3390/biologics1020006

Yoha, K. S., Nida, S., Dutta, S., Moses, J. A., & Anandharamakrishnan, C. (2022). Targeted delivery of probiotics: Perspectives on research and commercialization. *Probiotics and Antimicrobial Proteins*, *14*(1), 15–48. DOI: 10.1007/s12602-021-09791-7

Yunes, R. A., Poluektova, E. U., Vasileva, E. V., Odorskaya, M. V., Marsova, M. V., Kovalev, G. I., & Danilenko, V. N. (2020). A multi-strain potential probiotic formulation of GABA-producing Lactobacillus plantarum 90sk and Bifidobacterium adolescentis 150 with antidepressant effects. *Probiotics and Antimicrobial Proteins*, *12*(3), 973–979. DOI: 10.1007/s12602-019-09601-1

Zang, T., Han, L., Lu, Z., Tan, L., Liang, D., Shen, X., Liao, X., Liu, Y., Ren, H., & Sun, J. (2024). The History and Prediction of Prebiotics and Postbiotics: A Patent Analysis. *Nutrients*, *16*(3), 380. DOI: 10.3390/nu16030380

Zhang, W., Sadeghi, A., Karaca, A. C., Zhang, J., & Jafari, S. M. (2024). Carbohydrate polymer-based carriers for colon targeted delivery of probiotics. *Critical Reviews in Food Science and Nutrition, 64*(33), 12759–12779. DOI: 10.1080/10408398.2023.2257321

Żółkiewicz, J., Marzec, A., Ruszczyński, M., & Feleszko, W. (2020). Postbiotics—A step beyond pre-and probiotics. *Nutrients, 12*(8), 2189. DOI: 10.3390/nu12082189

Zommiti, M., Feuilloley, M. G. J., & Connil, N. (2020). Update of Probiotics in Human World: A Nonstop Source of Benefactions till the End of Time. *Microorganisms, 8*(12), 1907. DOI: 10.3390/microorganisms8121907

Chapter 4
Epigenetic Biomarkers in Microbiome-Driven Nutrition Therapy

Aneesh Nair
https://orcid.org/0009-0003-9687-2398
Noorul Islam Centre for Higher Education, India

Sruthi Mariam George
Noorul Islam Centre for Higher Education, India

Arumugam Vijaya Anand
https://orcid.org/0000-0001-7485-1586
Bharathiar University, India

Rakesh Kumar Yadav
KU Leuven, Belgium

ABSTRACT

The convergence of epigenomic and microbiome research marks a transformative step in precision medicine. The human microbiome, a diverse ecosystem shaping digestion, immunity, and metabolism, interacts with epigenetic mechanisms such as DNA methylation, histone modifications, and non-coding RNAs influenced by diet and microbial metabolites. Compounds like short-chain fatty acids, folate, and bile acid derivatives regulate key epigenetic enzymes (DNMTs, HATs, HDACs), modulating chromatin accessibility and gene expression tied to metabolic and immune functions. Epigenetic biomarkers, being reversible and environmentally responsive, offer dynamic insight into nutritional status and disease trajectories. Integrating metagenomic and epigenomic data enables stratification of microbiota-dependent

DOI: 10.4018/979-8-3373-4382-2.ch004

epigenetic phenotypes, supporting personalized nutrition strategies. This chapter discusses mechanistic, clinical, and methodological advances shaping microbiome-driven precision nutrition.

1. INTRODUCTION TO EPIGENETIC BIOMARKERS IN NUTRITION SCIENCE

Epigenetic biomarkers represent quantifiable changes in the regulation of gene expression that occur without alterations to the underlying DNA sequence, instead reflecting the influence of environmental factors such as diet and gut microbiome on gene expression. Within the field of nutrition, epigenetic biomarkers can provide a dynamic readout of how nutritional exposures and microbial metabolites alter biological processes, and may potentially predict health outcomes, guide dietary intervention, and influence personalized nutrition recommendations. Epigenetic regulation occurs through several coordinated, pathway-based mechanisms, with DNA methylation, histone modifications, and non-coding RNA, especially microRNAs all being important contributors. These pathways can respond to dietary components and microbial metabolites (including short-chain fatty acids, bile acids, and vitamins) as well as host-microbe interactions, subsequently leading to changes in transcriptional activity that ultimately affect metabolism, inflammation, and energy homeostasis.(Lopomo et al., 2016; Tiffon, 2018)

1.1 Definition and classification of epigenetic biomarkers (DNA methylation, histone markers, and miRNA expression)

DNA methylation marks are the most well-characterized epigenetic marks in nutrition science, and are generally located on cytosine-phosphate-guanine (CpG) dinucleotides, and can modulate gene expression by changing transcriptional accessibility. Diet- and microbiome-related alterations in methylation patterns have been associated with metabolic traits, inflammatory profiles, and aging processes, and the profiling of methylation can be performed on methylation arrays or by whole-genome bisulfite sequencing (Table 1). Histone modifications are the result of post-translational modifications to histones, including acetylation, methylation, phosphorylation, and ubiquitination, which can alter the structure of chromatin and gene accessibility. Histone marks respond to metabolite diets (e.g. acetyl-CoA or S-adenosylmethionine), establishing a mechanistic link between nutrition and transcriptional programs. miRNA expression evaluates the expression of microRNAs that modulate gene expression post-transcriptionally through targeted mRNA degradation and translational repression. miRNA profiles can change in response to dietary components and microbiome-derived signals, serving as sensitive indicators of nutritional status and host–microbiome interactions (Deiuliis, 2016).

Table 1. Classification and Features of Epigenetic Biomarkers

Epigenetic Biomarker Type	Mechanism of Action	Detection Methods	Nutritional Influence	Clinical Relevance
DNA Methylation	Addition of methyl group to CpG sites	Bisulfite sequencing, MS-PCR	Folate, B12, choline	Gene silencing; metabolic regulation
Histone modifications	Acetylation, methylation, phosphorylation	ChIP-seq, Western blot	SCFAs (butyrate), polyphenols	Chromatin remodelling
miRNA expression	Post-transcriptional gene regulation	qRT-PCR, RNA-seq	Omega-3, curcumin	Inflammation, metabolism

In nutrition therapy driven by the microbiome, epigenetic biomarkers serve as a mechanistic link connecting dietary changes and microbiota-produced metabolites with physiological response by the host. Dietary practices and microbiome interactions can alter patterns of DNA methylation in signaling pathways related to energy expenditure, lipid handling, and inflammatory response, which, in turn, affect disease risk and response to nutrition therapy (Mahmoud, 2022). Microbial metabolites, including butyrate, propionate, and other short-chain fatty acids, can, either directly or indirectly, alter acetylation of histones and DNA methylation patterns through changes in availability of substrates and cofactors for epigenetic enzymes (Shock et al., 2021a). Dietary patterns can appear to affect miRNA networks in response to caloric load, or increased fiber or probiotic and fermented food intake, which is expressed in gut–liver signaling and central or systemic metabolism (Yu et al., 2021).

1.2 Rationale for their use in Personalized Nutrition: Dynamic Responsiveness, Environmental Sensitivity, and Clinical Utility

Personalized nutrition refers to a customized approach to dietary advice that aims to maximize health improvement by taking into account individual differences and uniqueness, including genetics, physiology, lifestyle, environment and the gut microbiome. Rather than a one-size-fits-all dietary paradigm, personalized nutrition recognizes that what is beneficial for one person may be less effective or even harmful for another. The promise for this paradigm lies in three core principles: dynamic responsiveness, contextual sensitivity and clinical relevance. A fourth dimension which is a growing evidence of host–microbe–epigenome interactions adds a mechanistic layer of complexity that may further refine our understanding of a personalized perspective, and, similarly, why there is such a difference in response from person to person to the same dietary exposure.

Dynamic responsiveness refers to a feedback loop between the diet and phenotype driven by variation in metabolism and physiology among individuals. The need for and absorption and use of nutrients is not a static process; factors like age, sex, body composition, hormonal status, and the presence of metabolic diseases will all influence the way the body consumes macronutrients, micronutrients, and bioactive compounds. This view states that dietary interventions will adapt over time when considering that a given diet can elicit different responses at different life stages or with a change in health status. For example, individual tolerance to carbohydrates can change with physical activity levels, sensitivity to insulin, and composition of the gut microbiome; or, the need for protein may change with change in muscle mass or disease state. On a practical level, personalization means continually assessing and adjusting underlying macronutrient balance, micronutrient sufficiency, and functional outcomes like glycemic response, lipid profiles, or inflammatory markers by utilizing real-time, or near real-time physiological data (Turnbaugh & Gordon, 2009). Tailoring diet to physiological state can optimize energy balance or health outcomes to a greater degree than static recommendations.

Environmental sensitivity prioritizes the diet within a context of real-world exposures, noting that diet does not exist in isolation. The same nutrient can have different effects depending on context; fat quality may interact with a person's level of physical activity and gut health to impact cardiovascular risk, while fiber may have different effects on glycemic control and microbiota composition, depending on the gut microbiome dynamics of the consumer and their habitual dietary intakes (Subhan & Chan, 2016). From a practical perspective, personalization must occur with regards to one's lifestyle practices and environmental exposures. This framework also increases adherence and translates to more real-world effectiveness by personalizing recommendations for feasible, manageable and sustainable dietary habit change within each consumer's context.

Clinical utility grounds personalization in important health outcomes. The ultimate goal of any diet is reduction of risk of disease, disease prevention, and promotion of overall health and well-being; clinical utility is the showing that the personalized approach makes a meaningful difference in outcomes that exceed those possible from the recommendations to the general population. Clinical utility depends on valid phenotyping, actionable targets, and evidence based/modifiable strategies for intervention. Important issues in clinical utility consideration include predictive value (what extent does a biomarker or metabolomic profile do in predicting the response to the diet), decision usefulness (to what extent will the information change decision making), and cost-effectiveness.

1.3 Emerging role of host–microbe–epigenome interactions.

Host genetics, the gut microbiome, and the epigenome interact to influence nutritional responses in ways that go beyond host-related aspects. The gut microbiota plays an important role in the metabolism of dietary components, converting them into bioactive metabolites, such as short-chain fatty acid derivatives, that affect insulin sensitivity, inflammation, and gut barrier integrity. Although all individuals have distinct microbial communities, each person responds uniquely to food. Therefore, their individual postprandial physiology and health trajectories are influenced by their microbial composition. Microbiome-informed personalization could help predict glycemic responses to foods, fat-storing behaviors, and micronutrient status to support health-related decisions, some people provide more or less efficient fermentation of fermentable fibers provide metabolites that may positively or negatively alter metabolic health, depending on microbial characteristics. Epigenetic processes could then change gene expression in metabolic pathways that were previously triggered by dietary or microbiome-related nutrients with specific bioactive components and/or metabolites - embedding life experiences of diet or diet-related, specifically from microbial sources into ontological dietary modifications that then regulate weight gain or metabolic adjustment to the diet. From a systems biology perspective, data collected could form a incorporation of host genetics, microbial modulation of dietary responses, and epigenetic transmission to create meaningful interpretations of variability related to appetite regulation, energy expenditure, and disease risk, which host genetics alone do not fully explain. Practically, the evidence of an integrated approach could help efficiency stratification for specific interventions, guide microbiome-informed nutritional choices, promote epigenome-informed food-selection decision making, and help guide practicing health and nutrition professionals in devising planning recommendations for better nutrition, while also considering intergenerational aspects and life-course nutrition (Wang et al., 2022).

This promise comes with many challenges. The quality and consistency of evidence varies between domains, and further strong, replicated trials and real-world studies are needed to create clear causal and generalizable conclusions. Integrating and interpreting data will include complex multi-omics data, as well as behavioral and environmental data, which will require advanced analytics, standardized measures, and transparent decision-support tools that both clinicians and individuals will find trustworthy. In order to avoid increasing health equity gaps, there will also need to be a focus on accessibility and equity and costs of personalized nutrition programs will need to be considered; the programs need to be cost-effective, and culturally and ethnically responsive in order to be inclusive for diverse populations and their social determinants of health. Privacy and ethics are a crucial consideration, as genetic and microbiome and various lifestyle data will be collected, thus requiring strong governance, informed consent process, and data protection framework.

A dynamic responsiveness ensures that individuals' recommendations are able to truly adapt as their physiology changes; an environmental sensitivity ensures that recommendations are congruent with their actual patterns in the world to enhance feasibility and ultimate adherence; and clinical utility ensures that there will be an ultimately demonstrated direct application to their health. The emergence of the field of host–microbe–epigenome interactions demonstrates a newly developed potential mechanistic understanding for individual variability in response to dietary patterns, therefore allowing us to proceed to personalized nutrition approaches that could be not only personalized, but mechanistically informed, with the potential for durability throughout life.

2. MICROBIAL METABOLITES AS EPIGENETIC MODULATORS

2.1 Biochemical pathways of microbial fermentation (e.g., SCFA synthesis via fiber metabolism)

Microbial metabolites have proven to be an important portion of the regulation of the epigenetic landscape of the host related to diet, gut microbiome composition and physiology of the host. In this regard, short-chain fatty acids (SCFAs) such as butyrate, acetate and propionate, are valuable for their role as an energy source for colonocytes and as signaling metabolites that can alter gene expression via epigenetic mechanisms.

SCFA production is dependent on the microbial fermentation of dietary fiber in luminal gut contents. Anaerobic fermentation of complex carbohydrates by fiber-degrading bacteria that belong to the two dominant phyla, Firmicutes and Bacteroidetes, generates SCFA profiles that will have contextual effects on the epigenetic landscape by altering histone modification and DNA methylation while remaining within the structure of chromatin (Fig.1). Butyrate is produced primarily by the butyrogenic bacteria including Roseburia, *Faecalibacterium prausnitzii*, and *Eubacterium rectale*, and is considered the primary energy source for colonocytes and a signaling metabolite that can modulate host gene expression patterns (Krautkramer et al., 2017). Fiber metabolism can modify epigenetic regulation through the balance and flux of SCFAs produced during metabolic fermentation that may be altered via dietary input, microbial ecology and physiology (Hullar & Fu, 2014).

Fig.1. Biochemical pathway linking fiber fermentation to epigenetic regulation

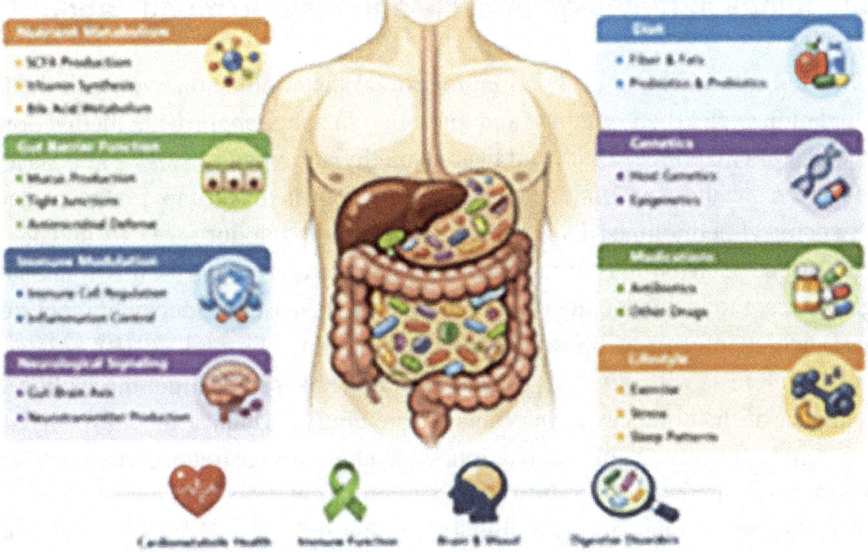

2.2 Functional effects of butyrate as an HDAC inhibitor: Impact on gene expression and chromatin remodeling

Butyrate is mostly known for its roles as an epigenetic modulator by acting as a histone deacetylase (HDAC) inhibitor. HDACs are enzymes that remove acetyl chains from lysine residues on histone tails, which leads to a closed conformation of chromatin and transcriptional repression. Physiologically relevant concentrations of butyrate inhibit class I and IIa HDACs, which results in increased histone acetylation, a more open chromatin conformation, and increased accessibility of transcription (Davie, 2003). This HDAC-inhibitory effect of butyrate results in broad changes in gene transcription, including differential expression of genes involved in cell cycle arrest, differentiation, apoptosis, and anti-inflammatory responses affected by the cell type. Additionally, inhibition of HDACs by butyrate can affect chromatin remodeling complexes and the recruitment of transcription factors, further driving varied cellular programs in the intestinal epithelial cells, immune cells, and tissues located beyond the gut (Bultman, 2014). Valuable to manage is that the epigenetic effects of butyrate are not limited to increased histone acetylation. Butyrate also alters non-histone protein acetylation and the modulation of signaling pathways that eventually converge at epigenetic regulators, facilitating the overall enhancement of gene regulatory networks.

2.3 Role of microbial folate, biotin, and tryptophan metabolites in methylation cycle and histone modification

In addition to histone acetylation, microbial metabolites interact with the host methylation cycle; dietary inputs and microbial metabolism provide methyl donors and cofactors that direct DNA and histone methylation patterns. As a key player in one-carbon metabolism, folate (vitamin B9) provides methyl groups for the formation of S-adenosylmethionine (SAM), the universal methyl donor for DNA and histone methylation. Contributions from microbial folate production and the host folate status together react to influence the ratio of intracellular SAM:S-adenosylhomocysteine (SAH), which informs methyltransferase activity (Engevik et al., 2019). Folate metabolism interacts with other B-vitamins and elements from methionine cycling, and the impact of disturbances in microbial folate could influence global methylation or gene specific patterns of methylation, which have downstream consequences for gene expression, genome stability, and differentiation processes.

Another metabolite, biotin (vitamin B7), is also influenced by the gut microbiota, and it plays a role in carboxylation and carboxyl-mation reactions, both of which are necessary for fatty-acid synthesis and energy metabolism. In addition to its metabolic activities, biotin status might indirectly impact epigenetic regulation via its role in histone biotinylation and possible interactions with chromatin-modifying enzymes (Zempleni et al., 2008).

While the precise contribution of microbially derived biotin to host chromatin states is an area of active investigation, biotin availability can influence gene expression programs by supporting the function of biotin-dependent carboxylases and possibly affecting transcriptional regulation through chromatin-associated processes.

The metabolism of tryptophan by gut microbes results in a variety of metabolites synthesized from tryptophan and indole, such as indole-3-acetic acid, indole-3-propionic acid, and metabolites from the kynurenine pathway. These metabolites can affect host epigenetic regulation through either direct or indirect means. For example, several indole derivatives activate aryl hydrocarbon receptor (AhR) signaling, which interacts with chromatin modifiers and transcriptional programs in gut epithelial and immune cells. In addition, changes in the catabolism of tryptophan alter the activity of the NAD+-dependent sirtuin family of deacetylases (e.g., SIRT1) that connect microbial metabolism to energy status and remodeling of chromatin. Kynurenine pathway products are also associated with methylation dynamics by altering cellular NAD+ levels and redox status, with effects on histone and DNA modification enzymes. Overall, microbial metabolites of tryptophan participate in an epigenetic regulatory network that links microbial signals with host metabolic status and immune responses (Agus et al., 2018; Seo & Kwon, 2023).

3. NUTRIENT–MICROBIOME–EPIGENOME AXIS IN HEALTH AND DISEASE

The human gut is inhabited by a complex microbial ecosystem in a balanced eubiosis state, maintaining mutualistic associations and providing beneficial functions (Al-Rashidi, 2022). These microbes play essential roles in the regulation of various biological functions such as nutrient metabolism, biosynthesis of micronutrients like vitamins, and immune processes, thus impacting health in several ways (*MicroRNAs as Regulators of Metabolic Disease: Pathophysiologic Significance and Emerging Role as Biomarkers and Therapeutics | International Journal of Obesity*, n.d.) (Li et al., 2022) (Table 2). The human gut microbiome mainly comprises six bacterial phyla, including Bacteroidetes, Firmicutes, Actinobacteria, Proteobacteria, Verrucomicrobia, and Fusobacteria (*Microbiota in Health and Diseases | Signal Transduction and Targeted Therapy*, n.d.-a). Increasing evidence suggests that, along with other factors such as physical activity, age, and lifestyles, diet has a pivotal role in the modulation of these gut microbiomes and their functions (De Filippo et al., 2010; *Modulation of the Gut Microbiota by Nutrition and Its Relationship to Epigenetics*, n.d.). The type of macronutrient intake, such as carbohydrates, proteins, and fats, influences the selection and persistence of these diverse bacterial groups, which in turn is a decisive factor for positive or adverse effects. For instance, the metabolism of indigestible carbohydrates by members of the Bacteroidetes and Bifidobacterium phyla produces short-chain fatty acids (SCFAs), which are generally beneficial for human health (Zhang, 2022).

Table 2. Nutrient-Microbiome-Epigenome Interactions in Common Diseases

Condition	Key Nutrient/ Metabolite	Epigenetic Marker Altered	Microbial Involvement	Outcome
Obesity	SCFAs, polyphenols	DNA Methylation of adipogenic genes	*Firmicutes/Bacteriodetes* ratio	Altered metabolism
Type 2 diabetes	Butyrate, folate	Hypomethylation of insulin-related genes	*Faecalibacterium spp.*	Improved glucose control
Cancer	Butyrate, phytochemicals	Histone acetylation of tumor suppressor genes	*Clostridium spp.*	Apoptosis induction
Neurodegeneration	Tryptophan metabolites	miRNA and histone changes	*Lactabacillus spp.*	Neuroprotection

In contrast, the western diet is often associated with the reduced microbiome diversity due to high calorie content and saturated fats (Frioux et al., 2023). Likewise, a diet with low fibre could lead to an increased risk of colon cancer and type 2 diabetes (*The Interplay between Diet and the Gut Microbiome: Implications for Health and Disease | Nature Reviews Microbiology*, n.d.). Further, the microbial metabolites produced by gut microbes could directly affect several enzymes, such as DNA methyltransferase 1 (DNMT1), which are involved in epigenetic modifications. Such epigenetic changes control the expression at the gene level and determine which proteins need to be synthesised (*Heterogeneity in VEGFR3 Levels Drives Lymphatic Vessel Hyperplasia through Cell-Autonomous and Non-Cell-Autonomous Mechanisms | Nature Communications*, n.d.). These epigenetic changes are considered vital for normal health and development. However, some diet-induced microbial metabolites can also influence and disrupt various epigenetic processes, which could lead to microbial dysbiosis, resulting in a diseased state (*Microbiota in Health and Diseases | Signal Transduction and Targeted Therapy*, n.d.-b). These epigenetic mechanisms, characterised by DNA methylation, histone modification, and non-coding RNA (involved in posttranscriptional gene regulation) are fundamental in various health conditions and diseases (Kim et al., 2024). All these processes are significantly affected by the epigenetically active microbial metabolites produced from different diets. For instance, folate, mainly produced by *Bifidobacterium spp*, is a methyl donor and is essential for the production of S-adenosylmethionine (SAM), which acts as a methyl-donating substrate for DNA methyltransferases. The process is crucial for important processes like DNA replication and repair (*Influences of Diet and the Gut Microbiome on Epigenetic Modulation in Cancer and Other Diseases | Clinical Epigenetics*, n.d.). Further, butyrate produced by various Firmicutes has been shown to reduce the expression of pro-angiogenic factors such as EGF and thus play a crucial role in preventing cancer. Therefore, microbial metabolites can have significant epigenetic influence that can lead to a healthy or disease state, indirectly controlled by the diet type. The epigenetic modifications induced by microbial metabolites are increasingly recognised as pivotal contributors to human diseases such as insulin resistance, cancers, and cardiovascular diseases (Carson & Lawson, 2018). Insulin resistance is a condition where cells become less responsive to insulin, which is often linked to diets rich in complex carbs and high fibre content, ultimately leading to metabolic illnesses like type 2 diabetes. Gut-microbes-derived metabolites such as SCFAs and bile acids play a significant role in insulin signalling by affecting the cell receptors involved in insulin sensitivity and glucose uptake, such as farnesoid X receptor (FXR) and G protein-coupled receptor TGR5 (*Synergistic Interplay of Diet, Gut Microbiota, and Insulin Resistance: Unraveling the Molecular Nexus - Gopal - 2024 - Molecular Nutrition & Food Research - Wiley Online Library*, n.d.).

Recent studies have also implicated a bidirectional relationship between heart failure and gut microbes and their metabolites. Heart failure generally involves remodelling the myocardium, a complex process requiring transcriptional changes such as DNA methylation. Growing evidence suggested the role of gut microbe-derived metabolites such as trimethylamine N-oxide (TMAO), SCFAs, and secondary bile acids as external factors influencing these complex mechanisms (*The Role of the Gut Microbiota in the Onset and Progression of Heart Failure: Insights into Epigenetic Mechanisms and Aging | Clinical Epigenetics*, n.d.). Further, the microbial metabolites are also linked to prevalence of colorectal cancer (CRC). A study showed (Krautkramer et al., 2016) that the Western-type diet prevented many of the microbiota-dependent chromatin changes that occur in a polysaccharide-rich diet, leading to increased risk of CRC. Such a diet and gut microbiome-metabolite-induced epigenetic modifications can exacerbate several risks of metabolic diseases. These metabolic changes are not only restricted to one generation but can also be transmitted; therefore, they require an appropriate diet, lifestyle, and therapeutic interventions.

4. TECHNOLOGIES FOR EPIGENETIC BIOMARKER DISCOVERY

4.1 Overview of epigenome-wide association studies (EWAS) and targeted approaches

The identification of epigenetic biomarkers is one of the foundational pillars of precision medicine, adding to our understanding of genetic variability, to explain the role of environmental exposures, lifestyle and the mechanisms and processes of disease in the regulation of genes. Epigenome-wide association studies (EWAS) have become a common strategy in the field of epigenetics similar to genome-wide association studies (GWAS), except focused on heritable or reversible epigenetic marks such as DNA methylation, histone modifications, and chromatin accessibility. EWAS studies inquiry the association of epigenetic features across the epigenome with phenotypes of interest including complex diseases, aging, exposure history, and treatment response.

Through the use of EWAS designs we can tap into the power of integrated biomarker signals from genetics, environment and stochastic processes to identify important biomarkers of overall biological effects and shed light on potential mechanistic pathways that could become therapeutic targets. Previous EWAS studies provided the foundation linking methylation patterns in regions of CpG-density, along with methylation density in terms of promoter-associated methylation as likely important mechanisms in the transmission of transcriptional changes that may lead to cancer, cardiovascular disease, neurodegeneration and more consequences of epigenetic processes. It is critical to keep study design strong (e.g., matched case–control or longitudinal cohorts) and to be careful in the consideration of the relevant tissues for the biomarkers of interest for consistently replicating EWAS in diverse cohorts which may also include replication of diverse cohorts for inclusion of different epigenetic processes from lifestyle and/or exposure, in order to converge epigenetic processes likely due to confounding variables of age, cell-type composition or smoking (Skinner, 2024). EWAS have methodologically progressed, through robust preprocessing and assessment of batch effects, cellular heterogeneity, and other technical artifacts, to improve reproducibility and comparability across cohorts. The field is still working on better causal inference, using methods such as Mendelian randomization and co-localization analyses, which may more accurately assess correlation versus possible causation with epigenetic associations.

EWAS investigates the epigenome for identifying differential epigenetic marks associated with a phenotype without pre-existing hypotheses and allows for the discovery of novel loci and pathways. EWAS can identify unexpected regulatory elements, temporally dynamic enhancer methylation, and tissue or cell-type specific epigenetic signals that are suggestive of new mechanisms or therapeutic targets. However, there are challenges due to the breadth of EWAS with respect to multiple testing correction, the regional aggregation of signals, and the interpretation of distal regulatory effects. Independent cohort replication and meta-analytic synthesis across studies are required to generate reliable biomarkers, as well as integrative analyses that connect methylation changes to gene expression and chromatin state. In contrast, targeted approaches are focused on predefined candidate regions or biomarkers, likely with some basis in prior knowledge related to gene regulation, known mechanisms of disease, or prior EWAS hits. Targeted approaches may have greater statistical power, improved interpretability, and greater feasibility for clinical translation, particularly in the presence of resource limitations or sample availability constraints precluding genome-scale analyses. As a result, they represent tools for validation studies, development of clinical assays (e.g., methylation panels for prognosis or therapy response), or instances where biological sampling is limited. The choice between EWAS and targeted approaches ultimately depends on the aims of the study, sample considerations, and the anticipated stability of the biomarker across tissues and over time.

4.2 High-resolution techniques included whole-genome bisulfite sequencing (WGBS), reduced representation bisulfite sequencing (RRBS), ChIP-seq, and ATAC-seq

The advent of high-resolution epigenomic approaches has vastly improved our capacity to map regulatory landscapes at unprecedented detail. Whole-genome bisulfite sequencing (WGBS) interrogates DNA methylation with single-base resolution across the genome, allowing for the identification of differentially methylated regions and allelic methylation patterns in a comprehensive manner (Guanzon et al., 2024). WGBS is especially powerful for capturing methylation at non-CpG contexts and in regions of repetitive nature, yet it is highly resource demanding from both the standpoints of sequencing depth and data processing. Along with the need for significant bioinformatic infrastructure, there are also considerable challenges around alignment methods for bisulfite-converted reads and interpreting methylation in heterogeneous tissues.

Reduced representation bisulfite sequencing (RRBS) represents a more cost-effective and practical, albeit biased, approach by pre-enriching for CpG-dense regions providing high-CpG coverage of promoter and enhancer elements to alleviate the overall sequencing demands required by WGBS. While RRBS sacrifices the genome-wide approach characterizing a WGBS strategy, it is very well positioned for large-scale studies and comparative studies across samples and between groups in cases where the specific study question focuses on promoter regions and regulatory elements with high-CpG content. Furthermore, RRBS may often represent the most pragmatic balance between depth and breadth for clinically-scaled projects (Fig.2.) (Meissner et al., 2005).

Fig.2. Schematic representation of steps involved in Reduced representation bisulfite sequencing (RRBS)

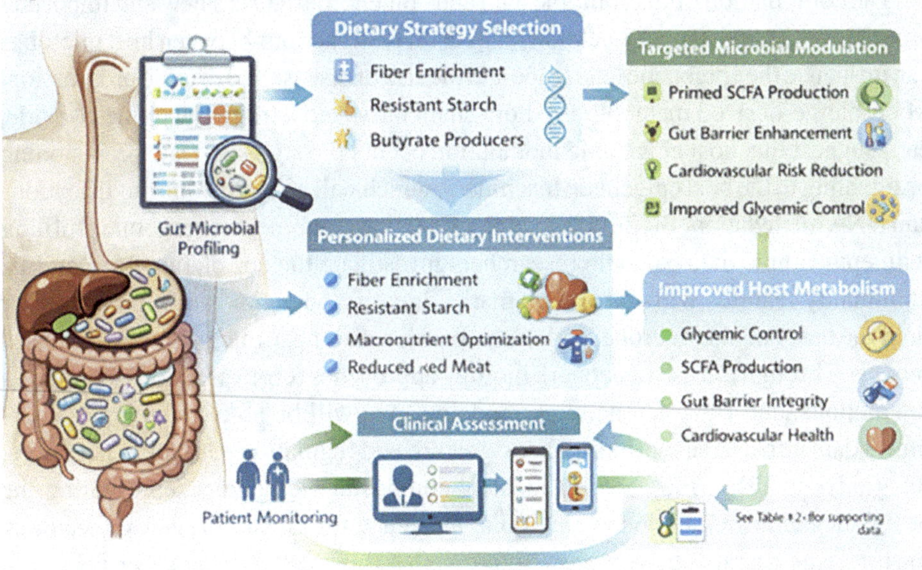

Chromatin immunoprecipitation sequencing (ChIP-seq) maps histone modifications and transcription factor binding sites, revealing the regulatory architecture of gene expression and linking specific patterns of methylation to functional chromatin states (Nakato & Sakata, 2021). ChIP-seq can identify domains with active enhancers, poised promoters, and repressive marks, giving functional meaning to epigenetic changes identified through EWAS.

Assay for Transposase-Accessible Chromatin using sequencing (ATAC-seq) profiles chromatin accessibility that understands open regulatory regions, which may be involved in the higher-order regulatory networks associated with disease. ATAC-seq uses small amounts of input material and quickly profiles the openness of chromatin to provide a mapping of accessible promoters and enhancers that are correlated with transcriptional activity. Combining these technologies provides an understanding of many levels of the epigenome - from DNA methylation to chromatin state to accessibility - giving a much richer context for biomarker discovery and mechanistic interpretation (Grandi et al., 2022). Furthermore, integrative analyses that connect methylation patterns with histone marks and accessibility landscapes allow us to carry functional meaning to epigenetic changes, enhancing our understanding of how regulatory disruptions lead to disease.

4.3 Integration of microbiome and epigenome data through bioinformatics pipelines and network biology

The combination of microbiome data and epigenome data is a new and important area of biomarker discovery, acknowledging that interactions between host microbes can influence the epigenetic landscape and the risk of disease and disease progression. Microbiome-derived metabolites (short-chain fatty acids, trimethylamine N-oxide, etc.) suggest that host epigenetic modulation occurs through substrate provisioning or signaling to the host epigenetic machinery, which will affect histone modifications and DNA methylation. Bioinformatics pipelines that combine metagenomic profiling with epigenomic data can help researchers investigate the correlation of microbial community features with epigenetic marks, identify potential causal pathways for both the host and the microbe, and develop interactive host-microbe network-based models. Through the use of network biology approaches (co-expressions, chromatin interactions, and Bayesian network modeling) we will be able to integrate multi-omics data into a cohesive biomarker signature and regulation networks. Therefore, integrative analyses may help to identify composite biomarkers representing the host endogenous regulation or microbial influence for greater predictive accuracy in stratifying therapeutic response. Examples of this include associations between methylation of inflammatory gene regulation and gut microbiota-derived metabolites, or associations of immune cell chromatin accessibility based on microbial diversity (Muhammad et al., 2024). Although that science is rapidly emerging there remains a pressing need for robust study designs that account for diet, antibiotic exposure, ethnicity, and importantly, other environmental confounders to be able to untangle and delineate direct epigenetic effects from secondary associations.

In practical terms, the workflow for epigenome-wide association studies (EWAS) and the evaluation of epigenetic biomarkers involves several key steps: study design and cohort specification, biospecimen acquisition (taking into consideration tissue type relevance and cell-type composition), and careful preprocessing with correction for batch effects, cell-type heterogeneity, and technical artifacts. The tissue selection choice could be consequential; for example, peripheral blood is easily attainable and useful for identification of systemic biomarker, but may not reflect epigenetic changes in tissues, like brain or liver, relevant to a specific pathobiological condition, and buccal swabs or saliva may have the advantage of being simple to collect, but these biospecimens have a different landscape of methylation. Therefore, deconvolution methods to provide estimates of cell-type proportions or, where possible, actual assessment of cell types of interest, are advantageous. The statistical analysis, as a general approach, will usually use a mixed-model framework, or some form of regression model to control for covariates, for example, age, sex, smoking status, BMI, ethnicity, or estimated cell-type proportions. More advanced methods, including linear mixed models or Bayesian hierarchical models, or machine learning feature selection approaches, allow for handling of high dimensional data or complex confounding structures. Replicating findings in independent cohorts and conducting meta-analytic summaries provide additional credibility of reported findings when developing biomarkers. Functional annotation and pathway analyses provide a means to convert epigenetic signals into biologically relevant hypotheses about connections between changes in methylation and gene repression, enhancer function, or chromatin structure. Validation of the biological relevance of epigenetic base modifications into a pathway can include comparative longitudinal measurements to provide a measure of temporal stability and cross-tissue comparisons to consider the potentially tissue-specific role for epigenetic modifications and ultimately functional validation in cellular or animal models when operational. Specific to studies of microbiome and epigenome interactions, models will need to consider confounding factors such as diet, exposure to antibiotic and environmental influences that could potentially influence both the microbiota composition and the epigenome. Longitudinal sampling, paired multi-omics and careful harmonization of sequencing apparatus are all approaches that will assist in elucidating causal pathways from simple associations.(Rakyan et al., 2011)

Innovative computational and experimental technologies are likely to further the reliability and translatability of epigenetic biomarkers. Single-cell epigenomics, such as single-cell ATAC-seq and single-cell bisulfite sequencing, can resolve epigenetic states at single cell resolution (e.g., for each cell type) in heterogeneous tissues, and improve the specificity of biomarker signatures while diminishing confounding due to cellular composition. This level of resolution can identify subpopulations of cells with specific regulatory states that may be important drivers of disease progression or response to treatment. Longitudinal multi-omics studies can utilize time-series data and causal inference methods to disentangle time-dependent regulatory processes and provide clues into timing of interventions. Integrative modeling approaches, such as multi-omics factor analysis and network-based priors, allow panels of biomarkers to be designed that simultaneously include levels of methylation, chromatin state, gene expression, and taxonomy of microbes (Liu, 2024). While this sophistication is exciting, translating such comprehensive analyses into clinically-usable biomarkers must be cognizant of test feasibility, cost, standardization, and regulatory pathways, emphasizing the importance of cross-disciplinary research teams comprising biologists, bioinformaticians, clinicians, and statisticians. Sharing data freely, transparently reporting statistics, and developing reproducible pipelines are essential for promotion of validation and clinical implementation .

5. APPLICATION OF EPIGENETIC BIOMARKERS IN PRECISION NUTRITION

Epigenetic biomarkers have a great potential to further develop precision nutrition by assessing the ways that individuals' dietary exposures are related to inheritable and fluctuating changes in gene expression. By creating an epigenetic profile such as DNA methylation, histone modification, and non-coding RNA, we can obtain a readout of the cumulative impact of diet, lifestyles, and environment, while not directly altering the genome itself. Epigenetic biomarkers can be either directly or indirectly used in precision nutrition to classify people into responder and non-responder groups based on specific dietary interventions and may offer better-targeted and more effective dietary strategies. For example, baseline methylation signatures in specific genes involved in lipid metabolism, inflammation, or glucose tolerance/glycemic response, or other related metabolic process may predict who is more likely to respond favorably to a Mediterranean-style diet, a high-fiber diet, or caloric restriction (Allison et al., 2021; Picó et al., 2019). Individuals' potential for dietary response could be classified using early attitudes of the relationship between epigenetic markers and specific dietary interventions, while assuming that heritable behavior, acquired epigenetic marks would, of each individual's current nutritional status, which includes long-term dietary on genomic state, establish a landscape in which variable epigenetic responses to interventions emerge (Ramos-Lopez, 2023). On more than linear predictions, integration of multiple-omics analyses indicates that collections of methylate marks, small RNA signatures, and chromatin accessibility signatures, each singling isolated individual markers could inform new classifications of responder, by not being able to account for tissue specify and context utility of each marker.

5.1 Use of epigenetic profiling to stratify responders vs. non-responders to dietary interventions

Personalized nutritional recommendations based on an individual's methylation signature conceptually shift away from traditional guidelines of nutrient provision. By conducting methylation interviews at loci associated with nutrient sensing, energy homeostasis, and inflammatory signaling pathways, clinicians and scientists alike can choose and structure macronutrient composition, micronutrient intake, and feeding frequency around the individual's methylation profile. For example, the methylation status of genes involved in one-carbon metabolism, or in oxidative stress responses may reveal increased preferences for food sources rich in folate, choline, or antioxidants, in order to maximize methyl donor availability, or tendency towards redox balance. Likewise, methylation indicators of insulin signaling or lipid-related processes such as lipogenesis may also be relevant to carbohydrate selection or fiber intakes. In addition, it must be acknowledged that methylation signatures are dynamic; they integrate both the individual's genetics and environmental exposures, thus suggesting that personalized plans can adapt and change iteratively over time as epigenetic readouts change with adherence to new dietary patterns and/or changes in lifestyle factors (Asif et al., 2025; Ramos-Lopez et al., 2022). In practice, implementation of personalized nutritional advice based on methylation signatures will need to consider systems of decision rules, plans of standardized panels of biomarkers, and also allow for transparency and clear communication to patients around the implications and limitations of their epigenetic data for planning nutrition and health.

5.2 Personalized nutritional plans based on individual methylation signatures

Tracking the effects of diet over time utilizing epigenetic tracking adds a new dynamic component to the study of nutrition. Tracking epigenomic changes over time may provide a trajectory of methylation changes in response to dietary interventions, flagging early signs of response or resistance before treatments become evident in clinical phenotypes. For instance, methylation changes within the promoter region of genes related to glucose metabolism or inflammatory pathways may precede measurable improvements in fasting glucose levels or inflammatory biomarkers, thus allowing for timely adjustments to dietary implications. Ongoing monitoring of epigenetic change will require consideration of potential confounding effects (age, sex, medications, changes to gut microbiome) and a robust data analytics pipeline to differentiate epigenetic change that occurs due to the intervention from natural variation or drift. Furthermore, epigenetic response would likely also depend on the tissue sampled, as easily accessible tissue surrogates (blood, saliva) may not effectively capture differences in metabolically relevant tissues (liver, adipose). Time-resolved epigenetic data does have the potential to transform outcome assessment in nutrition from a static endpoint measurement to a fluid systems-based approach and continuous feedback to optimize dietary changes (Zeb et al., 2023).

5.3 Time-course tracking of dietary efficacy through epigenetic monitoring

The ability to make real-time changes to nutritional approaches depends on the combination of fast epigenetic readouts, decision-support systems, and patient-facing technologies (Bhuiyan et al., 2025). Developments in minimally invasive sampling techniques (such as assays to detect circulating cell-free DNA methylation and saliva or buccal swabs to allow for methylation profiling) and high-throughput methylation assays now make the possibility of getting epigenetic updates in near-real-time a possibility. Coupling these fast epigenetic readouts with machine learning systems that include omics baseline data, dietary intake, physical activity and anthropometric changes, this system could suggest in-the-moment modifications to dietary prescriptions and recommend changes to macronutrient ratios, timing of meals, and micronutrient supplementation to get an epigenetic readout towards a desired health outcome. Further advances in ethical and pragmatic considerations (such as data privacy, interpretability of epigenetic changes, appealing to clinicians, etc.) will be essential for this vision to transition into the clinic and consumer applications. Similarly, user-centered design and education for clinicians will be part of the task of translating difficult epigenetic information into actionable recommendations for diet, without losing patient confidence or overwhelming patients.

5.4 Potential for real-time adaptation of nutritional strategies

The ability to modify nutritional strategies in real-time will depend on the convergence of rapid epigenetic readouts, decision-support systems and knowledge systems for patients. Novel minimally invasive sampling that captures epigenetic readouts (i.e., circulating cell-free DNA methylation assays, methylation profiling through saliva or buccal swab methods) and high-throughput processing provide the opportunity for near real-time epigenetic assessments (Birknerova et al., 2022). Coupling epigenetic assessments with machine learning algorithms that factor in baseline omics data, food intake, physical activity, and anthropometric data could then produce a therapeutic recommendations such as a diet plan modification (e.g., macronutrient ratios, meal timing, micronutrient recommendations, etc.) to shift the epigenetic response toward a targeted outcome based on intended health improvements. Ethics and practical implications that include things like data privacy, knowledge about impacted epigenetic modifications, clinical relevancy will need to be taken into consideration as we go from this vision of clinical applicability and applicability for consumers. At the same time, user-centered design and a clinician education approach will be worthwhile in modifying sequencing of epigenetic readouts to dietary modifications without overwhelming the patient and creating mistrust.

Recognizing both limitations and opportunities is a key component of working with epigenetic biomarkers in precision nutrition. DNA methylation records the history of exposure (i.e., stable), as well as subsequent gene regulation and risk for disease, or a loss of regulation. However, we should note DNA methylation is malleable and changes in response to the aging process, environmental exposure, and changes to the microbiome. It is therefore essential to put changes in DNA methylation into context based on considerations of tissue specificity, time from the exposure, and whether the changes can be functionally linked to metabolic outcomes. The rising popularity of combining multiple -omics data streams (epigenomics, transcriptomics, metabolomics, and microbiomics) can place dietary exposures into an even more nuanced framework to understand how dietary changes are mediating change in biological pathways as well as facilitate even stronger predictive models (Rakyan et al., 2011; Singh, 2023). While the consortiums that develop standardization across platforms, cohorts, and analytic pipelines is extensive and overwhelming, so too, is the need for large, diverse study populations that can increase generalizability of the findings. Additionally, social and ethical implications (e.g. access to epigenetic testing, avoiding deterministic messages about diet and health) must be taken into consideration to prevent misinformation or exacerbating health disparities. Collaborative consortia and data-sharing initiatives could offer reasonable solutions to expedite replication and translation endeavors while maintaining the rigor across studies.

6. INTEGRATION OF MULTI-OMICS AND ARTIFICIAL INTELLIGENCE

By integrating artificial intelligence (AI) with multi-omics data we can provide a robust framework to better understand the complex biology underlying host–microbiome–diet interactions. The integration of metagenomics (profiling microbial composition and potential functions), epigenomics (capturing regulatory responses of the host), transcriptomics (tracking gene expression dynamic), and metabolomics (number of small molecules produced by the host and microbiota) enables a transition from studying a single-omics link to a more holistic view of host–microbiome–diet interactions on a systems-level (Chetty & Blekhman, 2024; Hasin et al., 2017). The conceptual models proposed in this space aim to connect what happens with dietary input and migration of microbial communities, what metabolites from microbial metabolism can do to the epigenetic and transcriptional landscape on the host side, and how the host transcriptional and epigenetic landscape can re-program what occurs with metabolic pathways. The integration of this data layer will allow a more accurate description of causal chains and study how they connect into a robust biomarker and mechanistic pathway that underlies health and disease phenotypes. These models will have to consider specificity of tissue, temporal context, and inter-individual variability to minimize overgeneralizing and deceive the capture of context dependent effects.

6.1 Conceptual models for combining metagenomics, epigenomics, transcriptomics, and metabolomics

Metagenomics provides a foundation by describing microbial taxa and gene content and, thereby, allows for inferences of functional potential and community-averaged metabolic capabilities. Coupled with epigenomics, the models can connect microbial signals with host regulatory modifications, including DNA methylation and histone marks that may indicate exposure to microbial metabolites (e.g., short-chain fatty acids, bile acid derivatives). Transcriptomics produces dynamic readouts of the host gene expression response to both dietary and microbial cues, which typifies context-specific regulatory programs that static metagenomic profiles cannot reveal. Metabolomics rounds out the analyses by quantifying the end-products and intermediates generated in host and microbial metabolism, yielding direct readouts of biochemical perturbation (Q. Wang et al., 2019). Collectively, the various layers of data provide the opportunity to develop interaction networks and causal diagrams that describe how diet alters the microbiome and microbiome alters host biology via epigenetic and transcriptional means, which is in turn manifest in metabolic phenotypes. A major challenge in this work is to align data across scales and timeframes indicative of biological processes with embedded sampling time that is different among microbes and host tissues.

6.2 Machine learning approaches for biomarker discovery and predictive modeling

The extraction of meaningful patterns from high-dimensional, multi-omic datasets relies heavily on machine learning (ML) methods. Supervised learning methods, such as support vector machines, random forests, gradient boosting, elastic net, etc., have been utilized to find multi-omic signatures predicting health outcomes, dietary response, or risk of disease, etc (Babu & Snyder, 2023). However, due to the complexity and heterogeneity within multi-omic datasets, various sophisticated approaches are required, including deep learning models, graph-based approaches, and multi-view learning to handle multiple data modalities and missing data values. Cross-omics feature engineering, which essentially refers to changing features to make scales and biological meanings comparable across omics dataset types, is another very important step in model performance and interpretability. Examples of this have included multimodal variational autoencoders, integrative network analysis, and regularized regression on a combination of omic features which have promised to identify robust biomarkers and to assess non-linear relationships among host gene regulation, microbiome communities and metabolic outputs. The interpretability of multi-omic approaches is still an important consideration, thus the models that link model decisions back to known pathways and network modules would be preferred for outcome feasibility.

6.3 System-level modeling of host–microbiome–diet interactions

Modeling the system-level interactions among host, microbiome, and diet is often mechanistic and dynamic, using a model to assess how perturbations flow through biological networks and change over time. The methods can vary from mechanistic ordinary differential equation (ODE) models to flux balance analysis (FBA) of metabolic networks along with Bayesian networks or dynamic causal modeling that utilize prior knowledge and uncertainty (Gerber, 2014; Heinken & Thiele, 2015). Hybrid frameworks typically combine data-driven machine learning with mechanistic modules, allowing for both prediction and testing of scenarios (i.e., dietary interventions, antibiotic perturbations, or probiotic delivery), while also maintaining interpretable pathways. Time-series modeling is particularly useful in these types of scenarios to capture time-sensitivity and responses to dietary changes or shifts in the microbiome so that researchers can assess causality, as well as predict tipping points or resilient states (Gerber, 2014). The potential for using multi-omics in concert with system-level models shows the power of identifying dietary inputs and understanding the downstream effects on microbial metabolism, along with how microbial metabolites impact host epigenetic and transcriptional states, and how all of these inputs might lead to observable clinical outcomes. However, supporting computational discoveries and interpretations in biology will require cross-disciplinary validation across the sciences, including experimental perturbations in model organisms, or human studies of interventional or observational designs.

7. CHALLENGES, LIMITATIONS, AND FUTURE PROSPECTS

7.1 Biological and technical variability in epigenetic assays

Variability on both biologic and technical levels in measuring epigenetics remains a fundamental challenge to moving epigenetic biomarkers in a precision nutrition and clinical context. On a technical level, samples may differ (blood, tissue biopsies, or saliva), procedures may differ (some run as industry standards, while others as a research protocol), batch effects, and measuring technologies (array-based vs. sequencing-based methylation assays) introduce measurement noise that can camouflage true biological signals (Ross et al., 2022) . On a biological level, there are adequate biological sources of variability to introduce uncertainty into interpreting methylation or histone modifications potentially related to treatment. Cell type composition, circadian fluctuations, age, sex, medication use, and recent dietary exposures could all influence the biological state of the sample and, when possible, need to be incorporated into the analytic process. Strong analytic procedures (e.g., deconvolution of cell type mixtures, use of robust batch-correction, and replication using independent methods) are critical for differentiating meaningful epigenetic changes caused by an intervention from noise caused by technical processing or loss of susceptibility on the behalf of the sample.

7.2 Interindividual differences in microbiota composition and host epigenetic responsiveness

Variability in microbiota composition and differential host epigenetic response among individuals adds even more complexity to the picture. The human gut microbiome has high variability depending on a variety of factors such as genetics, early exposures, diet, history of antibiotic use and other environmental influences (Shock et al., 2021b). Thus, two individuals receiving the same diet may have different microbial ratifications and metabolite production, leading to different epigenetic and transcriptional responses in the host. Compounding this variability is tissue-specific epigenetic response; for example, a methylation event in peripheral blood may not reflect changes occurring in metabolically relevant tissues (i.e. adipose or liver). For this reason, variability makes it difficult to identify biomarkers that will be broadly generalizable, and points to the need for personalized biomarker panels that will include the baseline microbiome population, host genomics and epigenetic maps in the relevant tissues. Longitudinal sampling could assist in separating stable microbiome elements from responsive elements, but in the meantime, capturing variability from cross-sectional sampling in diverse populations will continue to be an important pursuit.

7.3 Standardization of biomarker validation pipelines

The standardization of biomarker validation pipelines is a fundamental impediment toward clinical translation. Valid biomarkers must undergo distinct discovery, validation, and replication stages, which include harmonized definitions of performance metrics (e.g., sensitivity, specificity, and predictive value) (Santaló & Berdasco, 2022). This requires standardization of the timing of sample collection (e.g., baseline and follow-up), assays platform, data normalization, and transparency regarding analytical methods employed. Furthermore, external responsibility in multi-center cohorts of heterogeneous strata (e.g., ethnicities and/or dietary habits) is needed to support robustness and generalizability. Finally, regulation and ethics must also consider the implications regarding data privacy, incidental findings, and access to epigenetic testing, among other considerations of fairness. Without standardized validation and reporting, the field can become vulnerable to fragmentation of evidence and slow clinical uptake, even for biomarkers that demonstrate evidence for valid use in challenging contexts.

7.4 Need for longitudinal, population-scale studies to support clinical translation

Longitudinal, population-scale studies are necessary to facilitate the clinical translation of multi-omic and epigenetic markers of diet. Repeated measures of a large, diverse cohort allow for the modeling of temporal trajectories to assess both test-retest reliability, and to investigate how age, life stage, and change in various environmental factors influence epigenetic signatures. Population-scale designs also facilitate the exploration of gene–diet–microbiome interactions across varying dietary patterns and cultural contexts, which amplifies the external validity of biomarkers. Pragmatic considerations include standardized dietary assessment measures, harmonized metadata schemas, and scalable sampling methods that minimize participant burden while maximizing richness of data (Zeevi et al., 2015). Funding biobanks, and platforms for data sharing, will be central to promoting the pace of replication, multi-cohort meta-analysis, and translation of research into personalized dietary guidance and public health recommendations.

Furthermore, practical translation requires considering health equity and health disparities and health access. Where epigenetic testing and multi-omics profiling are resource-intense, they may also widen health divides within and between populations who access healthcare differently. Implementation should happen with scalable and affordable workflow in mind, as well as community-engaged research to ensure predictive models accurately represent various dietary patterns and populations' health outcomes. Providing clinicians and nutritionists training on interpreting the outputs of omics work will be essential to avoid overinterpretation and deterministic messaging about diet and health. Being transparent about uncertainty, particularly on effect sizes, and communicating the inherently probabilistic approach of prediction to nurture trust in health contexts will be paramount.

8. CONCLUSION

Interdisciplinary cooperation will be pivotal for translating multi-omics knowledge into relevance in nutrition and health at the bedside. Moving from discovery to validation, and then from biomarkers to clinical use will necessitate shared goals, common methods, and a commitment to open-data sharing. When scientists and practitioners come together and leverage their individual expertise, we can translate complex dietary pathways which interrelate diet, the microbiome, host regulatory networks and metabolic outcomes into precise risk stratification, efficacious dietary recommendations and targeted interventions aimed to improve the health of all populations.

Developing a translational pipeline to take discoveries from bench to bedside will require strong regulatory and ethical foundations that promote transparency in how analytical methods and results are reported and communicated to clinicians and patients. Cross-disciplinary training models can develop a workforce who understands omics technologies, bioinformatics, nutritional science, and clinical care to ensure innovative approaches are rigorous and impactful in clinical practice. Involving patients and communities in the co-design of studies and translational tools will help align research interests with real-world needs and promote trust and uptake.

Adaptive nutrition platforms that combine microbiota and the host epigenome provide a novel vision for precision health. Adaptive nutrition platforms will integrate continuous or near-real-time data inputs, including dietary intake, physical activity, and longitudinal microbiome and epigenomic readouts of the host, into data-based personalized nutrition or dietary recommendations with the help of AI. This means users could receive recommendations and guidance when things change, concerning their microbiota composition, epigenetic state, and metabolic profiles, along with decision support for clinicians and dietitians. Practically, this could mean personalized dynamic meal plans, optimally dosing micronutrients, or time-restricted or aligned feeding strategies with targeted probiotic or prebiotic supplementation to help steer host–microbiome–diet relationships toward a more favorable trajectory for health.

9. REFERENCES

Agus, A., Planchais, J., & Sokol, H. (2018). Gut Microbiota Regulation of Tryptophan Metabolism in Health and Disease. *Cell Host & Microbe*, *23*(6), 716–724. DOI: 10.1016/j.chom.2018.05.003 PMID: 29902437

Al-Rashidi, H. E. (2022). Gut microbiota and immunity relevance in eubiosis and dysbiosis. *Saudi Journal of Biological Sciences*, *29*(3), 1628–1643. DOI: 10.1016/j.sjbs.2021.10.068 PMID: 35280528

Allison, J., Kaliszewska, A., Uceda, S., Reiriz, M., & Arias, N. (2021). Targeting DNA Methylation in the Adult Brain through Diet. *Nutrients*, *13*(11), 3979. DOI: 10.3390/nu13113979 PMID: 34836233

Asif, R., Liu, R., de Souza, R. J., Azab, S., Chong, M., Anand, S. S., & Deng, W. Q. (2025). A Scoping Review of Epigenetic Signatures of Diet and Diet-related Metabolites: Insights from Epigenome-Wide Association Studies and Their Implications for Cardiometabolic Health and Diseases. *The Yale Journal of Biology and Medicine*, *98*(2), 203–225. DOI: 10.59249/BDGN2070 PMID: 40589935

Babu, M., & Snyder, M. (2023). Multi-Omics Profiling for Health. *Molecular & Cellular Proteomics*, *22*(6), 100561. DOI: 10.1016/j.mcpro.2023.100561 PMID: 37119971

Bhuiyan, M. N. I., Saha, B. K., & Satter, M. A. (2025). Harnessing Artificial Intelligence and Precision Diets for Brain Health and Cognitive Resilience. *The Journal of Nutrition*, *155*(10), 3179–3190. Advance online publication. DOI: 10.1016/j.tjnut.2025.08.007 PMID: 40812476

Birknerova, N., Mancikova, V., Paul, E. D., Matyasovsky, J., Cekan, P., Palicka, V., & Parova, H. (2022). Circulating Cell-Free DNA-Based Methylation Pattern in Saliva for Early Diagnosis of Head and Neck Cancer. *Cancers (Basel)*, *14*(19), 4882. DOI: 10.3390/cancers14194882 PMID: 36230805

Bultman, S. J. (2014). Molecular pathways: Gene-environment interactions regulating dietary fiber induction of proliferation and apoptosis via butyrate for cancer prevention. *Clinical Cancer Research*, *20*(4), 799–803. DOI: 10.1158/1078-0432.CCR-13-2483 PMID: 24270685

Carson, C., & Lawson, H. A. (2018). Epigenetics of metabolic syndrome. *Physiological Genomics*, *50*(11), 947–955. DOI: 10.1152/physiolgenomics.00072.2018 PMID: 30240346

Chetty, A., & Blekhman, R. (2024). Multi-omic approaches for host-microbiome data integration. *Gut Microbes*, *16*(1), 2297860. DOI: 10.1080/19490976.2023.2297860 PMID: 38166610

Davie, J. R. (2003). Inhibition of Histone Deacetylase Activity by Butyrate. *The Journal of Nutrition*, *133*(7), 2485S–2493S. DOI: 10.1093/jn/133.7.2485S PMID: 12840228

De Filippo, C., Cavalieri, D., Di Paola, M., Ramazzotti, M., Poullet, J. B., Massart, S., Collini, S., Pieraccini, G., & Lionetti, P. (2010). Impact of diet in shaping gut microbiota revealed by a comparative study in children from Europe and rural Africa. *Proceedings of the National Academy of Sciences of the United States of America*, *107*(33), 14691–14696. DOI: 10.1073/pnas.1005963107 PMID: 20679230

Deiuliis, J. A. (2016). MicroRNAs as regulators of metabolic disease: Pathophysiologic significance and emerging role as biomarkers and therapeutics. *International Journal of Obesity*, *40*(1), 88–101. DOI: 10.1038/ijo.2015.170 PMID: 26311337

Deiuliis, J. A. (2016). MicroRNAs as regulators of metabolic disease: Pathophysiologic significance and emerging role as biomarkers and therapeutics. *International Journal of Obesity*, *40*(1), 88–101. DOI: 10.1038/ijo.2015.170 PMID: 26311337

Engevik, M. A., Morra, C. N., Röth, D., Engevik, K., Spinler, J. K., Devaraj, S., Crawford, S. E., Estes, M. K., Kalkum, M., & Versalovic, J. (2019). Microbial Metabolic Capacity for Intestinal Folate Production and Modulation of Host Folate Receptors. *Frontiers in Microbiology*, *10*, 2305. DOI: 10.3389/fmicb.2019.02305 PMID: 31649646

Frioux, C., Ansorge, R., Özkurt, E., Nedjad, C. G., Fritscher, J., Quince, C., Waszak, S. M., & Hildebrand, F. (2023). Enterosignatures define common bacterial guilds in the human gut microbiome. *Cell Host & Microbe*, *31*(7), 1111–1125.e6. DOI: 10.1016/j.chom.2023.05.024 PMID: 37339626

Gerber, G. K. (2014). The dynamic microbiome. *FEBS Letters*, *588*(22), 4131–4139. DOI: 10.1016/j.febslet.2014.02.037 PMID: 24583074

Grandi, F. C., Modi, H., Kampman, L., & Corces, M. R. (2022). Chromatin accessibility profiling by ATAC-seq. *Nature Protocols*, *17*(6), 1518–1552. DOI: 10.1038/s41596-022-00692-9 PMID: 35478247

Guanzon, D., Ross, J. P., Ma, C., Berry, O., & Liew, Y. J. (2024). Comparing methylation levels assayed in GC-rich regions with current and emerging methods. *BMC Genomics*, *25*(1), 741. DOI: 10.1186/s12864-024-10605-7 PMID: 39080541

Hasin, Y., Seldin, M., & Lusis, A. (2017). Multi-omics approaches to disease. *Genome Biology, 18*(1), 83. DOI: 10.1186/s13059-017-1215-1 PMID: 28476144

Heinken, A., & Thiele, I. (2015). Systems biology of host–microbe metabolomics. *Wiley Interdisciplinary Reviews. Systems Biology and Medicine, 7*(4), 195–219. DOI: 10.1002/wsbm.1301 PMID: 25929487

Heterogeneity in VEGFR3 levels drives lymphatic vessel hyperplasia through cell-autonomous and non-cell-autonomous mechanisms | Nature Communications. (n.d.). Retrieved October 18, 2025, from https://www.nature.com/articles/s41467-018-03692-0

Hullar, M. A. J., & Fu, B. C. (2014). Diet, the Gut Microbiome, and Epigenetics. *Cancer Journal (Sudbury, Mass.), 20*(3), 170–175. DOI: 10.1097/PPO.0000000000000053 PMID: 24855003

Influences of diet and the gut microbiome on epigenetic modulation in cancer and other diseases | Clinical Epigenetics. (n.d.). Retrieved October 18, 2025, from https://link.springer.com/article/10.1186/s13148-015-0144-7

Kim, B., Song, A., Son, A., & Shin, Y. (2024). Gut microbiota and epigenetic choreography: Implications for human health. *Revista de Medicina (São Paulo), 103*(29), e39051. DOI: 10.1097/MD.0000000000039051 PMID: 39029010

Krautkramer, K. A., Dhillon, R. S., Denu, J. M., & Carey, H. V. (2017). Metabolic programming of the epigenome: Host and gut microbial metabolite interactions with host chromatin. *Translational Research; the Journal of Laboratory and Clinical Medicine, 189*, 30–50. DOI: 10.1016/j.trsl.2017.08.005 PMID: 28919341

Krautkramer, K. A., Kreznar, J. H., Romano, K. A., Vivas, E. I., Barrett-Wilt, G. A., Rabaglia, M. E., Keller, M. P., Attie, A. D., Rey, F. E., & Denu, J. M. (2016). Diet-Microbiota Interactions Mediate Global Epigenetic Programming in Multiple Host Tissues. *Molecular Cell, 64*(5), 982–992. DOI: 10.1016/j.molcel.2016.10.025 PMID: 27889451

Li, D., Li, Y., Yang, S., Lu, J., Jin, X., & Wu, M. (2022). Diet-gut microbiota-epigenetics in metabolic diseases: From mechanisms to therapeutics. *Biomedicine and Pharmacotherapy, 153*, 113290. DOI: 10.1016/j.biopha.2022.113290 PMID: 35724509

Liu, H. (2024). Integrative Approaches in Computational Genomics: Combining Omics Data to Study Gene Evolution. Computational Molecular Biology, 14(0). https://bioscipublisher.com/index.php/cmb/article/view/3990

Lopomo, A., Burgio, E., & Migliore, L. (2016). Chapter Six—Epigenetics of Obesity. In Tao, Y.-X. (Ed.), *Progress in Molecular Biology and Translational Science* (Vol. 140, pp. 151–184). Academic Press., DOI: 10.1016/bs.pmbts.2016.02.002

Lopomo, A., Burgio, E., & Migliore, L. (2016). Chapter Six—Epigenetics of Obesity. In Tao, Y.-X. (Ed.), *Progress in Molecular Biology and Translational Science* (Vol. 140, pp. 151–184). Academic Press., DOI: 10.1016/bs.pmbts.2016.02.002

Mahmoud, A. M. (2022). An Overview of Epigenetics in Obesity: The Role of Lifestyle and Therapeutic Interventions. *International Journal of Molecular Sciences*, *23*(3), 1341. DOI: 10.3390/ijms23031341 PMID: 35163268

Mahmoud, A. M. (2022). An Overview of Epigenetics in Obesity: The Role of Lifestyle and Therapeutic Interventions. *International Journal of Molecular Sciences*, *23*(3), 1341. DOI: 10.3390/ijms23031341 PMID: 35163268

Meissner, A., Gnirke, A., Bell, G. W., Ramsahoye, B., Lander, E. S., & Jaenisch, R. (2005). Reduced representation bisulfite sequencing for comparative high-resolution DNA methylation analysis. *Nucleic Acids Research*, *33*(18), 5868–5877. DOI: 10.1093/nar/gki901 PMID: 16224102

Microbiota in health and diseases | Signal Transduction and Targeted Therapy. (n.d.-a). Retrieved October 18, 2025, from https://www.nature.com/articles/s41392-022-00974-4

Microbiota in health and diseases | Signal Transduction and Targeted Therapy. (n.d.-b). Retrieved October 18, 2025, from https://www.nature.com/articles/s41392-022-00974-4

MicroRNAs as regulators of metabolic disease: Pathophysiologic significance and emerging role as biomarkers and therapeutics | International Journal of Obesity. (n.d.). Retrieved October 18, 2025, from https://www.nature.com/articles/ijo2015170

Modulation of the Gut Microbiota by Nutrition and Its Relationship to Epigenetics. (n.d.). Retrieved October 18, 2025, from https://www.mdpi.com/1422-0067/25/2/1228

Muhammad, A. Y., Amonov, M., Baig, A. A., & Alvi, F. J. (2024). Gut Microbiome: An Intersection between Human Genome, Diet, and Epigenetics. *Advanced Gut & Microbiome Research*, *2024*(1), 6707728. DOI: 10.1155/2024/6707728

Nakato, R., & Sakata, T. (2021). Methods for ChIP-seq analysis: A practical workflow and advanced applications. *Methods (San Diego, Calif.)*, *187*, 44–53. DOI: 10.1016/j.ymeth.2020.03.005 PMID: 32240773

Picó, C., Serra, F., Rodríguez, A. M., Keijer, J., & Palou, A. (2019). Biomarkers of Nutrition and Health: New Tools for New Approaches. *Nutrients, 11*(5), 1092. DOI: 10.3390/nu11051092 PMID: 31100942

Rakyan, V. K., Down, T. A., Balding, D. J., & Beck, S. (2011). Epigenome-wide association studies for common human diseases. *Nature Reviews. Genetics, 12*(8), 529–541. DOI: 10.1038/nrg3000 PMID: 21747404

Ramos-Lopez, O. (2023). Epigenetic Biomarkers of Metabolic Responses to Lifestyle Interventions. *Nutrients, 15*(19), 4251. DOI: 10.3390/nu15194251 PMID: 37836535

Ramos-Lopez, O., Martinez, J. A., & Milagro, F. I. (2022). Holistic Integration of Omics Tools for Precision Nutrition in Health and Disease. *Nutrients, 14*(19), 4074. DOI: 10.3390/nu14194074 PMID: 36235725

Ross, J. P., van Dijk, S., Phang, M., Skilton, M. R., Molloy, P. L., & Oytam, Y. (2022). Batch-effect detection, correction and characterisation in Illumina HumanMethylation450 and MethylationEPIC BeadChip array data. *Clinical Epigenetics, 14*(1), 58. DOI: 10.1186/s13148-022-01277-9 PMID: 35488315

Santaló, J., & Berdasco, M. (2022). Ethical implications of epigenetics in the era of personalized medicine. *Clinical Epigenetics, 14*(1), 44. DOI: 10.1186/s13148-022-01263-1 PMID: 35337378

Seo, S.-K., & Kwon, B. (2023). Immune regulation through tryptophan metabolism. *Experimental & Molecular Medicine, 55*(7), 1371–1379. DOI: 10.1038/s12276-023-01028-7 PMID: 37394584

Shock, T., Badang, L., Ferguson, B., & Martinez-Guryn, K. (2021a). The interplay between diet, gut microbes, and host epigenetics in health and disease. *The Journal of Nutritional Biochemistry, 95*, 108631. DOI: 10.1016/j.jnutbio.2021.108631 PMID: 33789148

Shock, T., Badang, L., Ferguson, B., & Martinez-Guryn, K. (2021b). The interplay between diet, gut microbes, and host epigenetics in health and disease. *The Journal of Nutritional Biochemistry, 95*, 108631. DOI: 10.1016/j.jnutbio.2021.108631 PMID: 33789148

Singh, V. (2023). Current challenges and future implications of exploiting the omics data into nutrigenetics and nutrigenomics for personalized diagnosis and nutrition-based care. *Nutrition (Burbank, Los Angeles County, Calif.), 110*, 112002. DOI: 10.1016/j.nut.2023.112002 PMID: 36940623

Skinner, M. K. (2024). Epigenetic biomarkers for disease susceptibility and preventative medicine. *Cell Metabolism, 36*(2), 263–277. DOI: 10.1016/j.cmet.2023.11.015 PMID: 38176413

Subhan, F. B., & Chan, C. B. (2016). Review of Dietary Practices of the 21st Century: Facts and Fallacies. *Canadian Journal of Diabetes, 40*(4), 348–354. DOI: 10.1016/j.jcjd.2016.05.005 PMID: 27497150

Subhan, F. B., & Chan, C. B. (2016). Review of Dietary Practices of the 21st Century: Facts and Fallacies. *Canadian Journal of Diabetes, 40*(4), 348–354. DOI: 10.1016/j.jcjd.2016.05.005 PMID: 27497150

Synergistic Interplay of Diet, Gut Microbiota, and Insulin Resistance: Unraveling the Molecular Nexus—Gopal—2024—Molecular Nutrition & Food Research—Wiley Online Library. (n.d.). Retrieved October 18, 2025, from https://onlinelibrary.wiley.com/doi/abs/10.1002/mnfr.202400677

The interplay between diet and the gut microbiome: Implications for health and disease | Nature Reviews Microbiology. (n.d.). Retrieved October 18, 2025, from https://www.nature.com/articles/s41579-024-01068-4

The role of the gut microbiota in the onset and progression of heart failure: Insights into epigenetic mechanisms and aging | Clinical Epigenetics. (n.d.). Retrieved October 18, 2025, from https://link.springer.com/article/10.1186/s13148-024-01786-9

Tiffon, C. (2018). The Impact of Nutrition and Environmental Epigenetics on Human Health and Disease. *International Journal of Molecular Sciences, 19*(11), 3425. DOI: 10.3390/ijms19113425 PMID: 30388784

Tiffon, C. (2018). The Impact of Nutrition and Environmental Epigenetics on Human Health and Disease. *International Journal of Molecular Sciences, 19*(11), 3425. DOI: 10.3390/ijms19113425 PMID: 30388784

Turnbaugh, P. J., & Gordon, J. I. (2009). The core gut microbiome, energy balance and obesity. *The Journal of Physiology, 587*(17), 4153–4158. DOI: 10.1113/jphysiol.2009.174136 PMID: 19491241

Turnbaugh, P. J., & Gordon, J. I. (2009). The core gut microbiome, energy balance and obesity. *The Journal of Physiology, 587*(17), 4153–4158. DOI: 10.1113/jphysiol.2009.174136 PMID: 19491241

Wang, L., Zhang, W., Wu, X., Liang, X., Cao, L., Zhai, J., Yang, Y., Chen, Q., Liu, H., Zhang, J., Ding, Y., Zhu, F., & Tang, J. (2022). MIAOME: Human microbiome affect the host epigenome. *Computational and Structural Biotechnology Journal, 20*, 2455–2463. DOI: 10.1016/j.csbj.2022.05.024 PMID: 35664224

Wang, Q., Wang, K., Wu, W., Giannoulatou, E., Ho, J. W. K., & Li, L. (2019). Host and microbiome multi-omics integration: Applications and methodologies. *Biophysical Reviews*, *11*(1), 55–65. DOI: 10.1007/s12551-018-0491-7 PMID: 30627872

Yu, Y., Zhang, J., Wang, J., & Sun, B. (2021). MicroRNAs: The novel mediators for nutrient-modulating biological functions. *Trends in Food Science & Technology*, *114*, 167–175. DOI: 10.1016/j.tifs.2021.05.028

Yu, Y., Zhang, J., Wang, J., & Sun, B. (2021). MicroRNAs: The novel mediators for nutrient-modulating biological functions. *Trends in Food Science & Technology*, *114*, 167–175. DOI: 10.1016/j.tifs.2021.05.028

Zeb, F., Osaili, T., Obaid, R. S., Naja, F., Radwan, H., Cheikh Ismail, L., Hasan, H., Hashim, M., Alam, I., Sehar, B., & Faris, M. E. (2023). Gut Microbiota and Time-Restricted Feeding/Eating: A Targeted Biomarker and Approach in Precision Nutrition. *Nutrients*, *15*(2), 259. DOI: 10.3390/nu15020259 PMID: 36678130

Zeevi, D., Korem, T., Zmora, N., Israeli, D., Rothschild, D., Weinberger, A., Ben-Yacov, O., Lador, D., Avnit-Sagi, T., Lotan-Pompan, M., Suez, J., Mahdi, J. A., Matot, E., Malka, G., Kosower, N., Rein, M., Zilberman-Schapira, G., Dohnalová, L., Pevsner-Fischer, M., & Segal, E. (2015). Personalized Nutrition by Prediction of Glycemic Responses. *Cell*, *163*(5), 1079–1094. DOI: 10.1016/j.cell.2015.11.001 PMID: 26590418

Zempleni, J., Chew, Y. C., Hassan, Y. I., & Wijeratne, S. S. (2008). Epigenetic regulation of chromatin structure and gene function by biotin. *Nutrition Reviews*, *66*(Suppl 1), S46–S48. DOI: 10.1111/j.1753-4887.2008.00073.x PMID: 18673490

Zhang, P. (2022). Influence of Foods and Nutrition on the Gut Microbiome and Implications for Intestinal Health. *International Journal of Molecular Sciences*, *23*(17), 9588. DOI: 10.3390/ijms23179588 PMID: 36076980

Chapter 5
Feeding Your Microbes: Why What You Eat Matters

Richa Sharma
https://orcid.org/0009-0006-1174-2888
AAFT University of Media and Arts, India

Pankaj Singh Chandel
https://orcid.org/0000-0002-4135-8194
AAFT University of Media and Arts, India

ABSTRACT

The gut microbiome plays a pivotal role in shaping human metabolic health through complex interactions with diet. Dietary components influence microbial composition and activity, which in turn regulate nutrient metabolism and the production of microbial metabolites such as short-chain fatty acids, bile acid derivatives, and indoles. These metabolites act as signaling molecules affecting insulin sensitivity, inflammation, energy balance, and gut integrity. Inter-individual differences in gut microbiota partly explain variable responses to identical diets, highlighting the limitations of generalized dietary recommendations. This has led to the emergence of personalized and precision nutrition approaches that integrate microbiome profiles with dietary patterns to optimize metabolic outcomes. By linking diet–microbe interactions to metabolic health, nutrition science is shifting toward targeted, microbiome-informed strategies for disease prevention and health promotion.

1. INTRODUCTION: DIET AS A PRIMARY MODULATOR OF THE GUT MICROBIOME

The human gastrointestinal tract harbors a dense and diverse population of microorganisms collectively known as the gut microbiome. These microbial communities

DOI: 10.4018/979-8-3373-4382-2.ch005

coexist in a dynamic relationship with the host and play a central role in digestion, metabolism, immune regulation, and overall physiological balance. Over the past two decades, advances in molecular sequencing technologies have revealed that the gut microbiome is not a static entity; rather, it is highly responsive to environmental influences, with diet emerging as one of the most powerful and modifiable determinants of microbial composition and function.

Diet provides the primary substrates that fuel microbial growth and metabolic activity in the gut. While host enzymes digest a portion of consumed nutrients, a significant fraction particularly dietary fibers, resistant starches, and certain polyphenols escapes digestion and reaches the colon. Here, these compounds serve as energy sources for gut microbes, shaping their abundance, diversity, and metabolic outputs. Consequently, habitual dietary patterns exert long-term effects on microbial ecosystems, influencing health outcomes ranging from metabolic regulation to immune resilience (Singh et al., 2017).

Emerging evidence suggests that shifts in dietary intake can rapidly alter microbial composition, sometimes within days. Diets rich in plant-based foods tend to support a diverse microbiome dominated by beneficial fermentative bacteria, whereas diets high in saturated fats, refined carbohydrates, and low fiber are often associated with reduced microbial diversity and dysbiosis. Such imbalances have been linked to chronic conditions including obesity, type 2 diabetes, inflammatory bowel disease, and cardiovascular disorders (Valdes et al., 2018). These observations highlight the pivotal role of diet not only in maintaining microbial homeostasis but also in disease prevention and management.

Understanding diet as a primary modulator of the gut microbiome has transformed nutritional science. Rather than viewing nutrients solely through the lens of host requirements, modern nutrition increasingly recognizes the microbiome as an intermediary that modifies nutrient bioavailability, produces bioactive metabolites, and communicates with host systems. This perspective has laid the foundation for personalized nutrition strategies that consider individual microbial profiles to optimize health outcomes.

1.1 Overview of the Human Gut Microbiome

The human gut microbiome comprises trillions of microorganisms, including bacteria, archaea, viruses, and fungi, residing predominantly in the large intestine. Among these, bacteria represent the most extensively studied group and are mainly distributed across a limited number of dominant phyla, including *Firmicutes*, *Bacteroidetes*, *Actinobacteria*, and *Proteobacteria*. Although these phyla are common to most individuals, the relative abundance of microbial species varies widely, creating a unique microbial fingerprint for each person (Human Microbiome Project Consortium, 2012).

Microbial colonization begins at birth and evolves throughout early life, influenced by factors such as mode of delivery, infant feeding practices, antibiotic exposure, and early dietary patterns. By adulthood, the gut microbiome achieves relative stability, yet it remains adaptable to lifestyle and dietary changes. This adaptability allows the microbiome to respond to shifts in food availability, cultural dietary practices, and health status, reinforcing its role as an interface between external inputs and internal physiology.

Functionally, the gut microbiome contributes to host health through multiple mechanisms. It assists in the breakdown of complex carbohydrates, synthesizes essential vitamins such as vitamin K and certain B vitamins, and produces short-chain fatty acids (SCFAs) like acetate, propionate, and butyrate. These metabolites serve as energy sources for intestinal cells, regulate inflammatory pathways, and influence glucose and lipid metabolism. Additionally, the microbiome plays a critical role in educating and modulating the immune system, helping the host distinguish between harmless antigens and potential pathogens (Koh et al., 2016).

Collectively, the human gut microbiome represents a complex and metabolically active organ that extends host capabilities beyond human genetics alone. Its close interaction with dietary components positions nutrition as a key regulator of microbial health, reinforcing the concept that what we eat profoundly shapes not only our own physiology but also the microbial communities that support it.

1.2 Historical Perspective: From Digestion to Microbial Symbiosis

For much of scientific history, the human digestive system was viewed primarily as a mechanical and chemical apparatus responsible for breaking down food into absorbable nutrients. Early physiological studies focused on gastric acids, digestive enzymes, and intestinal motility, with microorganisms largely regarded as incidental passengers or, in some cases, harmful contaminants. The presence of bacteria in the gut was acknowledged, but their role was often underestimated and confined to fermentation of indigestible residues (Cummings & Macfarlane, 1997).

The late nineteenth and early twentieth centuries marked the first shift in this perspective, largely driven by the pioneering work of scientists such as Élie Metchnikoff. Metchnikoff proposed that certain intestinal bacteria could exert health-promoting effects and suggested that consumption of fermented foods might contribute to longevity. Although these ideas were initially met with skepticism, they laid the foundation for the concept of beneficial microbes and host–microbe cooperation (Metchnikoff, 1907).

A major transformation occurred with the advent of molecular biology and high-throughput sequencing technologies in the late twentieth and early twenty-first centuries. Culture-independent techniques revealed that the gut harbors an extraordinarily complex and diverse microbial ecosystem, far exceeding earlier estimates based on culture methods. Large-scale initiatives such as the Human Microbiome Project demonstrated that gut microbes are deeply integrated into host physiology, influencing metabolism, immune development, and even gene expression (Human Microbiome Project Consortium, 2012).

This growing body of evidence reframed the gut microbiota not as passive inhabitants, but as active symbiotic partners essential for human health. The modern understanding emphasizes mutualism, wherein the host provides nutrients and a stable environment, while microbes contribute metabolic functions that humans cannot perform independently. This historical shift from digestion-centered views to microbial symbiosis has fundamentally altered nutritional science and medical research, positioning the gut microbiome as a key determinant of health and disease.

1.3 Why "Feeding Microbes" Matters for Human Health

The concept of "feeding microbes" reflects a paradigm shift in nutrition, recognizing that dietary choices influence health not only by nourishing human cells but also by shaping microbial communities that regulate critical physiological processes. Gut microbes rely heavily on dietary substrates, particularly non-digestible carbohydrates, fibers, and phytochemicals, to sustain their growth and metabolic activity. When these substrates are abundant, beneficial microbes thrive and produce metabolites that support host health.

One of the most significant outcomes of microbial metabolism is the production of short-chain fatty acids (SCFAs), including acetate, propionate, and butyrate. These compounds play a central role in maintaining intestinal barrier integrity, modulating immune responses, reducing inflammation, and regulating glucose and lipid metabolism. Butyrate, in particular, serves as the primary energy source for colonocytes and has been shown to exert protective effects against colorectal cancer and inflammatory bowel diseases (Koh et al., 2016).

Conversely, diets low in fiber and rich in ultra-processed foods can deprive beneficial microbes of essential substrates, leading to reduced microbial diversity and functional capacity. Such dietary patterns have been associated with dysbiosis, increased intestinal permeability, and chronic low-grade inflammation hallmarks of many non-communicable diseases, including obesity, type 2 diabetes, cardiovascular disease, and certain autoimmune disorders (Sonnenburg & Sonnenburg, 2019).

Feeding microbes appropriately also has implications beyond physical health. Emerging research links gut microbial activity to brain function through the gut–

brain axis, influencing mood, stress response, and cognitive processes. Microbial metabolites and signaling molecules can interact with neural, endocrine, and immune pathways, suggesting that diet-mediated microbial modulation may play a role in mental well-being (Cryan et al., 2019). Thus, the act of "feeding microbes" represents a foundational strategy for promoting holistic health across the lifespan.

1.4 Scope and Objectives of the Chapter

This chapter aims to provide a comprehensive understanding of the relationship between diet and the gut microbiome, with a specific focus on how dietary components influence microbial composition, function, and metabolic outputs. Recognizing the microbiome as a critical mediator between food intake and health outcomes, the chapter integrates concepts from nutrition science, microbiology, and physiology to present an interdisciplinary perspective.

The scope of the chapter includes an examination of macronutrients, micronutrients, and bioactive food compounds such as dietary fibers and phytochemicals and their role in shaping microbial ecosystems. It also explores microbial metabolites and their systemic effects on host metabolism, immunity, and disease risk. Attention is given to both beneficial and adverse dietary patterns, highlighting how modern dietary transitions impact microbial diversity and health resilience.

The specific objectives of this chapter are to:

1. Explain the fundamental structure and functions of the human gut microbiome in relation to diet.
2. Analyze how different dietary components selectively nourish or suppress specific microbial populations.
3. Describe key microbial metabolites and their physiological significance for human health.
4. Highlight the relevance of microbiome-focused nutrition in disease prevention and personalized dietary strategies.

By addressing these objectives, the chapter seeks to equip readers with a clear conceptual framework for understanding why diet-driven microbial modulation is central to contemporary nutrition and personalized health approaches.

2. COMPOSITION AND FUNCTIONAL DYNAMICS OF THE GUT MICROBIOME

The gut microbiome represents a complex and dynamic ecological system composed of diverse microbial populations that interact continuously with the host and with one another. Beyond simple taxonomic composition, the functional capacity of the microbiome its ability to metabolize nutrients, produce bioactive compounds, and communicate with host systems defines its contribution to human health. These functions are not fixed; they evolve across the life span and respond to dietary patterns, environmental exposures, and physiological changes. Understanding both the composition and functional dynamics of the gut microbiome is therefore essential for interpreting its role in health and disease.

2.1 Major Microbial Phyla and Their Roles

Despite the immense diversity of microorganisms inhabiting the human gut, the majority of bacterial species belong to a relatively small number of dominant phyla. Among these, *Firmicutes* and *Bacteroidetes* account for nearly 90% of the adult gut microbiome, forming the functional backbone of microbial metabolism. These phyla perform essential roles in nutrient breakdown, energy harvest, immune modulation, and maintenance of intestinal integrity, thereby exerting a profound influence on host physiology (Human Microbiome Project Consortium, 2012).

The phylum *Firmicutes* includes a wide range of gram-positive bacteria such as *Lactobacillus*, *Clostridium*, *Ruminococcus*, and *Faecalibacterium*. Many members of this group are efficient fermenters of dietary fibers and resistant starches, producing short-chain fatty acids (SCFAs), particularly butyrate. Butyrate plays a critical role in maintaining colonic epithelial health by serving as the primary energy source for colonocytes, enhancing tight junction integrity, and exerting anti-inflammatory effects. Reduced abundance of butyrate-producing *Firmicutes* has been linked to inflammatory bowel disease and metabolic disorders (Louis & Flint, 2017).

Bacteroidetes are primarily involved in the degradation of complex carbohydrates, including plant-derived polysaccharides and host-derived glycans. Their extensive enzymatic repertoire allows them to adapt to varying dietary patterns, particularly diets rich in plant foods. Through polysaccharide fermentation, *Bacteroidetes* contribute to energy availability and SCFA production, especially acetate and propionate, which influence lipid metabolism and glucose homeostasis (Johnson et al., 2017).

Other phyla, although less abundant, play equally important roles. *Actinobacteria*, particularly the genus *Bifidobacterium*, are prominent in early life and are associated with immune maturation, vitamin synthesis, and protection against pathogenic bacteria. These microbes are known to metabolize oligosaccharides efficiently and contribute to gut barrier function. In contrast, *Proteobacteria* include a diverse group of gram-negative bacteria, some of which are opportunistic pathogens. An increased abundance of *Proteobacteria* is often considered a marker of microbial imbalance and intestinal inflammation (Shin et al., 2015).

Together, these microbial phyla operate as a coordinated metabolic network. Their balance and functional interactions, rather than the dominance of any single group, determine the overall health-promoting potential of the gut microbiome.

2.2 Microbial Diversity, Stability, and Resilience

Microbial diversity is a defining characteristic of a healthy gut microbiome and reflects the richness and evenness of microbial species present within the intestinal ecosystem. High diversity is associated with enhanced metabolic flexibility, improved immune regulation, and greater resistance to pathogenic invasion. From an ecological perspective, diversity allows multiple microbial species to perform overlapping functions, ensuring that essential metabolic processes are maintained even when environmental conditions fluctuate (Le Chatelier et al., 2013).

Stability refers to the ability of the gut microbiome to maintain a relatively consistent structure over time under normal physiological conditions. In healthy adults, the microbiome demonstrates a stable core composition, despite daily variations in food intake. This stability supports predictable metabolic outputs, such as SCFA production and vitamin synthesis, which are crucial for maintaining intestinal and systemic homeostasis. However, stability does not imply rigidity; a healthy microbiome retains the capacity to adapt to short-term dietary changes without losing functional integrity.

Resilience describes the ability of the gut microbiome to recover following disturbances, such as antibiotic exposure, acute illness, infection, or drastic dietary shifts. A resilient microbiome can return to its baseline composition and function after disruption, thereby limiting long-term adverse effects on host health. Reduced resilience may result in persistent dysbiosis, characterized by loss of beneficial microbes and overgrowth of opportunistic species, increasing the risk of chronic inflammation and metabolic dysfunction (Sommer et al., 2017).

Diet plays a central role in shaping microbial diversity and resilience. Diets rich in a wide variety of plant-based foods provide diverse fermentable substrates that support multiple microbial niches. In contrast, low-fiber, high-fat, and ultra-processed diets tend to reduce microbial diversity and weaken resilience, making the ecosystem more vulnerable to perturbations. Repeated disturbances in such contexts may lead to long-term loss of key microbial functions.

Importantly, diversity alone does not guarantee health. Functional diversity the range of metabolic activities performed by the microbiome is equally important.

Two individuals may harbor distinct microbial species yet exhibit similar metabolic outputs if functional redundancy is preserved. Therefore, a resilient and functionally diverse microbiome is better equipped to support host health across changing environmental and physiological conditions.

2.3 Development of the Gut Microbiome Across the Life Span

The human gut microbiome develops dynamically across the life span, beginning at birth and continuing to evolve in response to physiological, dietary, and environmental influences. Early microbial colonization represents a critical window of development, as initial microbial exposures play a foundational role in shaping immune function and metabolic programming. Mode of delivery significantly influences early colonization patterns; vaginally delivered infants are exposed to maternal vaginal and intestinal microbes, whereas cesarean-delivered infants often exhibit delayed microbial diversification (Penders et al., 2006).

Infant feeding practices further modulate microbial development. Breast milk contains human milk oligosaccharides (HMOs), which selectively nourish beneficial bacteria such as *Bifidobacterium*. These microbes contribute to immune maturation, pathogen resistance, and gut barrier development. Formula-fed infants typically show a more diverse but less *Bifidobacterium*-dominant microbiome, reflecting differences in substrate availability.

During childhood, microbial diversity increases steadily as dietary patterns expand and environmental exposures accumulate. The introduction of solid foods, particularly fiber-rich plant foods, supports the growth of fermentative bacteria and enhances functional complexity. By adolescence and early adulthood, the gut microbiome reaches a relatively stable state, although it remains responsive to long-term dietary habits and lifestyle factors.

In older adulthood, the gut microbiome often undergoes notable changes. Aging is associated with reduced microbial diversity, decreased abundance of beneficial SCFA-producing bacteria, and increased representation of pro-inflammatory taxa. These changes may be driven by altered dietary intake, reduced physical activity, medication use, and age-related immune decline. Such microbial shifts have been linked to frailty, inflammation, and metabolic dysfunction in the elderly population (O'Toole & Jeffery, 2015).

Understanding life-stage-specific microbial dynamics highlights the importance of targeted nutritional strategies. Supporting microbial development in early life, maintaining diversity in adulthood, and preserving resilience in older age may collectively contribute to long-term health and disease prevention.

2.4 Factors Influencing Microbial Composition (Diet, Age, Lifestyle, Medications)

Multiple interrelated factors shape the composition and function of the gut microbiome, with diet representing the most influential and modifiable determinant. Long-term dietary patterns determine the availability of substrates for microbial fermentation, thereby selectively promoting the growth of specific microbial populations. Diets rich in dietary fiber, whole grains, fruits, vegetables, and legumes support beneficial fermentative bacteria and SCFA production. In contrast, high-fat, high-sugar, and low-fiber diets are associated with reduced microbial diversity and increased abundance of inflammatory taxa (Singh et al., 2017).

Age-related physiological changes also influence microbial composition. Digestive efficiency, immune function, and hormonal regulation evolve across the life span, altering the intestinal environment in which microbes reside. These changes can modify microbial interactions and metabolic outputs, contributing to age-specific health outcomes.

Lifestyle factors such as physical activity, sleep quality, stress, and smoking further modulate the gut microbiome. Regular physical activity has been associated with increased microbial diversity and enhanced SCFA production, while chronic stress may disrupt microbial balance through neuroendocrine and immune pathways. Sleep disturbances and circadian rhythm disruption have also been linked to altered microbial composition.

Medications exert some of the most profound effects on gut microbial communities. Antibiotics, while essential for treating infections, can cause substantial and sometimes long-lasting reductions in microbial diversity. Non-antibiotic drugs, including proton pump inhibitors, antidiabetic agents, and non-steroidal anti-inflammatory drugs, have also been shown to alter microbial growth and metabolism (Maier et al., 2018).

These factors rarely act in isolation; rather, they interact continuously to shape microbial ecosystems. Recognizing this complexity underscores the need for integrative approaches that combine dietary strategies with lifestyle modification to support microbial health and resilience.

3. DIET–MICROBIOME INTERACTIONS: A BIDIRECTIONAL RELATIONSHIP

Diet and the gut microbiome exist in a dynamic, bidirectional relationship in which food choices shape microbial communities, and microbial metabolism, in turn, modifies the nutritional and physiological effects of the diet. Unlike traditional nutrition models that consider nutrients acting directly on host tissues, the microbiome-centered perspective recognizes gut microbes as active intermediaries. Dietary components provide substrates that determine microbial composition and metabolic activity, while microbial-derived metabolites influence host digestion, immunity, energy balance, and disease risk. This continuous feedback loop explains why identical diets may produce different health outcomes across individuals and highlights the microbiome's central role in personalized nutrition.

3.1 How Diet Shapes Microbial Composition and Function (≈400 words)

Diet is the most powerful external factor shaping the composition and functional capacity of the gut microbiome. While host genetics exert some influence, dietary patterns determine which microbial populations are selectively nourished or suppressed by regulating substrate availability in the gut. Non-digestible carbohydrates, particularly dietary fibers, resistant starches, and certain oligosaccharides, reach the colon intact and serve as primary energy sources for gut microbes. Regular consumption of these substrates promotes the growth of fermentative bacteria capable of producing short-chain fatty acids (SCFAs), which are central to gut and systemic health (Koh et al., 2016).

Macronutrient composition significantly alters microbial profiles. Diets rich in plant-based foods tend to increase microbial diversity and favor beneficial taxa such as *Bifidobacterium*, *Faecalibacterium*, and *Roseburia*. In contrast, high-fat, high-protein, and low-fiber diets particularly those rich in animal fats and processed foods have been associated with reduced microbial diversity and increased abundance of bile-tolerant and potentially pro-inflammatory species (Singh et al., 2017). Excessive protein intake, especially from animal sources, may also increase microbial production of potentially harmful metabolites such as ammonia and phenolic compounds.

Beyond composition, diet strongly influences microbial function. Microbes adapt their metabolic pathways in response to available nutrients, altering fermentation patterns, enzyme expression, and metabolite production. Polyphenol-rich foods such as fruits, tea, coffee, and cocoa interact with the microbiome in a reciprocal manner: microbes convert polyphenols into bioactive compounds, while polyphenols selectively modulate microbial growth (Cardona et al., 2013).

Micronutrients, including iron, zinc, and vitamins, also shape microbial ecosystems by influencing microbial growth dynamics and host–microbe interactions. Overall, diet determines not only which microbes are present, but also what they do metabolically. This functional modulation is crucial, as microbial metabolites rather than microbial identity alone largely determine health outcomes.

3.2 Microbial Adaptation to Dietary Patterns

Gut microbes possess remarkable metabolic flexibility, allowing them to adapt rapidly to changes in dietary intake. This adaptability reflects the evolutionary relationship between humans and their microbial partners, shaped by fluctuations in food availability across time and geography. Microbial genomes encode a wide range of carbohydrate-active enzymes, transporters, and metabolic pathways that enable efficient utilization of diverse dietary substrates (Flint et al., 2012).

When dietary patterns change, microbial populations adjust both in composition and functional gene expression. For example, increased intake of complex carbohydrates promotes expansion of polysaccharide-degrading bacteria, while reduced fiber availability shifts microbes toward alternative energy sources, including host-derived mucus glycans. Such shifts may compromise gut barrier integrity and increase susceptibility to inflammation if sustained over time (Sonnenburg & Sonnenburg, 2019).

Habitual dietary patterns exert stronger and more lasting effects than occasional meals. Long-term adherence to plant-based or traditional diets supports stable microbial communities adapted to fiber fermentation, whereas prolonged consumption of Western-style diets encourages microbes specialized in fat and simple sugar metabolism. These adaptations influence not only microbial growth but also cross-feeding interactions, in which metabolic by-products of one species serve as substrates for another, reinforcing ecosystem-level changes.

Microbial adaptation also extends to circadian feeding patterns. Irregular meal timing and disrupted circadian rhythms alter microbial oscillations, affecting metabolic outputs and host glucose regulation. This highlights how not only food composition but also eating behaviors shape microbial adaptation.

Importantly, microbial adaptability has limits. Chronic deprivation of fermentable substrates may lead to irreversible loss of certain microbial taxa across generations, as observed in industrialized populations. Such losses reduce functional redundancy and resilience, potentially increasing vulnerability to metabolic and inflammatory diseases. Thus, while the microbiome is adaptable, sustained dietary quality is essential to preserve its long-term functional capacity.

3.3 Short-Term vs Long-Term Dietary Influences

Dietary influences on the gut microbiome operate across multiple time scales, with both short-term and long-term effects contributing to microbial dynamics. Short-term dietary interventions can induce rapid changes in microbial composition and metabolic activity, often within days. Controlled feeding studies have demonstrated that shifts from plant-based to animal-based diets quickly alter microbial gene expression, bile acid metabolism, and fermentation patterns (David et al., 2014).

These short-term changes primarily reflect functional adaptation rather than permanent restructuring of the microbiome. Microbial populations adjust enzyme activity and substrate utilization in response to immediate nutrient availability, but core community structure often remains relatively stable. Once the dietary intervention ends, the microbiome typically reverts toward its baseline state, particularly in healthy individuals with high microbial resilience.

In contrast, long-term dietary habits exert deeper and more sustained effects. Habitual diets shape microbial diversity, stability, and functional specialization over months and years. Populations consuming traditional high-fiber diets consistently exhibit greater microbial diversity and higher SCFA production compared to individuals consuming Westernized diets. These long-term patterns influence immune tone, metabolic efficiency, and inflammation risk (De Filippo et al., 2010).

The distinction between short- and long-term effects has important implications for dietary interventions. While short-term dietary changes may yield temporary metabolic benefits, lasting improvements in microbial health require sustained dietary quality. Repeated cycles of dietary restriction and excess may also reduce microbial resilience, leading to incomplete recovery after disturbances such as antibiotic use.

Therefore, effective microbiome-focused nutrition strategies should prioritize long-term dietary patterns rather than short-lived interventions. Consistency in fiber intake, plant diversity, and minimally processed foods supports durable microbial adaptations that translate into long-term health benefits.

3.4 Interindividual Variability in Microbial Responses to Diet (≈400 words)

One of the most significant insights from microbiome research is the substantial interindividual variability in microbial responses to identical diets. While general dietary principles apply at the population level, individual microbiomes differ in composition, functional capacity, and metabolic responsiveness. These differences arise from variations in early-life microbial exposure, genetics, habitual diet, lifestyle, and prior medication use (Zeevi et al., 2015).

As a result, the same food may produce distinct metabolic outcomes across individuals. For example, identical carbohydrate-rich meals can lead to different postprandial glucose responses depending on microbial composition. Certain microbes enhance glucose tolerance through SCFA production, while others may contribute to insulin resistance via inflammatory pathways. This variability challenges one-size-fits-all dietary recommendations and underscores the need for personalized nutrition approaches.

Microbial functional capacity plays a critical role in this variability. Two individuals may harbor different microbial species yet possess similar metabolic pathways, leading to comparable responses. Conversely, individuals with similar taxa may differ in gene expression and metabolite production depending on dietary context. This functional heterogeneity explains why microbial composition alone does not always predict dietary response.

Emerging evidence suggests that microbiome-based stratification can improve dietary guidance by identifying responders and non-responders to specific interventions. Personalized diets that consider microbial profiles have shown promise in improving glycemic control and metabolic health.

Recognizing interindividual variability shifts nutrition science toward precision approaches, where dietary recommendations are tailored not only to human physiology but also to microbial ecology. This bidirectional understanding reinforces the central role of the microbiome in translating diet into health outcomes.

4. ROLE OF MACRONUTRIENTS IN MODULATING THE GUT MICROBIOME

Macronutrients majorly carbohydrates, proteins, and fats form the primary interface between diet and the gut microbiome. While these nutrients are traditionally evaluated based on their caloric contribution and effects on host metabolism, their influence on gut microbial composition and function is equally significant. Each macronutrient category provides distinct substrates that shape microbial growth, metabolic pathways, and metabolite production. The balance and quality of macronutrients consumed over time determine whether the gut microbial ecosystem supports health-promoting functions or shifts toward dysbiosis and disease risk.

4.1 Carbohydrates: Dietary Fiber, Resistant Starch, and Non-Digestible Oligosaccharides

Carbohydrates represent the most influential macronutrient group in shaping the gut microbiome, particularly those that escape digestion in the small intestine and reach the colon intact. Dietary fibers, resistant starches, and non-digestible oligosaccharides serve as the primary energy sources for many beneficial gut microbes. These compounds undergo microbial fermentation, leading to the production of short-chain fatty acids (SCFAs), including acetate, propionate, and butyrate, which play critical roles in gut and systemic health (Koh et al., 2016).

Dietary fiber encompasses a diverse group of plant-derived carbohydrates such as cellulose, hemicellulose, pectins, and beta-glucans. Different fiber types selectively stimulate the growth of specific microbial taxa, thereby enhancing microbial diversity. High-fiber diets are consistently associated with increased abundance of SCFA-producing bacteria such as *Faecalibacterium prausnitzii* and *Roseburia*, which contribute to anti-inflammatory signaling and intestinal barrier integrity (Flint et al., 2012).

Resistant starch, found in foods such as cooked-and-cooled rice, potatoes, legumes, and whole grains, resists enzymatic digestion and is preferentially fermented in the colon. Its fermentation strongly promotes butyrate production, supporting colonocyte health and reducing intestinal inflammation. Regular consumption of resistant starch has been shown to improve insulin sensitivity and metabolic outcomes through microbiome-mediated mechanisms.

Non-digestible oligosaccharides, including fructo-oligosaccharides (FOS) and galacto-oligosaccharides (GOS), act as prebiotics by selectively stimulating beneficial bacteria such as *Bifidobacterium* and *Lactobacillus*. These microbes contribute to immune modulation, pathogen inhibition, and vitamin synthesis. Importantly, carbohydrate diversity rather than total fiber quantity alone appears critical for maintaining a resilient and functionally diverse microbiome.

In contrast, diets high in refined carbohydrates and low in fiber deprive beneficial microbes of fermentable substrates, leading to reduced SCFA production and increased reliance on host-derived mucus as an energy source. Over time, this shift may compromise gut barrier integrity and promote low-grade inflammation, emphasizing the central role of complex carbohydrates in microbial health.

4.2 Proteins: Animal vs Plant Proteins and Microbial Metabolism

Proteins contribute significantly to gut microbial metabolism, particularly when consumed in amounts exceeding host digestive capacity. While most dietary protein is digested and absorbed in the small intestine, undigested protein residues reach the colon and undergo microbial fermentation. This process produces a range of metabolites that can exert both beneficial and harmful effects on host health, depending on protein source and dietary context (Windey et al., 2012).

Animal-based proteins are rich in sulfur-containing amino acids and aromatic compounds, which, when fermented by gut microbes, can generate metabolites such as ammonia, hydrogen sulfide, phenols, and indoles. Excessive production of these compounds has been associated with intestinal irritation, impaired barrier function, and increased inflammatory risk. Diets high in red and processed meats have been linked to microbial profiles associated with colorectal cancer and cardiovascular disease risk (Binns et al., 2015).

In contrast, plant-based proteins are typically consumed alongside dietary fiber, polyphenols, and complex carbohydrates, which modulate microbial fermentation patterns. Plant proteins tend to promote the growth of beneficial bacteria and favor SCFA production over proteolytic fermentation. Legumes, nuts, and whole grains support microbial diversity while minimizing the accumulation of harmful nitrogenous metabolites.

Microbial metabolism of protein-derived amino acids also produces bioactive compounds with regulatory functions. For example, certain indole derivatives derived from tryptophan metabolism strengthen intestinal barrier function and modulate immune responses. Thus, protein fermentation is not inherently harmful but becomes problematic when excessive protein intake is combined with low fiber availability.

The overall impact of dietary protein on the gut microbiome depends on protein quality, quantity, and the presence of fermentable carbohydrates. Balanced diets that emphasize plant-based protein sources and adequate fiber intake support favorable microbial metabolism and reduce the risk of proteolytic dysbiosis.

4.3 Dietary Fats: Saturated, Unsaturated, and Omega Fatty Acids

Dietary fats influence the gut microbiome both directly and indirectly through alterations in bile acid secretion, intestinal transit time, and inflammatory signaling. High-fat diets, particularly those rich in saturated fats, have been associated with reduced microbial diversity and increased abundance of bile-tolerant and pro-inflammatory bacteria. Saturated fats stimulate bile acid production, which selectively favors microbes capable of surviving in bile-rich environments, potentially contributing to dysbiosis (Devkota et al., 2012).

In contrast, unsaturated fats especially monounsaturated and polyunsaturated fatty acids appear to exert more favorable effects on microbial composition. Diets rich in olive oil, nuts, seeds, and fatty fish have been associated with increased abundance of beneficial taxa and improved microbial diversity. These fats may reduce inflammation and modulate bile acid profiles in ways that support microbial balance.

Omega-3 fatty acids, found in fatty fish and certain plant sources, have received particular attention for their microbiome-modulating effects. Omega-3 intake has been linked to increased abundance of SCFA-producing bacteria and reduced markers of intestinal inflammation. These effects may be mediated through both direct microbial interactions and host immune modulation (Watson et al., 2018).

Conversely, excessive intake of omega-6 fatty acids, particularly when not balanced with omega-3s, may promote pro-inflammatory microbial profiles. Thus, the ratio of dietary fats appears more important than total fat intake alone.

Overall, the quality and balance of dietary fats play a critical role in shaping gut microbial ecosystems. Replacing saturated fats with unsaturated and omega-3-rich fats may support microbial diversity, reduce inflammation, and improve metabolic health through microbiome-mediated pathways.

4.4 Macronutrient Balance and Microbial Dysbiosis

Macronutrient balance is a key determinant of gut microbial homeostasis. While individual macronutrients influence microbial composition and function, their combined effects determine whether the gut ecosystem remains balanced or shifts toward dysbiosis. Diets disproportionately high in one macronutrient such as high-fat, low-fiber or high-protein, low-carbohydrate diets can disrupt microbial interactions and metabolic outputs.

Low-carbohydrate diets that severely restrict fermentable fibers reduce SCFA production and promote microbial reliance on host-derived substrates, weakening gut barrier integrity. Similarly, excessive protein intake in the absence of adequate fiber increases proteolytic fermentation, leading to accumulation of potentially harmful metabolites. High-fat diets rich in saturated fats further exacerbate these effects by promoting inflammatory microbial profiles.

Dysbiosis is characterized by reduced microbial diversity, loss of beneficial taxa, and expansion of opportunistic species. This altered state has been associated with chronic low-grade inflammation, insulin resistance, obesity, and gastrointestinal disorders. Importantly, dysbiosis is often reversible through dietary modification, highlighting the therapeutic potential of macronutrient rebalancing (Singh et al., 2017).

Balanced diets that include adequate complex carbohydrates, moderate high-quality protein, and healthy fats provide complementary substrates that support microbial diversity and functional resilience. Such dietary patterns promote SCFA production, regulate immune responses, and maintain intestinal barrier integrity.

Understanding macronutrient balance from a microbiome perspective reinforces the need to move beyond calorie-focused dietary models. Instead, dietary strategies should aim to nourish both the host and its microbial partners, thereby supporting long-term metabolic and inflammatory health.

5. MICRONUTRIENTS AND THEIR INFLUENCE ON MICROBIAL HEALTH

Micronutrients, though required in relatively small amounts, play a critical role in shaping gut microbial composition and function. Vitamins and minerals influence microbial growth, enzyme activity, and metabolic interactions within the gut ecosystem. At the same time, gut microbes actively participate in micronutrient synthesis, transformation, and bioavailability, creating a complex, bidirectional relationship between micronutrient status and microbial health. Disruptions in micronutrient intake or absorption can therefore alter microbial ecology, with significant implications for host metabolism, immunity, and disease risk.

5.1 Vitamins and Microbial Synthesis

Vitamins are essential organic compounds that support numerous metabolic processes in both the host and the gut microbiome. Several vitamins, particularly water-soluble B-complex vitamins and vitamin K, are synthesized or modified by gut microbes, highlighting the microbiome's role as a metabolic partner rather than a passive consumer of nutrients. Microbial synthesis of vitamins contributes to host nutritional status, especially in the colon, where microbial metabolites can be absorbed and utilized (Rowland et al., 2018).

B-vitamins such as folate (B9), riboflavin (B2), biotin (B7), and cobalamin (B12) are synthesized by specific gut bacteria, including species of *Bifidobacterium*, *Lactobacillus*, and *Bacteroides*. These vitamins function as cofactors in energy metabolism, DNA synthesis, and neurotransmitter production. While dietary intake remains the primary source, microbial production may help buffer deficiencies, particularly when dietary supply is marginal.

Vitamin K, particularly menaquinones (vitamin K2), is largely produced by gut microbes and plays a crucial role in blood coagulation, bone health, and cardiovascular function. Reduced microbial diversity or antibiotic use can impair vitamin K synthesis, increasing the risk of deficiency-related complications.

Conversely, vitamin availability also shapes microbial composition. Certain microbes depend on exogenous vitamin sources for growth, while others synthesize vitamins and share them within microbial communities through cross-feeding interactions. Diets deficient in vitamins may therefore selectively disadvantage beneficial microbes, reducing microbial diversity and functional capacity.

Fat-soluble vitamins such as vitamins A and D influence microbial ecology indirectly through immune modulation. Vitamin D, in particular, has been shown to regulate antimicrobial peptide expression and intestinal barrier integrity, thereby shaping microbial composition. Thus, vitamins act not only as nutrients but also as regulators of host–microbe interactions, reinforcing the importance of adequate vitamin intake for maintaining microbial balance and resilience.

5.2 Minerals and Microbial Enzyme Activity

Minerals serve as essential cofactors for numerous microbial enzymes involved in fermentation, redox reactions, and energy metabolism. Elements such as magnesium, selenium, copper, and manganese support microbial enzymatic activity and influence microbial growth dynamics within the gut. Adequate mineral availability is therefore crucial for maintaining functional microbial ecosystems.

Magnesium is required for ATP-dependent reactions and nucleic acid synthesis in both host cells and microbes. Insufficient magnesium intake may impair microbial metabolic efficiency, leading to reduced fermentation capacity and altered SCFA production. Selenium, although required in trace amounts, supports antioxidant enzymes such as glutathione peroxidase, influencing microbial redox balance and resistance to oxidative stress.

Minerals also influence microbial competition and ecological balance. For example, copper and zinc possess antimicrobial properties at high concentrations, which can suppress pathogenic bacteria but may also disrupt beneficial microbes if intake exceeds physiological needs. Thus, mineral homeostasis is essential to prevent unintended microbial imbalance.

Microbes, in turn, regulate mineral bioavailability. Certain gut bacteria enhance mineral absorption by modifying gut pH, producing organic acids, or converting minerals into more bioavailable forms. SCFA production lowers colonic pH, increasing solubility and absorption of minerals such as calcium and magnesium. This reciprocal interaction highlights the microbiome's role in mineral metabolism and nutritional status.

Excessive mineral supplementation may disturb microbial ecology by favoring resistant or opportunistic species. Therefore, balanced mineral intake rather than excessive supplementation is essential for sustaining microbial enzyme activity, metabolic efficiency, and ecological stability within the gut.

5.3 Iron, Zinc, and Calcium: Dual Effects on Host and Microbes

Iron, zinc, and calcium exemplify micronutrients with dual and sometimes competing effects on host health and microbial ecology. Iron is essential for oxygen transport and cellular metabolism but also serves as a critical growth factor for many gut microbes, including pathogenic species. High luminal iron availability can promote the expansion of opportunistic bacteria while suppressing beneficial taxa, contributing to dysbiosis and inflammation (Zimmermann et al., 2010).

Iron supplementation, particularly in populations with anemia, has been associated with reduced microbial diversity and increased abundance of pathogenic *Entero-*

bacteriaceae. This highlights the need for careful iron management strategies that balance host requirements while minimizing adverse microbial effects.

Zinc plays a vital role in immune function, antioxidant defense, and enzyme activity. Adequate zinc supports gut barrier integrity and immune regulation, indirectly shaping microbial composition. However, excessive zinc intake can exert antimicrobial effects, disrupting microbial balance and reducing diversity. Zinc deficiency, on the other hand, compromises immune defenses and may allow pathogenic overgrowth.

Calcium influences microbial health primarily through interactions with bile acids and intestinal pH. Calcium can bind bile acids and fatty acids, reducing their antimicrobial effects and supporting beneficial microbial growth. Additionally, calcium-induced changes in luminal pH may favor SCFA-producing bacteria, contributing to anti-inflammatory effects.

These micronutrients illustrate the delicate balance required in micronutrient nutrition. Both deficiency and excess can alter microbial ecology, emphasizing the importance of context-specific, microbiome-aware micronutrient interventions.

5.4 Micronutrient Deficiencies and Altered Microbial Ecology

Micronutrient deficiencies can profoundly disrupt gut microbial composition and function, often amplifying the health consequences of nutrient inadequacy. Deficiencies in vitamins and minerals alter the intestinal environment, influencing microbial growth, metabolic activity, and resilience. In many cases, microbial alterations both result from and contribute to micronutrient deficiencies, creating a self-reinforcing cycle of dysbiosis and malnutrition.

Vitamin deficiencies, such as low folate or vitamin D status, have been associated with reduced microbial diversity and impaired immune–microbiome interactions. Vitamin D deficiency, in particular, is linked to increased intestinal permeability and inflammatory microbial profiles. Similarly, inadequate B-vitamin availability may impair microbial metabolic pathways, reducing SCFA production and energy efficiency.

Mineral deficiencies also reshape microbial ecosystems. Iron deficiency may reduce microbial diversity, while zinc deficiency compromises gut barrier integrity and immune defenses, facilitating pathogenic colonization. Calcium deficiency may indirectly affect microbial fermentation by altering intestinal pH and bile acid metabolism.

These microbial shifts can worsen nutrient absorption and metabolic efficiency, perpetuating deficiency states. In vulnerable populations such as infants, pregnant women, and older adults, micronutrient-related dysbiosis may have long-term health consequences.

Addressing micronutrient deficiencies through diet diversification, food-based approaches, and microbiome-supportive strategies may restore microbial balance more effectively than isolated supplementation. Recognizing the interdependence of micronutrient status and microbial ecology is essential for developing sustainable nutrition interventions.

6. PHYTOCHEMICALS, POLYPHENOLS, AND BIOACTIVE COMPOUNDS

Phytochemicals are naturally occurring bioactive compounds present in plant-based foods such as fruits, vegetables, whole grains, legumes, nuts, seeds, herbs, and beverages like tea and coffee. Although not classified as essential nutrients, phytochemicals exert profound effects on gut microbial composition and metabolic activity. Many phytochemicals escape digestion in the upper gastrointestinal tract and reach the colon, where they interact directly with gut microbes. Through microbial biotransformation, these compounds generate metabolites that influence host metabolism, immune regulation, and inflammatory pathways. Thus, phytochemicals act as key mediators in diet–microbiome–health interactions.

6.1 Plant-Based Bioactives and Microbial Biotransformation

A defining feature of phytochemicals is their limited absorption in the small intestine, which allows substantial quantities to reach the colon intact. In the large intestine, gut microbes play a central role in transforming these compounds into smaller, bioactive metabolites through processes such as hydrolysis, reduction, demethylation, and dehydroxylation (Rowland et al., 2018). This microbial biotransformation is essential for unlocking the biological activity of many plant-based bioactives.

Polyphenols, glucosinolates, lignans, and other phytochemicals often exist in complex, conjugated forms that are poorly bioavailable. Gut bacteria possessing specific enzymatic capabilities convert these compounds into metabolites with enhanced absorption and biological potency. For example, microbial metabolism of lignans produces enterolignans, which exhibit estrogen-modulating and cardioprotective effects. Similarly, the microbial conversion of soy isoflavones into equol has been associated with improved metabolic and cardiovascular outcomes.

Microbial biotransformation is highly individualized and depends on microbial composition, enzyme expression, and ecological interactions. As a result, individuals consuming identical diets may generate different metabolite profiles, leading to variable physiological responses. This interindividual variability highlights the importance of the microbiome in determining the functional impact of plant-based diets.

In addition to producing beneficial metabolites, phytochemicals also shape microbial ecology by selectively stimulating or inhibiting microbial growth. Many bioactives exert antimicrobial effects against pathogenic species while supporting beneficial taxa such as *Bifidobacterium* and *Lactobacillus*. This selective pressure promotes a more balanced microbial ecosystem.

Overall, microbial biotransformation represents a critical link between plant-based bioactives and host health. The health benefits attributed to phytochemical-rich diets cannot be fully understood without considering the metabolic contributions of the gut microbiome.

6.2 Polyphenols as Selective Microbial Modulators

Polyphenols constitute one of the most extensively studied classes of phytochemicals in relation to the gut microbiome. Found abundantly in fruits, vegetables, tea, coffee, cocoa, and red wine, polyphenols include flavonoids, phenolic acids, stilbenes, and tannins. These compounds act as selective microbial modulators, influencing microbial composition, diversity, and metabolic output (Selma et al., 2009).

Unlike broad-spectrum antimicrobial agents, polyphenols tend to exert selective inhibitory effects on pathogenic or opportunistic bacteria while promoting the growth of beneficial microbes. Studies have demonstrated that polyphenol-rich diets increase the abundance of SCFA-producing bacteria, contributing to anti-inflammatory and metabolic benefits. At the same time, polyphenols may suppress bacteria associated with dysbiosis and endotoxin production.

The interaction between polyphenols and microbes is reciprocal. While polyphenols shape microbial communities, microbial metabolism determines polyphenol bioavailability and activity. Microbial-derived metabolites such as urolithins, produced from ellagitannins, exhibit potent anti-inflammatory and antioxidant properties. However, only individuals with specific microbial profiles can produce these metabolites, underscoring the personalized nature of polyphenol responses.

Polyphenols also influence microbial gene expression and metabolic pathways. They can modulate bacterial enzymes involved in carbohydrate and lipid metabolism, indirectly affecting host energy balance. Additionally, polyphenols may enhance gut barrier integrity and reduce intestinal inflammation by promoting beneficial microbial functions.

Through their selective and modulatory actions, polyphenols function as diet-derived regulators of microbial ecology rather than simple antimicrobial agents. Their consistent consumption through diverse plant foods supports microbial diversity, resilience, and functional efficiency.

6.3 Flavonoids, Carotenoids, and Phenolic Acids (≈400 words)

Flavonoids, carotenoids, and phenolic acids represent key subclasses of phytochemicals with distinct yet overlapping effects on the gut microbiome. Flavonoids, including flavonols, flavanols, flavones, and anthocyanins, are widely distributed in fruits, vegetables, tea, and cocoa. These compounds reach the colon in substantial amounts, where they undergo microbial degradation into smaller phenolic metabolites with systemic biological activity (Williamson & Clifford, 2017).

Flavonoids have been shown to promote beneficial bacteria while inhibiting pathogenic species. Their metabolites influence inflammatory signaling, oxidative stress, and vascular function. Anthocyanins, in particular, have been associated with increased microbial diversity and improved metabolic profiles.

Carotenoids, such as beta-carotene and lycopene, are best known for their antioxidant properties. Although their interaction with the microbiome is less direct, emerging evidence suggests that carotenoids may influence microbial composition through immune modulation and antioxidant effects within the gut environment. Microbial metabolism may also affect carotenoid bioavailability and conversion to vitamin A.

Phenolic acids, including caffeic acid and ferulic acid, are abundant in whole grains, coffee, and fruits. These compounds are readily metabolized by gut microbes and contribute to SCFA production and anti-inflammatory effects. Their consistent intake supports microbial metabolic activity and gut barrier function.

Together, these phytochemical subclasses contribute to a diverse chemical environment within the gut, supporting microbial cross-feeding interactions and metabolic flexibility. Their combined presence in whole plant foods reinforces the importance of dietary diversity for optimal microbiome function.

6.4 Synergistic Effects of Phytochemicals and Dietary Fiber

Phytochemicals and dietary fiber often coexist within the same plant foods, creating synergistic effects on gut microbial health. While dietary fiber serves as a primary substrate for microbial fermentation, phytochemicals modulate microbial composition and metabolic pathways, enhancing the overall functional output of the microbiome (Gibson et al., 2017).

Fiber fermentation produces SCFAs that lower gut pH, creating favorable conditions for beneficial microbes. This acidic environment also enhances the stability and activity of certain phytochemical metabolites. In turn, phytochemicals may influence the types of microbes involved in fiber fermentation, promoting efficient SCFA production and reducing gas-producing or pathogenic species.

Whole foods such as fruits, vegetables, legumes, and whole grains provide a complex matrix in which fiber and phytochemicals interact dynamically. This food matrix effect explains why isolated supplements often fail to replicate the benefits of whole plant foods. The combined intake of fiber and phytochemicals supports microbial diversity, resilience, and metabolic adaptability.

Synergistic interactions also extend to immune modulation. SCFAs derived from fiber fermentation work alongside phytochemical metabolites to regulate inflammatory pathways, enhance gut barrier integrity, and support immune tolerance. These combined effects are particularly relevant in the prevention of chronic diseases such as obesity, diabetes, cardiovascular disease, and inflammatory bowel disorders.

Recognizing the synergy between phytochemicals and dietary fiber reinforces the value of plant-rich dietary patterns. From a microbiome perspective, the health benefits of plant foods arise not from single compounds but from complex, interactive networks of bioactives that nourish and regulate microbial ecosystems.

7. MICROBIAL METABOLITES AND HOST PHYSIOLOGICAL OUTCOMES

Microbial metabolites represent the functional output of gut microbiome activity and are key mediators linking diet to host physiology. These compounds influence metabolic regulation, immune balance, and neuroendocrine signaling. Among the most studied microbial metabolites are short-chain fatty acids, secondary bile acids, and neuroactive compounds, all of which translate dietary inputs into biological responses that shape health and disease risk.

7.1 Short-Chain Fatty Acids (SCFAs): Acetate, Propionate, and Butyrate

Short-chain fatty acids (SCFAs) are produced through microbial fermentation of dietary fibers and resistant starches in the colon. Acetate, propionate, and butyrate collectively account for the majority of SCFAs and play essential roles in host metabolism and gut health (Koh et al., 2016).

Acetate is the most abundant SCFA and circulates systemically, contributing to lipid metabolism, cholesterol synthesis, and appetite regulation. Propionate is primarily utilized by the liver, where it influences gluconeogenesis and inhibits cholesterol synthesis. It also stimulates the release of satiety hormones, thereby supporting metabolic regulation.

Butyrate serves as the primary energy source for colonocytes and is critical for maintaining intestinal barrier integrity. It enhances tight junction protein expression and exhibits strong anti-inflammatory properties through epigenetic and immune-modulating mechanisms. Reduced SCFA production, often associated with low-fiber diets, is linked to dysbiosis, inflammation, and metabolic disorders.

Through receptor-mediated signaling, SCFAs influence immune function, insulin sensitivity, and energy balance, highlighting their central role in diet–microbiome–host interactions.

7.2 Secondary Bile Acids and Lipid Metabolism

Bile acids are synthesized in the liver from cholesterol and released into the intestine to aid lipid digestion. Gut microbes convert primary bile acids into secondary bile acids through enzymatic reactions such as deconjugation and dehydroxylation (Ridlon et al., 2016). These microbial transformations significantly influence host lipid and glucose metabolism.

Secondary bile acids act as signaling molecules by activating receptors such as FXR and TGR5, which regulate bile acid synthesis, lipid homeostasis, insulin sensitivity, and energy expenditure. Through these pathways, microbial bile acid metabolism contributes to systemic metabolic regulation.

Bile acids also shape microbial composition due to their antimicrobial properties. Balanced bile acid pools support microbial diversity, whereas dysbiosis may promote the accumulation of pro-inflammatory secondary bile acids. Diets high in fat and low in fiber can disrupt bile acid metabolism, increasing disease risk.

Thus, secondary bile acids function as a critical interface between microbial activity, dietary patterns, and host metabolic health.

7.3 Microbial-Derived Neuroactive Compounds

The gut microbiome produces a range of neuroactive compounds that influence the gut–brain axis. These include gamma-aminobutyric acid (GABA), serotonin precursors, dopamine-related metabolites, and SCFAs with neuromodulatory properties (Cryan & Dinan, 2012).

Certain gut bacteria synthesize GABA, which plays a role in stress regulation and anxiety modulation. Microbes also influence serotonin production by regulating tryptophan metabolism in the gut, affecting mood, gut motility, and stress responses. Although many microbial neurotransmitters do not directly cross the blood–brain barrier, they communicate with the brain through immune, endocrine, and neural pathways, including the vagus nerve.

Alterations in microbial composition have been associated with mental health conditions such as anxiety, depression, and cognitive dysfunction. Diets rich in fiber, polyphenols, and fermented foods support microbial populations involved in beneficial neurochemical production.

These findings highlight the microbiome's role as a key contributor to neurophysiological regulation and mental well-being.

7.4 Metabolite-Mediated Immune and Inflammatory Regulation

Microbial metabolites are essential regulators of immune function and inflammatory balance. SCFAs, bile acid derivatives, and tryptophan metabolites interact with immune cells to maintain immune tolerance and prevent excessive inflammation (Kau et al., 2011).

Butyrate and other SCFAs promote the differentiation of regulatory T cells and suppress pro-inflammatory cytokine production. They also strengthen the intestinal barrier, reducing microbial translocation and systemic inflammation. Tryptophan-derived metabolites activate aryl hydrocarbon receptors that support mucosal immunity and epithelial integrity.

Secondary bile acids further regulate immune responses by modulating macrophage activity and inflammatory signaling pathways. Dysregulated microbial metabolism can shift immune responses toward chronic inflammation, contributing to metabolic and autoimmune disorders.

Diet-induced changes in microbial metabolite production therefore play a decisive role in immune homeostasis. Supporting metabolite diversity through balanced, fiber-rich diets is essential for maintaining immune resilience and inflammatory control.

8. DIETARY PATTERNS AND THEIR IMPACT ON MICROBIAL ECOLOGY

Diet is a key determinant of gut microbial composition and activity. Different dietary patterns can either enhance beneficial microbes, produce important metabolites, or induce dysbiosis. These microbial changes influence immune response, metabolism, and overall health. Understanding how diet shapes microbial ecology helps develop personalized nutrition strategies to improve health outcomes.

8.1 Plant-Based and Vegetarian Diets

Plant-based and vegetarian diets are rich in fiber, resistant starch, and polyphenols, which nourish beneficial gut bacteria like *Bifidobacterium* and *Faecalibacterium*. Fermentation of these compounds produces short-chain fatty acids (SCFAs), promoting gut barrier integrity and reducing inflammation. A diverse plant diet increases microbial richness and supports metabolic health. Limiting animal protein and saturated fats further favors a resilient gut ecosystem. Regular consumption of such diets is linked with lower risk of cardiovascular diseases, obesity, and chronic metabolic conditions (De Filippis et al., 2016; Singh et al., 2017).

8.2 Mediterranean Diet and Microbial Diversity

The Mediterranean diet includes whole grains, legumes, fruits, vegetables, olive oil, and moderate fish. Its high fiber and polyphenol content support beneficial microbes like *Faecalibacterium prausnitzii* and *Roseburia*, enhancing SCFA production. Omega-3 fatty acids from fish reduce gut inflammation, while dietary variety increases microbial richness. Long-term adherence improves metabolic health, reduces dysbiosis, and supports immune function. This diet exemplifies how culturally adaptable, whole-food-based patterns promote gut microbial diversity and host wellbeing (De Filippis et al., 2016; Ghosh et al., 2020).

8.3 Western Diet and Microbial Dysbiosis

Western diets, high in refined carbohydrates, saturated fats, and low fiber, decrease microbial diversity and SCFA-producing bacteria. They favor pro-inflammatory species, increase gut permeability, and contribute to metabolic disorders such as obesity and insulin resistance. Short-term intake can rapidly alter the microbiome, showing its sensitivity to diet. Chronic consumption leads to microbial imbalance and loss of beneficial taxa, emphasizing the detrimental effect of processed foods on gut microbial ecology (David et al., 2014; Sonnenburg & Sonnenburg, 2019).

8.4 Traditional and Indigenous Diets

Traditional and indigenous diets are rich in whole foods, tubers, wild plants, and fermented products, which support diverse and functional microbiomes. Fermented foods introduce beneficial microbes, while high-fiber plant foods enhance SCFA production. Seasonal dietary variation strengthens microbial adaptability. Populations consuming ancestral diets often show low prevalence of metabolic and inflammatory disorders. Studying these diets offers insights into restoring gut microbial diversity and informs modern nutritional strategies for sustainable health (Smits et al., 2017; Sonnenburg & Sonnenburg, 2019).

9. PROBIOTICS, PREBIOTICS, SYNBIOTICS, AND POSTBIOTICS

Microbiome-targeted interventions such as probiotics, prebiotics, synbiotics, and postbiotics are emerging tools for promoting gut health. These agents modulate microbial composition, enhance beneficial metabolites, and support host immunity. Understanding their mechanisms, applications, and limitations is critical for designing effective nutrition strategies and functional foods.

9.1 Definitions and Mechanisms of Action

Probiotics are live microorganisms that confer health benefits when administered in adequate amounts. Prebiotics are non-digestible compounds that selectively stimulate growth of beneficial microbes. Synbiotics combine probiotics and prebiotics to synergistically enhance microbial function. Postbiotics are bioactive metabolites produced by microbes, such as short-chain fatty acids and peptides. Probiotics compete with pathogens, modulate immune responses, and strengthen the gut barrier. Prebiotics serve as substrates for fermentation, increasing SCFA production. Together, these agents influence microbial balance and host physiology through metabolic, immunological, and signaling pathways (Markowiak & Śliżewska, 2017; Salminen et al., 2021).

9.2 Evidence-Based Benefits and Limitations

Clinical studies show probiotics can improve gut health, reduce diarrhea, alleviate IBS symptoms, and support immunity. Prebiotics enhance SCFA production, improve mineral absorption, and modulate inflammation. Synbiotics may offer additive or synergistic effects. Postbiotics show potential anti-inflammatory and metabolic benefits. However, effects are strain- and dose-specific, and variability exists between individuals. Not all formulations are equally effective, and evidence in some conditions is limited. Personalized approaches are necessary to maximize benefits and minimize inefficacy (Sanders et al., 2019; Plaza-Diaz et al., 2019).

9.3 Food-Based vs Supplement-Based Approaches

Food-based approaches deliver probiotics and prebiotics via fermented foods, yogurt, kefir, kimchi, and high-fiber diets, promoting natural microbial diversity. Supplements offer standardized doses and targeted strains but may lack the complexity of whole foods. Synbiotic foods combine prebiotics and probiotics in a convenient matrix, enhancing efficacy. Choice between food and supplement-based approaches depends on dietary habits, health status, and specific therapeutic goals. A combination of both strategies often ensures optimal microbial modulation (Zawistowska-Rojek & Zaręba, 2020; Gibson et al., 2017).

9.4 Safety, Regulation, and Future Directions

Probiotics and prebiotics are generally safe for healthy individuals, though caution is required in immunocompromised patients. Regulatory frameworks vary globally, with labeling and health claims strictly monitored in some regions. Postbiotics may offer safer alternatives as they are non-viable but bioactive. Future research focuses on personalized microbiome interventions, next-generation probiotics, precision synbiotics, and engineered postbiotics. Integrating these approaches into functional foods and medical nutrition therapy holds promise for preventive and therapeutic strategies (Hill et al., 2014; Aguilar-Toalá et al., 2018).

10. PERSONALIZED NUTRITION: MICROBIOME-GUIDED DIETARY INTERVENTIONS

Personalized nutrition considers individual variability in genetics, microbiome composition, and metabolism to optimize dietary strategies. Microbiome-guided interventions aim to tailor diet based on an individual's gut microbial profile, enhancing nutrient utilization, metabolic health, and disease prevention.

10.1 Interindividual Differences in Nutrient Metabolism

Individuals exhibit significant variability in nutrient metabolism due to differences in gut microbial composition and enzymatic activity. Some microbes efficiently ferment dietary fibers into short-chain fatty acids, while others metabolize polyphenols differently, affecting nutrient bioavailability and host responses. These interindividual differences explain why identical diets can produce variable glycemic responses, lipid profiles, or inflammatory outcomes. Accounting for microbial variability allows more precise dietary interventions, improving efficacy for weight management, metabolic regulation, and gastrointestinal health (Zeevi et al., 2015; Kovatcheva-Datchary et al., 2015).

10.2 Microbiome Profiling Techniques and Biomarkers

Microbiome profiling employs next-generation sequencing, 16S rRNA gene analysis, metagenomics, metabolomics, and metatranscriptomics to identify microbial taxa and functional capabilities. Biomarkers such as microbial diversity, SCFA production, and bile acid metabolism provide insights into gut health and dietary responsiveness. These techniques enable mapping of microbial signatures associated with disease risk, nutrient metabolism efficiency, and response to dietary interventions, forming the basis for microbiome-guided nutrition plans (Knight et al., 2018; Johnson et al., 2019).

10.3 Integration of Genetics, Metabolomics, and Microbial Data

Combining genomic, metabolomic, and microbial data offers a holistic view of individual metabolic capacities. Host genetics influence nutrient absorption, enzyme expression, and microbial interactions, while metabolomics captures functional outcomes of diet-microbe interactions. Integrating these datasets facilitates identification of personalized dietary targets, predicting responses to specific foods or nutrients, and developing interventions that optimize metabolic pathways, gut health, and overall well-being (Zeevi et al., 2015; David et al., 2014).

10.4 Personalized Diet Planning for Metabolic and Gut Health

Microbiome-guided personalized diets aim to improve metabolic markers, glycemic control, lipid profile, and gut microbial balance. Intervention strategies may include tailored fiber intake, specific probiotics, polyphenol-rich foods, or reduced fermentable sugars, depending on microbial composition and functional capacity. By leveraging individual microbiome and metabolic data, these diets enhance nutrient utilization, reduce inflammation, and support sustainable health outcomes. Evidence supports their potential for preventing metabolic syndrome, obesity, and gastrointestinal disorders (Berry et al., 2020; Zmora et al., 2019).

11. CLINICAL AND PUBLIC HEALTH IMPLICATIONS

The human gut microbiome plays a central role in health and disease. Alterations in microbial composition can contribute to chronic metabolic, immune, and inflammatory disorders. Understanding these relationships enables microbiome-targeted nutritional strategies for disease prevention, personalized interventions, and public health initiatives.

11.1 Role of the Microbiome in Obesity, Diabetes, and Cardiovascular Disease

The gut microbiome influences energy harvest, glucose metabolism, and lipid homeostasis. Dysbiosis can increase susceptibility to obesity, insulin resistance, type 2 diabetes, and atherosclerosis. Reduced microbial diversity, lower SCFA-producing bacteria, and expansion of pro-inflammatory taxa are commonly observed in these conditions. Diet, antibiotics, and lifestyle interact with microbiota to modulate disease risk. Microbiome-guided interventions, including prebiotics, probiotics, and personalized diets, can improve metabolic profiles, reduce inflammation, and support cardiovascular health (Tilg et al., 2020; Zhao et al., 2018).

11.2 Gut Microbiome and Immune-Mediated Disorders

The gut microbiome shapes immune system development and regulation. Dysbiosis is linked with autoimmune disorders such as inflammatory bowel disease, rheumatoid arthritis, and allergies. Beneficial microbes modulate T-cell responses, produce anti-inflammatory metabolites, and enhance barrier function. Microbiome-targeted interventions, including probiotics and postbiotics, show promise in restoring immune homeostasis, reducing inflammation, and mitigating disease severity. Personalized microbial strategies can complement conventional therapy in immune-mediated disorders (Belkaid & Hand, 2014; Honda & Littman, 2016).

11.3 Microbiome-Targeted Nutrition in Preventive Healthcare

Targeting the gut microbiome through diet and functional foods is emerging as a preventive healthcare strategy. High-fiber, polyphenol-rich diets, fermented foods, and pre/probiotic supplementation enhance microbial diversity and metabolic resilience. Early-life microbiome modulation can reduce risk of obesity, allergies, and metabolic syndrome. Population-level interventions, such as nutrition education and public health campaigns, can promote microbiome-friendly diets to prevent chronic diseases and improve overall health outcomes (Valdes et al., 2018; Thursby & Juge, 2017).

11.4 Challenges in Translating Research into Practice

Despite promising evidence, translating microbiome research into clinical practice faces challenges. Interindividual variability, strain-specific effects, lack of standardized guidelines, and regulatory issues complicate implementation. Longitudinal studies and robust clinical trials are needed to establish causal relationships. Cost, accessibility, and patient adherence further limit widespread adoption. Integrating microbiome data with genetics, metabolomics, and lifestyle factors is critical to develop actionable, evidence-based interventions for public health and clinical settings (Zmora et al., 2019; Sanders et al., 2019).

12. ETHICAL, TECHNOLOGICAL, AND PRACTICAL CONSIDERATIONS

Personalized microbiome-guided nutrition raises ethical, technological, and practical issues. While promising for improving health, challenges include data privacy, accessibility, cultural appropriateness, and limitations in scientific evidence. Addressing these concerns is essential for safe, equitable, and effective implementation of personalized dietary strategies.

12.1 Data Privacy and Microbiome Testing

Microbiome profiling generates sensitive personal data, including health status and metabolic patterns. Ensuring secure storage, consent, and ethical use is critical. Unauthorized sharing of microbial data may lead to discrimination or privacy breaches. Clear regulatory frameworks, robust data anonymization, and participant awareness are necessary to maintain trust. Transparency in how microbiome data is collected, stored, and applied is crucial for ethical personalized nutrition programs (Cani et al., 2019; Lynch & Pedersen, 2016).

12.2 Accessibility and Cost of Personalized Nutrition

High costs of microbiome sequencing, analysis, and tailored interventions limit accessibility, particularly in low-resource settings. Personalized nutrition requires integration of dietary counseling, technology, and continuous monitoring, which may not be universally feasible. Strategies to reduce costs, simplify testing, and integrate affordable dietary guidance are essential for equitable public health impact (Zeevi et al., 2015; Joyner et al., 2019).

12.3 Cultural and Dietary Diversity Considerations

Cultural practices, dietary preferences, and local food availability must be considered when designing personalized nutrition. Standardized interventions may not align with traditional diets or ethical/religious food restrictions. Tailoring recommendations to respect cultural diversity enhances adherence, sustainability, and health outcomes. Inclusion of culturally appropriate foods can maintain microbial diversity and promote community acceptance of microbiome-based strategies (De Filippis et al., 2016; Tomlinson et al., 2019).

12.4 Limitations of Current Evidence

Although microbiome research has advanced rapidly, many findings are observational and strain-specific. Interindividual variability, short study durations, and limited long-term data hinder generalization. Evidence gaps exist regarding causal links between microbial changes and clinical outcomes. Caution is needed in translating research into dietary recommendations, emphasizing the need for large-scale, randomized, and longitudinal studies (Zmora et al., 2019; Vangay et al., 2018).

13. FUTURE PERSPECTIVES AND EMERGING RESEARCH

The field of microbiome-guided nutrition is rapidly evolving, with technological advances and novel interventions offering opportunities for precision health. Future research focuses on integrating AI, next-generation probiotics, and dietary microbiome modulation to optimize personalized dietary strategies.

13.1 AI and Machine Learning in Microbiome-Based Nutrition

Artificial intelligence (AI) and machine learning (ML) enable the analysis of complex microbiome datasets, predicting individual responses to foods and dietary interventions. By integrating microbial composition, metabolomics, and clinical parameters, AI models can personalize nutrition, optimize health outcomes, and identify novel biomarkers. These technologies accelerate hypothesis generation, enhance predictive accuracy, and facilitate real-time dietary recommendations, making microbiome-guided interventions more precise and actionable (Zeevi et al., 2015; Johnson et al., 2019).

13.2 Precision Fermentation and Next-Generation Probiotics

Next-generation probiotics and precision fermentation involve engineering microbes with targeted functions, such as SCFA production, bile acid metabolism, or pathogen inhibition. These approaches aim to restore microbial balance, enhance metabolic capacity, and support immune regulation. Fermented functional foods with designer microbes can provide controlled health benefits, bridging the gap between conventional probiotics and personalized nutrition. Ongoing research focuses on safety, efficacy, and strain-specific optimization for clinical and preventive applications (Sanders et al., 2019; Aguilar-Toalá et al., 2018).

13.3 Microbiome Editing Through Diet

Dietary interventions can selectively modulate microbial composition and function, a concept known as microbiome editing. Specific fibers, polyphenols, or fermented foods can enhance beneficial taxa while suppressing pathogenic microbes. Combined with personalized approaches, this strategy can optimize metabolic, immune, and gastrointestinal health. Integrating microbiome editing with lifestyle and environmental factors offers a practical, non-invasive method to influence microbial ecology and promote long-term well-being (Valdes et al., 2018; Ghosh et al., 2020).

13.4 Research Gaps and Directions for Future Studies

Despite advancements, knowledge gaps remain regarding causal relationships between microbial changes and health outcomes. Longitudinal, multi-omics, and interventional studies are needed to validate predictive models. Population diversity, strain-specific effects, and long-term safety of engineered microbes require exploration. Future research should focus on integrating microbiome, metabolome, and genetic data, expanding access to microbiome-guided nutrition, and developing standardized protocols for clinical translation (Zmora et al., 2019; Knight et al., 2018).

14. CONCLUSION: TOWARD PRECISION FEEDING OF THE GUT MICROBIOME

The human gut microbiome is a central mediator of nutrition, metabolism, and health. Precision feeding—tailoring diet to individual microbial profiles—represents the frontier of personalized nutrition, offering opportunities to prevent and manage chronic diseases.

14.1 Summary of Key Insights

Dietary patterns, including plant-based, Mediterranean, and traditional diets, significantly shape microbial diversity and function. Probiotics, prebiotics, synbiotics, and postbiotics modulate host metabolism and immunity. Microbiome-guided personalized nutrition leverages individual variability in microbial composition, genetics, and metabolomics. Emerging technologies, AI, and precision fermentation enable targeted interventions, while ethical, cultural, and practical considerations must guide implementation. Collectively, these strategies highlight the potential to optimize health through microbiome-focused dietary approaches (Zeevi et al., 2015; Valdes et al., 2018).

14.2 Implications for Nutrition Science and Personalized Healthcare

Precision microbiome nutrition advances nutrition science by integrating multi-omics data and individual response profiles. Clinical applications include managing obesity, diabetes, cardiovascular disease, and immune-mediated disorders. Public health strategies can incorporate microbiome-friendly diets to reduce disease prevalence. By translating microbiome research into evidence-based, personalized interventions, healthcare can become proactive, preventive, and patient-centered, fostering long-term metabolic and gut health (Berry et al., 2020; Zmora et al., 2019).

14.3 Final Remarks on Feeding Microbes for Lifelong Health

Feeding the gut microbiome through tailored diet and functional foods offers a sustainable approach to lifelong health. Maintaining microbial diversity, supporting SCFA production, and reducing dysbiosis are key to preventing chronic disease and enhancing immunity. Future research, technological integration, and culturally appropriate strategies will enable microbiome-centered precision nutrition to become an actionable cornerstone in healthcare, promoting resilience, vitality, and well-being across the lifespan (Sanders et al., 2019; Ghosh et al., 2020).

REFERENCES

Aguilar-Toalá, J. E., Garcia-Varela, R., Garcia, H. S., Mata-Haro, V., González-Córdova, A. F., Vallejo-Cordoba, B., & Hernández-Mendoza, A. (2018). Postbiotics: An evolving term within the functional foods field. *Trends in Food Science & Technology*, *75*, 105–114. DOI: 10.1016/j.tifs.2018.03.009

Aguilar-Toalá, J. E., Garcia-Varela, R., Garcia, H. S., Mata-Haro, V., González-Córdova, A. F., Vallejo-Cordoba, B., & Hernández-Mendoza, A. (2018). Postbiotics: An evolving term within the functional foods field. *Trends in Food Science & Technology*, *75*, 105–114. DOI: 10.1016/j.tifs.2018.03.009

Belkaid, Y., & Hand, T. W. (2014). Role of the microbiota in immunity and inflammation. *Cell*, *157*(1), 121–141. DOI: 10.1016/j.cell.2014.03.011 PMID: 24679531

Berry, S. E., Valdes, A. M., Drew, D. A., Asnicar, F., Mazidi, M., Wolf, J., & Segal, E. (2020). Human postprandial responses to food and potential for precision nutrition. *Nature Medicine*, *26*(6), 964–973. DOI: 10.1038/s41591-020-0934-0 PMID: 32528151

Berry, S. E., Valdes, A. M., Drew, D. A., Asnicar, F., Mazidi, M., Wolf, J., & Segal, E. (2020). Human postprandial responses to food and potential for precision nutrition. *Nature Medicine*, *26*(6), 964–973. DOI: 10.1038/s41591-020-0934-0 PMID: 32528151

Binns, N., Lee, M. K., & Lee, A. (2015). The relationship between gut microbiota and protein digestion. *Nutrition Research Reviews*, *28*(2), 121–135. DOI: 10.1017/S0954422415000100 PMID: 26650242

Cani, P. D., Van Hul, M., & Delzenne, N. M. (2019). Microbiome and metabolic health: From mechanisms to therapeutic perspectives. *Nature Reviews. Endocrinology*, *15*(2), 69–85. DOI: 10.1038/s41574-018-0143-9 PMID: 30602737

Cardona, F., Andrés-Lacueva, C., Tulipani, S., Tinahones, F. J., & Queipo-Ortuño, M. I. (2013). Benefits of polyphenols on gut microbiota and implications in human health. *The Journal of Nutritional Biochemistry*, *24*(8), 1415–1422. DOI: 10.1016/j.jnutbio.2013.05.001 PMID: 23849454

Cryan, J. F., & Dinan, T. G. (2012). Mind-altering microorganisms: The impact of the gut microbiota on brain and behaviour. *Nature Reviews. Neuroscience*, *13*(10), 701–712. DOI: 10.1038/nrn3346 PMID: 22968153

Cryan, J. F., O'Riordan, K. J., Cowan, C. S. M., Sandhu, K. V., Bastiaanssen, T. F. S., Boehme, M., Codagnone, M. G., Cussotto, S., Fulling, C., Golubeva, A. V., Guzzetta, K. E., Jaggar, M., Long-Smith, C. M., Lyte, J. M., Martin, J. A., Molinero-Perez, A., Moloney, G., Morelli, E., Morillas, E., & Dinan, T. G. (2019). The microbiota–gut–brain axis. *Physiological Reviews*, *99*(4), 1877–2013. DOI: 10.1152/physrev.00018.2018 PMID: 31460832

Cummings, J. H., & Macfarlane, G. T. (1997). Role of intestinal bacteria in nutrient metabolism. *Clinical Nutrition (Edinburgh, Lothian)*, *16*(1), 3–11. DOI: 10.1016/S0261-5614(97)80252-X PMID: 9406136

David, L. A., Maurice, C. F., Carmody, R. N., Gootenberg, D. B., Button, J. E., Wolfe, B. E., Ling, A. V., Devlin, A. S., Varma, Y., Fischbach, M. A., Biddinger, S. B., Dutton, R. J., & Turnbaugh, P. J. (2014). Diet rapidly and reproducibly alters the human gut microbiome. *Nature*, *505*(7484), 559–563. DOI: 10.1038/nature12820 PMID: 24336217

David, L. A., Maurice, C. F., Carmody, R. N., Gootenberg, D. B., Button, J. E., Wolfe, B. E., Ling, A. V., Devlin, A. S., Varma, Y., Fischbach, M. A., Biddinger, S. B., Dutton, R. J., & Turnbaugh, P. J. (2014). Diet rapidly and reproducibly alters the human gut microbiome. *Nature*, *505*(7484), 559–563. DOI: 10.1038/nature12820 PMID: 24336217

David, L. A., Maurice, C. F., Carmody, R. N., Gootenberg, D. B., Button, J. E., Wolfe, B. E., Ling, A. V., Devlin, A. S., Varma, Y., Fischbach, M. A., Biddinger, S. B., Dutton, R. J., & Turnbaugh, P. J. (2014). Diet rapidly and reproducibly alters the human gut microbiome. *Nature*, *505*(7484), 559–563. DOI: 10.1038/nature12820 PMID: 24336217

De Filippis, F., Pellegrini, N., Vannini, L., Jeffery, I. B., La Storia, A., Laghi, L., Serrazanetti, D. I., Di Cagno, R., Ferrocino, I., Lazzi, C., Turroni, S., Cocolin, L., Brigidi, P., Neviani, E., Gobbetti, M., O'Toole, P. W., & Ercolini, D. (2016). High-level adherence to a Mediterranean diet beneficially impacts the gut microbiota and associated metabolome. *Gut*, *65*(11), 1812–1821. DOI: 10.1136/gutjnl-2015-309957 PMID: 26416813

De Filippis, F., Pellegrini, N., Vannini, L., Jeffery, I. B., La Storia, A., Laghi, L., Serrazanetti, D. I., Di Cagno, R., Ferrocino, I., Lazzi, C., Turroni, S., Cocolin, L., Brigidi, P., Neviani, E., Gobbetti, M., O'Toole, P. W., & Ercolini, D. (2016). High-level adherence to a Mediterranean diet beneficially impacts the gut microbiota and associated metabolome. *Gut*, *65*(11), 1812–1821. DOI: 10.1136/gutjnl-2015-309957 PMID: 26416813

De Filippo, C., Cavalieri, D., Di Paola, M., Ramazzotti, M., Poullet, J. B., Massart, S., Collini, S., Pieraccini, G., & Lionetti, P. (2010). Impact of diet in shaping gut microbiota revealed by a comparative study in children from Europe and rural Africa. *Proceedings of the National Academy of Sciences of the United States of America*, *107*(33), 14691–14696. DOI: 10.1073/pnas.1005963107 PMID: 20679230

Devkota, S., Wang, Y., Musch, M. W., Leone, V., Fehlner-Peach, H., Nadimpalli, A., Antonopoulos, D. A., Jabri, B., & Chang, E. B. (2012). Dietary-fat-induced taurocholic acid promotes pathobiont expansion and colitis in IL-10−/− mice. *Nature*, *487*(7405), 104–108. DOI: 10.1038/nature11225 PMID: 22722865

Flint, H. J., Scott, K. P., Duncan, S. H., Louis, P., & Forano, E. (2012). Microbial degradation of complex carbohydrates in the gut. *Gut Microbes*, *3*(4), 289–306. DOI: 10.4161/gmic.19897 PMID: 22572875

Flint, H. J., Scott, K. P., Duncan, S. H., Louis, P., & Forano, E. (2012). Microbial degradation of complex carbohydrates in the gut. *Gut Microbes*, *3*(4), 289–306. DOI: 10.4161/gmic.19897 PMID: 22572875

Ghosh, T. S., Rampelli, S., Jeffery, I. B., Santoro, A., Neto, M. C., Capri, M., & Candela, M. (2020). Mediterranean diet intervention alters the gut microbiome in older people reducing frailty and improving health status. *Gut*, *69*(7), 1218–1228. DOI: 10.1136/gutjnl-2019-319654 PMID: 32066625

Ghosh, T. S., Rampelli, S., Jeffery, I. B., Santoro, A., Neto, M. C., Capri, M., & Candela, M. (2020). Mediterranean diet intervention alters the gut microbiome in older people reducing frailty and improving health status. *Gut*, *69*(7), 1218–1228. DOI: 10.1136/gutjnl-2019-319654 PMID: 32066625

Ghosh, T. S., Rampelli, S., Jeffery, I. B., Santoro, A., Neto, M. C., Capri, M., & Candela, M. (2020). Mediterranean diet intervention alters the gut microbiome in older people reducing frailty and improving health status. *Gut*, *69*(7), 1218–1228. DOI: 10.1136/gutjnl-2019-319654 PMID: 32066625

Gibson, G. R., Hutkins, R., Sanders, M. E., Prescott, S. L., Reimer, R. A., Salminen, S. J., Scott, K., Stanton, C., Swanson, K. S., Cani, P. D., Verbeke, K., & Reid, G. (2017). Expert consensus document: The International Scientific Association for Probiotics and Prebiotics (ISAPP) consensus statement. *Nature Reviews. Gastroenterology & Hepatology*, *14*(8), 491–502. DOI: 10.1038/nrgastro.2017.75 PMID: 28611480

Gibson, G. R., Hutkins, R., Sanders, M. E., Prescott, S. L., Reimer, R. A., Salminen, S. J., Scott, K., Stanton, C., Swanson, K. S., Cani, P. D., Verbeke, K., & Reid, G. (2017). The International Scientific Association for Probiotics and Prebiotics (ISAPP) consensus statement. *Nature Reviews. Gastroenterology & Hepatology*, *14*(8), 491–502. DOI: 10.1038/nrgastro.2017.75 PMID: 28611480

Gibson, G. R., Hutkins, R., Sanders, M. E., Prescott, S. L., Reimer, R. A., Salminen, S. J., Scott, K., Stanton, C., Swanson, K. S., Cani, P. D., Verbeke, K., & Reid, G. (2017). Expert consensus document: The International Scientific Association for Probiotics and Prebiotics (ISAPP) consensus statement on the definition and scope of prebiotics. *Nature Reviews. Gastroenterology & Hepatology*, *14*(8), 491–502. DOI: 10.1038/nrgastro.2017.75 PMID: 28611480

Hill, C., Guarner, F., Reid, G., Gibson, G. R., Merenstein, D. J., Pot, B., Morelli, L., Canani, R. B., Flint, H. J., Salminen, S., Calder, P. C., & Sanders, M. E. (2014). Expert consensus document: The International Scientific Association for Probiotics and Prebiotics consensus statement on the scope and appropriate use of the term probiotic. *Nature Reviews. Gastroenterology & Hepatology*, *11*(8), 506–514. DOI: 10.1038/nrgastro.2014.66 PMID: 24912386

Honda, K., & Littman, D. R. (2016). The microbiome in infectious disease and inflammation. *Annual Review of Immunology*, *34*, 307–336. DOI: 10.1146/annurev-immunol-041015-055728 PMID: 22224764

Human Microbiome Project Consortium. (2012). Structure, function and diversity of the healthy human microbiome. *Nature*, *486*(7402), 207–214. DOI: 10.1038/nature11234 PMID: 22699609

Human Microbiome Project Consortium. (2012). Structure, function and diversity of the healthy human microbiome. *Nature*, *486*(7402), 207–214. DOI: 10.1038/nature11234 PMID: 22699609

Human Microbiome Project Consortium. (2012). Structure, function and diversity of the healthy human microbiome. *Nature*, *486*(7402), 207–214. DOI: 10.1038/nature11234 PMID: 22699609

Johnson, A. J., Vangay, P., Al-Ghalith, G. A., Hillmann, B. M., Ward, T. L., Shields-Cutler, R. R., Kim, A. D., Shmagel, A. K., Syed, A. N., Walter, J., Menon, R., Koecher, K., & Knights, D. (2019). Daily sampling reveals personalized diet-microbiome associations in humans. *Cell Host & Microbe*, *25*(6), 789–802. DOI: 10.1016/j.chom.2019.05.005 PMID: 31194939

Johnson, A. J., Vangay, P., Al-Ghalith, G. A., Hillmann, B. M., Ward, T. L., Shields-Cutler, R. R., Kim, A. D., Shmagel, A. K., Syed, A. N., Walter, J., Menon, R., Koecher, K., & Knights, D. (2019). Daily sampling reveals personalized diet-microbiome associations in humans. *Cell Host & Microbe*, *25*(6), 789–802. DOI: 10.1016/j.chom.2019.05.005 PMID: 31194939

Johnson, A. J., Vangay, P., Al-Ghalith, G. A., Hillmann, B. M., Ward, T. L., Shields-Cutler, R. R., & Knights, D. (2017). Daily sampling reveals personalized diet–microbiome associations. *Cell Host & Microbe*, *21*(6), 789–802. DOI: 10.1016/j.chom.2019.05.005 PMID: 31194939

Joyner, M. J., Paneth, N., & Ioannidis, J. P. A. (2019). What happens when underpowered studies are pooled? *Nature*, *569*(7758), 447–449. DOI: 10.1038/d41586-019-01409-7

Kau, A. L., Ahern, P. P., Griffin, N. W., Goodman, A. L., & Gordon, J. I. (2011). Human nutrition, the gut microbiome and the immune system. *Nature*, *474*(7351), 327–336. DOI: 10.1038/nature10213 PMID: 21677749

Kau, A. L., Ahern, P. P., Griffin, N. W., Goodman, A. L., & Gordon, J. I. (2011). Human nutrition, the gut microbiome and the immune system. *Nature*, *474*(7351), 327–336. DOI: 10.1038/nature10213 PMID: 21677749

Knight, R., Vrbanac, A., Taylor, B. C., Aksenov, A., Callewaert, C., Debelius, J., Gonzalez, A., Kosciolek, T., McCall, L.-I., McDonald, D., Melnik, A. V., Morton, J. T., Navas, J., Quinn, R. A., Sanders, J. G., Swafford, A. D., Thompson, L. R., Tripathi, A., Xu, Z. Z., & Dorrestein, P. C. (2018). Best practices for analysing microbiomes. *Nature Reviews. Microbiology*, *16*(7), 410–422. DOI: 10.1038/s41579-018-0029-9 PMID: 29795328

Knight, R., Vrbanac, A., Taylor, B. C., Aksenov, A., Callewaert, C., Debelius, J., Gonzalez, A., Kosciolek, T., McCall, L.-I., McDonald, D., Melnik, A. V., Morton, J. T., Navas, J., Quinn, R. A., Sanders, J. G., Swafford, A. D., Thompson, L. R., Tripathi, A., Xu, Z. Z., & Dorrestein, P. C. (2018). Best practices for analysing microbiomes. *Nature Reviews. Microbiology*, *16*(7), 410–422. DOI: 10.1038/s41579-018-0029-9 PMID: 29795328

Koh, A., De Vadder, F., Kovatcheva-Datchary, P., & Bäckhed, F. (2016). From dietary fiber to host physiology: Short-chain fatty acids as key bacterial metabolites. *Cell*, *165*(6), 1332–1345. DOI: 10.1016/j.cell.2016.05.041 PMID: 27259147

Koh, A., De Vadder, F., Kovatcheva-Datchary, P., & Bäckhed, F. (2016). From dietary fiber to host physiology: Short-chain fatty acids as key bacterial metabolites. *Cell*, *165*(6), 1332–1345. DOI: 10.1016/j.cell.2016.05.041 PMID: 27259147

Koh, A., De Vadder, F., Kovatcheva-Datchary, P., & Bäckhed, F. (2016). From dietary fiber to host physiology: Short-chain fatty acids as key bacterial metabolites. *Cell*, *165*(6), 1332–1345. DOI: 10.1016/j.cell.2016.05.041 PMID: 27259147

Koh, A., De Vadder, F., Kovatcheva-Datchary, P., & Bäckhed, F. (2016). From dietary fiber to host physiology: Short-chain fatty acids as key bacterial metabolites. *Cell*, *165*(6), 1332–1345. DOI: 10.1016/j.cell.2016.05.041 PMID: 27259147

Koh, A., De Vadder, F., Kovatcheva-Datchary, P., & Bäckhed, F. (2016). From dietary fiber to host physiology: Short-chain fatty acids as key bacterial metabolites. *Cell*, *165*(6), 1332–1345. DOI: 10.1016/j.cell.2016.05.041 PMID: 27259147

Kovatcheva-Datchary, P., Nilsson, A., Akrami, R., Lee, Y. S., De Vadder, F., Arora, T., Hallen, A., Martens, E., Björck, I., & Bäckhed, F. (2015). Dietary fiber-induced improvement in glucose metabolism is associated with increased abundance of *Prevotella*. *Cell Metabolism*, *22*(6), 971–982. DOI: 10.1016/j.cmet.2015.10.001 PMID: 26552345

Le Chatelier, E., Nielsen, T., Qin, J., Prifti, E., Hildebrand, F., Falony, G., & Bork, P. (2013). Richness of human gut microbiome correlates with metabolic markers. *Nature*, *500*(7464), 541–546. DOI: 10.1038/nature12506 PMID: 23985870

Louis, P., & Flint, H. J. (2017). Formation of propionate and butyrate by the human colonic microbiota. *Environmental Microbiology*, *19*(1), 29–41. DOI: 10.1111/1462-2920.13589 PMID: 27928878

Lynch, S. V., & Pedersen, O. (2016). The human intestinal microbiome in health and disease. *The New England Journal of Medicine*, *375*(24), 2369–2379. DOI: 10.1056/NEJMra1600266 PMID: 27974040

Maier, L., Pruteanu, M., Kuhn, M., Zeller, G., Telzerow, A., Anderson, E. E., & Typas, A. (2018). Extensive impact of non-antibiotic drugs on human gut bacteria. *Nature*, *555*(7698), 623–628. DOI: 10.1038/nature25979 PMID: 29555994

Markowiak, P., & Śliżewska, K. (2017). Effects of probiotics, prebiotics, and synbiotics on human health. *Nutrients*, *9*(9), 1021. DOI: 10.3390/nu9091021 PMID: 28914794

Metchnikoff, É. (1907). *The prolongation of life: Optimistic studies*. Heinemann. https://archive.org/details/prolongationofli00metc

O'Toole, P. W., & Jeffery, I. B. (2015). Gut microbiota and aging. *Science*, *350*(6265), 1214–1215. DOI: 10.1126/science.aac8469 PMID: 26785481

Penders, J., Thijs, C., Vink, C., Stelma, F. F., Snijders, B., Kummeling, I., & Stobberingh, E. E. (2006). Factors influencing the composition of the intestinal microbiota in early infancy. *Pediatrics, 118*(2), 511–521. DOI: 10.1542/peds.2005-2824 PMID: 16882802

Plaza-Diaz, J., Ruiz-Ojeda, F. J., Gil-Campos, M., & Gil, A. (2019). Mechanisms of action of probiotics. *Advances in Nutrition, 10*(S1), S49–S66. DOI: 10.1093/advances/nmy063 PMID: 30721959

Ridlon, J. M., Harris, S. C., Bhowmik, S., Kang, D. J., & Hylemon, P. B. (2016). Consequences of bile salt biotransformations by intestinal bacteria. *Gut Microbes, 7*(1), 22–39. DOI: 10.1080/19490976.2015.1127483 PMID: 26939849

Rowland, I., Gibson, G., Heinken, A., Scott, K., Swann, J., Thiele, I., & Tuohy, K. (2018). Gut microbiota functions: Metabolism of nutrients and other food components. *European Journal of Nutrition, 57*(1), 1–24. DOI: 10.1007/s00394-017-1445-8 PMID: 28393285

Rowland, I., Gibson, G., Heinken, A., Scott, K., Swann, J., Thiele, I., & Tuohy, K. (2018). Gut microbiota functions: Metabolism of nutrients and other food components. *European Journal of Nutrition, 57*(1), 1–24. DOI: 10.1007/s00394-017-1445-8 PMID: 28393285

Salminen, S., Collado, M. C., Endo, A., Hill, C., Lebeer, S., Quigley, E. M., & von Wright, A. (2021). The International Scientific Association of Probiotics and Prebiotics (ISAPP) consensus statement on the definition and scope of postbiotics. *Nature Reviews. Gastroenterology & Hepatology, 18*(9), 649–667. DOI: 10.1038/s41575-021-00440-6 PMID: 33948025

Sanders, M. E., Merenstein, D. J., Reid, G., Gibson, G. R., & Rastall, R. A. (2019). Probiotics and prebiotics in intestinal health and disease: From biology to the clinic. *Nature Reviews. Gastroenterology & Hepatology, 16*(10), 605–616. DOI: 10.1038/s41575-019-0173-3 PMID: 31296969

Sanders, M. E., Merenstein, D. J., Reid, G., Gibson, G. R., & Rastall, R. A. (2019). Probiotics and prebiotics in intestinal health and disease: From biology to the clinic. *Nature Reviews. Gastroenterology & Hepatology, 16*(10), 605–616. DOI: 10.1038/s41575-019-0173-3 PMID: 31296969

Sanders, M. E., Merenstein, D. J., Reid, G., Gibson, G. R., & Rastall, R. A. (2019). Probiotics and prebiotics in intestinal health and disease: From biology to the clinic. *Nature Reviews. Gastroenterology & Hepatology, 16*(10), 605–616. DOI: 10.1038/s41575-019-0173-3 PMID: 31296969

Sanders, M. E., Merenstein, D. J., Reid, G., Gibson, G. R., & Rastall, R. A. (2019). Probiotics and prebiotics in intestinal health and disease: From biology to the clinic. *Nature Reviews. Gastroenterology & Hepatology*, *16*(10), 605–616. DOI: 10.1038/s41575-019-0173-3 PMID: 31296969

Selma, M. V., Espín, J. C., & Tomás-Barberán, F. A. (2009). Interaction between phenolics and gut microbiota: Role in human health. *Journal of Agricultural and Food Chemistry*, *57*(15), 6485–6501. DOI: 10.1021/jf902107d PMID: 19580283

Shin, N. R., Whon, T. W., & Bae, J. W. (2015). Proteobacteria: Microbial signature of dysbiosis in gut microbiota. *Trends in Biotechnology*, *33*(9), 496–503. DOI: 10.1016/j.tibtech.2015.06.011 PMID: 26210164

Singh, R. K., Chang, H. W., Yan, D., Lee, K. M., Ucmak, D., Wong, K., Abrouk, M., Farahnik, B., Nakamura, M., Zhu, T. H., Bhutani, T., & Liao, W. (2017). Influence of diet on the gut microbiome and implications for human health. *Journal of Translational Medicine*, *15*(1), 73. DOI: 10.1186/s12967-017-1175-y PMID: 28388917

Singh, R. K., Chang, H. W., Yan, D., Lee, K. M., Ucmak, D., Wong, K., Abrouk, M., Farahnik, B., Nakamura, M., Zhu, T. H., Bhutani, T., & Liao, W. (2017). Influence of diet on the gut microbiome and implications for human health. *Journal of Translational Medicine*, *15*(1), 73. DOI: 10.1186/s12967-017-1175-y PMID: 28388917

Singh, R. K., Chang, H. W., Yan, D., Lee, K. M., Ucmak, D., Wong, K., Abrouk, M., Farahnik, B., Nakamura, M., Zhu, T. H., Bhutani, T., & Liao, W. (2017). Influence of diet on the gut microbiome and implications for human health. *Journal of Translational Medicine*, *15*(1), 73. DOI: 10.1186/s12967-017-1175-y PMID: 28388917

Singh, R. K., Chang, H. W., Yan, D., Lee, K. M., Ucmak, D., Wong, K., Abrouk, M., Farahnik, B., Nakamura, M., Zhu, T. H., Bhutani, T., & Liao, W. (2017). Influence of diet on the gut microbiome and implications for human health. *Journal of Translational Medicine*, *15*(1), 73. DOI: 10.1186/s12967-017-1175-y PMID: 28388917

Singh, R. K., Chang, H. W., Yan, D., Lee, K. M., Ucmak, D., Wong, K., & Liao, W. (2017). Influence of diet on the gut microbiome and implications for human health. *Journal of Translational Medicine*, *15*(1), 73. DOI: 10.1186/s12967-017-1175-y PMID: 28388917

Smits, S. A., Leach, J., Sonnenburg, E. D., Gonzalez, C. G., Lichtman, J. S., Reid, G., Knight, R., Manjurano, A., Changalucha, J., Elias, J. E., Dominguez-Bello, M. G., & Sonnenburg, J. L. (2017). Seasonal cycling in the gut microbiome of the Hadza hunter-gatherers of Tanzania. *Science*, *357*(6353), 802–806. DOI: 10.1126/science.aan4834 PMID: 28839072

Sommer, F., Anderson, J. M., Bharti, R., Raes, J., & Rosenstiel, P. (2017). The resilience of the intestinal microbiota influences health and disease. *Nature Reviews. Microbiology, 15*(10), 630–638. DOI: 10.1038/nrmicro.2017.58 PMID: 28626231

Sonnenburg, E. D., & Sonnenburg, J. L. (2019). The ancestral and industrialized gut microbiota and implications for human health. *Nature Reviews. Microbiology, 17*(6), 383–390. DOI: 10.1038/s41579-019-0191-8 PMID: 31089293

Sonnenburg, E. D., & Sonnenburg, J. L. (2019). The ancestral and industrialized gut microbiota and implications for human health. *Nature Reviews. Microbiology, 17*(6), 383–390. DOI: 10.1038/s41579-019-0191-8 PMID: 31089293

Sonnenburg, E. D., & Sonnenburg, J. L. (2019). *The good gut: Taking control of your weight, your mood, and your long-term health.* Penguin Press.

Thursby, E., & Juge, N. (2017). Introduction to the human gut microbiota. *The Biochemical Journal, 474*(11), 1823–1836. DOI: 10.1042/BCJ20160510 PMID: 28512250

Tilg, H., Zmora, N., Adolph, T. E., & Elinav, E. (2020). The intestinal microbiota fuelling metabolic inflammation. *Nature Reviews. Immunology, 20*(1), 40–54. DOI: 10.1038/s41577-019-0198-4 PMID: 31388093

Tomlinson, C., Khoury, J., & Dainty, K. N. (2019). Cultural competence in personalized nutrition: Integrating microbiome data. *Nutrients, 11*(10), 2410. DOI: 10.3390/nu11102410 PMID: 31600938

Valdes, A. M., Walter, J., Segal, E., & Spector, T. D. (2018). Role of the gut microbiota in nutrition and health. *BMJ (Clinical Research Ed.), 361*, k2179. https://www.bmj.com/content/361/bmj.k2179. DOI: 10.1136/bmj.k2179 PMID: 29899036

Valdes, A. M., Walter, J., Segal, E., & Spector, T. D. (2018). Role of the gut microbiota in nutrition and health. *BMJ (Clinical Research Ed.), 361*, k2179. DOI: 10.1136/bmj.k2179 PMID: 29899036

Valdes, A. M., Walter, J., Segal, E., & Spector, T. D. (2018). Role of the gut microbiota in nutrition and health. *BMJ (Clinical Research Ed.), 361*, k2179. DOI: 10.1136/bmj.k2179 PMID: 29899036

Valdes, A. M., Walter, J., Segal, E., & Spector, T. D. (2018). Role of the gut microbiota in nutrition and health. *BMJ (Clinical Research Ed.), 361*, k2179. DOI: 10.1136/bmj.k2179 PMID: 29899036

Vangay, P., Johnson, A. J., Ward, T. L., Al-Ghalith, G. A., Shields-Cutler, R. R., Hillmann, B. M., Lucas, S. K., Beura, L. K., Thompson, E. A., Till, L. M., Batres, R., Paw, B., Pergament, S. L., Saenyakul, P., Xiong, M., Kim, A. D., Kim, G., Masopust, D., Martens, E. C., & Knights, D. (2018). US immigration westernizes the human gut microbiome. *Cell, 175*(4), 962–972. DOI: 10.1016/j.cell.2018.10.029 PMID: 30388453

Watson, H., Mitra, S., Croden, F. C., Taylor, M., Wood, H. M., Perry, S. L., & Hold, G. L. (2018). A randomised trial of the effect of omega-3 polyunsaturated fatty acid supplements on the human intestinal microbiota. *Gut*, *67*(11), 1974–1983. DOI: 10.1136/gutjnl-2017-314968 PMID: 28951525

Williamson, G., & Clifford, M. N. (2017). Colonic metabolites of berry polyphenols: The missing link to biological activity? *British Journal of Nutrition*, *118*(4), 317–328. DOI: 10.1017/S0007114517001864 PMID: 20955650

Windey, K., De Preter, V., & Verbeke, K. (2012). Relevance of protein fermentation to gut health. *Molecular Nutrition & Food Research*, *56*(1), 184–196. DOI: 10.1002/mnfr.201100542 PMID: 22121108

Zawistowska-Rojek, A., & Zaręba, D. (2020). Food and supplement sources of probiotics and prebiotics. *Critical Reviews in Food Science and Nutrition*, *60*(1), 1–18. DOI: 10.1080/10408398.2019.1572683 PMID: 30277800

Zeevi, D., Korem, T., Zmora, N., Israeli, D., Rothschild, D., Weinberger, A., Ben-Yacov, O., Lador, D., Avnit-Sagi, T., Lotan-Pompan, M., Suez, J., Mahdi, J. A., Matot, E., Malka, G., Kosower, N., Rein, M., Zilberman-Schapira, G., Dohnalová, L., Pevsner-Fischer, M., & Segal, E. (2015). Personalized nutrition by prediction of glycemic responses. *Cell*, *163*(5), 1079–1094. DOI: 10.1016/j.cell.2015.11.001 PMID: 26590418

Zeevi, D., Korem, T., Zmora, N., Israeli, D., Rothschild, D., Weinberger, A., Ben-Yacov, O., Lador, D., Avnit-Sagi, T., Lotan-Pompan, M., Suez, J., Mahdi, J. A., Matot, E., Malka, G., Kosower, N., Rein, M., Zilberman-Schapira, G., Dohnalová, L., Pevsner-Fischer, M., & Segal, E. (2015). Personalized nutrition by prediction of glycemic responses. *Cell*, *163*(5), 1079–1094. DOI: 10.1016/j.cell.2015.11.001 PMID: 26590418

Zeevi, D., Korem, T., Zmora, N., Israeli, D., Rothschild, D., Weinberger, A., Ben-Yacov, O., Lador, D., Avnit-Sagi, T., Lotan-Pompan, M., Suez, J., Mahdi, J. A., Matot, E., Malka, G., Kosower, N., Rein, M., Zilberman-Schapira, G., Dohnalová, L., Pevsner-Fischer, M., & Segal, E. (2015). Personalized nutrition by prediction of glycemic responses. *Cell, 163*(5), 1079–1094. DOI: 10.1016/j.cell.2015.11.001 PMID: 26590418

Zeevi, D., Korem, T., Zmora, N., Israeli, D., Rothschild, D., Weinberger, A., Ben-Yacov, O., Lador, D., Avnit-Sagi, T., Lotan-Pompan, M., Suez, J., Mahdi, J. A., Matot, E., Malka, G., Kosower, N., Rein, M., Zilberman-Schapira, G., Dohnalová, L., Pevsner-Fischer, M., & Segal, E. (2015). Personalized nutrition by prediction of glycemic responses. *Cell, 163*(5), 1079–1094. DOI: 10.1016/j.cell.2015.11.001 PMID: 26590418

Zeevi, D., Korem, T., Zmora, N., Israeli, D., Rothschild, D., Weinberger, A., Ben-Yacov, O., Lador, D., Avnit-Sagi, T., Lotan-Pompan, M., Suez, J., Mahdi, J. A., Matot, E., Malka, G., Kosower, N., Rein, M., Zilberman-Schapira, G., Dohnalová, L., Pevsner-Fischer, M., & Segal, E. (2015). Personalized nutrition by prediction of glycemic responses. *Cell, 163*(5), 1079–1094. DOI: 10.1016/j.cell.2015.11.001 PMID: 26590418

Zhao, L., Zhang, F., Ding, X., Wu, G., Lam, Y. Y., Wang, X., & Zhao, Y. (2018). Gut bacteria selectively promoted by dietary fibers alleviate type 2 diabetes. *Science, 359*(6380), 1151–1156. DOI: 10.1126/science.aao5774 PMID: 29590046

Zimmermann, M. B., Chassard, C., Rohner, F., N'Goran, E. K., Nindjin, C., Dostal, A., Utzinger, J., Ghattas, H., Lacroix, C., & Hurrell, R. F. (2010). The effects of iron fortification on the gut microbiota in African children: A randomized controlled trial. *The American Journal of Clinical Nutrition, 92*(6), 1406–1415. DOI: 10.3945/ajcn.110.004564 PMID: 20962160

Zmora, N., Zeevi, D., Korem, T., Segal, E., & Elinav, E. (2019). Taking it personally: Personalized utilization of the human microbiome in health and disease. *Cell Host & Microbe, 25*(2), 324–330. DOI: 10.1016/j.chom.2019.01.017 PMID: 30763539

Zmora, N., Zeevi, D., Korem, T., Segal, E., & Elinav, E. (2019). Taking it personally: Personalized utilization of the human microbiome in health and disease. *Cell Host & Microbe, 25*(2), 324–330. DOI: 10.1016/j.chom.2019.01.017 PMID: 30763539

Zmora, N., Zeevi, D., Korem, T., Segal, E., & Elinav, E. (2019). Taking it personally: Personalized utilization of the human microbiome in health and disease. *Cell Host & Microbe, 25*(2), 324–330. DOI: 10.1016/j.chom.2019.01.017 PMID: 30763539

Zmora, N., Zeevi, D., Korem, T., Segal, E., & Elinav, E. (2019). Taking it personally: Personalized utilization of the human microbiome in health and disease. *Cell Host & Microbe*, *25*(2), 324–330. DOI: 10.1016/j.chom.2019.01.017 PMID: 30763539

Chapter 6
Microbial Metabolites and Their Role in Human Health

Sameel Hassan
https://orcid.org/0009-0001-7559-5550
University of Tuscia, Italy

Banzeer Ahsan Abbasi
https://orcid.org/0000-0003-3036-4481
Rawalpindi Women University, Pakistan

Wajeeha Zarwa
Quaid-i-Azam University, Islamabad, Pakistan

Tabassum Yaseen
Bacha Khan University, Charsadda, Pakistan

Maria Riaz
University of Agriculture, Faisalabad, Pakistan

Shumaila Ijaz
https://orcid.org/0009-0003-9614-9802
Shenzhen University, China

Muhammad Anas
https://orcid.org/0000-0001-5127-8043
Selçuk University, Turkey

Ayush Madan
https://orcid.org/0000-0001-5089-1794
People's University, India

Javed Iqbal
https://orcid.org/0000-0002-9032-2622
Bacha Khan University, Charsadda, Pakistan

ABSTRACT

Microbial metabolites are small molecules produced by microorganisms that have important effects on human health. Gut microbes synthesize different types of products from dietary fibers including SCFAs, vitamins, amino acids, neurotransmitters, antibiotics. Bacteria in digestive tract generate most of these substances when they

DOI: 10.4018/979-8-3373-4382-2.ch006

break up fiber and nutrient elements in food. Butyrate acetate and propionate as short-chain fatty acids safeguard digestive health through anti-inflammatory response and boost metabolic processes. The human body depends on vitamin B12 and vitamin K made by gut organisms to work properly. Some metabolites control mental health outcomes, fight microbes, destroy cancer cells. When gut microbiota changes because of bad eating habits and antibiotic use it will reduce beneficial product generation and result in weight problems, diabetes and neurological issues. This chapter explains the creation of microbial metabolites within the body plus their medical benefits and disease prevention methods.

TABLE OF CONTENTS

1. INTRODUCTION

In the human body, there are trillions of microorganisms, the so-called microbiota, which inhabit different bodily sites, such as the skin, mouth, respiratory tract, and most extensively, the gastrointestinal (GI) tract (Krautkramer et al., 2021). These microorganisms mainly bacteria but also include viruses, archaea and fungi have a dynamic relationship with its host which is mutualistic in nature. Among the most notable components of this relationship is the synthesis of the microbial-made metabolites, which are small, bioactive compounds created during the metabolic processes of microbes that have a dramatic effect on human physiology (Bhushan et al., 2019; Krautkramer et al., 2021).

The greatest quantity and diversity of microbial life occurs in the gastrointestinal tract, more commonly known as the gut, of the human body when compared to all other microbial habitats. This is because the gut microbiome is a powerful molecular workhouse with more than 100 trillion microbial cells, and thousands of other species. It acts more like a virtual organ and plays a vital role in digestion, immune modulation, and synthesis of nutrients and neurochemical communication. Microbial metabolites pose as the most worker of gut microbial action directing crosstalk among the gut and other owner systems, such as the immune, metabolic system as well as the nervous system (Noronha et al., 2019; Pires et al., 2024).

The microbial metabolites are more broadly classified into the primary and the secondary metabolites. Primary metabolites Components required by microbes to grow and include such compounds as short-chain fatty acids (SCFAs), vitamins and amino acids. The secondary metabolites, on the other hand, do not have direct relation to growth but have significant roles in microbe to microbe interaction and modulation by the host. These are alkaloids, bacteriocins, pigments and antibiotics. Both types of metabolites are essential players in the field of human health and the prevention of illness (Varshney et al., 2024).

Diet is a significant regulator of microbial metabolic products. Complex carbohydrates, polyphenols and fibers ingested by the host are also fermented by the microbiome within the colon, which results in the production of SCFAs such as butyrate, propionate, and acetate. These SCFAs promote the pH regulation of the colon, the growth of pathogenic bacteria, the enhancement of the intestinal barrier in addition to the regulation of inflammation. On the same note, the gut microbes also produce important vitamins like B-group vitamins and vitamin K which are critical to the process of energy metabolism, formation of red blood cells and coagulation (Zhang, 2022).

Moreover, the implications of microbial metabolites are vast as far as mental health and neurological performance are concerned. Gut-brain axis, the new domain of studies, revealed the role of metabolites, including gamma-aminobutyric acid (GABA), serotonin, and their derivatives, in the cognitive performance and mood stabilization, and even in neurodevelopment. Disturbances in the metabolite profiles of bacteria with an emphasis on psychiatrides and neurodegenerative disorders have been connected to several psychiatric and neurodegenerative disorders, such as anxiety, depression, and Parkinson disease (Maia et al., 2024).

The chapter also explores how microbial metabolites can be classified, how they are made and what is their physiological importance. It examines how they contribute to gut integrity, regulation of the immune system and to emotional health, as well as counteracting infections and neoplasia. The Presence of microbial imbalances and how they relate to the potential nutritional and medical interventions that could be used to utilize these powerful compounds to prevent disease and optimize human health are also discussed.

2. TYPES OF METABOLIC METABOLITES

Production of microbial metabolites, however, can be grouped into two major categories namely, primary metabolites and secondary metabolites. This is because of their functional roles in terms of microbial physiology and their effects on the host. Whereas primary metabolites are typically directly involved with the growth, development and reproduction of the microorganism, it is not part of the regulating or defensive response of the microorganism to the environment itself or the host organism (Thirumurugan et al., 2018).

2.1. Primary Metabolites

Primary metabolites are synthesized during the active growing period of microorganisms, and these metabolites, organic acids, amino acids, vitamins and short-chain fatty acids (SCFAs) are essential, not only to the survival of microorganisms but to the health of mankind as well. Among the SCFAs, there is a specific importance of acetate, propionate, and butyrate, due to the fact that the SCFAs are mostly produced in the gut by the fermentation of non-digestible carbohydrates, mostly dietary fibers by the gut bacteria (He et al., 2020). The most common SCFA is acetate which is transported into the blood stream to take part in cholesterol metabolism and lipogenesis. Propionate is mostly processed in liver and was associated with gluconeogenesis, as well as satiety signals. However, butyrate is the primary fuel of colonocytes and has strong anti-inflammatory and anticancer effects and is thus, essential in maintaining colonic health (Campos-Perez & Martinez-Lopez, 2021).

It is currently appreciated that a number of amino acids such as glutamate, lysine, and tryptophan are synthesized by the intestine microbial flora. Of these, tryptophan is of central importance to host neurophysiology since it is used to synthesize the two key molecules in the regulation of mood and immune responses, serotonin and kynurenine. Additionally, essential vitamins including vitamin B12 (cobalamin), biotin (B7), folate (B9), riboflavin (B2), and vitamin K are in part synthesized by microbes, which significantly enhances nutritional homeostasis of the host, especially in a susceptible population prone to dietary impoverishment or malabsorptive syndromes (Estrada & Contreras, 2019).

Further, hydrogen, lactate and succinate synthesis by microbes as intermediate products of metabolism further mediates the influence on the gut ecosystem with the pH, redox potential and competitive microbial interactions of the intestine. These primary metabolites may be significantly changed in both abundance and composition with microbial diversity, food sources and host genetics (Wang et al., 2020).

2.2. Secondary Metabolites

Secondary metabolites are normally produced when microbes are maintained in the stationary phase of growth and serve directly no role in the replication of cells. The compounds are, however, ecologically and therapeutically significant. Well-known instances are bacteriocins, non-ribosomal peptides, polyketides, alkaloids and phenazines. A big number of these molecules are either antimicrobial, immunomodulatory, or cytotoxic (Conrado et al., 2022).

Bacteriocins are produced ribosomally by microorganisms and have either a narrow spectrum or broad-spectrum antimicrobial effect, commonly employed by the bacteria in order to prevent the growth of competing organisms. Their production also adds to the gut microbial homeostasis and has the ability to inhibit pathogenic residence. Some of the most famous producers of bacteriocins with prospective probiotic use are the lactic acid bacteria such as Lactobacillus or Enterococcus (Anjana & Tiwari, 2022).

Streptomyces and other actinomycetes produce non-ribosomal peptides and polyketides which are the major building block of antibiotics, e.g., erythromycin, tetracycline, and rifamycin. Even though it was first identified in the microorganisms of soil, the bacteria that inhabits the gut can also possess genes coding to similar bioactive compounds indicating an untapped potential in terms of therapeutic agents. Other secondary metabolites have antitumor potential in addition to antimicrobial effect (Lozenov et al., 2023). An example of this is a metabolite commonly known as butyrate, which despite being a primary metabolite also demonstrates histone deacetylase inhibitor and may induce cancer cell growth arrest and apoptosis. Other secondary metabolites such as indole derivatives and phenazines regulate the immune responses of the host, oxidative stress pathways and cellular signalling pathways (Anwer et al., 2025).

Table 1. Classification of microbiota-derived primary and secondary metabolites, highlighting their microbial sources and key roles in human health. The table outlines crucial functions such as energy production, anti-inflammatory effects, immune modulation, lipid metabolism, and neurological regulation, emphasizing the metabolic versatility of gut microbes.

Type	Metabolite	Microbial Source	Function in Human Health	Citation
Primary Metabolite	Acetate	*Bacteroides, Firmicutes*	Energy source, lipid synthesis	(Yu et al., 2019)
	Propionate	*Bacteroides, Veillonella*	Glucose regulation, satiety	(Zhang & Huang, 2023)
	Butyrate	*Faecalibacterium, Roseburia*	Colonocyte fuel, anti-inflammatory	(Salvi & Cowles, 2021)
	Vitamin B12	*Propionibacterium, E. coli*	RBC formation, neurological function	(Tripathi et al., 2024)
	Folate (B9)	*Lactobacillus, Bifidobacterium*	DNA synthesis, methylation	(D'Aimmo et al., 2023)
	Biotin (B7)	*Bacteroides, Lactobacillus*	Fatty acid synthesis, enzyme cofactor	(Hossain et al., 2022)
	Riboflavin (B2)	*Bifidobacterium*	Redox reactions, energy production	(Solopova et al., 2020)
	Tryptophan derivatives	*Clostridium, Bacteroides*	Serotonin precursor, mood regulation	(Zhou et al., 2023)
	Indole-3-propionic acid	*Clostridium sporogenes*	Neuroprotection, antioxidant	(Li et al., 2024)
	SCFA (general)	Diverse anaerobes	Gut health, immune modulation	(Liu et al., 2023)
Secondary Metabolite	Bacteriocins	*Lactobacillus, Enterococcus*	Inhibits pathogens, maintains microbial balance	(Almeida-Santos et al., 2021)
	Reuterin	*Lactobacillus reuteri*	Broad-spectrum antimicrobial	(Niamah et al., 2020)
	Indole derivatives	*Bacteroides, Clostridium*	Immune modulation, epithelial protection	(Ye et al., 2022)
	Non-ribosomal peptides	*Streptomyces*, gut actinomycetes	Antibiotic, antitumor activity	(Rui et al., 2025)
	Polyketides	*Streptomyces*	Antibacterial, antifungal	(Risdian et al., 2019)
	Phenazines	*Pseudomonas spp.*	Redox-active, antimicrobial	(Kang et al., 2022)
	Conjugated linoleic acid	*Lactobacillus, Propionibacteria*	Anti-inflammatory, lipid regulation	(Salsinha et al., 2018)
	Secondary bile acids	*Clostridium, Bacteroides*	Host metabolism, receptor signaling	(Ramírez-Pérez et al., 2018)
	Urolithins	Polyphenol-converting bacteria	Antioxidant, anticancer	(Ercolini & Fogliano, 2018)

3. HOW MICROBIAL METABOLITES ARE PRODUCED

The production of microbial metabolites is a multigene reaction to environmental signals that are complex and tightly regulated, the production of which is made by microbial (largely bacterial) metabolism as they cooperate with one another based on diet input, micro-interaction, and in response to host accommodations. In the human gut (where host-microbe symbiosis is very integrated) the nature, structure and composition of the diet as the most significant control of biosynthesis by the microbes is the significant single regulator of the metabolic output (Du et al., 2025).

At the biochemical level, metabolites of microbes are created in the lower gastrointestinal system when dietary macronutrients that would not have been digested in the upper gastrointestinal system, that is undigested complex carbohydrates, proteins and lipids, are fermented. They ferment these substrates at the level of the colon using some of the microbial consortia. An example is that the species in phylum firmicutes (*Faecalibacterium prausnitzii* and *Eubacterium rectale*) are more skilled butyrate producers through acetyl-CoA or butyryl-CoA pathway, and Bacteroidetes species produce predominantly acetate and propionate via succinate or acrylate pathway (Oliphant & Allen-Vercoe, 2019).

Most fermentation activities on fibers are saccharolytic fermentation, on resistant starches and oligosaccharides. These intricate polysaccharides must subsequently require the enzymes they require to hydrolyse them, and these may or may not be grouped in so-called polysaccharide utilization loci (PULs). They are particularly abundant in Bacteroides species where they enable them to degrade an extremely wide and vast number of plant and host glycans. The ferment end products are monosaccharides that are further catalyzed by the addition of SCFAs and gaseous products such as hydrogen, methane and carbon dioxide (Cheng et al., 2022).

Proteolytic fermentation The escaped proteins degrade by proteolysis in the microbes of special interest to specific gut microbes and synthesise branched-chain fatty acids, ammonia, phenolic compounds and indole derivatives. Although neuroprotective and anti-inflammatory properties of production of some of such products, such as indole-3-propionic acid, are proven, the nature of some of the others, such as hydrogen sulfide and p-cresol, can be toxic, at least, when produced in large amounts. The shape and proportion of species of microorganisms thus determines which net effect will be left behind the protein fermentation be it positive or negative (Korpela, 2018).

Though it has been noted that gut microbiota controls the rate of lipid metabolism to a significant extent, this area of study is not very well studied yet. Specifically, one of such mechanisms is the conversion of bile acids and cholesterol by them. The bile acids that are produced by the liver and sent to the intestine will be discovered undergoing some chemical modification by the utilization of enzymes that belong to microbes that include bile salt hydrolase, 7a dehydroxylases. These secondary bile acids, produced as byproducts, e.g., deoxycholic acid and lithocholic acid affect the bile acid absorption, the receptor activity of essential bile acids, as well as systemic metabolism signaling pathways, and, as a result, once again the lipid homeostasis of the host, its inflammation, and intestinal homeostasis (Collins et al., 2023).

Vitamin synthesis is a significant feature of micro biology through which vitamin precursors in food can be converted to bio active vitamins. The most excellent one is that of the folate (vitamin B9) whose type Lactobacillus and Bifidobacterium species manufacture but when exposed to certain anaerobic conditions, cobalamin (vitamin B12) is produced by the Escherichia coli. The strong association of this metabolic process with microbial carriers is reflected in the observation that in most cases, biosynthetic gene clusters (BGCs) encoding the biochemical and regulation of the pathways necessary to produce the metabolite are also available (Das et al., 2019).

They typically respond to environmental stress, interspecies competition or quorum-sensing signals that cause them to produce secondary metabolites (Anas et al., 2025)

. When these stimuli bind, they induce the expression of inactive gene clusters in microbial genome that make structurally diverse pharmacologically active compounds. The recent developments of metagenomics and metabolomics revealed an immense amount of cryptic gene clusters in the worlds of gut microbial communities, and this reality states that there is much to be learned that has never been characterised under metabolites (Begani et al., 2018).

4. BENEFITS FOR GUT HEALTH

Microbiome contribute in integrity of gastrointestinal physiology in the sense that this phenomenon has capacity of offering metabolites that have been thought to be the main actants of this regulation. These metabolites have a direct activity with the components of the epithelial, immunological and neural components of the gut lumen and therefore physiological state is controlled. Among some of the known roles, there is the sustenance of the integrity of the intestinal barrier, regulation of inflammatory and safeguarding against pathogens. Among the microbial products of metabolism which have been discovered to exert an influence on gut health, the most thoroughly understood are the short-chain fatty acids (SCFAs) with their major actors being butyrate, acetate, and propionate which occupy much of the activity of the SCFAs (Gasaly, De Vos, et al., 2021).

4.1. Short-Chain Fatty Acids

The end-products of fermentation of carbohydrate indigestible to the microbiota are short-chain fatty acids (SCFAs), local energy sources increased with the necessities to act as modulators. There appeared to be large concentrations of acetate, propionate and butyrate in luminal colonic contents but butyrate qualifies as pre eminent position in colonic environment as key source of colonic- epithelial cells energy. Butyrate is the key factor in epithelial homeostasis and inhibitor of progression of dysplastic epithelial growth and is the only microecologic molecule to alter the energy metabolism and level of oxidative stress in the colon of colonocytes (Gasaly, Hermoso, et al., 2021).

SCFAs are powerful against inflammatory. To illustrate the case, butyrate inhibits the signaling of nuclear factor-kappa B (NF-kB) and promotes differentiation of regulatory T-cell (Treg) through histone deacetylase (HDAC) black. The properties enhance immune tolerance, and decrease long-term inflammatory diseases such as ulcerative colitis, Crohn disease and colorectal cancer. Propionate and acetate also possess anti-inflammatory properties and appetite, glucose homeostasis and lipid metabolism regulate the G-protein-coupled receptors (GPR) including GPR41 and GPR43 on intestinal and immune cells (Li et al., 2018).

Microbial fermentation of the indigestible components of the dietary fiber generates SCFA, which controls the gut ecosystem, as they reduce the pH of the gut lumen. This acidifies to the extent that it discourages growth of some pathogenic species which do not grow so well under low acidity levels but on the other hand it encourages the growth of both the desirable anaerobic strains of the microbes. This reduction of luminal pH serves further to increase the solubility of the minerals and as calcium and magnesium get absorbed more, this process has a fortifying effect on the bones and the net impact on the metabolism (Huang et al., 2023).

4.2. Gut Barrier Protection

The intestinal barrier consists of the monolayer of the epithelial cell that is compounded due to tight junctions and further the act of protection with mucus and secretory immunoglobulin A (IgA). The metabolite products of the intestinal microbiota, especially butyrate, increase tight junction proteins such as claudins and occludin and, thereby, enhances epithelial strength. The mechanism decreases intestinal permeability or what people tend to call leaky gut, which is directly associated with systemic inflammation, metabolic syndrome, and maladaptations in the immunoregulation field. Concurrently butyrate and other short-chain fatty acids enhance mucin secretion by the secretory cells (goblet cells) thus establishing the mucus layer constituting both a physical seclusion to pathogens and a niche in which commensal microorganisms specializing in mucin degradation proliferate over and thus ensure a high mucus turnover (Salvi & Cowles, 2021).

Besides structural and functional roles, the molecules of the metabolites that are made by microbes stimulate the release of antimicrobial peptides (AMPs) by Paneth cells. These AMPs differentiate between pathogens and commensals, thus leading to microbial homeostasis. Meanwhile, the short-chain fatty acids (SCFAs) stimulate IgA production in part of the lymphoid tissue in the presence of the gutt (GALT) that reinforces the immunological storage process and defends itself against the invading bacteria and viruses (Ma & Ma, 2019).

5. IMMUNE SYSTEM SUPPORT

Microbial metabolites play an essential role in the functioning of the human immune system, on local and systemic scales, as both a means of ensuring immune homeostasis of stomach fluid and to attempt to elicit immune reactions against pathogens. The human body has just about 70 percent of all immune cells in the gut, which is the largest immune organ. The bi-directional relationship between the immune components of the host and the gut microbiota is central to the balance of the tolerance predisposition to commensal microbes and robust immune response to the hazardous overcomers. Studies on the best known microbial metabolites, which have an impressive role in the coordination of this method, are short-chain fatty acids (SCFAs), tryptophan metabolites, and secondary bile acids (Wang et al., 2023).

Figure 1. Microbial metabolites modulate immune responses: Key compounds such as butyrate, propionate, acetate, indole derivatives, and bile acid metabolites enhance mucosal immunity, promote regulatory T cells, stimulate IL-22, and balance Th17/Treg activity, contributing to immune homeostasis

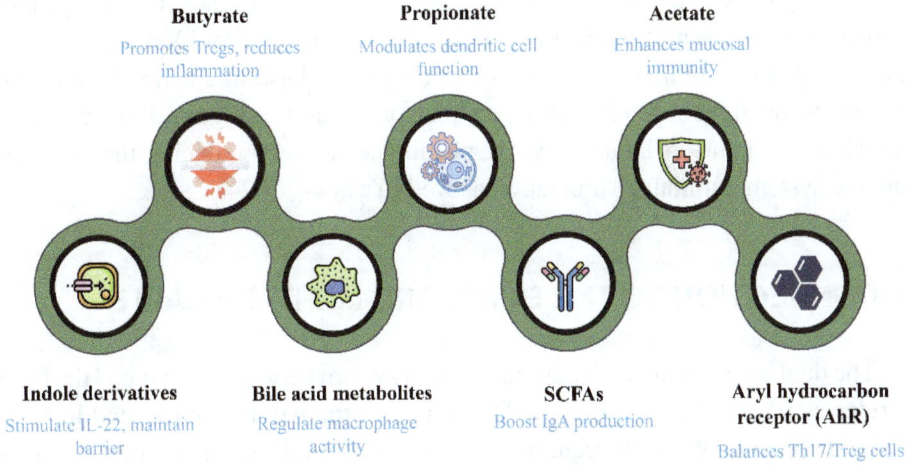

Examples of SCFAs that influence the behaviour of immune cells include butyrate, propionate and acetate. The well-known activity of SCFAs is histone acetyltransferases (HAT) that alters the way that genes are read through favoring or discouraging the expression of the genes of immune cells by suppressing histone deacetylases (HDACs)(Ratajczak et al., 2019). It is established that such epigenetic regulation is biased towards the development of naive T cells into regulatory T cells (Tregs), which in turn prevent the development of unwanted pathological overreactivity of the immune system, and thus prevent it with autoimmune diseases. Yet, butyrate supplementation has been shown to increase Treg in the intestine and, therefore, safeguard against experimental colitis in mice (Lv et al., 2025).

In dendritic cells, SCFAs mediated the synthesis of cytokines by inhibiting the pro-inflammatory factors like IL-6, IL-12 and TNF -alpha as well as stimulating the anti-inflammatory type of cytokines IL-10. This creates tolerogenic immune milieu in the bowel. G-protein coupled receptor (GPCR) such as GPR41, GPR43 and GPR109A located on immune cells are also sensitive to the SCFAs as they trigger cascades of signals that affect the migration of cells, release of cytokines and cell phagocytosis (Parada Venegas et al., 2019).

Besides SCFAs, dietary tryptophan apparently is converted by the microbes to form indole derivates, indole-3-aldehyde and indole-3 propionic acid. These chemicals are AhR ligands which are transcription factors, mounted on various immune cells. The activation of AhR leads to the production of interleukin-22 (IL-22) and increases epithelial barrier activity and release antimicrobial peptides thus providing mucosal immunity. The necessity of having a stable Th17/Treg immune system with the gut has also prompted indole metabolites to be implicated in the same (Li, 2023).

The other set of immune regulatory metabolic interventions involves bile acids, which are produced by the microbiome. The secondary bile acids like deoxycholic acid and lithocholic acid interact with nuclear receptors farnesoid X receptor (FXR) and Takeda G protein-coupled receptor 5 (TGR5). These interactions inhibit the signal transductions of pro-inflammatory phenotypes and reprogram the macrophage polarization to anti-inflammatory M2 phenotypes thereby reducing the intestinal and the systemic immune stimulation as well (Ye et al., 2024).

6. CONNECTION TO THE BRAIN AND MENTAL HEALTH

The dual interaction of the communication system between the gut and the brain is referred to as the gut-brain axis. The neural, hormonal, metabolic, and immune system is also between the central nervous system and the gastrointestinal tract. Most potent potential mediators of this axis are molecules produced by microbes, which influence the condition of the brain and psychological status through multiple mechanisms, including those involving modification of neurotransmitter synthesis, immune signaling, and activation of the vagus nerve (Arneth, 2018).

The microbial metabolites produced as part of the indole biosynthesis of tryptophan are one of the most studied forms of microbial metabolites pertaining to this area of concern. Tryptophan is essential amino acids and it is used in the production of serotonin which is one of the most vital neurotransmitters in regards to mood regulation, cognition and sleep. Even though a small percentage of serotonin is synthesized in the brain, the remaining 90 percent is synthesized in the principal by enterochromaffin cells within the gob through the process of conversion regulated by gut microbiota. The intake of tryptophan may be altered according to the concentration of some bacteria like Bifidobacterium and Lactobacillus which is able to induce tryptophan into serotonin and kynurenine compounds. These metabolites, separately, affect the signaling of the neurons, inflammation and neurogenesis (Waclawiková & El Aidy, 2018).

There are also some influences of the indol derivates such as the indole-3-propionic acid, and the indole-3 acetic acid that affect the brain. Indole-3-propionic acid is an example that exhibits neuroprotective effect because it reduces the level of oxidative stress and amyloid-beta aggregation which is a process mediated by diseases of neurodegeneration like Alzheimer s disease. Other indole compounds may mediate the effect of the activity of the microbes and the functioning of immune system in the brain by activation of microglia and control of production of cytokines in the brain (Konopelski & Mogilnicka, 2022).

Figure 2. Microbial metabolites and their neurological functions: Key compounds such as serotonin, indole-3-propionic acid, butyrate, and GABA influence brain activity through pathways that regulate mood, cognition, neuroprotection, neuroinflammation, and stress

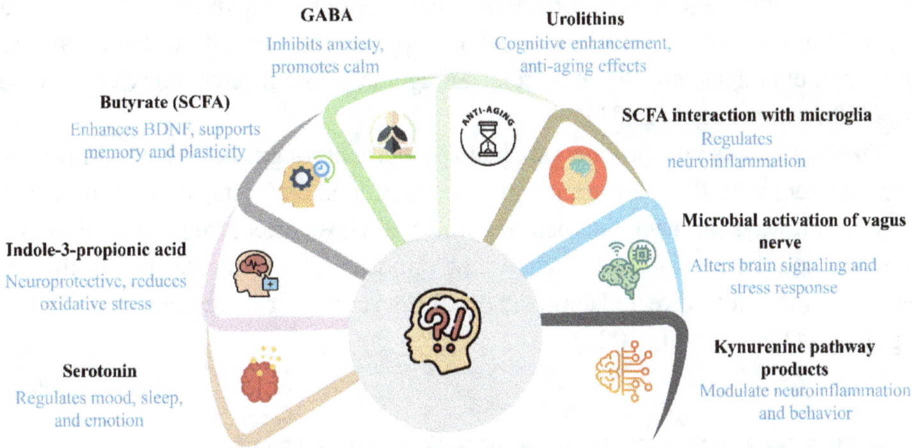

The SCFA short-chain fatty acids (SCFAs) (principally, butyrate and propionate) come across the blood-brain barrier and occupy neuroactive effects. Butyrate is a histone deacetylase (HDAC) inhibitor that can affect expression of genes in the brain, butyrate has been reported to increase synaptic plasticity, benefit memory formation, and lead to an antidepressant-like behavior in preclinical experiments. SCFAs have also been shown to regulate the secretion of the neurotrophic factor of brain (BDNF), which is a significant molecule in neuronal survival and plasticity (Alpino et al., 2024).

The resemblance of the manufacturing of both communications paths is the vagus nerve, which goes straight between the gut and the brain. The vagal afferents may be stimulated by microbial metabolites, resulting in adjustment of the central nervous system activities. As an example, in studies of animals, the intake of Lactobacillus rhamnosus has been linked to a decrease in anxiety and depression-like behaviors, which are eliminated upon a cut in the vagus nerve, evidence that shows that vagal pathways are involved in mediating microbiota-guided neurobehavioral consequences (Longo et al., 2023).

Besides, the systemic inflammatory and immune signaling modulated by microorganisms indirectly influence the health of the brain. Among other attributes, mood disorders like depression are often characterized by chronic low-grade inflammation and increased concentrations of pro-inflammatory cytokines. Microbial metabolites which antagonize this inflammatory burden to restore the balance of communication between immune systems and the human brain include SCFAs and secondary bile acids that encourage anti-inflammation (Patil et al., 2025).

The human studies continue to prove the gut-brain connection. Numerous psychiatric and neurological syndromes, such as depression and anxiety, autism spectrum disorder, and multiple sclerosis, have been associated with dysbiosis. The changes in microbial composition are frequently associated with changes in the fecal and serum metabolite profile and this fact supports the suggestion that microbial-generated chemicals are the most relevant agents of brain physiology (Averina et al., 2020; Morais et al., 2021).

Therefore, microbial products are main participants of gut-brain communication. They interact with the neurotransmitter production and effects, alter neuroinflammatory pathways, and activate neural pathways whose effects are mood, thinking, and conduct. These findings provide new opportunities in mental health therapy by using microbiota-directed approaches, like psychobiotics, prebiotics, and dietary regulation (Verma et al., 2024).

7. ROLE IN MAKING VITAMINS AND NUTRIENTS

The ability of the gut microbiota helps in producing some essential vitamins and nutrients that are vital to a human being, and this is an important but neglected role of the microbiota (Hossain et al., 2022). Besides providing supplementary nutrition of diet sources, these microbially produced compounds are essential in many body processes and include important energy metabolism in cells, red blood cell production, immune protection, and sex-related roles in blood coagulation. These vitamins have their biosynthesis concentrated in the colon a place where high population density of the microbes has the genetic and enzyme assembly to transform dietary precursors into the bioavailable form (Wan et al., 2022).

One of the most famous microbially produced vitamins is the vitamins of B-complex group. A number of species belonging to the Bacteroides, Lactobacillus and Bifidobacterium genera have been reported to be involved in the synthesis of folate (vitamin B9), biotin (B7), riboflavin (B2), pyridoxine (B6) and, pantothenic acid (B5) (Hrubša et al., 2022; Wang et al., 2021). These vitamins have been found as coenzymes in many of the metabolic pathways such as fatty acid synthesis, nucleotide and neurotransmitter synthesis. As an illustration, folate facilitates DNA repair and methylation and neural tube defects and cognitive impairments are related to deficiency. Riboflavin and niacin are also part of redox reactions and the energy metabolism in the mitochondrion (Mikkelsen & Apostolopoulos, 2019).

However, Vitamin B12 (cobalamin) is produced by a smaller number of microbes such as some anaerobic bacteria such as Propionibacterium and Lactobacillus reuteri. The human body does not produce this vitamin and it has to depend on external means. Even though B12 production by microbes primarily occurs in the colon, which is distal to the best location of absorption of B12 in the small intestine ileum, it could still play an indirect role by keeping the microbial community competitive and the ecosystem stable. Furthermore, the corrinoid compounds, through microbial synthesis, which are B12 analogs, can have regulatory roles in a microbial community and host signaling (Qi et al., 2023).

Another vital nutrient that is synthesized by the gut bacteria is the vitamin K especially the menaquinones (vitamin K2). The production involves Escherichia coli and a number of species of Bacteroides and Enterococcus. Vitamin K2 is also a key element in blood coagulation as a cofactor of the gamma-carboxylation of factors that mediate blood clotting. It also plays a role in strengthening the bones by controlling the lodging of calcium and osteocalcin stimulation (Camelo-Castillo et al., 2021).

Besides vitamins, there are other bioactive nutrients biosynthesized in the gut by microbes. As an example, conjugated linoleic acids (CLAs) which are formed during the isomerization of dietary polyunsaturated fatty acids by the microbes are anti-inflammatory and exert cholesterol-lowering effects. It is also reported that gut microbes produce key amino acids such as tryptophan and glutamine, which are precursors of neurotransmitters and immune regulators (Ma & Ma, 2019).

Nutrient synthesis by microbes is not a homogenous process and it is very dependent on the character of the microbiota and on availability of substrates. As an example, diets which contain insufficient fibre or contain excess processed food do not always contain the precursors required by microbes to produce the vitamins. Furthermore, taking antibiotics that are broad-spectrum may greatly upset the microbial world, disturbing the production process of such vital compounds and resulting in temporary insufficiencies, particularly of B vitamins (Kolodziejczyk et al., 2019).

Remarkably, there are also vitamin-producing probiotic strains that are specially chosen because of this. As an example, Lactobacillus plantarum and Bifidobacterium bifidum are well known producers of folate and they were used in fortified food and supplements to enhance nutritional results. The possibility of designing gut microbes to increase production of endogenous vitamins via synthetic biology or selective enrichment is also becoming a popular research angle with regards to solving malnutrition, particularly among one of the more vulnerable groups (Elazzazy et al., 2025; Patra, 2024).

8. ANTIMICROBIAL AND ANTICANCER EFFECTS

In addition to their use in metabolism and nutrition, microbial metabolites are also strong bioactive compounds that act as antimicrobial and anticancer agents. The gut microbes use these compounds (especially secondary metabolites) to form niches through oppression of rivals and pathogens. At the same time, they also play a part in host defense collective actions and modulate cell signaling pathways of tumor promotion and cell death. The twofold activity of these metabolites highlights their medicinal value in the treatment of infections and the prevention or abating of cancer advancement (Hashem, 2025).

Bacteriocins One of the most investigated antimicrobial microbial metabolites are the bacteriocins which are ribosomally produced peptides synthesized by different intestinal bacteria including members of Lactobacillus, Enterococcus and Bacillus. These peptides have been shown to have targeted killing mechanism, in the sense that they stimulate membrane disruption in competing microbes, or cannot allow them to complete key metabolic pathways (Bisht et al., 2024). Bacteriocins have the ability to resist major common intestinal diseases such as Clostridium difficile, Salmonella, and Listeria monocytogenes, which help maintain a balance between microbes and avoid excessive multiplication of dangerous ones. They are good subjects to be applied in probiotic products and food preservation due to their specificity and safety profile (O'Connor et al., 2020; Shafique et al., 2022).

Short chain fatty acids (SCFAs) and especially butyrate also have antimicrobial actions, butyric action is mainly acidification of the colon. SCFAs reduce the luminal pH to levels unfavorable to most pathogenic bacteria whereas the acid-tolerant beneficial species are favored. Butyrate has been demonstrated to have inhibiting capabilities on E. coli O157:HG and Salmonella enterica among others. Moreover, SCFAs have the ability to augment host defense via inducing antimicrobial peptide (AMP) production, as well as reinforcing the epithelial barrier, thus restricting the pathogen translocation across the intestinal lining (Li et al., 2022).

Microbial metabolites have also become key relevants in cancer defense with butyrate once again taking the center stage. Butyrate is a histone deacetylase (HDAC) inhibitor that affects the gene expression by mediating alterations in chromatin structure. This may cause cellular arrest of the cell cycle, apoptosis and decrease proliferation of the cancer cells (Chen et al., 2019). The key to chemoprevention of colorectal cancer using butyrate is its selective cytotoxicity against transformed colonocytes, and its promotion of normal epithelial differentiation. This has been backed by epidemiological studies whereby colorectal cancer was observed to have lower incidence in populations with high intake of dietary fiber which has been associated with increased butyrate production (Singh et al., 2025).

Additional anticancerous microbial metabolites are indole derivatives (metabolites of tryptophan), secondary bile acids (which have complicated context-dependent effects) and piscicides, reuterin (broad-salvage antimicrobial produced by Lactobacillus reuteri). Reuterin can prevent the growth of gram positive and negative bacteria and has been found to have cytotoxic effects on tumor cells due to the creation of reactive oxygen species (ROS) (Pattnaik et al., 2022). Moreover, metabolites that can be anti-inflammatory and antiproliferative may be formed by microbial metabolism of polyphenols and flavonoids, which are plant-derived substances contained in the diet. As an example, ellagic acid is degraded by microbes to produce urolithins, which are demonstrated to inhibit tumor growth and regulate pathways that lead to cancer development (Nakkarach et al., 2021).

Innovative approaches to the treatment of cancer include the therapeutic potential of metabolites that are produced by microbes. Recent developments in metagenomics and metabolomics, however, are starting to allow researchers to define tumor suppressing or promoting microbial signatures. Manipulation of the microbiome via probiotic, prebiotic, or fecal microbiota transplantation (FMT) has the potential to increase the endogenous supply of beneficial metabolites and decrease the levels of unfriendly ones (Mafe & Büsselberg, 2025).

9. HEALTH PROBLEMS LINKED TO MICROBIAL IMBALANCE

Optimum production of healthy microbial metabolites depends on having a balanced and diverse gut microbiota. Nevertheless, interference with this fragile ecosystem called dysbiosis may lead to dramatic reduction of the production of healthy compounds such as SCFAs, vitamins and anti-inflammatory metabolites. The causes of dysbiosis are such factors as poor food habits, regular intake of antibiotics, infections, chronic inflammation, and exposure to environmental toxins. The result of this alteration in microbial composition is frequently to shift the balance between commensal and the potentially helpful species in favor of pathogenic or opportunistic types, and this sets up a cascade of metabolic and immune disturbances (Das & Nair, 2019).

The gastrointestinal malfunction is one of the most immediate outcomes of microbial unfavorability: it includes such conditions as the inflammatory bowel disease (IBD), irritable bowel syndrome (IBS) and colorectal cancer. Epithelial barrier defects in IBD are characterized by reduced abundance of bacteria that produce butyrate, which increases intestinal permeability and improves intestinal inflammation. Equally, decreased production of indole derivatives by the microbes in the mucosal region compromises mucosal immunity, and increasing load of detrimental metabolism like hydrogen sulfide production and phenolic compounds enhances tissue injury (Chelakkot et al., 2018; Stolfi et al., 2022).

In addition to the gut, dysbiosis has been associated with other systemic diseases. Abnormal SCFA profiles and the elevated endotoxin load were closely associated with such metabolic disorders as insulin resistance, obesity, and type 2 diabetes. Neurological and psychiatric disorders (e.g. depression, autism spectrum disorder, and Parkinson disease) have also been linked to compromised gut-brain axis communication due to a lack of microbial metabolites conversion. These observations need to be highlighted; they are the importance of microbial metabolites in systemic homeostasis and the necessity of intervention strategies partially involving reestablishing microbiota balance (Kandpal et al., 2022; Sun & Shen, 2018).

10. MEDICAL AND DIETARY APPLICATIONS

The therapeutic relevance of microbial metabolites has led to growing interest in using dietary and clinical interventions to modulate their production. By promoting beneficial gut microbes through targeted strategies, such as dietary fiber enrichment, probiotic supplementation, and prebiotic intake, healthcare practitioners aim to restore optimal metabolite profiles. These approaches can help rebalance SCFA levels, reinforce intestinal barrier function, enhance vitamin biosynthesis, and suppress pro-inflammatory pathways. Clinically, therapies like fecal microbiota transplantation (FMT), metabolite-based supplements, and microbiome-targeted drugs are being explored for treating a broad range of disorders, from gastrointestinal inflammation to metabolic and neurological conditions (Missiego-Beltrán & Beltrán-Velasco, 2024).

10.1. Probiotics and Prebiotics

Probiotics and prebiotics offer practical tools to enhance microbial metabolite production and restore gut homeostasis. Probiotics introduce live beneficial bacteria that produce SCFAs, vitamins, and antimicrobial peptides, thereby improving gut integrity and immune modulation. Prebiotics, on the other hand, selectively fuel these probiotic strains by providing fermentable substrates such as inulin, galactooligosaccharides (GOS), and resistant starches. The combined use of both—synbiotics—has shown promise in boosting butyrate levels, enhancing mucosal immunity, and alleviating symptoms of gastrointestinal and metabolic disorders.

10.2. Future Uses in Medicine

Emerging medical applications are focused on designing next-generation therapeutics based on microbial metabolite pathways. These include engineered probiotics that deliver targeted metabolites, precision nutrition plans to shape the gut metabolome, and metabolite-based diagnostics for early disease detection. Advances in metagenomics and metabolomics now allow for personalized interventions, where specific microbial metabolites can be manipulated to manage chronic diseases such as cancer, diabetes, and neurodegeneration, signaling a shift toward microbiome-informed precision medicine.

11. CONCLUSION

Microbial metabolites serve as a critical link between the human host and its gut microbiota, influencing nearly every aspect of health—from digestion and immunity to brain function and disease resistance. These bioactive compounds, including short-chain fatty acids, vitamins, amino acids, neurotransmitter precursors, and antimicrobial agents, arise primarily from microbial fermentation of dietary substrates. Their functions extend far beyond the gut, regulating systemic inflammation, modulating neural circuits, and protecting against chronic diseases such as obesity, diabetes, cancer, and neurodegeneration.

Disruption of the gut microbial ecosystem—whether through poor dietary habits, antibiotic use, or illness—can significantly impair the production of these vital metabolites, leading to metabolic imbalances, immune dysregulation, and heightened disease risk. Restoring this balance through diet, probiotics, prebiotics, and emerging postbiotic therapies represents a promising frontier in personalized and preventive healthcare. With advancing tools in metabolomics and microbial genomics, future research will continue to uncover new metabolites, pathways, and therapeutic applications that harness the power of the human microbiome. Ultimately, a deeper understanding of microbial metabolites offers not only insights into fundamental human biology but also novel strategies to improve health outcomes through microbiota-centered interventions.

REFERENCES

Almeida-Santos, A. C., Novais, C., Peixe, L., & Freitas, A. R. (2021). Enterococcus spp. as a producer and target of bacteriocins: A double-edged sword in the antimicrobial resistance crisis context. *Antibiotics (Basel, Switzerland)*, *10*(10), 1215. DOI: 10.3390/antibiotics10101215 PMID: 34680796

Alpino, G. C. Á., Pereira-Sol, G. A., Dias, M. M., Aguiar, A. S., & Peluzio, M. C. G. (2024). Beneficial effects of butyrate on brain functions: A view of epigenetic. *Critical Reviews in Food Science and Nutrition*, *64*(12), 3961–3970. DOI: 10.1080/10408398.2022.2137776 PMID: 36287024

Anas, M., Khattak, W. A., Fahad, S., Alrawiq, N., Alrawiq, H. S., Abdelsalam, N. R., Jaremko, M., & Quraishi, U. M. (2025). Mitigating heavy metal pollution in agriculture: A multi-omics and nanotechnology approach to safeguard global wheat production. *Journal of Hazardous Materials Advances*, *17*, 100584. https://doi.org/https://doi.org/10.1016/j.hazadv.2024.100584. DOI: 10.1016/j.hazadv.2024.100584

Anjana, a., & Tiwari, S. K. (2022). Bacteriocin-producing probiotic lactic acid bacteria in controlling dysbiosis of the gut microbiota. *Frontiers in Cellular and Infection Microbiology, 12*, 851140.

Anwer, E. K., Ajagbe, M., Sherif, M., Musaibah, A. S., Mahmoud, S., ElBanbi, A., & Abdelnaser, A. (2025). Gut microbiota secondary metabolites: Key roles in GI tract cancers and infectious diseases. *Biomedicines*, *13*(1), 100. DOI: 10.3390/biomedicines13010100 PMID: 39857684

Arneth, B. M. (2018). Gut–brain axis biochemical signalling from the gastrointestinal tract to the central nervous system: Gut dysbiosis and altered brain function. *Postgraduate Medical Journal*, *94*(1114), 446–452. DOI: 10.1136/postgradmedj-2017-135424 PMID: 30026389

Averina, O. V., Zorkina, Y. A., Yunes, R. A., Kovtun, A. S., Ushakova, V. M., Morozova, A. Y., Kostyuk, G. P., Danilenko, V. N., & Chekhonin, V. P. (2020). Bacterial metabolites of human gut microbiota correlating with depression. *International Journal of Molecular Sciences*, *21*(23), 9234. DOI: 10.3390/ijms21239234 PMID: 33287416

Begani, J., Lakhani, J., & Harwani, D. (2018). Current strategies to induce secondary metabolites from microbial biosynthetic cryptic gene clusters. *Annals of Microbiology*, *68*(7), 419–432. DOI: 10.1007/s13213-018-1351-1

Bhushan, B., Singh, B. P., Saini, K., Kumari, M., Tomar, S. K., & Mishra, V. (2019). Role of microbes, metabolites and effector compounds in host–microbiota interaction: A pharmacological outlook. *Environmental Chemistry Letters*, *17*(4), 1801–1820. DOI: 10.1007/s10311-019-00914-9

Bisht, V., et al. (2024). Understanding of probiotic origin antimicrobial peptides: a sustainable approach ensuring food safety. *npj Science of Food*, *8*(1), 67.

Camelo-Castillo, A., Rivera-Caravaca, J. M., Orenes-Piñero, E., Ramírez-Macías, I., Roldán, V., Lip, G. Y. H., & Marín, F. (2021). Gut microbiota and the quality of oral anticoagulation in vitamin K antagonists users: A review of potential implications. *Journal of Clinical Medicine*, *10*(4), 715. DOI: 10.3390/jcm10040715 PMID: 33670220

Campos-Perez, W., & Martinez-Lopez, E. (2021). Effects of short chain fatty acids on metabolic and inflammatory processes in human health. *Biochimica et Biophysica Acta (BBA)-. Biochimica et Biophysica Acta. Molecular and Cell Biology of Lipids*, *1866*(5), 158900. DOI: 10.1016/j.bbalip.2021.158900 PMID: 33571672

Chelakkot, C., Ghim, J., & Ryu, S. H. (2018). Mechanisms regulating intestinal barrier integrity and its pathological implications. *Experimental & Molecular Medicine*, *50*(8), 1–9. DOI: 10.1038/s12276-018-0126-x PMID: 30115904

Chen, J., Zhao, K.-N., & Vitetta, L. (2019). Effects of intestinal microbial–elaborated butyrate on oncogenic signaling pathways. *Nutrients*, *11*(5), 1026. DOI: 10.3390/nu11051026 PMID: 31067776

Cheng, J., Hu, J., Geng, F., & Nie, S. (2022). Bacteroides utilization for dietary polysaccharides and their beneficial effects on gut health. *Food Science and Human Wellness*, *11*(5), 1101–1110. DOI: 10.1016/j.fshw.2022.04.002

Collins, S. L., Stine, J. G., Bisanz, J. E., Okafor, C. D., & Patterson, A. D. (2023). Bile acids and the gut microbiota: Metabolic interactions and impacts on disease. *Nature Reviews. Microbiology*, *21*(4), 236–247. DOI: 10.1038/s41579-022-00805-x PMID: 36253479

Conrado, R., Gomes, T. C., Roque, G. S. C., & De Souza, A. O. (2022). Overview of bioactive fungal secondary metabolites: Cytotoxic and antimicrobial compounds. *Antibiotics (Basel, Switzerland)*, *11*(11), 1604. DOI: 10.3390/antibiotics11111604 PMID: 36421247

D'Aimmo, M. R.. (2023). Folate-producing bifidobacteria: Metabolism, genetics, and relevance. *Microbiome Research Reports*, *3*(1), 11. PMID: 38455078

Das, B., & Nair, G. B. (2019). Homeostasis and dysbiosis of the gut microbiome in health and disease. *Journal of Biosciences*, *44*(5), 117. DOI: 10.1007/s12038-019-9926-y PMID: 31719226

Das, P., Babaei, P., & Nielsen, J. (2019). Metagenomic analysis of microbe-mediated vitamin metabolism in the human gut microbiome. *BMC Genomics*, *20*(1), 208. DOI: 10.1186/s12864-019-5591-7 PMID: 30866812

Du, W., Zou, Z.-P., Ye, B.-C., & Zhou, Y. (2025). Gut microbiota and associated metabolites: Key players in high-fat diet-induced chronic diseases. *Gut Microbes*, *17*(1), 2494703. DOI: 10.1080/19490976.2025.2494703 PMID: 40260760

Elazzazy, A. M., Baeshen, M. N., Alasmi, K. M., Alqurashi, S. I., Desouky, S. E., & Khattab, S. M. R. (2025). Where Biology Meets Engineering: Scaling up microbial nutraceuticals to bridge nutrition, therapeutics, and global impact. *Microorganisms*, *13*(3), 566. DOI: 10.3390/microorganisms13030566 PMID: 40142459

Ercolini, D., & Fogliano, V. (2018). Food design to feed the human gut microbiota. *Journal of Agricultural and Food Chemistry*, *66*(15), 3754–3758. DOI: 10.1021/acs.jafc.8b00456 PMID: 29565591

Estrada, J. A., & Contreras, I. (2019). Nutritional modulation of immune and central nervous system homeostasis: The role of diet in development of neuroinflammation and neurological disease. *Nutrients*, *11*(5), 1076. DOI: 10.3390/nu11051076 PMID: 31096592

Gasaly, N., de Vos, P., & Hermoso, M. A. (2021). Impact of bacterial metabolites on gut barrier function and host immunity: A focus on bacterial metabolism and its relevance for intestinal inflammation. *Frontiers in Immunology*, *12*, 658354. DOI: 10.3389/fimmu.2021.658354 PMID: 34122415

Gasaly, N., Hermoso, M. A., & Gotteland, M. (2021). Butyrate and the fine-tuning of colonic homeostasis: Implication for inflammatory bowel diseases. *International Journal of Molecular Sciences*, *22*(6), 3061. DOI: 10.3390/ijms22063061 PMID: 33802759

Hashem, Z. S. (2025). Bacterial Metabolites in Defense: A Crucial Aspect of Microbial Interaction and Host Protection. In *Metabolic Dynamics in Host-Microbe Interaction* (pp. 101-120). Springer. DOI: 10.1007/978-981-96-1305-2_5

He, J., Zhang, P., Shen, L., Niu, L., Tan, Y., Chen, L., Zhao, Y., Bai, L., Hao, X., Li, X., Zhang, S., & Zhu, L. (2020). Short-chain fatty acids and their association with signalling pathways in inflammation, glucose and lipid metabolism. *International Journal of Molecular Sciences, 21*(17), 6356. DOI: 10.3390/ijms21176356 PMID: 32887215

Hossain, K. S., Amarasena, S., & Mayengbam, S. (2022). B vitamins and their roles in gut health. *Microorganisms, 10*(6), 1168. DOI: 10.3390/microorganisms10061168 PMID: 35744686

Hrubša, M., Siatka, T., Nejmanová, I., Vopršalová, M., Kujovská Krčmová, L., Matoušová, K., Javorská, L., Macáková, K., Mercolini, L., Remião, F., Máťuš, M., & Mladěnka, P. (2022). Biological properties of vitamins of the B-complex, part 1: Vitamins B1, B2, B3, and B5. *Nutrients, 14*(3), 484. DOI: 10.3390/nu14030484 PMID: 35276844

Huang, S.-C., He, Y.-F., Chen, P., Liu, K.-L., & Shaukat, A. (2023). Gut microbiota as a target in the bone health of livestock and poultry: Roles of short-chain fatty acids. *Animal Diseases, 3*(1), 23. DOI: 10.1186/s44149-023-00089-5

Kandpal, M., Indari, O., Baral, B., Jakhmola, S., Tiwari, D., Bhandari, V., Pandey, R. K., Bala, K., Sonawane, A., & Jha, H. C. (2022). Dysbiosis of gut microbiota from the perspective of the gut–brain axis: Role in the provocation of neurological disorders. *Metabolites, 12*(11), 1064. DOI: 10.3390/metabo12111064 PMID: 36355147

Kang, J., Cho, Y.-H., & Lee, Y. (2022). Pyocyanin and 1-Hydroxyphenazine promote anaerobic killing of Pseudomonas aeruginosa via single-electron transfer with ferrous iron. *Microbiology Spectrum, 10*(6), e02312–e02322. DOI: 10.1128/spectrum.02312-22 PMID: 36321913

Kolodziejczyk, A. A., Zheng, D., & Elinav, E. (2019). Diet–microbiota interactions and personalized nutrition. *Nature Reviews. Microbiology, 17*(12), 742–753. DOI: 10.1038/s41579-019-0256-8 PMID: 31541197

Konopelski, P., & Mogilnicka, I. (2022). Biological effects of indole-3-propionic acid, a gut microbiota-derived metabolite, and its precursor tryptophan in mammals' health and disease. *International Journal of Molecular Sciences, 23*(3), 1222. DOI: 10.3390/ijms23031222 PMID: 35163143

Korpela, K. (2018). Diet, microbiota, and metabolic health: Trade-off between saccharolytic and proteolytic fermentation. *Annual Review of Food Science and Technology, 9*(1), 65–84. DOI: 10.1146/annurev-food-030117-012830 PMID: 29298101

Krautkramer, K. A., Fan, J., & Bäckhed, F. (2021). Gut microbial metabolites as multi-kingdom intermediates. *Nature Reviews. Microbiology*, *19*(2), 77–94. DOI: 10.1038/s41579-020-0438-4 PMID: 32968241

Li, L., Yang, C., Jia, M., Wang, Y., Zhao, Y., Li, Q., Gong, J., He, Y., Xu, K., Liu, X., Chen, X., Hu, J., & Liu, Z. (2024). Synbiotic therapy with Clostridium sporogenes and xylan promotes gut-derived indole-3-propionic acid and improves cognitive impairments in an Alzheimer's disease mouse model. *Food & Function*, *15*(15), 7865–7882. DOI: 10.1039/D4FO00886C PMID: 38967039

Li, M., van Esch, B. C. A. M., Henricks, P. A. J., Folkerts, G., & Garssen, J. (2018). The anti-inflammatory effects of short chain fatty acids on lipopolysaccharide-or tumor necrosis factor α-stimulated endothelial cells via activation of GPR41/43 and inhibition of HDACs. *Frontiers in Pharmacology*, *9*, 533. DOI: 10.3389/fphar.2018.00533 PMID: 29875665

Li, S. (2023). Modulation of immunity by tryptophan microbial metabolites. *Frontiers in Nutrition*, *10*, 1209613. DOI: 10.3389/fnut.2023.1209613 PMID: 37521424

Li, S., Heng, X., Guo, L., Lessing, D. J., & Chu, W. (2022). SCFAs improve disease resistance via modulate gut microbiota, enhance immune response and increase antioxidative capacity in the host. *Fish & Shellfish Immunology*, *120*, 560–568. DOI: 10.1016/j.fsi.2021.12.035 PMID: 34958920

Liu, X., Shao, J., Liao, Y.-T., Wang, L.-N., Jia, Y., Dong, P., Liu, Z., He, D., Li, C., & Zhang, X. (2023). Regulation of short-chain fatty acids in the immune system. *Frontiers in Immunology*, *14*, 1186892. DOI: 10.3389/fimmu.2023.1186892 PMID: 37215145

Longo, S., Rizza, S., & Federici, M. (2023). Microbiota-gut-brain axis: Relationships among the vagus nerve, gut microbiota, obesity, and diabetes. *Acta Diabetologica*, *60*(8), 1007–1017. DOI: 10.1007/s00592-023-02088-x PMID: 37058160

Lozenov, S., Krastev, B., Nikolaev, G., Peshevska-Sekulovska, M., Peruhova, M., & Velikova, T. (2023). Gut microbiome composition and its metabolites are a key regulating factor for malignant transformation, metastasis and antitumor immunity. *International Journal of Molecular Sciences*, *24*(6), 5978. DOI: 10.3390/ijms24065978 PMID: 36983053

Lv, J., Hao, P., Zhou, Y., Liu, T., Wang, L., Song, C., Wang, Z., Liu, Z., & Liu, Y. (2025). Role of the intestinal flora-immunity axis in the pathogenesis of rheumatoid arthritis-mechanisms regulating short-chain fatty acids and Th17/Treg homeostasis. *Molecular Biology Reports*, *52*(1), 1–11. DOI: 10.1007/s11033-025-10714-w PMID: 40544212

Ma, N., & Ma, X. (2019). Dietary amino acids and the gut-microbiome-immune axis: Physiological metabolism and therapeutic prospects. *Comprehensive Reviews in Food Science and Food Safety*, *18*(1), 221–242. DOI: 10.1111/1541-4337.12401 PMID: 33337014

Mafe, A. N., & Büsselberg, D. (2025). The Effect of Microbiome-Derived Metabolites in Inflammation-Related Cancer Prevention and Treatment. *Biomolecules*, *15*(5), 688. DOI: 10.3390/biom15050688 PMID: 40427581

Maia, J. M., Solon, I. G., Soriano, R. N., & Branco, L. G. S. (2024). Exploring the links between pro-inflammatory diets, gut dysbiosis, serotonin, and their implications for psychiatric and neurodegenerative disorders. *Brain Behavior and Immunity Integrative*, *8*, 100097. DOI: 10.1016/j.bbii.2024.100097

Mikkelsen, K., & Apostolopoulos, V. (2019). B vitamins and ageing. *Biochemistry and cell biology of ageing: Part I biomedical science*, 451-470.

Missiego-Beltrán, J., & Beltrán-Velasco, A. I. (2024). The Role of Microbial Metabolites in the Progression of Neurodegenerative Diseases—Therapeutic Approaches: A Comprehensive Review. *International Journal of Molecular Sciences*, *25*(18), 10041. DOI: 10.3390/ijms251810041 PMID: 39337526

Morais, L. H., Schreiber, H. L.IV, & Mazmanian, S. K. (2021). The gut microbiota–brain axis in behaviour and brain disorders. *Nature Reviews. Microbiology*, *19*(4), 241–255. DOI: 10.1038/s41579-020-00460-0 PMID: 33093662

Nakkarach, A., Foo, H. L., Song, A. A.-L., Mutalib, N. E. A., Nitisinprasert, S., & Withayagiat, U. (2021). Anti-cancer and anti-inflammatory effects elicited by short chain fatty acids produced by Escherichia coli isolated from healthy human gut microbiota. *Microbial Cell Factories*, *20*(1), 36. DOI: 10.1186/s12934-020-01477-z PMID: 33546705

Niamah, A. K., Abdulmuttaleb, A. M., & Hussain, N. A. (2020). Antibacterial spectrum of produced reuterin from new isolates of Lactobacillus reuteri. *Journal of Microbiology, Biotechnology and Food Sciences*, *10*(1), 134–139. DOI: 10.15414/jmbfs.2020.10.1.134-139

Noronha, A., Modamio, J., Jarosz, Y., Guerard, E., Sompairac, N., Preciat, G., Daníelsdóttir, A. D., Krecke, M., Merten, D., Haraldsdóttir, H. S., Heinken, A., Heirendt, L., Magnúsdóttir, S., Ravcheev, D. A., Sahoo, S., Gawron, P., Friscioni, L., Garcia, B., Prendergast, M., & Thiele, I. (2019). The Virtual Metabolic Human database: Integrating human and gut microbiome metabolism with nutrition and disease. *Nucleic Acids Research*, *47*(D1), D614–D624. DOI: 10.1093/nar/gky992 PMID: 30371894

O'Connor, P. M., Kuniyoshi, T. M., Oliveira, R. P. S., Hill, C., Ross, R. P., & Cotter, P. D. (2020). Antimicrobials for food and feed; a bacteriocin perspective. *Current Opinion in Biotechnology*, *61*, 160–167. DOI: 10.1016/j.copbio.2019.12.023 PMID: 31968296

Oliphant, K., & Allen-Vercoe, E. (2019). Macronutrient metabolism by the human gut microbiome: Major fermentation by-products and their impact on host health. *Microbiome*, *7*(1), 91. DOI: 10.1186/s40168-019-0704-8 PMID: 31196177

Parada Venegas, D., De la Fuente, M. K., Landskron, G., González, M. J., Quera, R., Dijkstra, G., Harmsen, H. J. M., Faber, K. N., & Hermoso, M. A. (2019). Short chain fatty acids (SCFAs)-mediated gut epithelial and immune regulation and its relevance for inflammatory bowel diseases. *Frontiers in Immunology*, *10*, 277. DOI: 10.3389/fimmu.2019.00277 PMID: 30915065

Patil, S., & Mehdi, S. F. S. (2025). The Gut-Brain Axis and Mental Health: How Diet Shapes Our Cognitive and Emotional Well-Being. *Cureus*, *17*(7). Advance online publication. DOI: 10.7759/cureus.88420 PMID: 40842787

Patra, D. (2024). Synthetic biology-enabled engineering of probiotics for precision and targeted therapeutic delivery applications. *Exon*, *1*(2), 54–66. DOI: 10.69936/en11y0024

Pattnaik, S., Imchen, M., Kumavath, R., Prasad, R., & Busi, S. (2022). Bioactive microbial metabolites in cancer therapeutics: Mining, repurposing, and their molecular targets. *Current Microbiology*, *79*(10), 300. DOI: 10.1007/s00284-022-02990-7 PMID: 36002695

Pires, L., Gonzalez-Paramás, A. M., Heleno, S. A., & Calhelha, R. C. (2024). Gut microbiota as an endocrine organ: Unveiling its role in human physiology and health. *Applied Sciences (Basel, Switzerland)*, *14*(20), 9383. DOI: 10.3390/app14209383

Qi, X., Zhang, Y., Zhang, Y., Luo, F., Song, K., Wang, G., & Ling, F. (2023). Vitamin B12 produced by Cetobacterium somerae improves host resistance against pathogen infection through strengthening the interactions within gut microbiota. *Microbiome*, *11*(1), 135. DOI: 10.1186/s40168-023-01574-2 PMID: 37322528

Ramírez-Pérez, O.. (2018). The role of the gut microbiota in bile acid metabolism. *Annals of Hepatology*, *16*(1), 21–26.

Ratajczak, W., Rył, A., Mizerski, A., Walczakiewicz, K., Sipak, O., & Laszczyńska, M. (2019). Immunomodulatory potential of gut microbiome-derived short-chain fatty acids (SCFAs). *Acta Biochimica Polonica*, *66*(1), 1–12. DOI: 10.18388/abp.2018_2648 PMID: 30831575

Risdian, C., Mozef, T., & Wink, J. (2019). Biosynthesis of polyketides in Streptomyces. *Microorganisms*, *7*(5), 124. DOI: 10.3390/microorganisms7050124 PMID: 31064143

Rui, S., Fengrui, G., Yining, Z., Hong, S., Xuewen, Y., Changping, W., & Chunjia, Y. (2025). Biological activity of secondary metabolites of actinomycetes and their potential sources as antineoplastic drugs: A review. *Frontiers in Microbiology*, *16*, 1550516. DOI: 10.3389/fmicb.2025.1550516 PMID: 40406345

Salsinha, A. S., Pimentel, L. L., Fontes, A. L., Gomes, A. M., & Rodríguez-Alcalá, L. M. (2018). Microbial production of conjugated linoleic acid and conjugated linolenic acid relies on a multienzymatic system. *Microbiology and Molecular Biology Reviews : MMBR*, *82*(4), 00019–00018. DOI: 10.1128/MMBR.00019-18 PMID: 30158254

Salvi, P. S., & Cowles, R. A. (2021). Butyrate and the intestinal epithelium: Modulation of proliferation and inflammation in homeostasis and disease. *Cells*, *10*(7), 1775. DOI: 10.3390/cells10071775 PMID: 34359944

Shafique, B., Ranjha, M. M. A. N., Murtaza, M. A., Walayat, N., Nawaz, A., Khalid, W., Mahmood, S., Nadeem, M., Manzoor, M. F., Ameer, K., Aadil, R. M., & Ibrahim, S. A. (2022). Recent trends and applications of nanoencapsulated bacteriocins against microbes in food quality and safety. *Microorganisms*, *11*(1), 85. DOI: 10.3390/microorganisms11010085 PMID: 36677377

Singh, V., Shirbhate, E., Kore, R., Vishwakarma, S., Parveen, S., Veerasamy, R., Tiwari, A. K., & Rajak, H. (2025). Microbial metabolites-induced epigenetic modifications for inhibition of colorectal cancer: Current status and future perspectives. *Mini-Reviews in Medicinal Chemistry*, *25*(1), 76–93. DOI: 10.2174/01138955753 20344240625080555 PMID: 38982701

Solopova, A., Bottacini, F., Venturi degli Esposti, E., Amaretti, A., Raimondi, S., Rossi, M., & van Sinderen, D. (2020). Riboflavin biosynthesis and overproduction by a derivative of the human gut commensal Bifidobacterium longum subsp. infantis ATCC 15697. *Frontiers in Microbiology*, *11*, 573335. DOI: 10.3389/fmicb.2020.573335 PMID: 33042083

Stolfi, C., Maresca, C., Monteleone, G., & Laudisi, F. (2022). Implication of intestinal barrier dysfunction in gut dysbiosis and diseases. *Biomedicines*, *10*(2), 289. DOI: 10.3390/biomedicines10020289 PMID: 35203499

Sun, M.-F., & Shen, Y.-Q. (2018). Dysbiosis of gut microbiota and microbial metabolites in Parkinson's Disease. *Ageing Research Reviews*, *45*, 53–61. DOI: 10.1016/j.arr.2018.04.004 PMID: 29705121

Thirumurugan, D., et al. (2018). An introductory chapter: secondary metabolites. *Secondary metabolites-sources and applications, 1*, 13.

Tripathi, A., Pandey, V. K., Panesar, P. S., Taufeeq, A., Mishra, H., Rustagi, S., Malik, S., Kovács, B., Suthar, T., & Shaikh, A. M. (2024). Fermentative production of vitamin B12 by Propionibacterium shermanii and Pseudomonas denitrificans and its promising health benefits: A review. *Food Science & Nutrition, 12*(11), 8675–8691. DOI: 10.1002/fsn3.4428 PMID: 39619983

Varshney, N.. (2024). Significance of microbial biomolecules, secondary metabolites, and their impact on the diverse aspects of human health. In *Industrial microbiology and biotechnology: an insight into current trends* (pp. 99–127). Springer. DOI: 10.1007/978-981-97-1912-9_6

Verma, A., Inslicht, S. S., & Bhargava, A. (2024). Gut-brain axis: Role of microbiome, metabolomics, hormones, and stress in mental health disorders. *Cells, 13*(17), 1436. DOI: 10.3390/cells13171436 PMID: 39273008

Waclawiková, B., & El Aidy, S. (2018). Role of microbiota and tryptophan metabolites in the remote effect of intestinal inflammation on brain and depression. *Pharmaceuticals (Basel, Switzerland), 11*(3), 63. DOI: 10.3390/ph11030063 PMID: 29941795

Wan, Z., Zheng, J., Zhu, Z., Sang, L., Zhu, J., Luo, S., Zhao, Y., Wang, R., Zhang, Y., Hao, K., Chen, L., Du, J., Kan, J., & He, H. (2022). Intermediate role of gut microbiota in vitamin B nutrition and its influences on human health. *Frontiers in Nutrition, 9*, 1031502. DOI: 10.3389/fnut.2022.1031502 PMID: 36583209

Wang, J., Zhu, N., Su, X., Gao, Y., & Yang, R. (2023). Gut-microbiota-derived metabolites maintain gut and systemic immune homeostasis. *Cells, 12*(5), 793. DOI: 10.3390/cells12050793 PMID: 36899929

Wang, S. P., Rubio, L. A., Duncan, S. H., Donachie, G. E., Holtrop, G., Lo, G., Farquharson, F. M., Wagner, J., Parkhill, J., Louis, P., Walker, A. W., & Flint, H. J. (2020). Pivotal roles for pH, lactate, and lactate-utilizing bacteria in the stability of a human colonic microbial ecosystem. *mSystems, 5*(5), 00645–00620. DOI: 10.1128/mSystems.00645-20 PMID: 32900872

Wang, Y., Liu, L., Jin, Z., & Zhang, D. (2021). Microbial cell factories for green production of vitamins. *Frontiers in Bioengineering and Biotechnology, 9*, 661562. DOI: 10.3389/fbioe.2021.661562 PMID: 34222212

Ye, D., He, J., & He, X. (2024). The role of bile acid receptor TGR5 in regulating inflammatory signalling. *Scandinavian Journal of Immunology, 99*(4), e13361. DOI: 10.1111/sji.13361 PMID: 38307496

Ye, X., Li, H., Anjum, K., Zhong, X., Miao, S., Zheng, G., Liu, W., & Li, L. (2022). Dual role of indoles derived from intestinal microbiota on human health. *Frontiers in Immunology, 13*, 903526. DOI: 10.3389/fimmu.2022.903526 PMID: 35784338

Yu, C., Liu, S., Chen, L., Shen, J., Niu, Y., Wang, T., Zhang, W., & Fu, L. (2019). Effect of exercise and butyrate supplementation on microbiota composition and lipid metabolism. *The Journal of Endocrinology, 243*(2), 125–135. DOI: 10.1530/JOE-19-0122 PMID: 31454784

Zhang, P. (2022). Influence of foods and nutrition on the gut microbiome and implications for intestinal health. *International Journal of Molecular Sciences, 23*(17), 9588. DOI: 10.3390/ijms23179588 PMID: 36076980

Zhang, S.-M., & Huang, S.-L. (2023). The commensal anaerobe Veillonella dispar reprograms its lactate metabolism and short-chain fatty acid production during the stationary phase. *Microbiology Spectrum, 11*(2), e03558–e03522. DOI: 10.1128/spectrum.03558-22 PMID: 36975840

Zhou, M., Fan, Y., Xu, L., Yu, Z., Wang, S., Xu, H., Zhang, J., Zhang, L., Liu, W., Wu, L., Yu, J., Yao, H., Wang, J., & Gao, R. (2023). Microbiome and tryptophan metabolomics analysis in adolescent depression: Roles of the gut microbiota in the regulation of tryptophan-derived neurotransmitters and behaviors in human and mice. *Microbiome, 11*(1), 145. DOI: 10.1186/s40168-023-01589-9 PMID: 37386523

Chapter 7
Microbiota in Food Sensitivities and Allergies

B. Lokeshwari
https://orcid.org/0009-0005-6612-5134
Department of Microbiology, Sacred Heart College, Tirupattur, India

K. Gayathri
https://orcid.org/0009-0007-3786-2009
Department of Microbiology, Sacred Heart College, Tirupattur, India

P. Saranraj
https://orcid.org/0000-0002-5052-6532
Department of Microbiology, Sacred Heart College, Tirupattur, India

K. Kesavardhini
https://orcid.org/0009-0005-8235-042X
Department of Microbiology, Sacred Heart College, Tirupattur, India

K. Arthi
Department of Microbiology, Sacred Heart College, Tirupattur, India

M. Manigandan
https://orcid.org/0000-0002-8115-2713
Department of Microbiology, Sacred Heart College, Tirupattur, India

ABSTRACT

Food allergy is known to result due to a highly intricate interplay between food antigens, host immunity, and intestinal microbe composition. Imbalances in these factors could result in hypersensitivity. Pathways in food allergy include alterations in epithelial cell/tissue regeneration, along with improper immunity against food antigens, which leads to a boosted T-helper cell type 2 (Th2) response. Intestinal epithelial cells, which include stem cells, Paneth cells, mucus secreting goblet cells, and tuft cells, have been analyzed in terms of epithelial integrity. Inclusion of intestinal microbe composition also discovers gut microbe roles in epithelial cell/pathophysiology, which underlines short-chain fatty acid-mediated functions, microbial lactate, which points to other microbe metabolites. Inclusion of gut mi-

DOI: 10.4018/979-8-3373-4382-2.ch007

crobe composition on gut epithelial cell/pathophysiology also underlines microbe functions in maintaining epithelial cell/pathophysiology, clues of which include microbe-mediated secure functioning of tight junction proteins.

1. INTRODUCTION

The human digestive tract also holds a complex population of microorganisms termed the human gut microbiota, comprising bacteria, viral, and eukaryotic organisms. These microbes have a wide array of physiological roles, which are essential in human physiology and health; hence, they biosynthesize important vitamin compounds and ferment non-digestible carbohydrates. Bacteria from the phyla Firmicutes and Bacteroidetes predominantly comprise the gut microbiota, while the less predominant ones are from phyla Actinobacteria and Verrucomicrobia. Food allergy constitutes a major concern both in the medical and general community, with a prevalence rate of up to 10% of the entire population in the United States of America (Ansaldo et al., 2021). IgE-mediated food allergy entails a detrimental health effect triggered by a particular immune response, which is regularly observed after measurable exposure to a distinct food.

Food Allergy is an immune-mediated disorder that appears repeatedly due to hypersensitivity to various allergens and can result in life-threatening reactions (Khan et al., 2022). About 10% of children and 4% of adults worldwide experience food allergies. These constitute one aspect of growing concerns in global health. Some clinical symptoms of food allergies include atopic dermatitis, vomiting, diarrhea. Sometimes food allergy results in life-threatening anaphylactic shock and even death. Some most common food allergens include shellfish, peanuts, soy foods, eggs, milk from cows, and shellfish (Wiersinga et al., 2020). The intestinal wall framework and the molecular reaction of the pro-inflammatory response caused by the admission of bacterial invaders due to enhanced permeability are some important factors in the development of immune responses. Exercise-related physical factors also affect permeability.

Certain diets and low-to-moderate-intensity exercise have been suggested as non-pharmacological treatments to assist preserve the integrity of the gut wall (Warren et al., 2020). Some therapeutic approaches address the gut microbiome to treat food allergies and associated disorders (Zimmermann et al., 2023). Probiotics, prebiotics, synbiotics, and Fecal Microbiota Transplantation (FMT) are a few of them. FMT consists of the transfer of microbiota from a healthy donor to a patient, intended to restore balance and relieve discomfort. Dysbiosis has also been shown to contribute to other conditions, like Irritable Bowel Syndrome (IBS), in which barrier defects and antimicrobial peptides/Toll-Like Receptors are upregulated (Wong et al., 2024).

2. MECHANISMS OF FOOD ALLERGY

2.1 Regulation of allergen uptake

Microfold (M) cells that carries allergens to Dendritic Cells (DCs) and other Antigen-Presenting Cells when they are activated by microbial signals. Additionally, the microbiota regulates the intake of allergens by promoting goblet cells to make mucus and Paneth cells to produce antimicrobial peptides (Muthukumar et al., 2020). Notably, CX3CR1+ cells are putative macrophages that are usually present in the intestinal lamina propria and are mainly involved in the uptake of allergens from the intestinal lumen. Nevertheless, these cells move in reaction to alterations in the composition of the gut microbiota, which lowers the absorption of allergens. By interacting with DCs, the intestinal microbiota can indirectly improve intestinal barrier integrity and control the intake of dietary allergens.

2.2 Regulation of signalling molecules involved in immune responses

Intestinal microbiota-derived metabolites play a crucial role in regulating immune responses and facilitating host communication. Short-chain fatty acids (SCFAs) promote the differentiation of Th0 cells into Foxp3+ regulatory T (Treg) cells through interactions with dendritic cells (DCs) via G-protein coupled receptors (GPRs). Clostridium strains reduce allergene sensitivity by modulating the permeability and innate lymphoid cells' functions. Foxp3+ Treg cells play crucial roles in immunological tolerance by modulating B cells to secrete IgA/IgG4, which further inhibits the functions and activities of the Th2 cells and their related cytokines. Pattern Recognition Receptors (PRRs), including Toll-Like Receptors (TLRs), play a critical part in the regulation of the immune system to food allergy by recognizing viral elements and inducing the inflammatory response (Perrier et al., 2011). TLR signaling further enhances the secretion of cytokines by different innate cells to safeguard the body from allergy. In addition to the previous mechanisms, the Aryl Hydrocarbon Receptor (AHR) signaling mechanism is critical for the regulation of the secretion of IL-22; however, the secretion of IL-22 is down-regulated due to the knockout of the AHR mechanism since AHR signaling enhances the secretion of CD103+ DCs and levels of food allergene tolerance by promoting the immune system's balance by adjusting the activities of the innate immune cells within the body by balancing the microbial signal for homeostatic feedback regulation between tolerance and sensitivity.

2.3 T Helper 2 (TH2) Cell–Mediated Food Allergy

TSLP, IL-25, and IL-33 are produced when pathogens like helminths and PAMPs such bacterial TLR2 ligands stimulate or activate IECs. This leads to damaged barriers, facilitating TH2 cell-mediated immunity (Esterházy et al., 2019). However, there is the helminth *Heligmosomoides polygyrus* can suppress food allergies through an IL-10-mediated pathway that efficiently suppresses TH2 cell responses. Mast cell granule-releasers release a variety of inflammatory mediators, including histamine and the cytokines TNF-α, IL-4, IL-13, and IL-6. Additionally, these products decrease the intestinal walls' ability to function. These products make up the helminth-stimulated TH2 cell response, along with the systemic levels of helminth antigen-stimulated IgE and IgG1 (Khodoun et al., 2018). Thus, colonization by the fungal pathogen *Candida albicans* has been found in murine studies to facilitate the passage of oral antigens through the gastrointestinal system, a mechanism mediated by the colonization-induced mucosal influx and mast cell degranulation. This represents the TH2 cell immune response provided by the microbes. In this case, it drives the progress of food allergy (Kayama et al., 2020). In Fig. 1, the mechanisms by which the gut microbial flora regulates the function of the barriers by ensuring the enhancement of epithelial barriers and the modulation or management of the immune pathway signals.

Figure 1. Gut Microbiota in Immune Tolerance and Allergic Inflammation via Intestinal Barrier Modulation

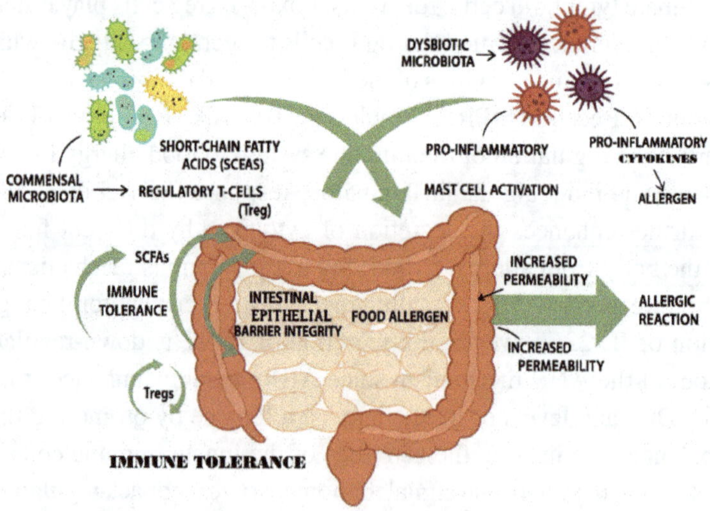

3. INTESTINAL EPITHELIAL CELLS AND BARRIER FUNCTION

Intestinal epithelial cells (IECs) form a selective barrier maintained by tight junction proteins like occludin and claudin, while mucins, the main components of the mucus barrier, are O-linked glycoproteins. Glycan-defective animals show increased intestinal permeability and altered microbiota, leading to higher susceptibility to Inflammatory Bowel Disease (IBD). The gut microbiota thrives in the mucus layer, which, influenced by dietary fibers, can thin out during fiber absence, allowing bacterial infiltration (Slifer et al., 2020). The Muc2 mutation in Immune signaling, genetics, and gut health intricately regulate mucus barrier maintenance, with dysregulated responses potentially predating intestinal inflammation (Turner et al., 2009).

3.1 Intestinal Barrier–Gut Microbiota Interactions

The gut microbiota plays a crucial role in regulating host physiology and immunity through food component metabolism and metabolite production. Dietary fiber, mainly from plant polysaccharides, supports gut flora, which ferment this fiber into Short-Chain Fatty Acids (SCFAs) like acetate, butyrate, and propionate. SCFAs regulate both mucosal and systemic immune functions, enhancing intestinal IgA responses via GPR43 and influencing bone marrow hematology through GPR41 (Bloemendaal et al., 2016). Butyrate is vital for Treg cell induction and immunological tolerance to dietary allergens through GPR109a. Intestinal epithelial cells engage with SCFAs via G-protein coupled receptors (GPRs) to activate inflammatory pathways and stimulate barrier defenses, including mucin production and tight junction protein expression. Gut microbiota also help enforce mucosal tolerance by modulating dendritic cell (DC) functions and promoting Treg development, thus maintaining gut health and homeostasis (Farin et al., 2016).

3.2 Features of subgroups of intestinal epithelial cells

The intestinal epithelium consists of specialized cells with distinct roles: enteroendocrine cells release hormones for gut regulation, microfold cells transport antigens, goblet cells produce mucins for a protective mucus layer, tuft cells detect helminths and trigger immune responses, paneth cells secrete antimicrobial peptides, and absorptive cells (enterocytes) are responsible for nutrient and water absorption (Koo et al., 2012, Shroyer et al., 2007).

3.2.1 Intestinal Stem Cells

Intestinal Stem Cells (ISCs) are the thin, undifferentiated cells that coexist with Paneth cells at the base of the crypts; this area is known as the crypt base columnar cells. All epithelial cell lineages, including as enterocytes, goblet cells, enteroendocrine cells, Paneth cells, and tuft cells, are produced by these intestinal stem cells via a hierarchy of proliferative transit-amplifying cells. The small intestinal crypt as a classic model for studying adult stem cell biology, characterized by continuous, rapid turnover driven by a resident stem cell population (Clevers and Bevins et al., 2013). LGR5+ cells divide quickly for epithelial renewal under normal conditions, while these cells are triggered by stress to replace intestinal cells that have been destroyed. These cell types are balanced by the crypt to promote self-renewal and repair. Several signaling pathways control the activity of stem cells. Paneth cells produce the majority of WNT3, which is vital, and R-spondin-1 promotes WNT signaling. Their appropriate self-renewal and differentiation are also aided by Notch and BMP signals (Eriguchi et al., 2012).

3.2.2 Paneth cells

The small intestinal crypts, paneth cells specialized secretory cells are dispersed amid intestinal stem cells. lysozymes and other antibacterial components found in large eosinophilic secretory granules (Sato et al., 2011). To improve the mucosal barrier, these granules are released into the intestinal lumen. Furthermore, maintaining the intestinal stem cell niche requires paneth cells (Clevers 2013).

3.2.3 Goblet cells

In the intestinal epithelial layer, the intestinal goblet cells are interspersed between the absorptive cells. Intestinal goblet cells are characterized by a goblet cell shape due to the thin cytoplasmic base and expanded Apical domain replete with secretion globules that contain mucin protein (Dekker et al., 2002). The protective and lubricating intestinal barrier is formed when the goblet cells secrete mucin, a mixture that combined with water creates mucus (Yan et al., 2017; Hou et al., 2017). In addition, goblet cells may protect gastrointestinal homeostasis through the secretion of other biologically active agents, including cytokines and antimicrobial peptides. WNT and Notch signaling pathway inhibition regulates the process of goblet cell differentiation (van der Post et al., 2019).

3.2.4 Tuft cells

Tuft cells that respond to the stimulus of hypoxia and infection of organs such as the lungs and intestine. Tuft cells employ a G protein-coupled receptor, a taste receptor, to control mucosal immunity. In response to infection with a helminth and allergens, there is a tremendous proliferation of tuft cells and goblet cells. In a response that is mediated through the STAT6 signaling pathway, type 2 innate lymphoid cells (ILC2s) trigger the proliferation of tuft and goblet cells by releasing the cytokines IL-4 and IL-13. Tuft cells promote the secretion of the cytokine IL-25, a response that mediates the innate immune response against the helminth through the promotion of the production and activation of type 2 innate lymphoid cells through a self-reinforcing loop (Sunaga et al., 2022). The regulation of gut microbiota by the various types of epithelial cells in the intestines is summarised in the Table 1, contributing to the maintenance of a healthy host-microbial symbiotic relationship through the regulation of microbial population, prevention of the entry and colonization of pathogens, and creation and maintenance of immune tolerance.

Table 1. Roles of Intestinal Epithelial Cells in the Regulation of Gut Microbiota

S. No	Cell Type	Characteristics	Mechanisms Regulating Gut Microbiota
1	Intestinal stem cells	Located at crpt base; regulated by WNT, Notch, BMP pathways.	Maintains continuous epithelial renewal, ensuring barrier integrity essential for controlling microbial access.
2	Paneth cells	Located at crypt base among stem cells; contain eosinophilic granules with lysozymes.	Secrete antimicrobial peptides directly restricting microbial growth, shape microbial composition.
3	Goblet cells	Dispersed among enterocytes; large mucin-filled granules.	Produces mucins forming the mucus layer that physically separate microbes from epithelium.
4	Tuft cells	Chemosensory sentinel cells responding to infection; express GPCRs	Detect helminths and initiate type 2 immune responses IL-25 to activate ILC2s and parasite burden.
5	Microfold (m) cells	Antigen- sampling epithelial cells	Transport luminal antigens to immune cells, supporting immune surveillance.
6	Enterocytes cells	Primary nutrient-absorbing cells	Regulate microbial growth indirectly by controlling nutrient availability;
7	Enteroendocrine cells	Hormone-secreting cells influences gut physiology	Secrete hormones that modulate motility, secretion and microbial habitat, condition, indirectly shaping microbiota composition.

4. INTESTINAL EPITHELIAL CELLS AFFECTED BY GUT MICROBIOTA

According to Kayama et al. (2020), the gut microbiota primarily interacts with intestinal epithelial cells through metabolic products, bacterial components, and intrinsic bacterial traits. The main metabolic products of bacteria are lactate, Bile Acids (BAs), Short-Chain Fatty Acids (SCFAs), and tryptophan; intrinsic bacterial characteristics include bacterial adhesion, which has also been demonstrated to be important in maintaining the integrity of the intestinal epithelium; and bacterial components include lipopolysaccharides and flagellin, among others. outlined the gut microbiome's regulatory signaling pathways in intestinal epithelial cells (Koh et al., 2016).

4.1 Intestinal cells and short-chain fatty acids (SCFAs)

Microbial fermentation of dietary The gut produces fiber and the SCFAs mostly as acetate, propionate, and butyrate, with minor levels of valerate, caproate, and isovalerate. In addition to providing the host with energy, particularly succinate or SCFA, also regulate the physiological processes of immune cells and intestinal epithelial cells. They are also essential for maintaining the integrity of the epithelial layer and for tissue healing after intestinal mucosal injury. By upregulating Claudin1, activating the HIF1 pathway, or this tight junction protein assembly by activating AMPK signaling pathways, butyrate may improve the function of the epithelial barrier. Furthermore, SCFAs promote goblet cells' mucus synthesis and discharge (Hodgkinson et al., 2023).

The chemical barrier in the intestine, enhance the transcription of MUC genes in goblet cells in the intestine. They also induce the release of α-defensin (Abdalkareem Jasim et al., 2022) in Paneth cells of the small intestine. Besides, certain pathogen-derived metabolites, including succinate or SCFAs, can be sensed by epithelial cells lining the intestine. Tuft cells in the intestine, for instance, recognize invasive pathogens like helminthes through succinate. To eliminate the helminth infection, tuft cells secrete IL-25 cytokine in response to the pathogen. To eliminate the parasite, the type 2 innate immune response is triggered. These clinical investigations hypothesize the role of butyrate in inflammatory bowel conditions such as Ulcerative Colitis. The intestinal barrier function promoted by microencapsulated sodium butyrate may correlate with improving the symptoms in patients with IBD or UC when given through the enema or oral route (Fekete and Buret, 2023).

4.2 Microbial lactate and epithelial cell responses

Microbial fermentation of dietary Fiber and other carbohydrates, including lactose and glucose, produces lactate, an organic acid. The primary lactate-producing bacteria in the neonatal gut microbiota are Bifidobacteria, Lactobacilli, and Enterococci, while certain types of Staphylococci can also make lactate (Lee et al., 2018). The lactate has special biological properties that include regulating immune responses and promoting intestinal mucosal tissue regeneration. Microbial fermentation can create lactate, which can decrease inflammatory responses in intestinal epithelium and bone marrow cells by reducing activation that is dependent on Toll-Like Receptors (TLRs) and IL-1β pathways. Clinical uses have also been investigated, probiotics containing *Bifidobacterium bifidum* and *Lactobacillus acidophilus* have been shown to be useful in reducing diarrhea in cancer patients receiving radiation therapy. According to these results, using lactobacilli symbionts or lactate salts may help shield human gut tissue from harm during radiation therapy (Rodríguez-Colman et al., 2017).

5. GUT BARRIER AND MICROBIOTA INTERACTIONS

One key feature of the intestinal wall is its selective permeability, allowing ions, water, and nutrients to pass while blocking pathogens. This permeability can be heightened by both endogenous factors, such as inflammation, and exogenous factors, including certain food ingredients, toxins, or medications, which can result in a leaky gut. Studies indicate that disruptions to the intestinal barrier are caused by hyperglycemia, a significant aspect of diabetes (Vanuytsel et al., 2021). When human colonic cells (Caco-2) are exposed to high glucose levels for extended periods, their structure becomes less organized, leading to decreased tight junction protein expression, increased intestinal barrier permeability, and disruption of the surrounding structural networks (Thaiss et al., 2018). Mucus and epithelium are critical for the intestinal barrier that prevents inflammation, featuring two sublayers in the mucous layer. The outer layer is loose and thick, supporting a healthy environment where harmful bacteria are unable to overgrow or penetrate due to the presence of commensal microorganisms (Dubois et al., 2023).

5.1 Microbiota influence on tight junction proteins

TJ proteins regulate the rate of paracellular transport, which includes the passage of consumed nutrients between neighbouring epithelial cells (Johansson et al., 2008). TJ proteins appear in electron micrographs as sites of membrane fusion between adjacent cells. They serve as environmental condition sensors that dynamically control solute transport within cells. Bacteria that change TJ protein expression and distribution can affect intestinal permeability (Pradhan et al., 2020). Some pathogenic strains of *Escherichia coli*, such the *E. coli* O157:H7 strain that causes bloody diarrhea, produce toxins like Shiga toxins (STx). Therefore, by reducing the expression of TJ proteins, non-pathogenic *E. coli* promotes the manufacture of the STx2a toxin by the *E. coli* O157:H7 strain (Gou et al., 2022).

Lactobacillus and Bifidobacterium species are frequently used as probiotics, notably *Lactobacillus reuteri*, which enhances the synthesis of Tight Junction (TJ) proteins critical for intestinal wall integrity. Additionally, *L. plantarum* facilitates the translocation of ZO-1 to the TJ region in human epithelial models, creating a paracellular seal between epithelial cells, though it does not significantly affect occludin expression (Caminero et al., 2023). Modulation typically normalizes intestinal permeability and maintains barrier integrity, rather than causing excessive permeability. Antibiotics can negatively affect gut microbiota, leading to dysbacteriosis through an imbalance of bacterial populations. Additionally, digestive proteases from gut flora, which break down host proteins, can harm the intestinal barrier by cleaving Tight Junction (TJ) proteins, thereby increasing paracellular permeability in the epithelial barriers (Xiaoli et al., 2018). Table 2 shows that different probiotic strains enhance intestinal barrier integrity by lowering epithelial permeability via the upregulation of tight junction proteins such as occludin, claudins, and ZO-1. These improvements are achieved through anti-inflammatory effects and the activation of protective signaling pathways, leading to better gut barrier function and mucosal homeostasis.

Table 2. Effects of Probiotic Strains on Intestinal Tight Junction Proteins and Barrier Integrity

S. No	Probiotic Strains	Proteins Affected	Effect on Protein	Intestinal Barrier	Mechanisms
1	*Lactobacillus rhamnosus*	ZO-1, Occludin, Claudin-1	Upregulation of Expression	Strengthens intestinal barrier integrity, reduces permeability.	• Reduces pro-inflammatory cytokines (TNF-α, IFN-γ). • Activates protective pathways (MAPK/ERK, PI3K/Akt). • Modulates gut immune response.
2	*Lactobacillus plantarum*	ZO-1, Occludin	Translocation & Assembly	Improves epithelial sealing and paracellular resistance.	• Promotes TJ protein translocation to cell junctions. • Enhances assembly of functional TJ complexes. • May trigger cytoskeletal reorganization via host receptors.
3	*Lactobacillus reuteri*	Occludin, Claudin-1	Upregulation & Stabilization	Enhances barrier stability and protects against episodic inflammatory insults.	• Upregulates TJ protein expression. • Produces bioactive factors (e.g., reuterin) to inhibit pathogens. • Protects against TNF-α/LPS-induced TJ protein internalization/degradation.
4	*Bifidobacterium breve*	ZO-1, Occludin	Enhanced Expression & Support	Supports mucosal repair and resilience against ongoing inflammation.	• Upregulates TJ protein gene/protein expression. • Secretes SCFAs (e.g., acetate) to nourish colonocytes and promote repair. • Competitively excludes pathogens, resists their toxins.
5	*Bifidobacterium infantis*	ZO-1, Occludin	Stabilization & Protection	Prevents endotoxin (e.g., LPS)-induced barrier impairment and systemic inflammation.	• Exerts anti-inflammatory effects via TLR/NF-κB modulation. • Binds/neutralizes endotoxins. • Enhances mucin production for a protective layer.

5.2 Microbiota in mucus layer biosynthesis & degradation

The mucous layer keeps the epithelium and gut microbes apart. Mucin proteins make up the remaining 95% of mucus, which is mostly water. The latter come together to form lengthy polymers that can contain a large number of germs in a gel-like structure. Due to their high glycosylation, mucins are able to keep the mucus's water content high. These enzymes often offer the gut microbial community a selective environment since only particular microorganisms can adhere to the mucin glycans in mucus (Wang et al., 2021). These mucin glycans are connected to by bacteria, which facilitates colonization. The gut microbiota can alter the mucus's composition and characteristics, which impacts the intestinal barrier's permeability and integrity (Qu et al., 2021). Furthermore, mucus that has been degraded by gut bacteria becomes less viscous and more porous to microorganisms and toxins, which might allow luminal bacteria to enter and trigger an increase in inflammatory reactions (Paone and Caniet al., 2020). Therefore, the growth of other bacteria that have lost the sites that allow them to bind to mucus can be inhibited by bacterial degradation of mucin glycans. Losing certain bacteria can then cause others to thrive excessively, which can lead to the development of dysbacteriosis (Schroeder, 2019).

5.3 Antioxidant roles of gut microorganisms

When the intestinal barrier malfunctions, oxidative stress frequently follows. There are several ramifications for cell physiology from the latter, which is an imbalance between the production and removal of ROS in favor of the former. ROS concentrations fluctuate with the physiological state of the host cells. Typically, when the mitochondrial electron transport chain is operating, far less than 10% of the oxygen that is ingested is transformed into ROS (Kunst et al., 2023). Hydrogen peroxide, for instance, interferes with the barrier function of Caco-2 cell monolayers in a dose-dependent manner. Moreover, a negative linear correlation has been demonstrated between the paracellular barrier's function and the production of additional ROS. The antioxidant defense system provides protection against ROS by reducing ROS levels and returning them to their original range.

Among the many positive impacts of probiotics are their antioxidant qualities. Bifidobacterium and Lactobacillus bacteria have the ability to boost antioxidant levels and neutralize ROS (Feng and Wang et al., 2020). Therefore, certain members of the gut microbiota can lower ROS levels and stop oxidative stress. The intestinal integrity is thus improved, and the immune system's activation is reduced. One major issue is the large oxygen gradient that exists across the gut wall. The apical mucosa nearest the lumen has been found to maintain in vivo oxygen concentrations of 0.1% to 1%, while the vascularized submucosa maintains oxygen concentrations of around 6% or more (Wu et al., 2022). At 7% to 10% oxygen content, the colonic muscle has the highest oxygen content. Because of this oxygen gradient, both host and microbial cells must be highly capable of adjusting to varying oxygen concentrations (Banan et al., 2000).

6. MECHANISMS IN FOOD SENSITIVITIES

The critical significance of as-yet-unidentified environmental factors as regulators of illness expression is highlighted by the incapacity of genetic drift to explain this increase in occurrence. Studies have linked food sensitivities to a variety of microbial signals that may be triggered by enteric infections or alterations in the commensal gut microbiota. Particularly, protein antigens may become substrates of the metabolism of gut microbes, leading to changes in antigenicity or the generation of metabolites that have a direct impact on tolerogenic reactions (Verbeke K et al., 2018).

6.1 Adverse reactions to food

One in five individuals globally is used to experience adverse reactions to food ingredients, with a diverse range of symptoms dependent on the specific underlying etiology and pathophysiological processes involved. Among these reactions are non-immune processes such as lactose maldigestion, which arises when the body is unable to adequately digest the disaccharide lactose. This inability is typically due to either a primary or secondary deficiency of the enzyme β-galactosidase, commonly known as lactase (Zevallos et al., 2017). IgE-mediated food allergies need sensitization, which is characterized by the production of IgE14 specific to dietary allergens.

Reexposure to the allergen causes allergen-specific IgE, which is associated to FcεRI (also called FCER1A) on mast cells and basophils, to crosslink and release mediators that induce acute symptoms, such as histamine (Kemppainen et al., 2017). Food protein-induced proctocolitis and protein-induced enterocolitis syndrome are types of non-IgE-mediated food allergies. In individuals with HLA-DQ2 and HLA-DQ8 genes, gluten intake can lead to celiac disease, a CD4+ T cell-mediated food sensitivity with autoimmune features. The prevalence of celiac disease is increasing globally alongside other autoimmune conditions. Environmental factors include the timing and frequency of gluten introduction, breastfeeding practices, dysbiosis, and infections, as genetic predisposition (Zevallos et al., 2017).

6.2 Microbial & environmental factors influencing sensitivity

Numerous organizations have connected food sensitivity to practices including early eating, antibiotic usage, and cesarean delivery that can change the intestinal microbiota's makeup (Karhus et al., 2018). Although results from prospective birth cohort studies on celiac disease have been published, there is no proof that early eating habits have a statistically significant effect on the development of celiac disease (Silvester et al., 2017). Furthermore, it has been shown that intestinal helminth infections might intensify the body's response to dietary antigens, potentially leading to food allergies.

Early-life gastrointestinal infections can hinder the immature immune system and mucosal integrity, potentially increasing vulnerability to food sensitivities. Dysbiosis linked to celiac disease displays Proteobacteria growth and opportunistic pathogens in the proximal small intestine (Crespo-Escobar et al., 2017). Animal studies have provided some mechanistic insight into how the microbial ecology of the intestine might alter responses to different antigens or allergens68. Most mechanistic information is derived from basic studies that explain how specific bacteria interact with the antigen or allergen itself, as well as how microorganisms imprint pro-inflammatory or tolerance induction in the host (Singh et al., 2018).

6.3 Microorganism–diet interactions

Gut microbiota acts as a metabolic organ, enhancing host metabolic functions. Bacteria can influence immune responses to food through antigen metabolism. Specifically, proteolytic-resistant gluten proteins are critical in T cell-mediated inflammation in celiac disease, as their partial digestion leads to high-molecular-mass oligopeptides that can provoke T cell responses associated with the conditions (David et al., 2014). When associated with Antigen-Presenting Cells (APCs), gluten peptides serve as appealing energy sources for gastrointestinal bacteria. Opportunistic infections, such as those caused by *Pseudomonas aeruginosa*, can further degrade gluten peptides via protease digestion, yielding shorter yet immunogenic sequences.

These bacterial modified peptides may cross the intestinal epithelial barrier more efficiently than those produced by human proteases, potentially impacting the host's immune response. Lactobacillus species, critical to the human duodenal microbiota, can decompose and eliminate gluten peptides generated by both human and pathogenic proteases. Notably, Lactobacillus species are typically more abundant and diverse in healthy individuals than in those with celiac diseases (Sonnenburg et al., 2016). The immunogenicity of food antigens is significantly regulated by these microbes. Since many food allergens, such as peanut and egg proteins, cannot be broken down by mammalian proteases, this may be relevant to a variety of food sensitivities (Zevallos et al., 2017).

6.4 Immunogenicity of food antigens

In the absence of tissue damage, mucosal CD103+ DCs that populate mesenteric lymph nodes and lamina propria of the small intestine present luminal dietary antigen to naive CD4+ T helper cells that differentiate into pTreg cells in a TGFβ-dependent, RA-dependent manner (Zhou et al., 2017). IRF8-dependent mucosal

CD103+CD11b– DC subset has the strongest inducers of pTreg cells and mucosal tolerance in steady-state conditions (Nistal et al., 2016). Retinal dehydrogenase 2 (RALDH2), an enzyme catalyzing Retinoic Acid (RA), highly expressed in CD103+CD11b DC subset, has a tolerogenic gene expression program. RALDH2 has been known to secrete IL-12 and trigger TH1 cell-mediated immunity in tissue stress conditions like infections by skin parasites Leishmania major in mices (Herran et al., 2017). DCs secrete pro-inflammatory IL-12, an inducer of TH1 cell-mediated responses to dietary antigenic proteins like gluten (IRF1-dependent). IRF1 was found to be indispensable for induction of TH1 responses but dispensable for repression of type I interferon-dependent pTreg cell induction (Koppel et al., 2017).

7. BIOLOGICAL BASIS OF FOOD SENSITIVITY FOR MICROBIOTA–IMMUNE AXIS

7.1 Microbial metabolites with immunomodulatory function

The intestinal microbiota plays a crucial role in maintaining a tolerogenic gut environment by preventing inflammation against foreign antigens. It enhances epithelial integrity and supports regulatory T cells through the production of immunomodulatory metabolites from bacterial metabolism of dietary substrates. During tissue distress, these metabolites help preserve the epithelial barrier integrity. In celiac disease, an increase in the pro-inflammatory cytokine IL-15 leads to dysbiosis, characterized by reduced butyrate levels and a decline in butyrate-producing bacteria. IL-15 is essential for gut homeostasis, influencing immune system maturation and barrier function maintenance (Schwarzer et al., 2017). AhR activation may protect against peanut allergy in rats by enhancing dendritic cell (DC) phenotype and function during allergic sensitization. While dietary interventions and gut microbiota effects on food sensitization remain clinically unfeasible, understanding beneficial bacterial compounds and their nutritional precursors (Bunyavanich et al., 2016).

7.2 TH1-Mediated immunity to food antigens

In the absence of tissue injury, mucosal CD103+ dendritic cells, abundant in mesenteric LNs and the lamina propria of the small intestine, present luminal dietary antigens to naive CD4+ T helper cells, leading to their conversion to pTreg cells via TGFβ/RA-mediated signaling (Luda et al., 2016). The mucosal IRF8-mediated CD103+CD11b- dendritic cell lineage is essential for pTreg cell generation and the induction of oral tolerance in the absence of tissue damage. The dendritic cell lineage has a specific gene expression signature, which is highly tolerogenic, particularly with high expression of genes encoding the production of retinal dehydrogenase 2 (RALDH2), an enzyme catalyzing the generation of Retinoic Acid (RA) (Moretto et al., 2015). Furthermore, during episodes of tissue stress, such as infections with the cutaneous parasite Leishmania major, the CD103+CD11b− DCs are capable of secreting interleukin-12 (IL-12), which enhances TH1 cell-mediated immune responses. However, it is important to note that intestinal inflammation can impede the ability of CD103+ DCs to promote differentiation into pTreg cells. Additionally, while IRF1 is not essential for the suppression of type I interferon-dependent pTreg cell generation, it is necessary for the initiation of TH1 cell responses to dietary antigens (Hall et al., 2011).

7.3 Reovirus-triggered TH1 response to dietary Antigens

There are two possibilities regarding an infectious aetiology of celiac disease: either reovirus-induced elevation of pro-inflammatory type I interferon or virus-mediated overexpression and release of the enzyme tissue transglutaminase (Bouziat et al., 2017). The pTreg cell response was repressed and a pathogenic TH1 cell response to gluten was instead activated as a result of interactions between the virus and the host, shifting these correlations toward causality. The viral genes that correlate with LOT will make it easy to understand the underlying mechanisms and concentrate on certain pathways by generating viral reassortants or mutants. By inhibiting the formation of pTreg cells via type I interferon pathways, T1L reovirus has been shown to generate a form of lasting immune tolerance (LOT). A noteworthy correlation was observed between the levels of anti-reovirus antibody titres and the expression of intestinal mucosal IRF1 in patients with celiac disease, indicating that prior virus–host interactions may trigger significant, enduring changes in immune homeostasis linked to increased expression of mucosal IRF1. Additionally, the levels of anti-reovirus antibodies were markedly higher in celiac disease patients compared to those conditions (Sollid et al., 2013).

7.4 Role of il-15 in th1 induction

This cytokine has been demonstrated to cause LOT106,173 and to be increased in response to double-stranded RNA174 or lipopolysaccharide stimulation. It's interesting to note that IL-15 is not linked to reovirus-mediated LOT5, indicating that it may be a separate inflammatory pathway that results in LOT (Zhernakova et al., 2010). More specifically, it has been shown that IL-15 confers RA adjuvant properties in mice and promotes the growth of intestinal CD103+ DCs with a pro-inflammatory phenotype that produce large levels of IL-12. Consequently, overexpression of IL-15 in the lamina propria suppresses the formation of pTreg cells and causes TH1 cell responses to dietary antigens. These findings are relevant to celiac disease, where polymorphisms in the gene that produces IL-12 are suggested as a genetic risk factor and IL-15 upregulation in the lamina propria is associated with an upregulation of IL-12 (Berni Canani et al., 2016).

8. FUTURE PERSPECTIVES ON MICROBIOTA-BASED THERAPIES

Probiotics are live microorganisms that provide various health benefits when consumed in sufficient quantities. They play a crucial role in maintaining the balance of microbial levels in the intestinal tract, inhibiting the growth of harmful pathogens. Additionally, probiotics support the gut's mucous lining in regulating the immune system. The primary categories of probiotics are: a) those from the genus Bifidobacterium, b) those derived from Saccharomyces yeast, and c) lactic acid probiotics, which are the most prevalent within these classifications (Plummer et al., 2020).

The most probiotics originate from the Lactobacillus and Bifidobacterium genera. These probiotics have vast potential for aiding human immune systems. Probiotics have been applied for the modulation and prevention of various allergy-related ailments. This application is based on promoting the gut barrier and modulating the levels of both Th1/Th2. Moreover, probiotics help in modulating the levels of Th1/Th2 balance. *Lacticaseibacillus rhamnosus* acts efficiently in accelerating the process for developing an oral tolerance approach in an individual suffering from a milk allergy (Zuo et al., 2021). *Lacticaseibacillus casei* strain associated with the probiotic genera Bifidobacterium. Moreover, this application has been validated to amplify the

Probiotics can boost the tolerogenic adaptability of the immune reaction to food allergens or enhance microbial lineages that induce tolerance (Mak et al., 2020). The connection between gut microbiota and food allergy is a rapidly evolving area with tremendous latent value for discovering new strategies (Anwar et al., 2021). These methods include probiotics, prebiotics, synbiotics, postbiotics, FMT, dietary therapy, and traditional Chinese medicines, which are focused on modulating gut microbiota. However, the gut flora associated with specific food allergies could differ, and the human trials, animal models are highly inconsistent. Bifidobacteria, yeast, and lactic-acid bacteria are the three major kinds of probioticic lactic-acid bacteria are the most abundant (Leviatan et al., 2020).

9. CONCLUSION

Gut microbiota, intestinal barrier integrity, and host immunity form a complex process, which is a critical basis on which food allergy/sensitivities, development, evolution, and management. Several alterations in gut microbial homeostasis, also known as dysbiosis, can impair intestinal barrier integrity in terms of reduced expression of junction proteins, mucus secretion, and increased oxidative stress, thus increasing passage of an allergen across epithelia to invoke autoimmune reactions. One of the most crucial roles of microbial metabolites, SCFAs, and Lactic acid has been shown to play a regulatory role in improving epithelial integrity, mucus secretion, stimulating regulatory T cell supporting tolerance, which is vital within oral tolerance. In contrast, dysbiosis can impact by functioning immunity to become Th2/Th1, respectively, which leads to food allergy/celiacs, respectively, which is often triggered by factors like diet, infection, use of antibiotics, and reovirus. However, intestinal epithelial cells, Paneth cells, goblet cells, tuft cells, microfold (M) cells, play a critical role in gut-associated microbia-host immunity roles, which is a regulatory mechanism seen on both sides of a defense, regulatory, regulatory cell. The management of the medical conditions using probiotics, prebiotics, Fecal Microbiota Transplant, there exist complexities for their variation in gut microbia.

10. REFERENCES

Abdalkareem Jasim, S., Jade Catalan Opulencia, M., Alexis Ramírez-Coronel, A., & Markov, A. (2022). The emerging role of microbiota-derived short-chain fatty acids in immunometabolism. *International Immunopharmacology, 110*, 108983. DOI: 10.1016/j.intimp.2022.108983

Ansaldo, E., Farley, T. K., & Belkaid, Y. (2021). Control of immunity by the microbiota. *Annual Review of Immunology, 39*(1), 449–479. DOI: 10.1146/annurev-immunol-093019-112348

Anwar, F., Altayb, H. N., Al-Abbasi, F. A., Al-Malki, A. L., Kamal, M. A., & Kumar, V. (2021). Antiviral effects of probiotic metabolites on COVID-19. *Journal of Biomolecular Structure & Dynamics, 39*(11), 4175–4184. DOI: 10.1080/07391102.2020.1775123

Banan, A., Fields, J. Z., Decker, H., Zhang, Y., & Keshavarzian, A. (2000). Nitric oxide and its metabolites mediate ethanol-induced microtubule disruption and intestinal barrier dysfunction. *The Journal of Pharmacology and Experimental Therapeutics, 294*(3), 997–1008. DOI: 10.1016/S0022-3565(24)39164-5

Berni Canani, R., Sangwan, N., Stefka, A. T., Nocerino, R., Paparo, L., Aitoro, R., Calignano, A., Khan, A. A., Gilbert, J. A., & Nagler, C. R. (2016). *Lactobacillus rhamnosus* GG-supplemented formula expands butyrate-producing bacterial strains in food allergic infants. *The ISME Journal, 10*(3), 742–750. DOI: 10.1038/ismej.2015.151

Bloemendaal, A. L., Buchs, N. C., George, B. D., & Guy, R. J. (2016). Intestinal stem cells and intestinal homeostasis in health and in inflammation. *Surgery, 159*(5), 1237–1248. DOI: 10.1016/j.surg.2016.01.014

Bouziat, R., Hinterleitner, R., Brown, J. J., Stencel-Baerenwald, J. E., Ikizler, M., Mayassi, T., Meisel, M., Kim, S. M., & Jabri, B. (2017). Reovirus infection triggers inflammatory responses to dietary antigens and development of celiac disease. *Science, 356*(6333), 44–50. DOI: 10.1126/science.aah5298

Bunyavanich, S., Shen, N., Grishin, A., Jones, S. M., Leung, D. Y. M., Sampson, H., Sicherer, S., & Clemente, J. C. (2016). Early-life gut microbiome composition and milk allergy resolution. *The Journal of Allergy and Clinical Immunology, 138*(4), 1122–1130. DOI: 10.1016/j.jaci.2016.03.041

Caminero, A., Guzman, M., Libertucci, J., & Lomax, A. E. (2023). The emerging roles of bacterial proteases in intestinal diseases. *Gut Microbes, 15*(1), 2181922. DOI: 10.1080/19490976.2023.2181922

Clevers, H. (2013). The intestinal crypt, a prototype stem cell compartment. *Cell, 154*(2), 274–284. DOI: 10.1016/j.cell.2013.07.004

Clevers, H. C., & Bevins, C. L. (2013). Paneth cells: Maestros of the small intestinal crypts. *Annual Review of Physiology*, *75*(1), 289–311. DOI: 10.1146/annurev-physiol-030212-183744

Crespo-Escobar, P., Mearin, M. L., Hervás, D., Auricchio, R., Castillejo, G., Gyimesi, J., Martínez-Ojinaga, E., Werkstetter, K., & Koletzko, S. (2017). The role of gluten consumption at an early age in celiac disease development: A further analysis of the prospective PreventCD cohort study. *The American Journal of Clinical Nutrition*, *105*(4), 890–896. DOI: 10.3945/ajcn.116.144352

David, L. A., Maurice, C. F., Carmody, R. N., Gootenberg, D. B., Button, J. E., Wolfe, B. E., Ling, A. V., Devlin, A. S., & Turnbaugh, P. J. (2014). Diet rapidly and reproducibly alters the human gut microbiome. *Nature*, *505*(7484), 559–563. DOI: 10.1038/nature12820

Dekker, J., Rossen, J. W., Büller, H. A., & Einerhand, A. W. (2002). The MUC family: An obituary. *Trends in Biochemical Sciences*, *27*(3), 126–131. DOI: 10.1016/S0968-0004(01)02052-7

Dubois, N., Muñoz-Garcia, J., Heymann, D., & Renodon-Cornière, A. (2023). High glucose exposure drives intestinal barrier dysfunction by altering its morphological, structural and functional properties. *Biochemical Pharmacology*, *216*, 115765. DOI: 10.1016/j.bcp.2023.115765

Eriguchi, Y., Takashima, S., Oka, H., Shimoji, S., Nakamura, K., & Teshima, T. (2012). Graft-versus-host disease disrupts intestinal microbial ecology by inhibiting Paneth cell production of α-defensins. *Blood*, *120*(1), 223–231. DOI: 10.1182/blood-2011-12-401166

Esterházy, D., Canesso, M. C. C., Mesin, L., Muller, P. A., de Castro, T. B. R., Lockhart, A., ElJalby, M., Faria, A. M. C., & Mucida, D. (2019). Compartmentalized gut lymph node drainage dictates adaptive immune responses. *Nature*, *569*(7754), 126–130. DOI: 10.1038/s41586-019-1125-3

Farin, H. F., Jordens, I., Mosa, M. H., Basak, O., Korving, J., Tauriello, D. V., de Punder, K., Angers, S., Peters, P. J., Maurice, M. M., & Clevers, H. (2016). Visualization of a short-range Wnt gradient in the intestinal stem-cell niche. *Nature*, *530*(7590), 340–343. DOI: 10.1038/nature16937

Fekete, E., and Buret, A. G. (2023). The role of mucin O-glycans in microbiota dysbiosis, intestinal homeostasis, and host-pathogen interactions. *American Journal of Physiology-Gastrointestinal and Liver Physiology, 324*(5), G452–G465. DOI: 10.1152/ajpgi.00261.2022

Feng, T., & Wang, J. (2020). Oxidative stress tolerance and antioxidant capacity of lactic acid bacteria as probiotic: A systematic review. *Gut Microbes*, *12*(1), 1801944. DOI: 10.1080/19490976.2020.1801944

Gou, H. Z., Zhang, Y. L., & Zhang, L. (2022). How do intestinal probiotics restore the intestinal barrier? *Frontiers in Microbiology*, *13*, 929346. DOI: 10.3389/fmicb.2022.929346

Hall, J. A., Grainger, J. R., Spencer, S. P., & Belkaid, Y. (2011). The role of retinoic acid in tolerance and immunity. *Immunity*, *35*(1), 13–22. DOI: 10.1016/j.immuni.2011.07.002

Herran, A. R., Pérez-Andrés, J., Caminero, A., Nistal, E., Vivas, S., Ruiz de Morales, J. M., Casqueiro, J., & Sollid, L. M. (2017). Gluten-degrading bacteria are present in the human small intestine of healthy volunteers and celiac patients. *Research in Microbiology*, *168*(7), 673–684. DOI: 10.1016/j.resmic.2017.04.008

Hodgkinson, K., El Abbar, F., Dobranowski, P., Manoogian, J., Butcher, J., Figeys, D., Mack, D., & Stintzi, A. (2023). Butyrate's role in human health and the current progress towards its clinical application to treat gastrointestinal disease. *Clinical Nutrition (Edinburgh, Lothian)*, *42*(1), 61–75. DOI: 10.1016/j.clnu.2022.10.024

Hou, Q., Ye, L., Huang, L., & Yu, Q. (2017). The research progress on intestinal stem cells and its relationship with intestinal microbiota. *Frontiers in Immunology*, *8*, 599. DOI: 10.3389/fimmu.2017.00599

Johansson, M. E., Phillipson, M., Petersson, J., Velcich, A., Holm, L., & Hansson, G. C. (2008). The inner of the two Muc2 mucin-dependent mucus layers in colon is devoid of bacteria. *Proceedings of the National Academy of Sciences of the United States of America*, *105*(39), 15064–15069. DOI: 10.1073/pnas.0803124105

Karhus, L. L., Gunnes, N., Størdal, K., & Ludvigsson, J. F. (2018). Influenza and risk of later celiac disease: A cohort study of 2.6 million people. *Scandinavian Journal of Gastroenterology*, *53*(1), 15–23. DOI: 10.1080/00365521.2017.1362464

Kayama, H., Okumura, R., & Takeda, K. (2020). Interaction between the microbiota, epithelia, and immune cells in the intestine. *Annual Review of Immunology*, *38*(1), 23–48. DOI: 10.1146/annurev-immunol-070119-115104

Kemppainen, K. M., Lynch, K. F., Liu, E., Lönnrot, M., Simell, V., Briese, T., Koletzko, S., Hagopian, W., Rewers, M., She, J.-X., Simell, O., Toppari, J., Ziegler, A.-G., Akolkar, B., Krischer, J. P., Lernmark, Å., Hyöty, H., Triplett, E. W., & Agardh, D. (2017). Factors that increase risk of celiac disease autoimmunity after a gastrointestinal infection in early life. *Clinical Gastroenterology and Hepatology*, *15*(5), 694–702. DOI: 10.1016/j.cgh.2016.10.033

Khan, I., Bai, Y., Ullah, N., Liu, G., Rajoka, M. S. R., & Zhang, C. (2022). Differential susceptibility of the gut microbiota to DSS treatment interferes in the conserved microbiome association in mouse models of colitis and is related to the initial gut microbiota difference. *Advanced Gut & Microbiome Research*, *2022*, 7813278. Advance online publication. DOI: 10.1155/2022/7813278

Khodoun, M. V., Tomar, S., Tocker, J. E., Wang, Y. H., & Finkelman, F. D. (2018). Prevention of food allergy development and suppression of established food allergy by neutralization of thymic stromal lymphopoietin, IL-25, and IL-33. *The Journal of Allergy and Clinical Immunology*, *141*(1), 171–179. DOI: 10.1016/j.jaci.2017.02.046

Koh, A., De Vadder, F., Kovatcheva-Datchary, P., & Backhed, F. (2016). From dietary fiber to host physiology: Short-chain fatty acids as key bacterial metabolites. *Cell*, *165*(6), 1332–1345. DOI: 10.1016/j.cell.2016.05.041

Koo, B.-K., Spit, M., Jordens, I., Low, T. Y., Stange, D. E., van de Wetering, M., van Es, J. H., & Clevers, H. (2012). Tumour suppressor RNF43 is a stem-cell E3 ligase that induces endocytosis of Wnt receptors. *Nature*, *488*(7413), 665–669. DOI: 10.1038/nature11308

Koppel, N., Maini Rekdal, V., & Balskus, E. P. (2017). Chemical transformation of xenobiotics by the human gut microbiota. *Science*, *356*(6344), eaag2770. Advance online publication. DOI: 10.1126/science.aag2770

Kunst, C., Schmid, S., Michalski, M., Tümen, D., Buttenschön, J., Müller, M., Gülow, K., & Falk-Paulsen, M. (2023). The influence of gut microbiota on oxidative stress and the immune system. *Biomedicines*, *11*(5), 1388. DOI: 10.3390/biomedicines11051388

Lee, Y. S., Kim, T. Y., Kim, Y., Lee, S. H., Kim, S., Kang, S. W., Yang, J.-Y., Baek, I.-J., Sung, Y. H., Park, Y.-Y., & Kweon, M.-N. (2018). Microbiota-derived lactate accelerates intestinal stem-cell-mediated epithelial development. *Cell Host & Microbe*, *24*(6), 833–846.e6. DOI: 10.1016/j.chom.2018.11.002

Leviatan, S., & Segal, E. (2020). Identifying gut microbes that affect human health. *Nature*, *587*(7834), 373–374. DOI: 10.1038/d41586-020-03069-8

Luda, K. M., Joeris, T., Persson, E. K., Rivollier, A., Demiri, M., Sitnik, K. M., Pool, L., Holm, J. B., Melo-Gonzalez, F., & Agace, W. W. (2016). IRF8 transcription-factor-dependent classical dendritic cells are essential for intestinal T cell homeostasis. *Immunity, 44*(4), 860–874. DOI: 10.1016/j.immuni.2016.02.008

Mak, J. W. Y., Chan, F. K. L., & Ng, S. C. (2020). Probiotics and COVID-19: One size does not fit all. *The Lancet. Gastroenterology & Hepatology, 5*(7), 644–645. DOI: 10.1016/S2468-1253(20)30122-9

Moretto, M. M., Harrow, D. I., Hawley, T. S., & Khan, I. A. (2015). Interleukin-12-producing CD103+CD11b−CD8+ dendritic cells are responsible for eliciting gut intraepithelial lymphocyte response against *Encephalitozoon cuniculi. Infection and Immunity, 83*(12), 4719–4730. DOI: 10.1128/IAI.00820-15

Muthukumar, J., Selvasekaran, P., Lokanadham, M., and Chidambaram, R. (2020). Food and food products associated with food allergy and food intolerance—An overview. *Food Research International, 138*(Part B), 109780. DOI: 10.1016/j.foodres.2020.109780

Nistal, E., Caminero, A., Herran, A. R., Arias, L., Vivas, S., de Morales, J. M. R., Calleja, S., de Miera, L. E. S., Arroyo, P., & Casqueiro, J. (2016). Study of duodenal bacterial communities by 16s rRNA gene analysis in adults with active celiac disease versus non celiac disease controls. *Journal of Applied Microbiology, 120*(6), 1691–1700. DOI: 10.1111/jam.13111

Paone, P., & Cani, P. D. (2020). Mucus barrier, mucins and gut microbiota: The expected slimy partners? *Gut, 69*(12), 2232–2243. DOI: 10.1136/gutjnl-2020-322260

Perrier, C., & Corthésy, B. (2011). Gut permeability and food allergies. *Clinical and Experimental Allergy, 41*(1), 20–28. DOI: 10.1111/j.1365-2222.2010.03639.x

Plummer, E. L., Lozinsky, A. C., Axelrad, C., Garland, S. M., Jacobs, S. E., & Tang, M. L. K. (2020). Postnatal probiotics and allergic disease in very preterm infants: Sub-study to the ProPrems randomized trial. *Allergy, 75*(1), 83–88. DOI: 10.1111/all.14088

Pradhan, S., Karve, S. S., Weiss, A. A., Hawkins, J., Poling, H. M., Helmrath, M. A., Wells, J. M., & McCauley, H. A. (2020). Tissue responses to Shiga toxin in human intestinal organoids. *Cellular and Molecular Gastroenterology and Hepatology, 10*(1), 171–190. DOI: 10.1016/j.jcmgh.2020.02.006

Qu, D., Wang, G., Yu, L., Tian, F., Chen, W., & Zhai, Q. (2021). The effects of diet and gut microbiota on the regulation of intestinal mucin glycosylation. *Carbohydrate Polymers, 258*, 117651. DOI: 10.1016/j.carbpol.2021.117651

Rodríguez-Colman, M. J., Schewe, M., Meerlo, M., Pras-Raves, M., Sacchetti, A., & Burgering, B. M. (2017). Interplay between metabolic identities in the intestinal crypt supports stem cell function. *Nature*, *543*(7645), 424–427. DOI: 10.1038/nature21673

Sato, T., van Es, J. H., Snippert, H. J., Stange, D. E., Barker, N., Shroyer, N. F., & Clevers, H. (2011). Paneth cells constitute the niche for Lgr5 stem cells in intestinal crypts. *Nature*, *469*(7330), 415–418. DOI: 10.1038/nature09637

Schroeder, B. O. (2019). Fight them or feed them: How the intestinal mucus layer manages the gut microbiota. *Gastroenterology Report*, *7*(1), 3–12. DOI: 10.1093/gastro/goy052

Schwarzer, M., Hermanova, P., Srutkova, D., Hudcovic, T., Akgün, J., Wiedermann, U., & Kozakova, H. (2017). Diet matters: Endotoxin in the diet impacts the level of allergic sensitization in germ-free mice. *PLoS One*, *12*(1), e0167786. DOI: 10.1371/journal.pone.0167786

Shroyer, N. F., Helmrath, M. A., Wang, V. Y.-C., Antalffy, B., Henning, S. J., & Zoghbi, H. Y. (2007). Intestine-specific ablation of mouse atonal homolog 1 (Math1) reveals a role in cellular homeostasis. *Gastroenterology*, *132*(7), 2478–2488. DOI: 10.1053/j.gastro.2007.03.047

Silvester, J. A., & Leffler, D. A. (2017). The effect of gastrointestinal viral infections and vaccination on risk of celiac disease autoimmunity. *Clinical Gastroenterology and Hepatology*, *15*(5), 703–705. DOI: 10.1016/j.cgh.2016.12.014

Singh, P., Arora, A., Strand, T. A., Leffler, D. A., Catassi, C., Green, P. H., Kelly, C. P., Ahuja, V., & Makharia, G. K. (2018). Global prevalence of celiac disease: Systematic review and meta-analysis. *Clinical Gastroenterology and Hepatology*, *16*(6), 823–836. DOI: 10.1016/j.cgh.2017.06.037

Slifer, Z. M., & Blikslager, A. T. (2020). The integral role of tight junction proteins in the repair of injured intestinal epithelium. *International Journal of Molecular Sciences*, *21*(3), 972. DOI: 10.3390/ijms21030972

Sollid, L. M., & Jabri, B. (2013). Triggers and drivers of autoimmunity: Lessons from coeliac disease. *Nature Reviews. Immunology*, *13*(4), 294–302. DOI: 10.1038/nri3407

Sonnenburg, J. L., & Bäckhed, F. (2016). Diet–microbiota interactions as moderators of human metabolism. *Nature*, *535*(7610), 56–64. DOI: 10.1038/nature18846

Sunaga, S., Tsunoda, J., Teratani, T., Mikami, Y., & Kanai, T. (2022). Heterogeneity of ILC2s in the intestine; homeostasis and pathology. *Frontiers in Immunology*, *13*, 867351. DOI: 10.3389/fimmu.2022.867351

Thaiss, C. A., Levy, M., Grosheva, I., Zheng, D., Soffer, E., Blacher, E., Braverman, S., Tengeler, A. C., Serradas, P., & Elinav, E. (2018). Hyperglycemia drives intestinal barrier dysfunction and risk for enteric infection. *Science*, *359*(6382), 1376–1383. DOI: 10.1126/science.aar3318

Turner, J. R. (2009). Intestinal mucosal barrier function in health and disease. *Nature Reviews. Immunology*, *9*(11), 799–809. DOI: 10.1038/nri2653

van der Post, S., Jabbar, K. S., & Hansson, G. C. (2019). Structural weakening of the colonic mucus barrier is an early event in ulcerative colitis pathogenesis. *Gut*, *68*(12), 2142–2151. DOI: 10.1136/gutjnl-2018-317571

Vanuytsel, T., Tack, J., & Farre, R. (2021). The role of intestinal permeability in gastrointestinal disorders and current methods of evaluation. *Frontiers in Nutrition*, *8*, 717925. DOI: 10.3389/fnut.2021.717925

Verbeke, K. (2018). Nonceliac gluten sensitivity: What is the culprit? *Gastroenterology*, *154*(3), 471–473. DOI: 10.1053/j.gastro.2018.01.013

Wang, B. X., Wu, C. M., & Ribbeck, K. (2021). Home, sweet home: How mucus accommodates our microbiota. *The FEBS Journal*, *288*(6), 1789–1799. DOI: 10.1111/febs.15504

Warren, C. M., Jiang, J., & Gupta, R. S. (2020). Epidemiology and burden of food allergy. *Current Allergy and Asthma Reports*, *20*(2), 6. DOI: 10.1007/s11882-020-0898-7

Wiersinga, W. J., Rhodes, A., Cheng, A. C., Peacock, S. J., & Prescott, H. C. (2020). Pathophysiology, transmission, diagnosis, and treatment of coronavirus disease 2019 (COVID-19): A review. *Journal of the American Medical Association*, *324*(8), 782–793. DOI: 10.1001/jama.2020.12839

Wong, G. W.-K. (2024). Food allergies around the world. *Frontiers in Nutrition*, *11*, 1391631. DOI: 10.3389/fnut.2024.1373110

Wu, L., Xie, X., Li, Y., Liang, T., Zhong, H., Yang, L., Li, Y., & Liu, S. (2022). Gut microbiota as an antioxidant system in centenarians associated with high antioxidant activities of gut-resident *Lactobacillus*. *NPJ Biofilms and Microbiomes*, *8*(1), 102. DOI: 10.1038/s41522-022-00366-0

Xiaoli, L., Figler, H. M., Banerjee, K. G., Hayes, C. S., Dudley, E. G., & Moxley, R. A. (2018). Non-pathogenic *Escherichia coli* enhance Stx2a production of *E. coli* O157:H7 through both bamA-dependent and independent mechanisms. *Frontiers in Microbiology*, *9*, 1325. DOI: 10.3389/fmicb.2018.01325

Yan, K. S., Janda, C. Y., Chang, J., Zheng, G. X. Y., Larkin, K. A., Luca, V. C., Chia, L. A., Mah, A. T., Han, A., Terry, J. M., Ootani, A., Roelf, K., Lee, M., Yuan, J., Li, X., Bolen, C. R., Wilhelmy, J., Davies, P. S., Ueno, H., & Kuo, C. J. (2017). Non-equivalence of Wnt and R-spondin ligands during Lgr5+ intestinal stem-cell self-renewal. *Nature*, *545*(7653), 238–242. DOI: 10.1038/nature22313

Zevallos, V. F., Raker, V., Tenzer, S., Jimenez-Calvente, C., Ashfaq-Khan, M., Rüssel, N., Pickert, G., Schild, H., Steinbrink, K., & Schuppan, D. (2017). Nutritional wheat amylase-trypsin inhibitors promote intestinal inflammation via activation of myeloid cells. *Gastroenterology*, *152*(5), 1100–1113. DOI: 10.1053/j.gastro.2016.12.006

Zhernakova, A., Elbers, C. C., Ferwerda, B., & Oosting, M. (2010). Evolutionary and functional analysis of celiac risk loci reveals SH2B3 as a protective factor against bacterial infection. *American Journal of Human Genetics*, *86*(6), 970–977. DOI: 10.1016/j.ajhg.2010.05.004

Zhou, L., Hörmann, S., & Schuppan, D. (2017). Abrogation of immunogenic properties of gliadin peptides through transamination by microbial transglutaminase is acyl-acceptor dependent. *Journal of Agricultural and Food Chemistry*, *65*(34), 7542–7552. DOI: 10.1021/acs.jafc.7b02557

Zimmermann, P. (2023). The immunological interplay between vaccination and the intestinal microbiota. *NPJ Vaccines*, *8*(1), 24. DOI: 10.1038/s41541-023-00627-9

Zuo, T., Zhang, F., Lui, G. C. Y., & Ng, S. C. (2021). Alterations in gut microbiota of patients with COVID-19 during time of hospitalization. *Gastroenterology*, *159*(3), 944–955. DOI: 10.1053/j.gastro.2020.05.048

Chapter 8
Microbial Dysbiosis and Metabolic Disorder

K. Kesavardhini
https://orcid.org/0009-0005-8235-042X
Department of Microbiology, Sacred Heart College, Tirupattur, India

P. Saranraj
https://orcid.org/0000-0002-5052-6532
Department of Microbiology, Sacred Heart College, Tirupattur, India

U. Subhalakshmi
https://orcid.org/0009-0007-8989-5486
Department of Microbiology, Sacred Heart College, Tirupattur, India

K. Gayathri
https://orcid.org/0009-0007-3786-2009
Department of Microbiology, Sacred Heart College, Tirupattur, India

B. Lokeshwari
https://orcid.org/0009-0005-6612-5134
Department of Microbiology, Sacred Heart College, Tirupattur, India

ABSTRACT

Microbial dysbiosis, defined as an imbalance in the composition and functional activity of microbial communities, has emerged as a major factor influencing host metabolic health. The human microbiota, which is mostly located in the Gut, Oral Cavity, Skin, and Vagina, is essential for nutrition metabolism, homeostasis, and immune system control. Changes in microbial abundance and diversity are linked to metabolic illnesses such as type 2 Diabetes, Obesity, Non-Alcoholic Fatty Liver Disorder, and even Metabolic Syndrome. These changes can be attributed to either an

DOI: 10.4018/979-8-3373-4382-2.ch008

increase in opportunistic (e.g., Escherichia coli, Staphylococcus aureus, Prevotella) or decreased beneficial pathogens. The breakdown of intestinal barrier function, systemic inflammation, endotoxemia, changes in the production of Short-Chain Fatty Acids (SCFA), and distortion of the metabolism of glucose and fats are among the processes of dysbiosis. Additionally, microbial compounds such as Trimethylamine-N-Oxide (TMAO) promote insulin resistance with cardiovascular risk.

1. INTRODUCTION

Over the years, research on the host's genetics, diet, and even physical inactivity has helped to clarify the pathophysiology of various metabolic disorders, including Non-Alcoholic Fatty Liver Disease, type 2 Diabetes, and Obesity. With billions of bacteria, viruses, fungi, and archaea in the human gastrointestinal tract is a complex ecosystem whose metabolism has been greatly underestimated and is often restricted to digesting. However, the last 20 years have seen a paradigm shift brought about by groundbreaking advancements in bioinformatics and DNA sequencing technologies. Because the gut microbiota is an active state and an integrated metabolite organ that actively participates in host physiology, scientists now view it as an essential participant as opposed to a passive observer. This vast shared genome provides the host with access to an extensive repertoire of enzymes and biochemical pathways that are absent from the human genome, thereby greatly expanding the functional coding and proteomic capacity beyond that of the host alone. At the intersection of host and microbial complexity, emerging insights into metabolic health and disease have been carefully elucidated, redefining the concepts of host–microbe reciprocity, dysfunction, and therapeutic intervention, and fundamentally reshaping our understanding of these prevalent disorders (Javdan et al., 2020).

The functional features of the microbiome and ecological balance, called eubiosis, define the proper functioning of the microbiome than its concrete composition. This advantageous scenario is marked by significant taxonomic diversity and evolutionary variation, which promote functional redundancy and resilience to environmental disturbances. The majority of the microbiome is made up of eubiotic, required anaerobic microbes from the phyla *Bacteroidetes* and *Firmicutes*, which support the host's vital physiological processes and preserve a healthy anaerobic balance. The community structure is effective at fermenting indigestible dietary fibers in addition to generating Short-Chain Fatty Acids (SCFAs), that regulate host metabolism which include acetate, propionate, and also butyrate- all vital energy sources for colonocytes. A healthy microbiome is essential for the growth and control of the immune system of the host in addition to aiding in the production of essential vitamins such vitamin K and B vitamins, as guarantees proper inflammatory responses. A healthy gut barrier, a complex structure made up of a thick layer, antimicrobial peptides, as well as proteins that create tight connections between epithelial cells, is essential to the symbiotic interaction. These proteins work together to preserve metabolic equilibrium by preventing the unchecked passage of microbial components into the systemic circulation (Rowland et al., 2018).

Dysbiosis, the disruption of this advantageous symbiotic association, is now recognized as a primary cause of metabolic disorders and is an indication of a serious decline in a good biological state. Dysbiosis is not an endpoint but a pathway to imbalance, which can be described by the loss of beneficial microbial taxa, decreased overall microbial diversity, as well as a relative increase in pathobionts and the commensal microbes capable of causing pathology under specific circumstances. The causes of this ecological shift are numerous and they include the excessive amounts of saturated fat and refined sugar, but deficient in dietary fiber, over and improper use of antibiotics, ongoing mental stress and toxins in the environment which can lead to this ecological change. The effects of this disturbance are far reaching and they go beyond the gut lumen. An altered dysbiotic microbiome has functional capacity changes such as reduced ability to generate beneficial SCFAs and increased ability to derive energy at the diet, importantly leading to positive energy balance. At the same time, it may facilitate the destruction eroding the protective mucosa layer and undermine the integrity of the tight junctions of intestinal walls, popularly known as leaky gut. The violation of the body's primary defense enables the subsequent release of microbial compounds within the system, triggering a series of responses that lead to chronic metabolic inflammatory (Borgeraas et al., 2018).

Dysbiosis is one of the reasons contributing to the growing understanding of the molecular relationships between a metabolic disorder, systemic inflammation, and leaky gut. Metabolic endotoxemia is a persistent low-grade systemic inflammatory state brought on by bacterial endotoxins, especially Gram-negative Lipopolysaccharide (LPS), which are transported through the portal circulation. Through the action of endotoxemia, the innate immune response activates pattern recognition receptors such as TLR4, which causes the generation of cytokines that promote inflammation, such as TNF and IL-6. By raising the Serine Phosphorylation of the sugar receptor substrate proteins, these inflammatory mediators directly affect insulin signaling in metabolically important organs such Adipose, Hepatic, and Muscle Tissues, leading to insulin resistance. Dysbiosis, with inflammation, alters host bile acid metabolic processes, transforming the bile acid pool into a more hydrophobic and pro-inflammatory state, hence affecting metabolic signaling through the FXR and TGR5 receptors. Furthermore, metabolites produced in the gut, including Trimethylamine N-Oxide (TMAO) and imidazole propionate, have been documented to directly influence the progression of atherosclerosis and glucose intolerance, respectively. Microbial dysbiosis is pointed as a causative agent in the pathological processes of the most widespread metabolic disorders on an world, being identified as an overall systemic threat to the metabolic homeostasis through the complex mechanisms characterized by a breakdown of Barrier Functionality, Chronic Inflammation, and Non-Specific Metabolite Signaling (Salem et al., 2018).

2. GUT MICROBIOTA CONTROLS THE HOST'S METABOLIC PHYSIOLOGICAL STATES

Complex food proteins and carbohydrates are broken down by the bacteria in the GI tract through enzymatic activities. The gut microbiota provides leucine, isoleucine, valine, and various other branched-chain amino acids. However, because it is necessary for the production of glutathione, the primary intracellular antioxidant, and detoxifier that the host requires for numerous biological processes, glycine is particularly important. Intestinal bacteria create small molecular weight signaling molecules, including gases, methane, Hydrogen Sulfide (HS), as well as non-gaseous metabolites. These compounds have the ability to regulate host genome expression, microbial pathogenicity, and metabolic genes. Additionally, microbes differentiate their gene expression and adapt to specific niches in response to a range of environmental cues, such as host hormones and nutrients. Diets robust in entire plant-based foods, especially those high in fiber, are necessary to maintain a robust, fermentation-producing gut microbiota.

Short Chain Fatty Acids (SCFA) are anaerobically converted into volatile fatty acids by members of the *Lactobacillaceae*, *Clostridaceae*, and *Bacteroides* genera, especially *Citrobacter* and *Serratia* species. These volatile fatty acids can enter monocarboxylate transporters to cross the Blood-Brain Barrier (BBB). GI tract bacteria use enzymes such as glycoside hydrolases or as polysaccharide lyases to preferentially conjugate these substrates, producing polyamines, polyphenols, antioxidants, and vitamins B and K. SCFAs (C-2 acetate, C-3 propionate, as well as C-4 butyrate) can colonize gut microbiota-factors at molar ratios between 3:1:1 and 10:2:1. Following the metabolism of short-chain fatty acids (SCFAs), a major proportion is ultimately converted to CO_2. Butyrate exerts profound effects on goblet cells, Paneth cells, and colonocytes, serving as a primary energy source for cellular metabolism. It plays a critical role in regulating apoptosis, cellular differentiation, and post-translational modifications of proteins and nucleic acids. In contrast, acetate and propionate enter the bloodstream and are taken up by the liver and other peripheral organs, where they function as key substrates for gluconeogenesis and lipid synthesis (Meijer et al., 2010)

The receptors associated with G-proteins GPR41 and GPR43 are expressed in a number of tissues, including inflammatory cells, gut enteroendocrine cell types, and even obese tissue commonly referred to as free fatty acid receptors three and two (FFARs 2/3), which are essential Short-Chain Fatty Acid (SCFA) receptors. Under some physiological circumstances, SCFAs cause the release of PYY and GLP-1 (and even GLP-2). In the first, PYY prevents intestinal lumen nutritional absorption, which impacts eating, while GLP-1 depolarizes β cells, which eventually reside in islets in the pancreas, to release insulin. In order to regulate fat deposition, gut microbiota alters the hepatic cellular production of bile acids and their storage in hepatic triglycerides is regulated by the Farnesoid X Receptors (FXR), a type of bile acid receptor. Deoxycholic acid and other bile acids have antimicrobial properties that affect the gut microbiome and help intestinal epithelial cells produce antimicrobial peptides (Ridlon et al., 2014). Additionally, bacteria changed choline but not carnitine into trimethylamine, which impacted choline's bioavailability and indirectly decreased the liver's triglyceride build up. The diet of the Geile Lemur 73 supplies iron, magnesium, and vitamin C to its intestinal flora. Numerous Dysregulation of the Short-Chain Fatty Acids (SCFAs), metabolites generated from tryptophan, and neuropsychiatric disorders are linked to inflammatory and metabolites, Aminobutyric Acid (GABA), nor-adrenaline, and DA, as well as acetate and 5-HT. Several of its components are important neurotransmitters and modulators that influence the brain-gut axis, according to Collins et al. (2012).

Serotonin is specifically involved in sexuality, drug misuse, hunger, emotion-related behaviors, and the stress response. It is now believed that a large number of recognized and unknown substances that come from gut bacteria make up the human metabolome. Large quantities of physiologically active metabolites, such as the two B vitamins (riboflavin [B2], niacin [B3], pantothenic acid [B5], pyridoxine [B6], folate [B9], and cobalamin [B12]), are produced by the bacteria in the gastrointestinal system. These metabolites affect genetic reactions to environmental stimuli by further regulating the activity of the chromatin-modifying enzymes in the human host. Acetyl-CoA is created by several metabolic processes when histone acetyltransferase carries out histone changes (acetylation and deacetylation) serves as the acetyl donor. DNA methylation and demethylation enzymes utilize glycine, serine, and methionine as substrates. Therefore, through epigenomic modifications, alterations in the gut microbiota can impact both distant cell lineages (such hepatocytes and adipocytes) and proximal intestinal cells. According to Miller and Bassler (2001), bacteria can limit competition and control the density of commensals and efface-pathogens by using quorum sense peptides and persistent microbial signal transduction *via* molecule release.

3. MODULATION OF GUT MICROBIOTA

The global obesity pandemic has stimulated research into targeted therapeutic approaches, including investigations into obesity and the health-promoting properties of specific gut bacteria and their metabolic byproducts. A nutritional planning intervention that alters the microbiota in addition to diet would be less affordable and cost-effective than medical or surgical interventions (Aronsson et al., 2010).

3.1 Probiotics

These relationships between the microbiota of the gut and obesity suggest that probiotic-induced microbiome modulation may lower body weight, BMI, fat mass, serving as a preventative or therapeutic measure against the inclination toward obesity. Probiotics are characterized as live bacteria that, when taken in sufficient quantities as a food or supplement, enhance the host organism's health. *Saccharomyces*, *Bifidobacterium*, and *Lactobacillus* have been shown to influence fat deposition and/or weight loss in overweight people (Rastall et al., 2005). In more than 60% of the *Lactobacillus* strain studies, body fat and/or body weight dropped. *Lactobacillus gasseri* and *Lactobacillus amylovorus*; *Lactobacillus plantarum* and *Lactobacillus rhamnosus* in a hypocaloric diet; *Lactobacillus plantarum* in conjunction with the pure strain its use in Anti-Obesity therapy 15 antibacterial *plantarum curvatus* bacilli or less acidophilus; and even *Lactobacillus casei* or poliphenolic compounds (Borgeraas et al., 2018).

Obese (mean BMI = 28.3) adult subjects with no known medical conditions ingested either *L. gasseri* or unsupplemented milk that was fermented for 12 weeks and followed up after study week 24. Dietary intake, anthropometry: body weight, BMI, and waist and hip circumference, and abdominal visceral and subcutaneous fat percentage by dual-energy ray absorptiometry were evaluated in these double-blind-placebo controlled intervention studies obese with fermented placebo group for a similar sex ratio to the supplemented one adding *Bifidobacterium lactis* and *Lactobacillus paracasei* F19 to a high-fat diet, but excluding *B. Thetaiotaomicron* lowers serum TAG concentration and hepatocellular fat deposition while increasing FIAF expression and providing the host organism with an overlapping anti-obesogenic benefit (Yin et al., 2010). However, intestinal endotoxin was much lower in mice treated with both *Bifidobacterium infantis* and *Bifidobacterium bifidum* for a month, however there was no increase in IL-6, TNF-α, or INF-γ *Bifidobacterium animalis* subspecies treatment. Lactis 420 prevents or reverses the movement of germs out of the stomach, improving overall inflammatory and metabolic condition. Furthermore, *A. Muciniphila*-enriched therapy correlated with improvement of the metabolic status and prevented HF-induced body weight increase, fasting hyperglycemia, metabolic endotoxemia, insulin resistance and inflammation of adipose tissue. Addition of extracellular vesicles from *A. muciniphila*, which boost the endocannabinoid tone in intestine, thereby promoting gut epithelial barrier function *via* augmented occludin expression and reduced intestinal permeability and controls the production of gut peptides and inflammation (Chelakkot et al., 2018).

3.2 Prebiotics

Non-digestible carbohydrates called prebiotics enhance host energy balance by specifically stimulating the microbiota, primarily *lactobacilli* and *bifidobacteria*. They improve dysbiosis and gut systemic disorders by restoring and/or maintaining Eubiosis, Normobiosis in the gut microbiota. The majority of fermentable dietary fibers, specifically non-digestible oligosaccharides (including fructo-, Galacto-, and resistant starch) found in various meals, are thought to be involved in the regulation of gut flora. By down-regulating ghrelin and up-regulating GLP-1 and PYY, it decreases food intake and increases satiety (Cani et al., 2009). After consuming 12 weeks of 21 g/d oligofructose for 48-year-old adults with a BMI more than 25 kg/m demonstrated Decreased Body Weight, Ghrelin Expression, and PYY Concentrations, as well as Low Calorie Consumption, Plasma Glucose, and Insulin Levels. Consuming oligofructose-rich syrup for 120 days (0–14 g Fructo-oligosaccharides/kg daily) caused overweight premenopausal women to lose up to 15 kg of body weight, along with corresponding decreases in fasting insulin and LDL cholesterol levels. When colonic bacteria ferment prebiotics, metabolically active SCFA are created. The anti-obesogenic effect of prebiotics is thought to be mediated by Butyrate, Propionate, and Acetate. Incorporate some butyrate-producing *Bifidobacterium* to enhance gut mucosal integrity and barrier function (Seganfredo et al., 2017).

3.3 Synbiotics and antibiotics

For improved results, synbiotics, a mix of probiotics and prebiotics may be utilized. The microbiota was altered by a combination, oligofructose-enriched inulin, *Lactobacillus rhamnosus*, and *B. lactis*, resulting in the decrease of *Clostridium perfringens* and the predominance of *Lactobacillus* and *Bifidobacterium*. It is more effective than probiotics or prebiotics alone, according to *in vitro* research (Saulnier et al., 2008); nonetheless, human trials are necessary (Beserra et al., 2015). Broad-spectrum antibiotics have also been shown to enhance the expression of gut tight junction proteins in mice, reduce inflammation brought on by Lipopolysaccharide (LPS), and lessen insulin resistance associated with obesity in the liver, muscle, and adipose tissue. The reduction in TLR4 and LPS activation may be the cause of these effects. Portal acetate, a potent activator of 50-AMP-activated kinase for protein, fatty acid oxidation, and energy use, is elevated by antibiotics. However, because of the issue of ongoing low-dose antibiotic usage, antibiotic resistance, the ability to change the commensal bacterial community, and weight gain are not transferred in human use (Carvalho and Abdalla Saad, 2013). Probiotic-induced gut microbiota modulatory effects are protective by decreasing the gut permeability challenges to fit epithelial cell tight junction-sealed, and it prevents translocation of whole bacteria with their products or metabolites, hence reducing LPS stimulation inflammation. Lower inflammation raises hypothalamic leptin and insulin sensitivity, leading to better satiety and glucose tolerance. Elevated GLP-1 and PYY as well as hypothalamic insulin sensitivity drive satiety and reduce food intake. Caloric restriction and high FIAF expression lead to decreased body weight and fat mass. Similarly, bariatric surgery increases gut microbiome diversity by reducing the F: B ratio of *Firmicutes* and increasing *Bacteroidetes*. This was confirmed by a recent systematic review of RYGB and LSG literature (Castanet et al., 2018).

4. CHANGES IN GUT MICROBIOTA IN METABOLIC DISORDERS AND GASTROINTESTINAL DYSMOTILITY

4.1 Changes in Gut Microbiota and Dysmotility of the Digestive System

Food cannot travel through the digestive tract without the waves of peristalsis. The peristaltic motor function is controlled by the Enteric Nervous System (ENS), GI cells in the smooth muscle, pacemaker cells known as interstitial of Cajal cells, Enterochromaffin (EC) as cells, and other components that synchronize the contraction and relaxation of the longitudinal and circular smooth muscles during the Muscularis Externa. Apart from host-specific genetics, nutrition and microbiota also play a role in GI physiology. An altered lumen and epithelial mucus microbiota are linked to the majority of GI disorders.

In view of the emerging knowledge regarding the gut microbiota, microbe-host interaction- immune and metabolic- GI motility disorders play a key pathogenic role. Previous research has shown that the gut flora in IBS patients is different from that in healthy individuals, which may result in abnormal bowel movements due to reduced colonic transit (Tap et al., 2017). Whether IBS patients and healthy controls harbor distinct GM profiles has not been established yet. According to prior publications, a "signature" microbial community would be reduced diversity and an overabundance of methanogenic or as *Clostridium spp*., which have been reported in relation to increased symptoms if suffering from diseases such as IBS. Because of their involvement in 5-hydroxytryptamine (5-HT, serotonin) synthesis

Clostridium spp. may inhibit GI activity, but this needs to be confirmed. Focusing on the microbiome-mediated pathogenesis of GI disease has been centered towards immune dysfunction, gut barrier breach, and flawed gut microbial signaling (Salem et al., 2018).

The association between SIBO and GI dysfunction further justifies the connection of a microbial-host interface and GI motility. Appropriate GI motility maintains the flow of luminal content through the GI tract, thereby preventing SIBO. Slow transit of luminal contents in GI dysmotility patients leads to SIBO. SIBO was secondary to the delayed upper-gut motility of patients by Malabsorption Syndrome. It is also responsible for gut defense dysfunction called SIBO. SIBO is kept at bay by secretory IgA, stomach acid, duodenal bile and defensins. As the host antimicrobial peptides with a role in gut innate immunity, Defensins limit pathogen organism colonisation and ensure commensal bacteria colonization at an optimal concentration. SIBO-induced GI problems are due to an over-zealous immunologic response and inflammation, impaired GI motility, the dysfunction of the intestinal epithelium barrier, dysregulated BA deconjugation as well as serotonergic modulation (Pimentel et al., 2004). Largely Gram-negative, carbohydrate fermenting facultative aerobes and anaerobe like *E. coli*, *K. pneumoniae*, *Enterococcus spp*., and *Proteus mirabilis* are commonly found in the colon of SIBO patients. Similarly, in a study on syndrome of malabsorption patients, elevations of total BAs, lactate and acetate and formate were detected compared to control patients. The levels of acetate and the SIBO symptoms were positively related in malabsorption syndrome patients. Researchers also demonstrated that unconjugated BAs were associated with steatorrhea, which is characterized by diminished intestinal fat utilization. This implies that excessive acetate and even deconjugated BA are resulted from the bacterial species in the small intestine of SIBO patients, on which fat malabsorption based. The small-intestine epithelial cells die if SFAs are not metabolized, which results in barriers loss, ileal brake, stasis, and an increase in bacteria into SI (Ghoshal et al., 2014).

4.2 Metabolic Disorders and Changes in Gut Microbiota

Numerous studies show that the gut microbiota plays a role in maintaining metabolic homeostasis, and that microbial dysbiosis can result from metabolic disorders and diseases by interacting with the gut barrier and causing metabolic inflammation. Furthermore, abundant evidences show that the microbiome controls weight and pathologically leads to T2D. Adding new gut bacteria to rats and humans *via* faecal transplants increases insulin sensitivity, resulting in weight loss (Nicholson et al., 2012). The dwellers of the guts control energy from indigestible carbohydrates enabling the host to synthesize and take up metabolites working as signaling molecules. Diet (including pre-, pro- and anti-biotics) does affect microbial metabolites and colonization but the core phyla in the healthy gut remain constant. To confirm that prebiotics and probiotics cause a gut flora change, further research is required. Antibiotics, with early life exposure or later in life can decimate microbiomes and drive metabolic disease (Kootte et al., 2017). Antibiotics might also enhance peripheral insulin sensitivity in the obese, and thus, metabolic function. Microbiota and obesity an enormous number of studies have shown the metabolism-manipulating possibility of microbiota inducing obesity. SIBO's been found in obese and diabetic patients. SIBO has been associated with slow gut transit in T2D patients, indicating the connection between dysbiosis of the gut microbiome and GI motility and metabolic disease. The impact of microbial activities on host metabolism is described in a small number was carefully monitored human research. These results suggest that alterations in gut microbiota may help treat metabolic problems associated with diabetes (Adamska et al., 2016). Table 1 presents the relationship between microbial dysbiosis and metabolic disorders by summarizing changes in key microbial groups and their associated metabolic conditions, including obesity, type 2 diabetes, insulin resistance, and metabolic syndrome. It also outlines the major biological mechanisms involved, such as altered energy extraction from the diet, compromised gut barrier integrity, persistent low-grade inflammation, disrupted bile acid metabolism, and hormonal imbalance, showing how microbiome alterations contribute to the development of metabolic diseases.

Table 1. Microbial Dysbiosis and Metabolic Disorder

S. No	Type of Dysbiosis	Key Microbes Affected	Associated Metabolic Disorder	Mechanism/Pathway
1	Gut dysbiosis	*Bacteroidetes, Firmicutes*	Obesity	Altered energy harvest from diet
2	Gut dysbiosis	*Akkermansia muciniphila*	Type 2 Diabetes	Impaired gut barrier and inflammation
3	Oral dysbiosis	*Porphyromonas gingivalis*	Insulin resistance	Systemic inflammation
4	Gut dysbiosis	*Lactobacillus*	Non-alcoholic fatty liver disease	Lipid metabolism disruption
5	Gut dysbiosis	*Clostridium cluster XIVa*	Obesity	SCFA reduction
6	Skin dysbiosis	*Staphylococcus aureus*	Atopic dermatitis → metabolic impact	Immune modulation
7	Gut dysbiosis	*Bifidobacterium*	Type 2 Diabetes	Glucose homeostasis alteration
8	Vaginal dysbiosis	*Lactobacillus*	Obesity-related insulin resistance	Inflammation and microbiota metabolites

continued on following page

Table 1. Continued

S. No	Type of Dysbiosis	Key Microbes Affected	Associated Metabolic Disorder	Mechanism/Pathway
9	Gut dysbiosis	*Faecalibacterium prausnitzii*	Metabolic syndrome	Anti-inflammatory SCFA loss
10	Gut dysbiosis	*Ruminococcus*	Obesity	Increased calorie extraction
11	Oral dysbiosis	*Treponema denticola*	Diabetes	Chronic inflammation
12	Gut dysbiosis	*Prevotella*	Insulin resistance	TMAO production and inflammation
13	Gut dysbiosis	*Methanobrevibacter smithii*	Obesity	Altered fermentation and energy harvest
14	Gut dysbiosis	*Escherichia coli*	Type 2 Diabetes	Endotoxemia and systemic inflammation
15	Gut dysbiosis	*Enterobacteriaceae*	Metabolic syndrome	Gut barrier disruption and LPS-induced inflammation

5. FOCUSING ON METABOLIC PATHWAYS AND GUT MICROBIOTA DYSBIOSIS

Currently available treatments for gut dysbiosis caused by bacteria include Antibiotics, Fecal Microbiota Transplantation (FMT), Dietary Modifications, and Probiotic Therapies.

5.1 Antibiotics

Antibiotics Neomycin and rifaximin poorly absorbed antibiotic, both promoted intestinal transit in IBS clinical trials. Additionally, multiple studies have demonstrated that a cocktail of antibiotics treatment for 4-8 weeks in obese mouse models or HFD fed mice improves metabolic features such as Improved Glucose Tolerance, Fat Mass Decline, limitation of Hepatic Steatosis with hepatic and systemic inflammation reduced, associated with changes in gut microbiota composition and integrity of the gut barrier along with metabolic endotoxemia (Reijnders et al., 2016). However, high-quality human clinical studies are urgently needed to address the question of whether such intervention can be similarly effective in humans, and whether gut microbiota could be manipulated this way to promote disturbed metabolism and metabolic diseases. Rifaximin, a non-systemic antibiotic was the most common treatment in individuals with SIBO. A meta-analysis and systematic review including 26 trials with rifaximin showed that SIBO was improved (or) disappeared in 70.8% of subjects with rifaximin treatment. It has been demonstrated that systemic antibiotics, like Norfloxacin, can eliminate SIBO. Normal hydrogen or methane breath tests were more often in treatments compared to placebos (51.1% versus 9.8%, respectively), according to a meta-analysis that included ten prospective clinical investigations of non-systemic antibiotics (Shah et al., 2013).

By potentially restoring "healthy" flora in recipients, Fecal Microbiota Transplantation (FMT) is believed to be helpful in reducing microbial dysbiosis. However, it is still debatable if FMT is a universal cure for IBS or just a placebo. A double-blind, randomized controlled research of 165 IBS patients showed that, while overall dysbiosis did not significantly change following FMT, the intensity of diarrhea significantly decreased in comparison to a placebo control group. According to a recent meta-analysis of five RCTs, FMT did not improve IBS symptoms more than a placebo (Ianiro et al., 2019). However, more extensive and sophisticated research is needed; the small-scale trials that were part of our meta-analysis have shown a significant risk of bias. In 71% of patients with resistant intestinal pseudo obstruction, SIBO was removed following FMT. Another study on metabolic syndrome in humans showed the impact of lean (allogenic) *versus* self-generated (autologous) FMT (Vrieze et al., 2012). Improvements in insulin resistance in the allogenic FMT trial group are attributed to the metabolism response, as seen by changes in blood plasma metabolic products such gamma-aminobutyric acid. The patient's initial limited fecal variety of germs at the beginning of the experiment is a prerequisite for this increase. Furthermore, alterations in gut microbiota composition- which can even be anticipated from fecal microbial communities prior to transplantation – are associated with the positive effects on the utilization of glucose shown in allogenic cohort patients (Vrieze et al., 2012).

5.2 Probiotics

Probiotics, which are live bacteria, are thought to improve intestinal flora. Only a few clinical trials have looked at this approach, and the outcomes have been inconsistent. According to a recent meta-analysis by Zhong et al. (2017), probiotic use was linked to better SIBO clearance. Probiotics have been demonstrated to help people with IBS, although it's still unknown how exactly they reduce symptoms. In another study utilizing a model of db/db T2D mice, probiotics derived from naturally fermented camel milk dramatically reduced blood-glucose and cholesterol levels (Wang et al., 2020). According to another study, when GPR43/41 was enhanced, probiotic-fed diabetic mice made more insulin. This, in turn, increased the release of glucagon-like peptide-1 in response to glucose (Wang et al., 2020). Overall, these findings suggest that therapeutic probiotics may be employed to manage metabolic disorders and gastrointestinal motility disturbances.

5.3 Dietary Intervention

Dietary intervention may be an effective approach to help patients correct their microbial dysbiosis. The colonic bacteria get translocated in the small intestine and ferment the carbohydrates. Gas is produced in excess which may leads to abdominal discomfort and bloating in the case of gut dysbiosis patients. Therefore, dietary restrictions, such as a low-FODMAPS diet, have been proposed to alleviate dysbiosis and IBS symptoms (Mehtab et al., 2019). Low FODMAP diets may play a major therapeutic role in managing SIBO or other dysbiotic disorders because they are also linked to a decreased absolute abundance of the bacteria. Furthermore, compared to diets heavy in fat or protein, a diet high in carbohydrates may encourage the growth of lesser pathogen organisms (Zmora et al., 2019).

5.4. Tiny Molecules

The three most important SCFAs that are eventually given as oral dietary supplements are Acetate, Butyrate, and Propionate. SCFAs are signal molecules that trigger a range of physiological responses in humans. GLP-1 and peptide YY are produced as a result of their impact on intestinal L cells through GPR 41, GPR 43 regions (free fatty acid 2-3, FFARs 2/3). It is noteworthy that GLP-1 peptide infused has been demonstrated to enhance insulin expression in white adipose tissue when adioposity is present. SCFAs encourage adipogenesis and the synthesis of leptin while reducing the breakdown of fat tissue. Bergman (1990) identified butyrate and acetate as hepatic lipogenic agents and propionate as a gluconeogenic substance in the liver (Adamska et al). On DC generated from human monocytes or bone marrow, butyrate inhibits nuclear NF-κB translocation, lowers the levels of costimuloatory molecules, and decreases the synthesis of IL-12. The ketone molecule βhydroxybutyrate (3-hydroxybutyrate), butyrate, and its structural homolog also promote the inhibition of HDACs. The modulation of gene expression is another function of HDACS, which alter certain histone modifications that control transcription, DNA replication, and repair. The cytokine also reduces inflammation by preventing NF-κB and STAT1 from being activated. Ten–eleven translocation (TET) methylcytosine dioxygenases and histone/DNA demethylases, which catalyze the oxidation of 5-methylcytosine and promote DNA demethylation, are strongly inhibited by succinate (Eisenstein, 2020).

6. CHANGES IN THE MICROBIOME LINKED TO TREATMENT OF MEDICAL INTERVENTION

Similar to its role in disease progression and manifestation, the gut microbiota is increasingly being integrated into pharmacological research and therapeutic strategies. The effects of medications or other treatments, including dietary restriction, physical activity, or surgery, can change the composition and activity of microbial consortia. Natural goods that include Probiotics, Synbiotics, or Prebiotics, such kimchi, sauerkraut, and live yogurt, can have an impact on the microbiome. Many people believe that these products are good for the digestive system. The research work focuses on widely utilized medical treatments that have been shown to be clinically beneficial. These are the best treatment approaches that have been established through clinical trials and research to produce the best outcomes (Dimidi et al., 2019).

Therefore, natural products fall outside the scope of this review, despite their potential benefits. The extent to which drugs alter the gut microbiota varies among individuals and can influence microbial composition down to the strain level. Additionally, they discovered that bacteria may play a part in medication metabolism. As a result, it is now clear that the gut microbiota plays a significant role in both medication and illness. Some drugs, like antibiotics, are made to specifically target bacteria, while others, like metformin, boost the production of SCFA linked to the microbiome, and still others, like PPIs, change its makeup or content. However, when these drugs are prescribed, their impact on the gut microbiota is not taken into account. The impact of medications or treatments on the gut microbiome has been the subject of recent research (Li et al., 2019).

6.1. Dietary and Exercise-Related Changes in the Gut Microbiome

The main causes of Type 2 Diabetes and obesity are inadequate physical exercise and excessive calorie intake. As a result, a calorie-deficit diet combined with increased physical activity is usually the main treatment for obesity. Dietary treatments for weight loss appear to improve the clinical features and composition of the microbiota. Numerous studies have found that the compositions of lean and obese individuals differ, and various research teams have demonstrated that lifestyle changes affect the composition of gut bacteria (Rodriguez-Castaño et al., 2017). Metagenomic research has begun to look at people who are overweight or obese in order to assess the functional effects of microbiome changes on obesity. Inflammation of low severity brought on by a bad diet is assumed to be the source of insulin resistance and Type 2 diabetes. Exercise has been shown to be an effective treatment or preventative measure for Type 2 diabetes. Interestingly, regular exercise also appears to affect the composition of the gut microbiota. Therefore, natural products are beyond the scope of this review, although they may be beneficial. The extent to which drugs influence the gut microbiota varies among individuals and can affect microbial composition at the strain level. Studies have investigated these lifestyle modifications by subjecting obese individuals to a 24-month low-calorie diet and physical activity routine or Type 2 Diabetes patients to a 6-month exercise program (Louis et al., 2016). Metagenomic studies of stool samples from these groups at baseline and at the conclusion of the experiment revealed that the abundance of *proteobacteria* was higher in both regimens. Nonetheless, increased numbers of *Proteobacteria* have been found to be a possible microbial indication of disease and have been connected to metabolic disorders. As a result, even while these therapies lessened the symptoms of some illnesses, their effects on the gut microbiota may not have been favorable (Pasini et al., 2019).

6.2. Changes in the Microbiome of the Gut of Metformin

Metformin, the first-line medication used to treat type 2 diabetes following lifestyle adjustment, functions as an anti-hyperglycemic by preventing hepatic gluconeogenesis and increasing glucose uptake in the tissue of skeletal muscles after being absorbed into the cell *via* Oct-3 (Bryrup et al., 2019). Nevertheless, it is still unclear how exactly metformin works. Additionally, research has shown that metformin therapy has a substantial impact on the microbiota, and multiple lines of evidence suggest that the medication acts in the gut. Ejtahed et al. (2019) examined the impact of glucophage on the composition of gut flora in obese non-diabetic individuals after observing weight loss in diabetics taking the medication. They showed that both before and after using metformin, there were notable structural changes in taxonomy and weight reduction. The phylum prosthetic bacteria, which includes the genera *Escherichia*, *Pseudomonas*, *Shigella*, and *Yersinia*, increased in every study. This result is in line with earlier research.

6.3. Changes in the Microbiome of the Gut Because of Cardiovascular Medicines

This plaque build-up frequently brought on by environmental factors like smoking, consuming a high-fat diet, and not exercising. Therefore, it should not be surprising that the recommended therapies for ACVD at the time of initial diagnosis are increased activity and a balanced diet. Atherosclerotic plaques surround the coronaries, and are blood-carrying arteries. This plaque build-up is frequently brought on by environmental factors like smoking, consuming a high-fat diet, and not exercising. Therefore, it should not be surprising that the recommended therapies for ACVD at the time of initial diagnosis are increased activity and a balanced diet. Pharmaceutical treatment is frequently advised to alleviate ACVD symptoms and slow the disease's progression. Maron and associates (2000) Often, hypercholesterolemia is treated with statins. In addition to lowering LDL cholesterol, these drugs may also have anti-inflammatory effects. Vieira-Silva et al. (2020) found an inverse relationship between statin use and an obese profile. They also talked about how statin medication might be used to treat microbes gut dysbiosis by altering the inflammatory state of the host. Patients with ACVD symptoms are advised to take more than just statins. Because Angiotensin-Converting Enzyme (ACE) medications manage high blood pressure and heart failure, β-blockers reduce irregular cardiac rhythms in ACVD. PPIs are known to trigger heart burn and indigestion, thus they may be advised in combination with drugs like ibuprofen other anti-platelets even though they are not directly used to address cardiovascular problems. It has been demonstrated that PPIs affect the microbiome by preventing the formation of acid in the digestive tract, which allows more bacteria to enter the intestine from the stomach (Clooney et al., 2016). Additionally, PPIs dramatically change the gut microbiota and raise *Actinobacteria* within the phylum level, which involves *bacillus*, one of the most common species in the human gut. Despite having diverse modes of action, these medications all have very comparable impacts on the composition of the microbiome, increasing the quantities of *Blautia* and *Streptococcus* (Vila et al., 2020).

6.4. Microbiome Changes Following Gastric Band Surgery

Diet and exercise are the main treatments for Obesity, however their efficacy varies widely, mostly due to patient adherence. However, people who simultaneously have diabetes with type 2 experience remission after bariatric surgery, which is now the most effective method of managing obesity. Rapid weight loss, improved insulin sensitivity, and improved glucose metabolism are possible outcomes of this method. The three most common procedures are gastric Roux-En-Y Bypass (RYGB), Vertical Sleeve Gastrectomy (VBG), and laparoscopic adjustable gastric bands. It has been demonstrated that gastric band surgery improves gut microbiota (Ülker and Yildiran, 2018). Most of these medically induced alterations are associated with improvements in metabolism. However, it should be noted that these changes may simply result from a change in the nature of the diet or from a reduced ability to consume. When comparing the changes in the microbiome composition associated with surgery to those reported with other types of intervention, they find that most of these gut genera overlap. Many of these genera experience significant changes following surgery compared to the pre-surgery baseline. Many studies have investigated the effects of Roux-en-Y Gastric Bypass (RYGB) surgery on the gut microbiome (Al Assal et al., 2020). Clinical cohort studies of RYGB have shown that the abundance of several genera belonging to the phyla Actinobacteria and Proteobacteria increases following surgery. The microbial profiles of patients who had RYGB and VBG procedures differed more than those of the patients' pre-surgery microbiomes. Tremaroli et al. (2015) also discovered that RYGB increased *Escherichia*, *Klebsiella*, and *Pseudomonas* all of which are *Proteobacteria*- much as the activity and diet therapies previously discussed (Tremaroli et al., 2015).

7. METABOLOMIC SIGNATURES IN METABOLIC DISEASES

Numerous metabolic illnesses have been studied using metabolomic profiling examination of small molecules and metabolites found in the host's cells, tissues, or biofluids. Researchers found some quite similar alterations (in levels of fecal and serum metabolites) as expected by studies, despite significant variations in the metabonomics technique and a considerable differentiation across disorders. Serum levels of number of metabolites, including uric acid, cholesterol, and inflammatory indicators like C- Reactive Protein Metabolite (CRPM), a biomarker for numerous disorders, exhibit notable time-related fluctuations. The disease progresses more quickly due to inflammation caused by high blood levels of certain substances (such as uric acid and cholesterol). Thus, the association between metabolic illness and increased levels of uric acid, cholesterol, and inflammatory markers was not surprising (Soletsky and Feig 2012).

All metabolic disorders have reduced indoles, according to serum metabolomics. Tryptophan is the building block for indoles, Aryl Hydrocarbon Receptor (AHR) receptors with anti-inflammatory and γ-δ T-cell-producing properties. Branch-Chain Amino Acids (BCAAs), that are more prevalent in disease, were linked to illness while other amino acids were not. Consequently, elevated plasma concentrations of BCAAs may represent a new biomarker for metabolic disorders. Additionally, there were some recurring patterns in the fecal metabolome. SCFAs including propionate, butyrate, and acetate were found to be higher in obese individuals but decreased in those with T2D and ACVD. Metabolic regulation of glucose, fat, and energy metabolism, bile acids, and cholesterol metabolites have been reported to be greater in obesity but lower in T2D and ACVD (Mietetinen and Gylling, 2000). Bile acids, however, have both beneficial and negative effects on human health, and an imbalance in them can make metabolic diseases worse (Hofmann, 1999). Metabolite levels typically fluctuate as a result of medical intervention. Following metformin treatment or gastric band surgery, uric acid, cholesterol, and other inflammatory markers all drop but indole levels increase, giving untreated patients a unique metabolite profile. Bile acid levels were also higher after the intervention than in the cohorts that received no treatment. Therapies have varying effects on fecal SCFAs (Jennis et al., 2017). Metformin raised levels as anticipated, however SCFA levels fell in T2D. In contrast, GBs lower SCFA levels to offset the elevated levels associated with obesity. Once more, there was no connection found between amino acids and the intervention. However, following GB surgery, BCAAs significantly dropped. Because various species create and consume different chemicals, the host and the shifting microbiome both have an impact on the metabolite levels. For instance, inflammatory markers and cholesterol are negatively correlated with Eubacterium, which is reduced in all disorders (Martinez et al., 2017).

8. METABOLIC DISEASES LINKED TO GUT DYSBIOSIS

Studies have revealed a complicated interaction between Host Diet, Genetics, and changes in the microbiome's composition in connection to Gut Bacteria, Obesity, Insulin Resistance, and Metabolic Syndrome (Harley and Karp, 2012). According to a number of studies, the release of gut bacterial LPS into the bloodstream start a chronic inflammatory process that eventually results in metabolic endotoxemia and obesity-related illnesses. The most significant consequences of the syndrome known as metabolic syndrome, and is defined by central obesity, a high blood sugar level, and elevated blood triglyceride levels, are the establishment of diabetes type 2, insulin resistance, hypertension, and fatty liver disease. People with high colonization levels of bacteria and archeae from the genera *Coprococcus*, *Bifidobacterium*, *Lactobacillus*, *Methanobrevibacter*, and *Faecalibacterium* are much less likely to experience inflammation and metabolic problems, which can lead to ischemic cardiovascular diseases and type 2 diabetes. These species create more SCFAs and hydrogen peroxides, which are known to prevent pathogenic species like *E. coli* and *Staphylococcus aureus* from forming biofilms (Arora and Backhed, 2016).

Obesity associated with behavioral and environmental factors, such as sedentary lifestyles and over indulgence in high-energy meals. The first evidence that microbes may contribute to maintaining energy balance and obesity came from experiments on germ-free animals. Many concerns remain regarding the intricate interaction between microbes and the host in the pathophysiology of obesity. Furthermore, compared to non-obese control animals, obese mice in genetic and diet-induced obesity models exhibited greater concentrations of *Firmicutes* to *Bacteroidetes* (De Filippo et al., 2010). In clinical trials involving healthy volunteers who were overweight or obese, a high proportion of bacteria related to Bacteroidetes was likewise associated with high total amounts of fecal SCFAs. Studies on mice and humans have shown that inflammation and *A. muciniphila* colonization are inversely correlated. Lower levels of *A. muciniphila* have also been seen in people with diabetes, cardiometabolic diseases, and morbidly obese individuals, which further supports their anti-obesity qualities (Cani and de Vos, 2017).

The role of the GI hypothalamic-pituitary-adrenalaxis in a person's susceptibility to obesity is still unknown. According to a recent study, rats fed a high-fat diet have higher levels of acetate produced by their gut microbiota (Perry et al., 2016) regulates the release of ghrelin, hyperphagia, and glucose-stimulated insulin. They concluded that obesity arises from a combination of these factors. Diet-induced obesity resulting from a high-fat (HF) diet activates microglia and astrocytes in the hypothalamus, leading to chronic low-grade inflammation. Acetate deposited in the hypothalamus, according to a study conducted on a mouse model. Researchers reported this drug has a central action and may have an anorectic effect that inhibits the growth of body mass. The neuroimmunendocrine system is essential for maintaining glucose homeostasis and avoiding adiposity in postprandial obesity following bariatric surgery. Both people and animals experience changes in their dietary preferences after bariatric surgery using Roux-En-Y Gastric Bypass (RYGB) operations. Usually, eating a fatty meal and oleic acid, a fatty acid metabolite, results in the production of OEA. PPARα receptors, which are known to activate the vagus nerve and release dopamine in the brain to induce satiety, may therefore be directly impacted by OEA. OEA levels in the brains of obese animals with dopamine inhibition are lower. After surgery, GI-brain axis signaling is altered in RYGB rats due to an increase in OEA and Dopamine 1 Receptor (D1R) expression. The outcome is observable alterations in feeding patterns in animals that refuse a low-fat diet. Furthermore, it is well known that RYGB significantly affects the secretion of a number of gut hormones, such as ghrelin and GLP-1. Exogenous GLP-1 or its analog aids in blood sugar regulation and weight loss in people with type 2 diabetes. Interestingly, by boosting butyrate-producing bacteria, the T2DM drug metformin may contribute to the restoration of a normal microbiota (Forslund et al., 2015).

9. MECHANISMS LINKING DYSBIOSIS TO METABOLIC DISORDERS

9.1 Hyperactivity of the Intestinal Permeability.

The mechanisms by which the gut–hypothalamic–pituitary–adrenal (HPA) axis influences an individual's susceptibility to obesity remain unclear. A recent study discovered a link between a high-fat diet and the quantity of acetate that rats' gut microbiome produces (Perry et al., 2016). They indicate that the system of parasympathetic neurons, which controls the release of ghrelin, hyperphagia, and glucose-stimulated insulin, is activated by continuous acetate turnover. Obesity brought on by an HF diet activates astrocytes and microglia in addition to creating persistent low-grade inflammation in the hypothalamus. Acetate was observed to accumulate in the hypothalamus in a study that used a mouse model. In addition to its central action, this drug may have an anorectic effect that inhibits the growth of body mass. Following bariatric surgery, the nervous system is essential for maintaining glucose homeostasis and avoiding postprandial obesity-related adiposity. Food preferences in people and animals alter following the Roux-en-Y gastric bypass (also known as RYGB) bariatric surgery. Eating a fatty meal or oleic acid, a fatty acid metabolite, usually results in the production of OEA. Therefore, PPARα receptors, which are known to activate the vagus nerve or release dopamine in the brain to induce satiety, may be directly impacted by OEA. Dopamine-inhibited obese animals had lower levels of OEA in their brains. After surgery, RYGB rats have elevated expression of Dopamine 1 Receptor(s) (D1R) and OEA, resulting in altered GI-brain axis signaling. Rejecting a low-fat diet causes animals to adjust their feeding patterns in observable ways. The release of various gut hormones, such as ghrelin and GLP-1, is also known to be significantly influenced by RYGB. In individuals with type 2 diabetes, endogenous GLP-1 or its analogs aid in blood glucose regulation and promote weight loss. Notably, the type 2 diabetes drug metformin may help restore a healthy gut microbiome by increasing the abundance of butyrate-producing bacteria (Forslund et al., 2015).

Numerous pathophysiological implications of a weakened intestinal barrier affect the start and potential complications of metabolic disorders. Bacterial LPS is a major contributor to the release of pro-inflammatory chemicals in a leaky gut. The main structural element of Lipopolysaccharide (LPS), a potent endotoxin found on the outer membrane of gram-negative bacteria, passes through the intestinal barrier and into the bloodstream, wherein lipoprotein carriers carry it to other areas of the human body (Moreira et al., 2012). Adhesion results in the constant creation and secretion of cytokines that are pro-inflammatory, including TNF-0, IL-1, and IL-6, which in turn promotes the NF-0-B and MAPK inflammatory pathway downstream. Because these inflammatory chemicals disrupt the signaling pathways that regulate insulin in Adipocytes, Hepatocytes, and Myocytes, low-grade and chronic systemic pathophysiology of insulin resistance is significantly influenced by inflammation (Shoelson et al., 2006). Consequently, dysbiosis-associated intestinal hyperpermeability remains not just a gut-related phenomenon; it has been found to be a critical early event through which alterations in gut microbiota result creates a systemic inflammatory response, which in turn encourages conditions including type 2 diabetes, obesity, and non-alcoholic fatty liver disease.

Type 3 diabetes mellitus (also called T3DM) is linked to chronic low-grade inflammation. An extended systemic reaction to low-grade inflammation that is persistent to immunological activation that takes place subclinically, as opposed to the acute or high-grade inflammatory response that follows infection or damage. Inflammatory flare-ups are caused by imbalances in gut microbial dysbiosis and are now identified as a primary feature of metabolic diseases (Hotamisligil, 2006). The system begins in the gut lamina propria, where alterations in the GM composition (often seen as Long-term, low-level stimulation for host innate immunity results from an increase in pathobiont populations and a drop in the ratio for *Firmicutes* to *Bacteroidetes*. Local immune cells, dendritic cells, and macrophages constantly come into contact with microbial-associated molecular patterns (MAMPs), such as lipopeptides and flagellin, which pass through the compromised intestinal barrier. The extended activation of PRRs, including TLRs and NLRs, continuously mobilizes a number of pro-inflammatory mediators. A self-sustaining loop of immune activation brought on by local inflammation underlies the pathophysiology of insulin resistance and metabolic syndrome. This cycle worsens gut epithelial injury and enhances immune cell migration into metabolic tissues (Lumeng and Saltiel, 2011). The systemic inflammation that results in tissue-specific deficits is caused by activated cells of the immune system and/or inflammatory cytokines moving from the gut to downstream metabolic organs. Macrophage infiltration in adipose tissue changes the previously described anti-inflammatory M2 cells type toward the pro-inflammatory M1 type form, enclosing deceased adipocytes in crown-shaped formations and generating high amounts of TNF-alpha and IL. These cytokines also directly suppress insulin signaling in a paracrine, endocrine way by causing the serine phosphorylation of IRS-1, which stops glucose absorption. Likewise, gut-derived endotoxins in the hepatic medium trigger the activation of Kupffer cells, which are liver-resident macrophages, leading to hepatic inflammation that lowers hepatic insulin clearance and promotes fibrosis and steatosis. Additionally, normal pancreatic 3-cells interact with the insulin-secreting machinery due to the cytokine environment, which also enhances apoptotic (Donath and Shoelson, 2011). Since the gut microbiota orchestrates the host immunological response and is believed to be at the vanguard of a continuous inflammatory symphony that causes metabolic disarray in most organ systems, it is therefore a primary target for treatment.

9.2 Metabolic Endotoxemia and Endotoxin Release

A two- to three-fold increase in the circulating endotoxin, Lipopolysaccharide (LPS), which originates from bacteria, is known as metabolic endotoxemia. According to Cani et al. (2007), it is a mechanism of sick microbiota in the gut that connects systemic metabolic inflammation. In addition to promoting the development of Gram-negative LPS-producing bacteria, a diet heavy in saturated fat also satisfies the requirements for permitting systemic absorption of endotoxin by stimulating intestinal chylomicron production. This condition is directly caused by changes in the gut environment as influenced by dietary and dysbiosis-induced modifications to the gut ecosystem. The hydrophobic components of LPS can be scavenged from the gut lumen by these enormous lipoprotein particles, which then carry the molecule into the lymphatic system and eventually the systemic circulation. Dysbiosis impairs this process, allowing endotoxins to enter the gut through the leaky mucous layer or tight junctions. When Lipopolysaccharide-Binding Protein (LPS) enters the bloodstream, it is mainly bound to sCD14 and Lipopolysaccharide-Binding Protein (LBP). These molecules then transport LPS to its main signaling receptor, Toll-like Receptors 4 (TLR4) is present in endothelium and immune cells all over the body. This results in a systemic inflammatory state (Moreira et al., 2012).

Both macrophages in the liver and adipose tissue bind the LPS-LBP complex with the CD14/TLR4/MD2 receptor complex, which sets off a strong intracellular signaling cascade that is a major contributor to metabolic illness. The MyD88-dependent pathway, which causes a The TRIF-dependent pathway, which produces the IFN response type I interferons and contributes to a protracted inflammatory response, and the rapid activation of NF-KB and consequent early pro-inflammatory cytokines genes like TNF-alpha and IL-1beta are the two different signaling pathways that are subsequently initiated by this complex (Kawasaki and Kawai, 2014). Due to the activation of kinases like JNK and IKK2, which phosphorylate IRS-1 at inhibitory serine sites, preventing normal tyrosine phosphorylation during signal transmission mediated by insulin, this cytokine storm has a detrimental effect on insulin activity. The cells in muscle, fat, and liver tissue no longer react to insulin as they should, which is a common feature of insulin resistance. Additionally, hepatic new lipogenesis and inhibition of fatty acid 2 oxidation are direct effects of endotoxemia that will lead to the development of hepatic steatosis (Saberi et al., 2009). Therefore, the imbalance within inflammation along with metabolism that defines obesity and type 2 diabetes can be directly induced by gut bacteria through a natural mechanism called metabolic endotoxemia.

9.2.1 Dysregulated Bile Acids Metabolism.

The liver converts cholesterol into bile acids, which are then converted to glutamate or glycine. It has long been known that bile acids have an impact on how dietary lipids are emulsified and absorbed in the small intestine. However, it is now recognized that they are powerful signaling molecules their metabolism is closely linked to the gut flora. This crucial host-microbe interaction is also referred to as the "gut-liver axis" (Wahlström et al., 2016). Following digestion, conjugated main bile acids are broken down by the enzyme bile salt hydrolase (BSH), which is created by "intestinal bacteria," which are primarily found in the colon and distal small intestine. BSH plays a role in the initial and most important stage of microbial transformations, which is the deconjugation of bile acids. Clostridium species carry out further bacterial dehydroxylation activities that convert primary bile acid compounds (cholate, chenodeoxycholate) into bile acids that are secondary (deoxycholate, lithocholate). This microbe-derived metabolism significantly alters the bile acid pool's chemical properties, signaling potential, and toxicity. Dysbiosis, which adversely affects host metabolism and inflammation, significantly modifies this intricate system (Jia et al., 2018).

They naturally bind to specific nuclear and membrane-based receptors, including TGR5 (G protein- coupled bile acid receptors 1) and the power sources farnesoid X receptor (FXR) mediates their overall metabolic effects. Hormone limits the production of bile acids by inhibiting the CYP7A1 enzyme, which is part of the recursive undesirable feedback circuit (Kuipers et al., 2014). This axis is upset by dysbiosis, and alterations in the typical pattern of bile acid composition can stop FXR from activating to stop the overproduction of BA, which leads to dyslipidemia and hepatic stress. Considering that some species of bile acids, including taurine linked beta-muricholic acid, have been demonstrated to be FXR antagonists, the dysbiosis may also impair feedback regulation. Additionally, alterations in microbiota have a comparable effect on the action of bile acids as ligands of the TGR5 receptor, an essential component of lipid metabolism and energy regulation. Insulin release and sensitivity are increased when enteroendocrine L- cells that activate TGR5 produce glucagon-like peptide-1 (GLP-1) (Thomas et al., 2009). Thus, under dysbiosis settings, alterations in the bile acid pool may directly regulate central metabolic pathways that lead to non-alcoholic fatty liver disease, glucose intolerance, and an imbalance in energy homeostasis.

9.3. Mitochondrial Mishap through Microbial Metabolites.

Mitochondria, also referred to as the cell's power plants, are crucial for preserving energy balance, and their dysfunction is a hallmark of metabolic diseases like obesity and insulin resistance. Compounds derived from the gut microbiota may directly influence neuronal bioenergetics, biogenesis, and dynamics as distant regulators of cellular metabolism, according to an increasing amount of studies (Bölhed et al., 2007). The short-chain fatty acid butyrate is one of these beneficial metabolites that usually enhance mitochondrial activity by providing an energy source and by upregulating mitochondrial biogenesis pathways like AMPK and fatty acid oxidation. When a situation of dysbiosis is achieved, however, the synthesis of toxic microbial molecules rises and the creation of helpful metabolites falls. H_2S, a potent inhibitor, Complex IV (cytochrome c oxidase) in human mitochondria, is overproduced by sulfate-reducing bacteria (*Desulfovibrio*) in the gut when it is ill. In the end, this blockage reduces the cell's ability to meet its energy and insulin response needs by causing it to make less ATP, produce fewer reactive oxygen species (ROS), and transition to an inefficient glycolytic metabolism (Carbonero et al., 2012).

Apart from hydrogen sulfide, mitochondrial health is directly impacted by a number of bacterial metabolic byproducts associated with dysbiosis. Gut bacteria like *Eggerthellalenta* create imidazole propionate, a histidine metabolite that inhibits insulin signaling at the IRS level prior to inflammatory cytokines (Koh et al. 2018). It causes hepatic and systemic insulin resistance by activating the mTORC1 pathway, which reduces insulin sensitivity. Moreover, high concentrations of Bent Chain Amino Acids (BCAAs), which are typically linked to dysbiotic microbiomes, may overwhelm the mitochondria's catabolic machinery. This might lead to the buildup of hazardous intermediates such acyl-CoAs. These intermediaries may enhance insulin resistance and impair mitochondrial function (Newgard et al., 2009). A cellular energy crisis and metabolic rigidity are caused by the interchange of these microbial metabolites, oxidative stress, change of insulin signaling, and limitation of electron transport. Microbes' direct attack on mitochondrial function is an attractive way that gut dysbiosis might lead to the energy needs of cells and the energy inefficiency that characterizes obesity and type 2 diabetes. Figure 1 illustrates how alterations in gut microbial composition contribute to metabolic disorders.

Figure 1. Gut Dysbiosis <> Metabolic Disorders: The Mechanistic Link

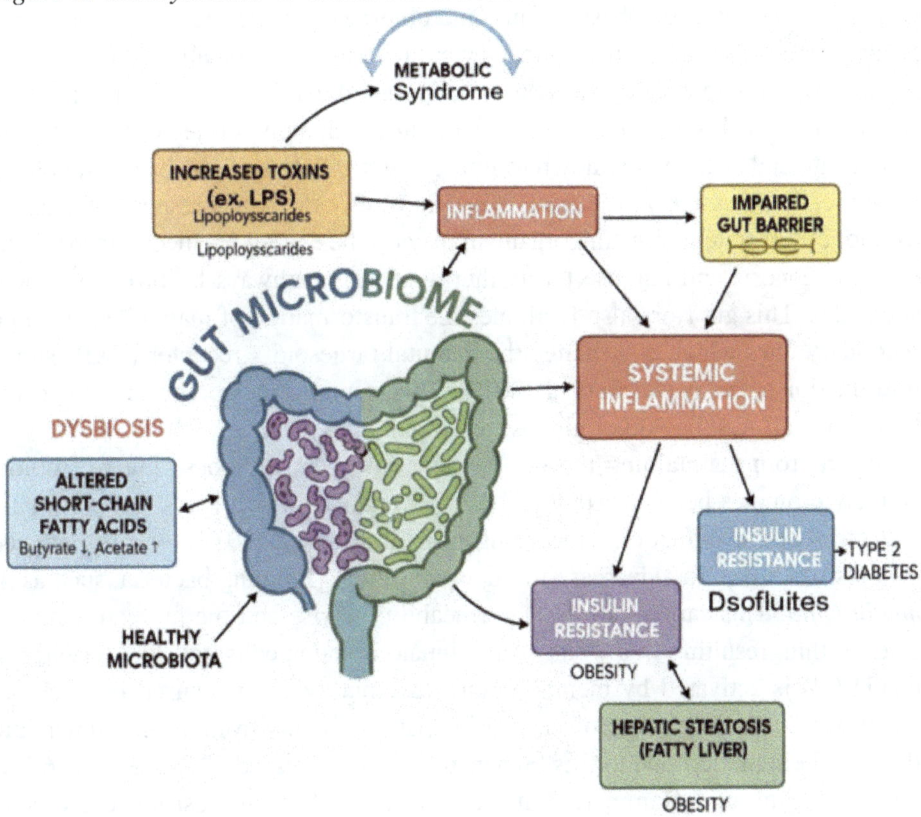

10. MICROBIAL DYSBIOSIS IN PARTICULAR METABOLIC DISORDERS.

10.1 Obesity

Furthermore, the gut microbiome of obese people differs, with a modified microbial ecology that includes a loss in total diversity and a modified ratio among the two major bacterial families, which frequently includes an increased ratio of *Firmicutes* to *Bacteroidetes* (Ley et al., 2006). As demonstrated by germ-free mice who remain lean when served a high-fat diet but quickly develop adiposity after obtaining microbiota from an obese mouse, this aberrant condition is not just a result of obesity but rather the cause of the illness (Turnbaugh et al., 2006). The underlying pathway involves an increased metabolic capacity of the microbiota, which is a hallmark of obesity. This microbiome's genetic arsenal breaks down foodstuff polysaccharides that humans would not normally be able to digest, leading to a more complete digestion process, a larger dietary intake of E, and a higher generation of SCFAs, or short-chain fatty acids. Although gut-derived SCFAs like propionate and acetate are known to improve gut satiety and glucose metabolism, systemically excessively producing these kinds of acids in the presence of a hyper-dysbiotic, substrate-harvesting organism may tip the energy balance in favor of the liver lipogenesis and adipose tissue thermogenesis pathways by providing more substrates. This gut flora also facilitates the transformation of main bile acids into secondary ones which can change the parental farnesoid x receptor (FXR) signal transduction pathway (Sayin et al., 2013). This results in fat storage and affects the body's overall metabolism of glucose and lipids.

Apart from maintaining the gut barrier's integrity, the obese gut microbiota actively promotes persistent low-grade inflammation, which leads to weight gain and metabolic dysfunction. According to Everard et al. (2013), obesity-induced dysbiosis is linked to a decrease in important mucus-foraging bacteria, such as *A. muciniphila*. This causes intestinal permeability to rise and the protective mucus layer to thin, resulting in a “leaky gut.” Innate immune cells' toll-like receptor 4, or (TLR4) is activated by metabolic endotoxemia, which is caused by bacterial endotoxins, especially Lipopolysaccharide (LPS), moving from the gut lumen into the portal circulation due to this breached barrier. Increased TNF-a and IL-6 levels in the resulting inflammation may be the cause of insulin resistance, a crucial aspect of the physiology of obesity. In metabolic systems such the liver, muscles, and adipose tissue, these drugs can also directly interfere with insulin signaling. Additionally, metabolites produced by microbes may affect the production of gut hormones including GLP-1 and even PYY, which regulate hunger and fullness and promote greater food intake. This is an example of how the dysbiotic microbiota may affect host metabolism and affect the gut-brain axis (Torres-Fuentes et al., 2017). A vicious cycle involving low-grade inflammation, hormonal imbalance, and excessive calorie intake makes it difficult to lose weight permanently.

10.2 Diabetes Mellitus Type 2

The intestinal microbiota of people with type 2 diabetes mellitus, or T2DM, differs from that in both healthy and simply obese people. Opportunistic infections and lactate-producing bacteria are more common in T2DM patients, who have an intermediately decreased microbial diversity (Qin et al., 2012). The most notable changes are the rise in genera involving *Clostridium hathewayi* and *Bacteroides caccae*, and the decline in genera that produce butyrate universally, such as *Rose-*

buria intestinalis and *Faecalibacterium prausnitzii*, which are implicated in insulin sensitivity and colon health. This dysbiotic ecosystem is a source of disease rather than a tourist attraction because transplanting the fecal microbiota from diabetic to mice lacking germs can transmit glucose intolerance (Kootte et al., 2017). In an informal sense, the T2DM microbiome can be characterized by decreased butyrate production and increased capacity for reactive stress resistance or sulfate reduction (an sign of gut inflammation). Butyrate deficiency is particularly detrimental since it improves gut integrity and lowers systemic inflammation, in part by blocking NF-0B signaling pathways, while also increasing insulin sensitivity by boosting L-cell production of GLP-1, or glucagon-like peptide (Canfora et al., 2015).

Insulin resistance and mitochondrial dysfunction are further exacerbated by the pathophysiological process of diabetic dysbiosis, which produces specific microbial chemicals that interfere with cellular energy consumption. For instance, Type 2 Diabetes (T2DM) has been causally linked to increased levels of the histidine compound imidazole sodium propionate, a compound catalyzed by gut microbes like *Eggerthellalenta.* This is because elevated levels of this metabolite activate mTORC1, which phosphorylates and degrades Insulin Receptor Substrate (IRS) and suppresses hormone signaling at the level of mitochondria (Koh et al., 2018). Additionally, there is a significant chance of dysbiosis, which could lead to an increase in the amount of branched-chain amino acids (BCAAs) in the blood. Since certain bacteria have been demonstrated to actively produce BCAAs, and a high level of BCAA amino acids is a risk factor for resistance to insulin (Pedersen et al., 2016). According to Aragon et al. (2018), the disruption of the intestinal-vascular axis is also influenced by the gut flora of diabetic patients. This is because whole-body glucose intolerance results from the endothelium's inability to react to insulin due to irregular microbial product generation and an altered bile acid balance. Due to this multifaceted attack on host metabolism through direct maladaptation in insulin signal transduction, induction of inflammation, and inhibition of gut hormone release (silence), the dysbiotic gut microbiome is an essential integrator of the Type 2 Diabetes Mellitus' intricate pathogenesis.

10.3 The Metabolic Syndrome

Central Obesity, High Blood Pressure, Hyperglycemia, and Dyslipidemia are among the diseases collectively referred to by the term Metabolic Syndrome (MetS). The gut microbiome is the most important and vital integrative site that links all of these different metabolic illnesses through a range of similar microbial activities (Cani et al., 2007). MetS's dysbiotic profile is frequently linked to a decline in both detrimental, anti-inflammatory bacteria and the total range of microbial genes that erode host indigestible fibers. These bacteria weaken the integrity of the ecosystem by upsetting the gut community. This maladaptive microbial population produces the crucial metabolites SCFA propionate and butyrate, which maintain endothelial integrity, regulate glucose homeostasis, and prevent hepatic gluconeogenesis. At the same time, inflammatory bacteria, including those that produce Lipopolysaccharide (LPS) and Trimethylamine (TMA), are on the rise. This ensuing systemic milieu, exacerbated by microbial dysbiosis, combines low-grade inflammation, hormonal imbalances, and disturbed lipid metabolism, all of which contribute to several diagnostic criteria associated with metabolic disorders (Le Chatelier et al., 2013).

Since the dysbiotic microbiota directly influences metabolism and cardiovascular disease risk factors, especially atherogenic dyslipidemia and hypertension, its activity may have an effect on the metabolic syndrome. Also, by affecting the synthesis of Vasoactive molecules, certain gut microorganisms might affect blood pressure. For example, the reduction of bacteria that produce SCFA inhibits the production of renin and vascular tone by the Gpr41 and olfr78 receptors in the kidney and blood vessels, hence increasing blood pressure (Pluznick et al., 2013). Furthermore, in the dysbiotic gut, microbial transitory catabolism of BA may produce a unique pool of bile acid molecules that cannot activate FXR and TGR5 receptors leading to elevated blood triglycerides and lower HDL cholesterol. Increased regulation of the supplementary choline and carnitine metabolite Trimethylamine N-Oxide (TMAO), which raises platelet reactivity, form cell migration, and early atherosclerosis, is linked to MetS (Tang et al., 2013). Therefore, among other aspects and components of this multifaceted/modal multifactorial disease, one important pathological metabolism component in Metabolic Syndrome is the gut flora. When it malfunctions, it produces atherogenic compounds, increased inflammatory stimuli, and decreased beneficial metabolites.

The growth of non-alcoholic fatty liver disease, or NAFLD, is significantly influenced by the gut-liver axis, a bidirectional communication pathway according to Henao-Mejia et al. (2012). Through the portal vein, gut-derived products- which are created by the intestinal microbiota are delivered to the liver. The underlying cause of NAFLD is dysbiosis, which is characterized by a relative depletion of beneficial butyrate producers from the phylum *Firmicutes*, such as *Ruminoccocaceae* and *Lachnospiraceae*, and an excess of endogenous Gram-negative *Bacteroidetes*. This specific microbiota composition has two main effects: it leads to a butyrate shortage, which is necessary to maintain the construction of the gastrointestinal barrier, and it encourages the growth of bacteria that could produce ethanol and other poisons on their own. Increased entrance of Microbe-Associated Molecular Patterns (MAMPs), particularly Lipopolysaccharide (LPS), through the portal system exacerbates gut barrier failure. Hepatic stellate cells and other Kupffer cells have Toll-Like Receptor 4 (TLR4) and liver macrophages, is activated when LPS enters the liver. Instead of producing a healthy liver condition like Alcoholic Fatty Kidney Disease, where ethanol-produced endotoxins stimulate TLRs, Instead of only steatosis and ultimately fibrosis, this causes a pro-inflammatory and pro-fibrogenic reaction that leads to Non-Alcoholic Steatohepatitis (NASH).

In addition to causing inflammation through the production of endotoxins, the gut microbiota linked to NAFLD promotes oxidative stress and the build-up of hepatic fat through a variety of other metabolism-related mechanisms. Dysbiosis alters bile acid metabolism toward an increasingly hydrophobic and cytotoxic bile acid profile that may result in hepatocyte destruction, in addition to exacerbating liver inflammation through FXR and TGR5 activation (Jia et al., 2018). Additionally, the gut microbiota affects choline metabolism because more bacteria that consume choline decrease it, which stops the liver from secreting VLDL and storing triglycerides in hepatocyte cytoplasm. By lowering hepatic antioxidants, the microbial synthesis of Trimethylamine (TMA) from phosphatidylcholine in food not only produces the proatherosclerotic TMAO but also directly contributes to hepatic oxidative stress. Moreover, oxidative stress caused by the cytochrome P450 2E1 (CYP2E1) channel can result in lipid peroxidation or hepatocyte damage, and microorganisms such as *Escherichia coli* create endogenous ethanol NAFLD is caused by a GM therapy is the main focus of target approaches due to a combination of elevated endogenous alcohol production, disruption to choline metabolism, altered bile acids signaling, and persistent endotoxemia (Spencer et al., 2011).

10.4 Gut microbiome-related cardiovascular disorders.

Because of the production of diet-dependent pro-atherogenic metabolites, the gut microbiota has become a significant non-traditional risk indicator for cardiovascular disease, or CVD (Tang et al., 2013). The most well-studied process is the transformation of dietary phosphatidylcholine, the amino acid choline, and even L-carnitine which can be found in red meat, eggs, and milk products into Trimethylamine (TMA), that is then oxidized by Flavin Monooxygenases (FMOs) in the liver to Trimethylamine N-Oxide (TMAO). Elevated plasma levels of TMAO have also been shown to have a possible correlation with an increased risk for severe cardiovascular problems (MI, stroke, and mortality), even in the absence of traditional risk factors. Inhibiting reworsal cholesterol transporters like ABCA1 and ABCG1 increases the conversion of macrophages to cholesterol-loaded foam cells (Xu and Wang, 2019); activating NLRP3 inflammasome signaling and NF-κB activity increases plasma thrombotic potential (Li et al., 2016); and causing endothelial dysfunction, which is associated with arterial inflammation, at least partially due to the production of reactive oxygen compounds that is dependent on NADPH oxidase (Wang et al., 2011).

In addition to the TMAO pathway, disruptions between the host and gut microbiota also impact immunological homeostasis, bile acid metabolism, and also systemic inflammation, all of which are factors in the growth of cardiovascular disease. As intestinal permeability rises, live bacteria and their immunogenic byproducts such as Lipopolysaccharide (LPS) translocate into the bloodstream. This plays a significant role in the "leaky gut syndrome" which is linked to a dysbiotic stool and frequently characterized by a poor fermenting flora that produces SCFA (Amar et al., 2011). Bacteremia and endotoxemia result in a persistent state of low-level inflammation, which is known to be linked to endothelial dysfunction and atherosclerosis. Furthermore, the gut microbiota is crucial for the metabolism of some antihypertensives, such as acetazolamide, which might impact its efficacy, and bacterial metabolites, such as phenylacetylglutamine, may bind adrenergic receptors and encourage platelet activation to induce thrombosis (Nemet et al., 2020). The cardiovascular system's FXR and TGR5 receptors are activated by secondary bile acids generated by gut bacteria, changing inflammation, lipid metabolism, and local vascular tone (Pols et al., 2011). As a result, the gut microbiota may influence cardiovascular disease in a number of ways, such as by directly metabolizing dangerous compounds like TMAO or indirectly influencing vascular biology, host inflammation, and medication metabolism. The gut microbiota becomes a crucial part of cardiovascular physiology during this phase.

11. MICROBIAL DYSBIOSIS DIAGNOSTIC TOOLS.

11.1 Metagenomics and 16S rRNA microbiome sequencing.

The foundation of microbiome research has been thought to be 16S ribosomal RNA, or rRNA, sequencing of DNA due to its low cost and high-throughput analysis for community characterisation (Kuczynski et al., 2012). According to reports, this technique makes use of the 16S rRNA genes, which has nine hypervariable regions (V1–V9). These sections produce genetic barcodes, or sequences, that enable differentiating between different species of bacteria and archaea. DNA is extracted from a sample, PCR is used to amplify the regions of interest, and the PCR amplicons are then sequenced on sequencers such as the Illumina MiSeq. For recommendations for taxonomic makeup, these sequences are then grouped into OTUs or Amplicon Sequence Variants (ASV). Bioinformatic pipelines (like QIIME 2 and MOTHUR) that use databases like SILVA or Green-genes to reference their sequences come next. Although 16S sequencing can only disclose creatures at the genus level, it is a great tool for revealing species in relative abundances and diversity. It only provides a general overview about the system structure and is unable to provide a trustworthy species- or strain-level annotation or any insight into the functional capabilities of the microbial community (Jovel et al., 2016).

Shotgun metagenomic sequencing overcomes the limitations of 16S sequencing and provides a complete view of the genetic composition of the entire microbiome by separating and reading each molecule in a sample (Qin et al., 2010). This non-specific approach allows for high-precision taxonomic resolution down to the species and even strain level and finds viruses, fungi, and archaea that are often missed by 16S. More importantly, since this catalog of all sequenced microbial genes includes all microbial genes, it can be utilized for functional profiling. Then, using databases like MetaCyT or KEGG, these genes can be overlaid into metabolic pathways. This suggests that the community's practicality with regard to bile acid metabolism, SCFA generation, and inflammatory potential. Nevertheless, this universal power has many disadvantages, such as high expenses, large data storage requirements, and complex bioinformatics requirements. Moreover, the degree of stochasticity for microbial composition may be affected by the degradation of microbial sequencing depth brought on by an excess of host DNA in feces, which is reflected in reliance on reference genome completeness (Quince et al., 2017). Metagenomics is essential to understand who is present as well as what they are doing in regard to metabolic health and dysbiosis.

11.2 Methods of Metabolomics

By bridging the gap between genetic capabilities or phenotypic host-microorganism interactions, the evaluation of tiny-molecule metabolites could identify the functional feedback that most closely resembles the gut microbiome as a whole (Wikoff et al., 2009). This method measures important bioactive molecules that result from the intricate relationship between microbial enzymes and dietary content, such as SCFAs, Bile Acids (BAs), TMAO, and indole derivatives. Nuclear Magnetic Resonance (NMR) spectroscopy, which has high accuracy and requires minimal sample preparation, and Mass Spectrometry (MS), which is typically used in combination with Gas or Liquid Chromatography (GC/LC-MS) for an outstanding level of sensitivity and selectivity of determining the quantity of numerous metabolites. To gain information into the condition of the gastrointestinal ecology, these metabolites can be analyzed in urine, blood, or stool samples. Indicators like a low Compared to taxonomic data alone, which only provides a dynamic and physiological picture of dysbiosis, the branched-chain amino acid to butyrate ratio in stool or a greater imidazole-propionate concentration in the blood provide a more direct assessment of metabolic abnormalities (Zhao et al., 2019).Metabolomics and sequencing data can be combined to create a causal model of microbiome influence that goes beyond correlation to mechanism by employing multimodal integration across complex omics

(Marcobal et al., 2013). Scientists can make a hypothesis about which bacterial taxa may be producing desirable or unwanted compounds by contrasting concentrations of most likely products of specific bacterial taxa (such 16S or metagenomics) with their presence of such bacteria. This integrative method can be used to identify a functional guild, such as a community of bacteria that work together to convert primary to secondary bile acids. Stable isotope probing can also directly verify metabolic flow and active participants and trace back the fate of labeled nutrients by utilizing microbial pathways. The metabolite profiles that are generated can also serve as a very precise biomarker of disease, such as in T2DM or NAFLD, with often superior diagnosis, as an alternative to depending only on microbial taxonomy. The metablome is quite complex and needs extensive spectral libraries to identify the molecule, thus there are still problems. Furthermore, because metabolite levels always fluctuate to some extent, they must be carefully controlled (Patti et al., 2012). However, metabolomics is a crucial method for transforming a list of bacteria into an insightful analysis of how they affect the host.

11.3 Dysbiosis Biomarkers

According to Weersma et al. (2020), dysbiosis biomarkers are measurable characteristics that go beyond taxonomic lists. They offer a numerical estimate rather than a list of abnormal gut ecosystem states and are typically linked to certain illness situations. These biomarkers may additionally be separated into a few categories. The first category is based on taxonomic ratios and indices, such as whether *Faecalibacterium praunitzii* has higher anti-inflammatory capability because its concentrations are lower than those of *Escherichia coli*. The richness and uniformity of species in a sample is known as alpha-diversity is the other important metric. Low diversities are a strong, widespread indicator of dysbiosis across a wide range of metabolic and inflammatory health conditions. Functional indicators are also crucial. For example, low levels of stool short-chain fatty acids, especially butyrate, may be a sign of poor gut health and fiber fermentation. Similarly, higher gastrointestinal permeability and metabolic endotoxemia can be inferred from high blood levels of soluble CD14 (sCD14) or Lipopolysaccharide-Binding Protein (LBP) (Amar et al., 2008). Compared to the presence or absence of a single microbial species, processing these measurements together produces a richer, more sensitive, and clinically relevant image.

Advanced biomarkers with a high predictive ability for customized nutrition and diagnostics are being produced *via* multi-omics-based applications. As an illustration, consider the microbiome's diagnostic potential, which is encoded in machine learning algorithms to forecast an individual's reaction to a particular diet according to metagenomic clusters of genes (Zeevi et al., 2015). Trimethylamine N-oxide

(TMAO) plasma concentration, which is astrong predictor of future cardiovascular risk and is directly formed from the metabolic product of particular gut bacteria, is another potent biomarker (Tang et al., 2013). Bile-acid ratios, such as the glycine/taurine conjugated ratio in blood or the primary/secondary bile-acid ratio in feces, are other particular indicators that may reliably point to a disruption in the gut-liver axis. A so-called dysbiosis index is created by combining these genetic data with clinical factors, and it can be used to cohort patients for therapies (Le Chatelier et al., 2013). In order to reestablish a robust, healthy microbiome, these biomarkers have the potential to be non-invasive, longitudinally monitored, and actionable in response to food counseling, probiotic selection guidance, and therapeutic efficacy evaluation.

11.4 Individualized Microbiome Assessment Panels.

Personalized Microbiome Analysis for Clinical and Real-World Applications Panels are the commercial and practical application of microbiome science with the goal of creating tools that patients and medical professionals may use, according to Zmora et al. (2016). Specific metabolomic assessments of significant fecal or serum compounds are frequently linked with the functional potential of a given gut microbiota and 16S or broad-band metagenomic sequencing of systematic connections. A customized "Microbiome Health Score" is then generated by applying proprietary algorithms to the collected data. These algorithms compare a person's microbiome to a sizable reference group of both healthy and sick people. Measures of variety, significant metabolite concentrations including butyrate, testosterone, propionate, and TMA, as well as the quantity of significant pathobiont and beneficial species, are frequently included in this score. The final report offers a window into each person's distinct microbial consequences to their own metabolic health, as it is a stratified risk assessment of illnesses including insulin resistance, inflammation, with increased intestinal permeability opposed to a straightforward diagnosis (Gupta et al., 2020).

The biggest benefit of these panels would be their capacity to provide individualized, evidence-based dietary and lifestyle recommendations as the cornerstone of a genuinely customized nutrition plan. Depending on the assessment, taking more fiber from different sources in order to stimulate the inactive butyrate production or eating more foods high in polyphenols it might be advised to encourage the development of advantageous Akkermansia (Asnicar et al., 2021). Dietary recommendations for individuals with an elevated TMAO level include reducing intake of dietary precursors like choline and carnitine, which are found in red meat as well as eggs, and recommending prebiotics to change the microbiological makeup of TMA-producing bacteria. Additionally, these panels can be utilized for longitudinal tracking, which allows the patient and physician to observe how certain dietary interventions, probiotics, or lifestyle modifications impact the gut ecology over time. However, there are still issues with the standards, interpretation, and regulatory framework (Kashyap et al., 2017). For avoidance and treatment of metabolic disorders, these panels are spearheading the shift from a general nutritional philosophy to data-driven, microbiome-informed, individualized nutritional modulation.

12. CONCLUSION

Microbial dysbiosis plays a significant role in the onset and progression of metabolic disorders such as obesity and type 2 diabetes. Alterations in gut microbial composition impair energy balance, glucose regulation, and lipid metabolism. The loss of beneficial microbes and enrichment of pro-inflammatory taxa promote gut barrier dysfunction and chronic low-grade inflammation. Dysbiosis also disrupts hormonal signaling and gut–brain communication, further aggravating metabolic imbalance. Dietary habits, lifestyle factors, and medications strongly influence microbial diversity and function. Emerging evidence suggests that microbiome-targeted interventions can improve metabolic health. However, the precise causal mechanisms remain incompletely defined. Advanced multi-omics and longitudinal studies are needed to clarify host–microbe interactions. Understanding these links may enable early diagnosis and personalized therapies. Overall, restoring microbial homeostasis represents a promising strategy for managing metabolic disorders.

13. REFERENCES

Adamska, A., Nowak, M., Piłaciński, S., Pilacinski, B., Adamska, B., Malewski, W., & Krętowski, A. (2016). Small intestinal bacterial overgrowth in adult patients with type 1 diabetes: Its prevalence and relationship with metabolic control and the presence of chronic complications of the disease. *Polish Archives of Internal Medicine, 126*(9), 628–634. DOI: 10.20452/pamw.3501 PMID: 27535109

Al Assal, K., Prifti, E., Belda, E., Sala, P. C., Clément, K., Dao, M.-C., Doré, J., Levenez, F., Taddei, C. R., Fonseca, D. C., Rocha, I. M., Balmant, B. D., Thomas, A. M., Santo, M. A., Dias-Neto, E., Setubal, J. C., Zucker, J.-D., Belarmino, G., Torrinhas, R. S., & Waitzberg, D. L. (2020). Gut Microbiota Profile of Obese Diabetic Women Submitted to Roux-en-Y Gastric Bypass and Its Association with Food Intake and Postoperative Diabetes Remission. *Nutrients, 12*(2), 278. DOI: 10.3390/nu12020278 PMID: 31973130

Amar, J., Burcelin, R., Ruidavets, J. B., Cani, P. D., Fauvel, J., Alessi, M. C., Chamontin, B., & Ferrières, J. (2008). Energy intake is associated with endotoxemia in apparently healthy men. *The American Journal of Clinical Nutrition, 87*(5), 1219–1223. DOI: 10.1093/ajcn/87.5.1219 PMID: 18469242

Amar, J., Chabo, C., Waget, A., Klopp, P., Vachoux, C., Bermúdez-Humarán, L. G., Smirnova, N., Bergé, M., Sulpice, T., Lahtinen, S., Ouwehand, A., Langella, P., Rautonen, N., Sansonetti, P. J., & Burcelin, R. (2011). Intestinal mucosal adherence and translocation of commensal bacteria at the early onset of type 2 diabetes: Molecular mechanisms and probiotic treatment. *EMBO Molecular Medicine, 3*(9), 559–572. DOI: 10.1002/emmm.201100159 PMID: 21735552

Aronsson, L., Huang, Y., Parini, P., Korach-André, M., Håkansson, J., Gustafsson, J. Å., Pettersson, S., Arulampalam, V., & Rafter, J. (2010). Decreased fat storage by Lactobacillus paracasei is associated with increased levels of angiopoietin-like 4 protein (ANGPTL4). *PLoS One, 5*(9), e13087. DOI: 10.1371/journal.pone.0013087 PMID: 20927337

Arora, T., & Bäckhed, F. (2016). The gut microbiota and metabolic disease: Current understanding and future perspectives. *Journal of Internal Medicine, 280*(4), 339–349. DOI: 10.1111/joim.12508 PMID: 27071815

Asnicar, F., Berry, S. E., Valdes, A. M., Nguyen, L. H., Piccinno, G., Drew, D. A., Leeming, E., Gibson, R., Le Roy, C., Khatib, H. A., Francis, L., Mazidi, M., Mompeo, O., Valles-Colomer, M., Tett, A., Beghini, F., Dubois, L., Bazzani, D., Thomas, A. M., & Segata, N. (2021). Microbiome connections with host metabolism and habitual diet from 1,098 deeply phenotyped individuals. *Nature Medicine*, *27*(2), 321–332. DOI: 10.1038/s41591-020-01183-8 PMID: 33432175

Bergman, E. N. (1990). Energy contributions of volatile fatty acids from the gastrointestinal tract in various species. *Physiological Reviews*, *70*(2), 567–590. DOI: 10.1152/physrev.1990.70.2.567 PMID: 2181501

Beserra, B. T. S., Fernandes, R., do Rosario, V. A., Mocellin, M. C., Kuntz, M. G. F., & Trindade, E. B. S. M. (2015). A systematic review and meta-analysis of the prebiotics and synbiotics effects on glycaemia, insulin concentrations and lipid parameters in adult patients with overweight or obesity. *Clinical Nutrition (Edinburgh, Lothian)*, *34*(5), 845–858. DOI: 10.1016/j.clnu.2014.10.004 PMID: 25456608

Borgeraas, H., Johnson, L. K., Skattebu, J., Hertel, J. K., & Hjelmesæth, J. (2018). Effects of probiotics on body weight, body mass index, fat mass and fat percentage in subjects with overweight or obesity: A systematic review and meta-analysis of randomized controlled trials. *Obesity Reviews*, *19*(2), 219–232. DOI: 10.1111/obr.12626 PMID: 29047207

Bryrup, T., Thomsen, C. W., Kern, T., Allin, K. H., Brandslund, I., Jørgensen, N. R., Vestergaard, H., Hansen, T., Hansen, T. H., Pedersen, O., & Nielsen, T. (2019). Metformin-induced changes of the gut microbiota in healthy young men: Results of a non-blinded, one-armed intervention study. *Diabetologia*, *62*(6), 1024–1035. DOI: 10.1007/s00125-019-4848-7 PMID: 30904939

Canfora, E. E., Jocken, J. W., & Blaak, E. E. (2015). Short-chain fatty acids in control of body weight and insulin sensitivity. *Nature Reviews. Endocrinology*, *11*(10), 577–591. DOI: 10.1038/nrendo.2015.128 PMID: 26260141

Cani, P. D., Amar, J., Iglesias, M. A., Poggi, M., Knauf, C., Bastelica, D., Neyrinck, A. M., Fava, F., Tuohy, K. M., Chabo, C., Waget, A., Delmée, E., Cousin, B., Sulpice, T., Chamontin, B., Ferrières, J., Tanti, J. F., Gibson, G. R., Casteilla, L., & Burcelin, R. (2007). Metabolic endotoxemia initiates obesity and insulin resistance. *Diabetes*, *56*(7), 1761–1772. DOI: 10.2337/db06-1491 PMID: 17456850

Cani, P. D., & de Vos, W. M. (2017). Next-generation beneficial microbes: The case of Akkermansia muciniphila. *Frontiers in Microbiology*, *8*, 1765. DOI: 10.3389/fmicb.2017.01765 PMID: 29018410

Cani, P. D., & de Vos, W. M. (2017). Next-generation beneficial microbes: The case of Akkermansia muciniphila. *Frontiers in Microbiology, 8*, 1765. DOI: 10.3389/fmicb.2017.01765 PMID: 29018410

Cani, P. D., Possemiers, S., Van de Wiele, T., Guiot, Y., Everard, A., Rottier, O., Geurts, L., Naslain, D., Neyrinck, A., Lambert, D. M., Muccioli, G. G., & Delzenne, N. M. (2009). Changes in gut microbiota control inflammation in obese mice through a mechanism involving GLP-2-driven improvement of gut permeability. *Gut, 58*(8), 1091–1103. DOI: 10.1136/gut.2008.165886 PMID: 19240062

Carbonero, F., Benefiel, A. C., & Gaskins, H. R. (2012). Contributions of the microbial hydrogen economy to colonic homeostasis. *Nature Reviews. Gastroenterology & Hepatology, 9*(9), 504–518. DOI: 10.1038/nrgastro.2012.85 PMID: 22585131

Carvalho, B. M., & Saad, M. J. A. (2013). Influence of gut microbiota on subclinical inflammation and insulin resistance. *Mediators of Inflammation, 986734*, 1–13. Advance online publication. DOI: 10.1155/2013/986734 PMID: 23840101

Chelakkot, C., Choi, Y., Kim, D.-K., Park, H. T., Ghim, J., Kwon, Y., Jeon, J., Kim, M.-S., Jee, Y.-K., Gho, Y. S., Park, H.-S., Kim, Y.-K., & Ryu, S. H. (2018). Akkermansia muciniphila-derived extracellular vesicles influence gut permeability through the regulation of tight junctions. *Experimental & Molecular Medicine, 50*(2), e450. DOI: 10.1038/emm.2017.282 PMID: 29472701

Clooney, A. G., Bernstein, C. N., Leslie, W. D., Vagianos, K., Sargent, M., Laserna-Mendieta, E. J., Claesson, M. J., & Targownik, L. E. (2016). A comparison of the gut microbiome between long-term users and non-users of proton pump inhibitors. *Alimentary Pharmacology & Therapeutics, 43*(9), 974–984. DOI: 10.1111/apt.13568 PMID: 26923470

Collins, S. M., Surette, M., & Bercik, P. (2012). The interplay between the intestinal microbiota and the brain. *Nature Reviews. Microbiology, 10*(11), 735–742. DOI: 10.1038/nrmicro2876 PMID: 23000955

De Filippo, C., Cavalieri, D., Di Paola, M., Ramazzotti, M., Poullet, J. B., Massart, S., Collini, S., Pieraccini, G., & Lionetti, P. (2010). Impact of diet in shaping gut microbiota revealed by a comparative study in children from Europe and rural Africa. *Proceedings of the National Academy of Sciences of the United States of America, 107*(33), 14691–14696. DOI: 10.1073/pnas.1005963107 PMID: 20679230

Dimidi, E., Cox, S. R., Rossi, M., & Whelan, K. (2019). Fermented Foods: Definitions and Characteristics, Impact on the Gut Microbiota and Effects on Gastrointestinal Health and Disease. *Nutrients, 11*(8), 1806. DOI: 10.3390/nu11081806 PMID: 31387262

Donath, M. Y., & Shoelson, S. E. (2011). Type 2 diabetes as an inflammatory disease. *Nature Reviews. Immunology, 11*(2), 98–107. DOI: 10.1038/nri2925 PMID: 21233852

Eisenstein, M. (2020). The hunt for a healthy microbiome. *Nature, 577*(7792), S6–S8. DOI: 10.1038/d41586-020-00193-3 PMID: 31996823

Ejtahed, H.-S., Tito, R. Y., Siadat, S.-D., Hasani-Ranjbar, S., Hoseini-Tavassol, Z., Rymenans, L., Verbeke, K., Soroush, A. R., Raes, J., & Larijani, B. (2019). Metformin induces weight loss associated with gut microbiota alteration in non-diabetic obese women: A randomized double-blind clinical trial. *European Journal of Endocrinology, 180*(3), 165–176. DOI: 10.1530/EJE-18-0826 PMID: 30540558

Everard, A., Belzer, C., Geurts, L., Ouwerkerk, J. P., Druart, C., Bindels, L. B., Guiot, Y., Derrien, M., Muccioli, G. G., Delzenne, N. M., de Vos, W. M., & Cani, P. D. (2013). Cross-talk between Akkermansia muciniphila and intestinal epithelium controls diet-induced obesity. *Proceedings of the National Academy of Sciences of the United States of America, 110*(22), 9066–9071. DOI: 10.1073/pnas.1219451110 PMID: 23671105

Forslund, K., Hildebrand, F., Nielsen, T., Falony, G., Le Chatelier, E., Sunagawa, S., Prifti, E., Vieira-Silva, S., Gudmundsdottir, V., Pedersen, H. K., Arumugam, M., Kristiansen, K., Voigt, A. Y., Vestergaard, H., Hercog, R., Costea, P. I., Kultima, J. R., Li, J., Jørgensen, T., & Pedersen, O. (2015). Disentangling type 2 diabetes and metformin treatment signatures in the human gut microbiota. *Nature, 528*(7581), 262–266. DOI: 10.1038/nature15766 PMID: 26633628

Ghoshal, U. C., & Srivastava, D. (2014). Irritable bowel syndrome and small intestinal bacterial overgrowth: Meaningful association or unnecessary hype. *World Journal of Gastroenterology, 20*(10), 2482–2491. DOI: 10.3748/wjg.v20.i10.2482 PMID: 24627585

Gupta, V. K., Kim, M., Bakshi, U., Cunningham, K. Y., Davis, J. M.III, Lazaridis, K. N., Nelson, H., Chia, N., & Sung, J. (2020). A predictive index for health status using species-level gut microbiome profiling. *Nature Communications, 11*(1), 4635. DOI: 10.1038/s41467-020-18476-8 PMID: 32934239

Harley, I. T. W., & Karp, C. L. (2012). Obesity and the gut microbiome: Striving for causality. *Molecular Metabolism, 1*(1-2), 21–31. DOI: 10.1016/j.molmet.2012.07.002 PMID: 24024115

Henao-Mejia, J., Elinav, E., Jin, C., Hao, L., Mehal, W. Z., Strowig, T., Thaiss, C. A., Kau, A. L., Eisenbarth, S. C., Jurczak, M. J., Camporez, J. P., Shulman, G. I., Gordon, J. I., Hoffman, H. M., & Flavell, R. A. (2012). Inflammasome-mediated dysbiosis regulates progression of NAFLD and obesity. *Nature*, *482*(7384), 179–185. DOI: 10.1038/nature10809 PMID: 22297845

Hofmann, A. F. (1999). Bile Acids: The Good, the Bad, and the Ugly. *Physiology (Bethesda, MD)*, *14*(1), 24–29. DOI: 10.1152/physiologyonline.1999.14.1.24 PMID: 11390813

Hotamisligil, G. S. (2006). Inflammation and metabolic disorders. *Nature*, *444*(7121), 860–867. DOI: 10.1038/nature05485 PMID: 17167474

Ianiro, G., Eusebi, L. H., Black, C. J., Gasbarrini, A., Cammarota, G., & Ford, A. C. (2019). Systematic review with meta-analysis: Efficacy of faecal microbiota transplantation for the treatment of irritable bowel syndrome. *Alimentary Pharmacology & Therapeutics*, *50*(3), 240–248. DOI: 10.1111/apt.15330 PMID: 31136009

Javdan, B., Lopez, J. G., Chankhamjon, P., Lee, Y.-C. J., Hull, R., Wu, Q., Wang, X., Chatterjee, S., & Donia, M. S. (2020). Personalized Mapping of Drug Metabolism by the Human Gut Microbiome. *Cell*, *181*(7), 1661–1679.e22. DOI: 10.1016/j.cell.2020.05.001 PMID: 32526207

Jennis, M., Cavanaugh, C. R., Leo, G. C., Mabus, J. R., Lenhard, J., & Hornby, P. J. (2017). Microbiota-derived tryptophan indoles increase after gastric bypass surgery and reduce intestinal permeability in vitro and in vivo. *Neurogastroenterology and Motility*, *30*(2), e13178. DOI: 10.1111/nmo.13178 PMID: 28782205

Jia, W., Xie, G., & Jia, W. (2018). Bile acid-microbiota crosstalk in gastrointestinal inflammation and carcinogenesis. *Nature Reviews. Gastroenterology & Hepatology*, *15*(2), 111–128. DOI: 10.1038/nrgastro.2017.119 PMID: 29018272

Jovel, J., Patterson, J., Wang, W., Hotte, N., O'Keefe, S., Mitchel, T., Perry, T., Kao, D., Mason, A. L., Madsen, K. L., & Wong, G. K. (2016). Characterization of the gut microbiome using 16S or shotgun metagenomics. *Frontiers in Microbiology*, *7*, 459. DOI: 10.3389/fmicb.2016.00459 PMID: 27148170

Kashyap, P. C., Chia, N., Nelson, H., Segal, E., & Elinav, E. (2017). Microbiome at the frontier of personalized medicine. *Mayo Clinic Proceedings*, *92*(12), 1855–1864. DOI: 10.1016/j.mayocp.2017.10.004 PMID: 29202942

Kawasaki, T., & Kawai, T. (2014). Toll-like receptor signaling pathways. *Frontiers in Immunology*, *5*, 461. DOI: 10.3389/fimmu.2014.00461 PMID: 25309543

Koh, A., Molinaro, A., Ståhlman, M., Khan, M. T., Schmidt, C., Mannerås-Holm, L., Wu, H., Carreras, A., Jeong, H., Olofsson, L. E., Bergh, P. O., Gerdes, V., Hartstra, A., de Brauw, M., Perkins, R., Nieuwdorp, M., Bergström, G., & Bäckhed, F. (2018). Microbially produced imidazole propionate impairs insulin signaling through mTORC1. *Cell*, *175*(4), 947–961.e17. DOI: 10.1016/j.cell.2018.09.055 PMID: 30401435

Kootte, R. S., Levin, E., Salojärvi, J., Smits, L. P., Hartstra, A. V., Udayappan, S. D., Hermes, G., Bouter, K. E., Koopen, A. M., Holst, J. J., Knop, F. K., Blaak, E. E., Zhao, J., Smidt, H., Harms, A. C., Hankemeijer, T., Bergström, G., & Nieuwdorp, M. (2017). Improvement of Insulin Sensitivity after Lean Donor Feces in Metabolic Syndrome Is Driven by Baseline Intestinal Microbiota Composition. *Cell Metabolism*, *26*(4), 611–619.e6. DOI: 10.1016/j.cmet.2017.09.008 PMID: 28978426

Kootte, R. S., Levin, E., Salojärvi, J., Smits, L. P., Hartstra, A. V., Udayappan, S. D., Hermes, G., Bouter, K. E., Koopen, A. M., Holst, J. J., Knop, F. K., Blaak, E. E., Zhao, J., Smidt, H., Harms, A. C., Hankemeijer, T., Bergström, G., Wu, G. D., Stoffels, M., & Nieuwdorp, M. (2017). Improvement of insulin sensitivity after lean donor feces in metabolic syndrome is driven by baseline intestinal microbiota composition. *Cell Metabolism*, *26*(4), 611–619.e6. DOI: 10.1016/j.cmet.2017.09.008 PMID: 28978426

Kuczynski, J., Stombaugh, J., Walters, W. A., González, A., Caporaso, J. G., & Knight, R. (2012). Using QIIME to analyze 16S rRNA gene sequences from microbial communities. *Current Protocols in Bioinformatics*, Chapter 10, Unit 10.7. DOI: 10.1002/0471250953.bi1007s36

Kuipers, F., Bloks, V. W., & Groen, A. K. (2014). Beyond intestinal soap–bile acids in metabolic control. *Nature Reviews. Endocrinology*, *10*(8), 488–498. DOI: 10.1038/nrendo.2014.60 PMID: 24821328

Le Chatelier, E., Nielsen, T., Qin, J., Prifti, E., Hildebrand, F., Falony, G., Almeida, M., Arumugam, M., Batto, J. M., Kennedy, S., Leonard, P., Li, J., Burgdorf, K., Grarup, N., Jørgensen, T., Brandslund, I., Nielsen, H. B., Juncker, A. S., Bertalan, M., & Pedersen, O. (2013). Richness of human gut microbiome correlates with metabolic markers. *Nature*, *500*(7464), 541–546. DOI: 10.1038/nature12506 PMID: 23985870

Ley, R. E., Turnbaugh, P. J., Klein, S., & Gordon, J. I. (2006). Microbial ecology: Human gut microbes associated with obesity. *Nature*, *444*(7122), 1022–1023. DOI: 10.1038/4441022a PMID: 17183309

Li, L., Abou-Samra, E., Ning, Z., Zhang, X., Mayne, J., Wang, J., Cheng, K., Walker, K., Stintzi, A., & Figeys, D. (2019). An in vitro model maintaining taxon-specific functional activities of the gut microbiome. *Nature Communications*, *10*(1), 4146. DOI: 10.1038/s41467-019-12087-8 PMID: 31515476

Louis, S., Tappu, R. M., Damms-Machado, A., Huson, D. H., & Bischoff, S. C. (2016). Characterization of the gut microbial community of obese patients following a weight-loss intervention using whole metagenome shotgun sequencing. *PLoS One*, *11*(2), e0149564. DOI: 10.1371/journal.pone.0149564 PMID: 26919743

Lumeng, C. N., & Saltiel, A. R. (2011). Inflammatory links between obesity and metabolic disease. *The Journal of Clinical Investigation*, *121*(6), 2111–2117. DOI: 10.1172/JCI57132 PMID: 21633179

Marcobal, A., Kashyap, P. C., Nelson, T. A., Aronov, P. A., Donia, M. S., Spormann, A., Fischbach, M. A., & Sonnenburg, J. L. (2013). A metabolomic view of how the human gut microbiota impacts the host metabolome using humanized and gnotobiotic mice. *The ISME Journal*, *7*(10), 1933–1943. DOI: 10.1038/ismej.2013.89 PMID: 23739052

Maron, D. J., Fazio, S., & Linton, M. F. (2000). Current perspectives on statins. *Circulation*, *101*(2), 207–213. DOI: 10.1161/01.CIR.101.2.207 PMID: 10637210

Martinez, K. B., Mackert, J. D., & McIntosh, M. K. (2017). Polyphenols and intestinal health. In Watson, R. R. (Ed.), *Nutrition and Functional Foods for Healthy Aging* (pp. 191–210). Elsevier., DOI: 10.1016/B978-0-12-805376-8.00018-6

Mehtab, W., Agarwal, A., Singh, N., Malhotra, A., & Makharia, G. (2019). All that a physician should know about FODMAPs. *Indian Journal of Gastroenterology*, *38*(5), 378–390. DOI: 10.1007/s12664-019-01002-0 PMID: 31802437

Meijer, K., de Vos, P., & Priebe, M. G. (2010). Butyrate and other short-chain fatty acids as modulators of immunity: What relevance for health? *Current Opinion in Clinical Nutrition and Metabolic Care*, *13*(6), 715–721. DOI: 10.1097/MCO.0b013e32833eebe5 PMID: 20823773

Miller, M. B., & Bassler, B. L. (2001). Quorum sensing in bacteria. *Annual Review of Microbiology*, *55*(1), 165–199. DOI: 10.1146/annurev.micro.55.1.165 PMID: 11544353

Newgard, C. B., An, J., Bain, J. R., Muehlbauer, M. J., Stevens, R. D., Lien, L. F., Haqq, A. M., Shah, S. H., Arlotto, M., Slentz, C. A., Rochon, J., Gallup, D., Ilkayeva, O., Wenner, B. R., Yancy, W. S.Jr, Eisenson, H., Musante, G., Surwit, R. S., Millington, D. S., & Svetkey, L. P. (2009). A branched-chain amino acid-related metabolic signature that differentiates obese and lean humans and contributes to insulin resistance. *Cell Metabolism*, *9*(4), 311–326. DOI: 10.1016/j.cmet.2009.02.002 PMID: 19356713

Nicholson, J. K., Holmes, E., Kinross, J., Burcelin, R., Gibson, G., Jia, W., & Pettersson, S. (2012). Host-gut microbiota metabolic interactions. *Science*, *336*(6086), 1262–1267. DOI: 10.1126/science.1223813 PMID: 22674330

Pasini, E., Corsetti, G., Assanelli, D., Testa, C., Romano, C., Dioguardi, F. S., & Aquilani, R. (2019). Effects of chronic exercise on gut microbiota and intestinal barrier in human with type 2 diabetes. *Minerva Medica*, *110*(1), 3–11. DOI: 10.23736/S0026-4806.18.05589-1 PMID: 30667205

Patti, G. J., Yanes, O., & Siuzdak, G. (2012). Innovation: Metabolomics: the apogee of the omics trilogy. *Nature Reviews. Molecular Cell Biology*, *13*(4), 263–269. DOI: 10.1038/nrm3314 PMID: 22436749

Pedersen, H. K., Gudmundsdottir, V., Nielsen, H. B., Hyotylainen, T., Nielsen, T., Jensen, B. A., Forslund, K., Hildebrand, F., Prifti, E., Falony, G., Le Chatelier, E., Levenez, F., Doré, J., Mattila, I., Plichta, D. R., Pöhö, P., Hellgren, L. I., Arumugam, M., Sunagawa, S., & Pedersen, O. (2016). Human gut microbes impact host serum metabolome and insulin sensitivity. *Nature*, *535*(7612), 376–381. DOI: 10.1038/nature18646 PMID: 27409811

Perry, R. J., Peng, L., Barry, N. A., Cline, G. W., Zhang, D., Cardone, R. L., Petersen, K. F., Kibbey, R. G., Goodman, A. L., & Shulman, G. I. (2016). Acetate mediates a microbiome-brain-β-cell axis to promote metabolic syndrome. *Nature*, *534*(7606), 213–217. DOI: 10.1038/nature18309 PMID: 27279214

Pimentel, M., Kong, Y., & Park, S. (2004). IBS subjects with methane on lactulose breath test have lower postprandial serotonin levels than subjects with hydrogen. *Digestive Diseases and Sciences*, *49*(1), 84–47. DOI: 10.1023/B:DDAS.0000011607.24171.c0 PMID: 14992440

Pluznick, J. L., Protzko, R. J., Gevorgyan, H., Peterlin, Z., Sipos, A., Han, J., Brunet, I., Wan, L. X., Rey, F., Wang, T., Firestein, S. J., Yanagisawa, M., Gordon, J. I., Eichmann, A., Peti-Peterdi, J., & Caplan, M. J. (2013). Olfactory receptor responding to gut microbiota-derived signals plays a role in renin secretion and blood pressure regulation. *Proceedings of the National Academy of Sciences of the United States of America, 110*(11), 4410–4415. DOI: 10.1073/pnas.1215927110 PMID: 23401498

Pols, T. W., Noriega, L. G., Nomura, M., Auwerx, J., & Schoonjans, K. (2011). The bile acid membrane receptor TGR5 as an emerging target in metabolism and inflammation. *Journal of Hepatology, 54*(6), 1263–1272. DOI: 10.1016/j.jhep.2010.12.004 PMID: 21145931

Qin, J., Li, R., Raes, J., Arumugam, M., Burgdorf, K. S., Manichanh, C., Nielsen, T., Pons, N., Levenez, F., Yamada, T., Mende, D. R., Li, J., Xu, J., Li, S., Li, D., Cao, J., Wang, B., Liang, H., Zheng, H., & Wang, J. (2010). A human gut microbial gene catalogue established by metagenomic sequencing. *Nature, 464*(7285), 59–65. DOI: 10.1038/nature08821 PMID: 20203603

Qin, J., Li, Y., Cai, Z., Li, S., Zhu, J., Zhang, F., Liang, S., Zhang, W., Guan, Y., Shen, D., Peng, Y., Zhang, D., Jie, Z., Wu, W., Qin, Y., Xue, W., Li, J., Han, L., Lu, D., & Wang, J. (2012). A metagenome-wide association study of gut microbiota in type 2 diabetes. *Nature, 490*(7418), 55–60. DOI: 10.1038/nature11450 PMID: 23023125

Quince, C., Walker, A. W., Simpson, J. T., Loman, N. J., & Segata, N. (2017). Shotgun metagenomics, from sampling to analysis. *Nature Biotechnology, 35*(9), 833–844. DOI: 10.1038/nbt.3935 PMID: 28898207

Rastall, R. A., Gibson, G. R., Gill, H. S., Guarner, F., Klaenhammer, T. R., Pot, B., Reid, G., Rowland, I. R., & Sanders, M. E. (2005). Modulation of the microbial ecology of the human colon by probiotics, prebiotics and synbiotics to enhance human health: An overview of enabling science and potential applications. *FEMS Microbiology Ecology, 52*(2), 145–152. DOI: 10.1016/j.femsec.2005.01.003 PMID: 16329901

Reijnders, D., Goossens, G. H., Hermes, G. D., Neis, E. P., van der Beek, C. M., Most, J., Holst, J. J., Lenaerts, K., Kootte, R. S., Nieuwdorp, M., Groen, A. K., Olde Damink, S. W., Boekschoten, M. V., Smidt, H., Zoetendal, E. G., Dejong, C. H. C., & Blaak, E. E. (2016). Effects of gut microbiota manipulation by antibiotics on host metabolism in obese humans: A randomized double-blind placebo-controlled trial. *Cell Metabolism, 24*(1), 63–74. DOI: 10.1016/j.cmet.2016.06.016 PMID: 27411009

Ridlon, J. M., Kang, D. J., Hylemon, P. B., & Bajaj, J. S. (2014). Bile acids and the gut microbiome. *Current Opinion in Gastroenterology*, *30*(3), 332–338. DOI: 10.1097/MOG.0000000000000057 PMID: 24625896

Rodriguez-Castaño, G. P., Caro-Quintero, A., Reyes, A., & Lizcano, F. (2017). Advances in Gut Microbiome Research, Opening New Strategies to Cope with a Western Lifestyle. *Frontiers in Genetics*, *7*, 224. DOI: 10.3389/fgene.2016.00224 PMID: 28119734

Rowland, I., Gibson, G., Heinken, A., Scott, K., Swann, J., Thiele, I., & Tuohy, K. (2018). Gut microbiota functions: Metabolism of nutrients and other food components. *European Journal of Nutrition*, *57*(1), 1–24. DOI: 10.1007/s00394-017-1445-8 PMID: 28393285

Saberi, M., Woods, N. B., de Luca, C., Schenk, S., Lu, J. C., Bandyopadhyay, G., Verma, I. M., & Olefsky, J. M. (2009). Hematopoietic cell-specific deletion of toll-like receptor 4 ameliorates hepatic and adipose tissue insulin resistance in high-fat-fed mice. *Cell Metabolism*, *10*(5), 419–429. DOI: 10.1016/j.cmet.2009.09.006 PMID: 19883619

Salem, A. E., Singh, R., Ayoub, Y. K., Khairy, A. M., & Mullin, G. E. (2018). The gut microbiome and irritable bowel syndrome: State of art review. *Arab Journal of Gastroenterology*, *19*(3), 136–141. DOI: 10.1016/j.ajg.2018.02.008 PMID: 29935865

Saulnier, D. M. A., Gibson, G. R., & Kolida, S. (2008). In vitro effects of selected synbiotics on the human faecal microbiota composition. *FEMS Microbiology Ecology*, *66*(3), 516–527. DOI: 10.1111/j.1574-6941.2008.00561.x PMID: 18673391

Sayin, S. I., Wahlström, A., Felin, J., Jäntti, S., Marschall, H. U., Bamberg, K., Angelin, B., Hyötyläinen, T., Orešič, M., & Bäckhed, F. (2013). Gut microbiota regulates bile acid metabolism by reducing the levels of tauro-beta-muricholic acid, a naturally occurring FXR antagonist. *Cell Metabolism*, *17*(2), 225–235. DOI: 10.1016/j.cmet.2013.01.003 PMID: 23395169

Seganfredo, F. B., Blume, C. A., Moehlecke, M., Giongo, A., Casagrande, D. S., Spolidoro, J. V. N., Padoin, A. V., Schaan, B. D., & Mottin, C. C. (2017). Weight-loss interventions and gut microbiota changes in overweight and obese patients: A systematic review. *Obesity Reviews*, *18*(8), 832–851. DOI: 10.1111/obr.12541 PMID: 28524627

Shah, S. C., Day, L. W., Somsouk, M., & Sewell, J. L. (2013). Meta-analysis: Antibiotic therapy for small intestinal bacterial overgrowth. *Alimentary Pharmacology & Therapeutics*, *38*(8), 925–934. DOI: 10.1111/apt.12479 PMID: 24004101

Shoelson, S. E., Lee, J., & Goldfine, A. B. (2006). Inflammation and insulin resistance. *The Journal of Clinical Investigation, 116*(7), 1793–1801. DOI: 10.1172/JCI29069 PMID: 16823477

Soletsky, B., & Feig, D. I. (2012). Uric Acid Reduction Rectifies Prehypertension in Obese Adolescents. *Hypertension, 60*(5), 1148–1156. DOI: 10.1161/HYPERTENSIONAHA.112.196980 PMID: 23006736

Spencer, M. D., Hamp, T. J., Reid, R. W., Fischer, L. M., Zeisel, S. H., & Fodor, A. A. (2011). Association between composition of the human gastrointestinal microbiome and development of fatty liver with choline deficiency. *Gastroenterology, 140*(3), 976–986. DOI: 10.1053/j.gastro.2010.11.049 PMID: 21129376

Tang, W. H., Wang, Z., Levison, B. S., Koeth, R. A., Britt, E. B., Fu, X., Wu, Y., & Hazen, S. L. (2013). Intestinal microbial metabolism of phosphatidylcholine and cardiovascular risk. *The New England Journal of Medicine, 368*(17), 1575–1584. DOI: 10.1056/NEJMoa1109400 PMID: 23614584

Tap, J., Derrien, M., Törnblom, H., Brazier, L., Cools-Portier, S., Doré, J., Störsrud, S., le Nevé, B., Öhman, L., & Simrén, M. (2017). Identification of an intestinal microbiota signature associated with severity of irritable bowel syndrome. *Gastroenterology, 152*(1), 111–123.e8. DOI: 10.1053/j.gastro.2016.09.049 PMID: 27725146

Thomas, C., Gioiello, A., Noriega, L., Strehle, A., Oury, J., Rizzo, G., Macchiarulo, A., Yamamoto, H., Mataki, C., Pruzanski, M., Pellicciari, R., Auwerx, J., & Schoonjans, K. (2009). TGR5-mediated bile acid sensing controls glucose homeostasis. *Cell Metabolism, 10*(3), 167–177. DOI: 10.1016/j.cmet.2009.08.001 PMID: 19723493

Torres-Fuentes, C., Schellekens, H., Dinan, T. G., & Cryan, J. F. (2017). The microbiota-gut-brain axis in obesity. *The Lancet. Gastroenterology & Hepatology, 2*(10), 747–756. DOI: 10.1016/S2468-1253(17)30147-4 PMID: 28844808

Tremaroli, V., Karlsson, F. H., Werling, M., Ståhlman, M., Kovatcheva-Datchary, P., Olbers, T., Fändriks, L., Le Roux, C. W., Nielsen, J., & Bäckhed, F. (2015). Roux-en-Y Gastric Bypass and Vertical Banded Gastroplasty Induce Long-Term Changes on the Human Gut Microbiome Contributing to Fat Mass Regulation. *Cell Metabolism, 22*(2), 228–238. DOI: 10.1016/j.cmet.2015.07.009 PMID: 26244932

Turnbaugh, P. J., Ley, R. E., Mahowald, M. A., Magrini, V., Mardis, E. R., & Gordon, J. I. (2006). An obesity-associated gut microbiome with increased capacity for energy harvest. *Nature, 444*(7122), 1027–1031. DOI: 10.1038/nature05414 PMID: 17183312

Ülker, I., & Yildiran, H. (2018). The effects of bariatric surgery on gut microbiota in patients with obesity: A review of the literature. *Bioscience of Microbiota, Food and Health, 38*(1), 3–9. DOI: 10.12938/bmfh.18-018 PMID: 30705797

Vieira-Silva, S., Falony, G., Belda, E., Nielsen, T., Aron-Wisnewsky, J., Chakaroun, R., Forslund, S. K., Assmann, K., Valles-Colomer, M., Nguyen, T. T. D., Proost, S., Prifti, E., Tremaroli, V., Pons, N., Le Chatelier, E., Andreelli, F., Bastard, J.-P., Coelho, L. P., Galleron, N., & Raes, J. (2020). Statin therapy is associated with lower prevalence of gut microbiota dysbiosis. *Nature, 581*(7808), 310–315. DOI: 10.1038/s41586-020-2269-x PMID: 32433607

Vila, A. V., Collij, V., Sanna, S., Sinha, T., Imhann, F., Bourgonje, A. R., Mujagic, Z., Jonkers, D. M. A. E., Masclee, A. A. M., Fu, J., Kurilshikov, A., Gacesa, R., & Weersma, R. K. (2020). Impact of commonly used drugs on the composition and metabolic function of the gut microbiota. *Nature Communications, 11*(1), 362. DOI: 10.1038/s41467-019-14177-z PMID: 31953381

Vrieze, A., Van Nood, E., Holleman, F., Salojärvi, J., Kootte, R. S., Bartelsman, J. F., Dallinga-Thie, G. M., Ackermans, M. T., Serlie, M. J., Oozeer, R., Derrien, M., Druesne, A., Van Hylckama Vlieg, J. E., Bloks, V. W., Groen, A. K., Heilig, H. G., Zoetendal, E. G., Stroes, E. S., de Vos, W. M., & Nieuwdorp, M. (2012). Transfer of intestinal microbiota from lean donors increases insulin sensitivity in individuals with metabolic syndrome. *Gastroenterology, 143*(4), 913–916.e7. DOI: 10.1053/j.gastro.2012.06.031 PMID: 22728514

Wahlström, A., Sayin, S. I., Marschall, H. U., & Bäckhed, F. (2016). Intestinal Crosstalk between Bile Acids and Microbiota and Its Impact on Host Metabolism. *Cell Metabolism, 24*(1), 41–50. DOI: 10.1016/j.cmet.2016.05.005 PMID: 27320064

Wang, Y., Dilidaxi, D., Wu, Y., Sailike, J., Sun, X., & Nabi, X. (2020). Composite probiotics alleviate type 2 diabetes by regulating intestinal microbiota and inducing GLP-1 secretion in db/db mice. *Biomedicine and Pharmacotherapy, 125*, 109914. DOI: 10.1016/j.biopha.2020.109914 PMID: 32035395

Wang, Z., Klipfell, E., Bennett, B. J., Koeth, R., Levison, B. S., Dugar, B., Feldstein, A. E., Britt, E. B., Fu, X., Chung, Y. M., Wu, Y., Schauer, P., Smith, J. D., Allayee, H., Tang, W. H., DiDonato, J. A., Lusis, A. J., & Hazen, S. L. (2011). Gut flora metabolism of phosphatidylcholine promotes cardiovascular disease. *Nature, 472*(7341), 57–63. DOI: 10.1038/nature09922 PMID: 21475195

Weersma, R. K., Zhernakova, A., & Fu, J. (2020). Interaction between drugs and the gut microbiome. *Gut, 69*(8), 1510–1519. DOI: 10.1136/gutjnl-2019-320204 PMID: 32409589

Wikoff, W. R., Anfora, A. T., Liu, J., Schultz, P. G., Lesley, S. A., Peters, E. C., & Siuzdak, G. (2009). Metabolomics analysis reveals large effects of gut microflora on mammalian blood metabolites. *Proceedings of the National Academy of Sciences of the United States of America, 106(10)*, 3698–3703. DOI: 10.1073/pnas.0812874106

Yin, Y.-N., Yu, Q.-F., Fu, N., Liu, X.-W., & Lu, F.-G. (2010). Effects of four bifidobacteria on obesity in high-fat diet induced rats. *World Journal of Gastroenterology, 16*(27), 3394–3401. DOI: 10.3748/wjg.v16.i27.3394 PMID: 20632441

Zeevi, D., Korem, T., Zmora, N., Israeli, D., Rothschild, D., Weinberger, A., Ben-Yacov, O., Lador, D., Avnit-Sagi, T., Lotan-Pompan, M., Suez, J., Mahdi, J. A., Matot, E., Malka, G., Kosower, N., Rein, M., Zilberman-Schapira, G., Dohnalová, L., Pevsner-Fischer, M., & Segal, E. (2015). Personalized Nutrition by Prediction of Glycemic Responses. *Cell, 163*(5), 1079–1094. DOI: 10.1016/j.cell.2015.11.001 PMID: 26590418

Zhao, L., Zhang, F., Ding, X., Wu, G., Lam, Y. Y., Wang, X., Fu, H., Xue, X., Lu, C., Ma, J., Yu, L., Xu, C., Ren, Z., Xu, Y., Xu, S., Shen, H., Zhu, X., Shi, Y., Shen, Q., & Zhang, W. (2019). Gut bacteria selectively promoted by dietary fibers alleviate type 2 diabetes. *Science, 359*(6380), 1151–1156. DOI: 10.1126/science.aao5774 PMID: 29590046

Zhong, C., Qu, C., Wang, B., Liang, S., & Zeng, B. (2017). Probiotics for preventing and treating small intestinal bacterial overgrowth: A meta-analysis and systematic review of current evidence. *Journal of Clinical Gastroenterology, 51*(4), 300–311. DOI: 10.1097/MCG.0000000000000814 PMID: 28267052

Zmora, N., Suez, J., & Elinav, E. (2019). You are what you eat: Diet, health and the gut microbiota. *Nature Reviews. Gastroenterology & Hepatology, 16*(1), 35–56. DOI: 10.1038/s41575-018-0061-2 PMID: 30262901

Zmora, N., Zeevi, D., Korem, T., Segal, E., & Elinav, E. (2016). Taking it Personally: Personalized Utilization of the Human Microbiome in Health and Disease. *Cell Host & Microbe, 19*(1), 12–20. DOI: 10.1016/j.chom.2015.12.016 PMID: 26764593

Chapter 9
Function of Gut Microbiota in Cancer as a Microbial Approach for Personalised Therapy

Sumira Malik
https://orcid.org/0000-0001-5077-1493
Amity University, Ranchi, India

Jutishna Bora
Amity University, Ranchi, India

Amrita Mishra
Amity University, Ranchi, India

Ayush Madan
https://orcid.org/0000-0001-5089-1794
People's University, India

ABSTRACT

The gut microbiota is a critical component in the complex interplay of processes underlying cancer formation, progression, and treatment, which is now receiving recognition due to the abundance of microbes, numbering in the trillions, within the human gut. Advancements in microbiota-targeted approaches, including faecal microbiota transplantation (FMT), probiotic therapy, and dietary modification, hold significant potential for restoring microbial homeostasis, enhancing immune-mediated anti-tumour responses, mitigating treatment side effects, and addressing existing challenges such as protocol uniformity in microbiota manipulation, safety,

DOI: 10.4018/979-8-3373-4382-2.ch009

long-term efficacy, and the complexity of microbial relationships. This review synthesises the cumulative insights into the dual role of gut microbiota as both an ally and an adversary in understanding cancer biology and treatment, serving as a salient biomarker and therapeutic target, and highlights research gaps that could be exploited to incorporate microbiome technology into personalised cancer management, aiming to maximise effectiveness.

INTRODUCTION

The term gut microbiota refers to a complex ecosystem that thrives in the human gastrointestinal tract, comprising billions of bacteria, viruses, fungi, and other microorganisms. These microorganisms work symbiotically to produce nutrients, aid digestion, support the immune system, and preserve health (Eissa, 2024). Diet, genetics, and involvement are some factors that influence the individual differences in gut microbiota composition and richness. According to estimates, there will be about 10 million deaths and 20 million new cases of Cancer worldwide in 2022, making it one of the leading causes of morbidity and mortality worldwide (Jang et al., 2025). The ageing population, lifestyle choices, and environmental exposures are some of the factors contributing to the increased incidence and mortality rates. Emerging scientific data have highlighted the gut microbiota in determining the initiation, progression, and post-response to cancer treatment, through mechanisms such as chronic inflammation, DNA damage, immunological regulation, metabolic changes, dysbiosis or tumorigenic processes. The relationship between gut microbiota and Cancer has promise for novel therapeutic, preventative, and diagnostic strategies showed in figure 1 (Eissa, 2024; Chigurupati, 2025).

Figure 1. Gut microbiota and its role in causing cancer

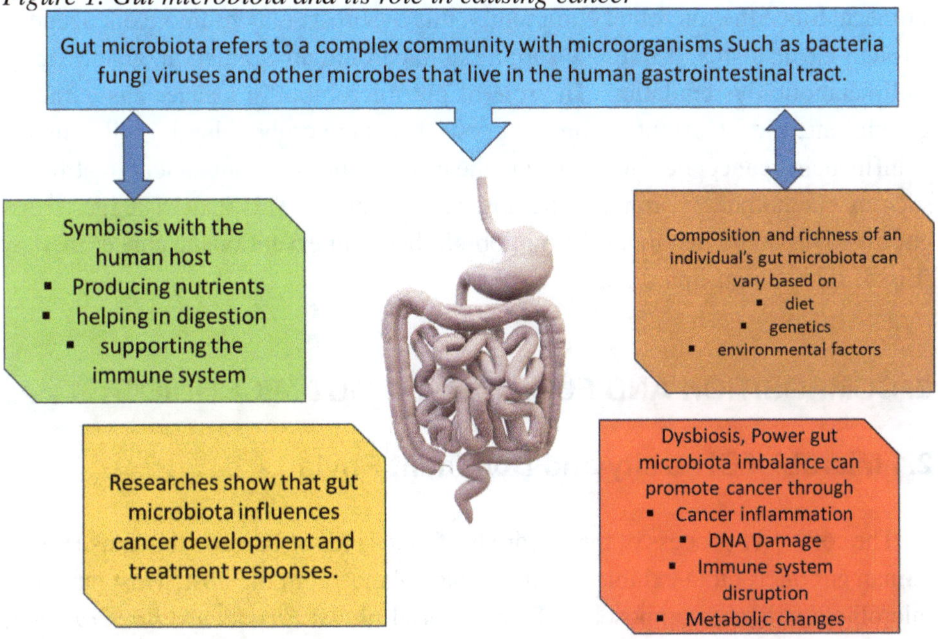

1.1 Overview of Gut Microbiota

The human gut microbiota, a highly complex microbial community comprising more than a thousand different species of bacteria, viruses, fungi, and other microorganisms, is a densely populated ecosystem of the gastrointestinal tract. Gut microbiota act as a dynamic metabolic organ, which breaks down dietary fiber, forms key vitamins, including B1, B9, B12, and K, breaks down bile acid, and balances immunological equilibrium. Several disorders are associated with disturbance in the symbiotic gut microbe-host connection that sustains gastrointestinal and general physiological function. Short-chain fatty acids, including butyrate, acetate, and propionate, are metabolic byproducts of the gut microbiota that are linked to preserving intestinal barrier function and controlling host metabolism (Eissa, 2024).

1.2 Global Burden of Cancer and Relevance of Microbiota

With about 20 million new cases and roughly 10 million cancer-related deaths globally in 2022, Cancer is a significant global health concern (Jang et al., 2025). The prevalence of Cancer is increasing, particularly in low and middle-income countries, where healthcare resources and preventive measures may be insufficient. The most prevalent malignancies are those of the lung, breast, colorectal, prostate, and stomach. Since the microbial community, this dysbiosis may promote oncogenesis through mechanisms of immune suppression, chronic inflammation, genotoxicity, and metabolic dysregulation. The role of gut microbiota in Cancer has garnered growing attention. Current research suggests that gut microbes play a significant role in influencing cancer development and the host's response to anticancer treatments, such as chemotherapy, immunotherapy, and radiation. This article suggests that gut microbes could be targets for microbiota-based interventions in cancer therapy (Eissa,2024; Chigurupati, 2025).

2. COMPOSITION AND FUNCTION OF GUT MICROBIOTA

2.1 Microbial Diversity and Dominant Phyla

The collective process of the hundreds of thousands of bacteria that make up the human gut microbiota exhibits a remarkable balance with the host. Most intestinal microbiota is likely composed of four bacterial phyla: *Firmicutes*, *Bacteroidetes, Proteobacteria,* and*Actinobacteria. Firmicutes* and *Bacteroidete*s comprise approximately 90% of the entire microbiota; however, the relative abundance of each varies significantly depending on factors that substantially influence the gut microbiome's composition, including diet, genetics, and environmental exposures. Due to an inverse interaction between *Firmicutes* and *Bacteroidetes* that controls the microbiome's diversity, the composition does not form distinct clusters but rather a continuum. Changes in the prevalence of these dominant phyla, associated with health and disease states, are prominent in dysbiosis, which is characterised by an increase in *Proteobacteria* and a decrease in the beneficial *Firmicutes*. Other microbes are purportedly classifying conditions through measurements of previously mentioned alpha-diversity, overlapping with a set of diseases such as colorectal Cancer and some metabolic disorders, suggesting a modular control on these phyla to maintain the well-functioning state of the gut. The relative abundance of such major phyla is also influenced by the constantly changing gut microbiota, which is influenced by the host’s diet, lifestyle, and medications (Manor et al., 2020).

2.2 Gut Microbiota Metabolic and Immunological Functions

The fermentation of dietary fibre into short-chain fatty acids (SCFAs), such as butyrate, propionate, and acetate, is one of the gut microbiota's crucial metabolic processes. These short-chain fatty acids (SCFAs) are vital energy substrates for colonocytes, regulating immunological responses and inflammation (Olofsson &

Bäckhed, 2022). SCFAs play a role in maintaining systemic regulation of immunity and metabolism, inhibiting inflammation, and regulating the function of the interstitial barrier (Li et al., 2024). In addition to fermentation, the metabolites of the microbiota may influence host functions by modulating the release of specific hormones and regulating metabolic pathways, including lipid and glucose metabolism, which are closely linked to cancer development (Olofsson & Bäckhed, 2022).

Immunologically, gut microbiota plays a central role in influencing immunologic host tolerance and activation. Facilitate immune system development, Treg cells, and signalling cascade inflammation (Li et al., 2024). Such interactions must be balanced because disruptions lead to persistent inflammation, a key factor in cancers like colorectal and stomach tumours. By strengthening the integrity of the epithelial barrier and competitively excluding harmful microorganisms, commensal bacteria help support intestinal immune homeostasis and mucosal immunity. Furthermore, it has been discovered that several bacterial species, such as *Bifidobacterium* and *Faecalibacterium*, are responsible for both modulating immune activity and eliciting anti-inflammatory responses (Manor et al., 2020).

2.3 Gut Microbiome and Host Interaction Mechanisms

Most of the gut's actions and those affecting the body's overall health are triggered by the numerous molecules and cells that connect the microbiome with the host. Gut microbes interact with epithelial cells by producing substances, particles, and metabolites that can transmit messages and oversee gut immunity (Li et al., 2024). Because of this, nutrients are shared, and the host's microbes and defence system are defined. Host genome also narrow the variety of microbes in the microbiome, leading to changes in the immune response and cellular energy usage. The sensation of bacteria, in addition to the release of extracellular vesicles, is described as a novel method through which bacteria and their hosts interact, influencing the microbial community and modulating the host's immune responses (Alberti et al., 2021).

In Cancer, a change in the host's microbiome and its interactions with the body contribute to tumorigenesis. Abnormal microbiota in the gut produce factors that cause inflammation, toxins that damage DNA, and materials that support the process of cancer formation and development (Li et al., 2024). In the opposite case, repairing or enhancing the balance of microbes can increase the effectiveness of immunotherapies by adjusting immune responses and overall levels of inflammation. It is essential to know these interactions when making microbiota-based therapies for Cancer.

3. GUT MICROBIOTA AND TUMORIGENESIS

Since the gut microbiota plays a vital part in the development of tumours, it has become essential in tumour studies. Not only does it contribute to local cancers of the digestive system, but it can also impact other parts of the body and the entire system in various ways. Research now recognises that when the gut is out of balance, known as dysbiosis, it plays a significant role in cancer risk, primarily through pathways involving inflammation, alterations to a cell's DNA, and the body's food processing (Kim & Lee, 2022; Ağagündüz et al., 2023). This text investigates the various roles gut microbiota plays in tumorigenesis and explains the pathways it affects, using cancer development as an example.

3.1 Role in Local Gastrointestinal Cancers

The gut microbiota is essential because the gastrointestinal tract contains the most microbes in the human body, and these microbes often play a role in the development of colon-related cancers, mainly colorectal Cancer. When microbes in the gut change, dysbiosis is closely tied to CRC's development and growth (Wong & Yu, 2023), it has been found through several studies that people with CRC have a lower microbiome diversity than healthy people, together with an increased level of bacteria linked to Cancer, namely *Fusobacterium nucleatum, Bacteroides fragilis*, and *Escherichia coli*. They participate in cancer formation by stimulating local inflammation, generating genotoxins, and compromising the epithelial barrier, thereby increasing the likelihood of Cancer (Kim & Lee, 2022).

More than CRC, gut microbiota is also involved in other gastrointestinal tumours, for example, gastric carcinoma, and *Helicobacter pylori* is the best understood risk-related microbe (Ağagündüz et al., 2023). CagA, VacA, ROS, and continuous inflammation are all factors that contribute to the development of cancerous changes caused by H. pylori. It is worth noting that other gut bacteria changes contribute to gastric Cancer by affecting the immune system on the mucosa and creating an inflammatory environment. Due to the influence of microbial metabolites and bacterial components, the local immune environment changes, which alters the tumour formation process and progression in the gut (Wong & Yu, 2023).

3.2 Impact on Extraintestinal and Systemic Cancers

Besides affecting Cancer of the digestive tract, gut microbiota has been associated with the development of breast, pancreatic, and lung cancers. Alterations in microbes nearby can impact other organs by influencing the immune system, altering metabolism, and allowing bacteria to enter the bloodstream. Breast cancer patients have abnormal gut microbiota showing fewer healthy species and more pathogenic ones, which change oestrogen levels and weaken the immune response in a way that increases their risk of Cancer. These interactions between microbiota and the host include enzymes, such as β-glucuronidase, that help increase the amount of estrogen available, contributing to hormone receptor-positive breast cancer (He et al., 2025).

Similar to bladder cancer, changes in the gut microbiome in pancreatic Cancer are linked to the disease's development and its response to therapy, affecting both systemic and local immunity. Additionally, lung cancer develops when microbes trigger inflammation in the body, thereby altering the immune system. The effect on the lungs is mediated by microbes in the gut and their metabolic products. They demonstrate that gut microbiota should be considered when discussing the causes and treatments of cancers in other parts of the body (Aghamajidi & Malenki Vareki, 2022).

3.3 Microbial Dysbiosis and Cancer Risk

A smaller and balanced range of microbes is a prominent feature of cancer-related changes in the microbiome. It fosters the formation of tumours through inflammation, problems with the immune barrier, and the growth of cancer-causing bacteria. Studying how different bacteria in the intestinal tract led to Cancer, researchers found that certain bacteria initiate the carcinogenic processes, while others affect the growth of tumours. Typically, the abnormal composition of bacteria results from a diet high in sugar, obesity, the use of antibiotics, and chronic inflammation, and is influenced by both genetic factors and immune system function. Besides, dysbiosis can modify the performance and safety of drugs used to treat Cancer, so changing the microbiome might improve the treatment results. It may be possible to detect Cancer earlier and categorise risk by studying bacterial profiles in the faces or biopsies of the gut (Kim & Lee, 2022).

3.4 Molecular Mechanisms: Inflammation, Genotoxicity, Metabolism, Metabolites

Cancer is more likely to develop in the gut because of complex mechanisms associated with inflammation, DNA damage, faulty metabolism, and the production of certain substances. When these pathways work together, they create a setting that allows tumours to form, affect the cells' DNA, alter their metabolism, and manipulate the immune system, which supports tumour formation, development, and response to various treatments.

Inflammation is a primary connection between changes in the gut bacteria and the development of tumours. An inflamed state caused by specific microbes creates an environment that is likely to support cancer development by releasing cytokines such as IL-6, IL-1β, TNF-α, and IL-17. Bacteria such as *Fusobacterium nucleatum*, Enterotoxigenic Bacteroides fragilis (ETBF), and Helicobacter pylori trigger inflammation by engaging specific receptors, activating NF-κB signalling, and modulating STAT3. This relationship results in frequent epithelial damage, increased immune system cell infiltration, and the support of processes such as new blood vessel growth, tissue spread to other parts of the body, and the avoidance of immune responses that would otherwise fight cancer cells. A good example is lipopolysaccharide (LPS), an endotoxin found in Gram-negative bacteria, which triggers the production of inflammatory substances by macrophages and epithelial cells, thereby enhancing the expression of hypoxia-inducible factor 1 alpha (HIF-1α) and vascular endothelial growth factor (VEGF), to increase angiogenesis in tumours. The chronic inflammation that follows makes it possible for Cancer to develop from genetic mutations and promotes tumour development (Chen et al., 2023)

Gut microbes may also contribute to carcinogenesis by damaging a person's DNA through genotoxicity. Sometimes, bacteria produce genotoxins that alter the host DNA, leading to mutations and inaccurate genetic information. In particular, Escherichia coli strains carrying the pks island can produce colibactin, which breaks the DNA in colonic epithelial cells and leads to many harmful outcomes. Furthermore, Campylobacter jejuni develops cytolethal distending toxin (CDT), leading to the destruction of DNA by DSBs and stopping the cell cycle, thus helping Cancer to develop (Chen et al., 2023; Zechner & Kienesberger, 2024).

Additionally, microbial activity in host cells can induce the production of reactive oxygen and nitrogen species, leading to DNA oxidation and breakage. Helicobacter pylori's control over MLH1 and MSH2 genes through microRNA leads to more genetic instability in gastric Cancer. As a result of a weak DNA damage response, harmful mutations accumulate, contributing to cancer development (Zechner & Kienesberger, 2024).

Our body's bacteria are linked to metabolic pathway modifications that enhance cancer risk. Microbial metabolites alter the energy consumption of immune cells, tumour cells, and cells involved in cancer genesis and treatment. Butyrate, propionate, and acetate are short-chain fatty acids frequently produced in the gut by certain bacteria from dietary fibres and have varying effects on the growth of tumours. For example, by modifying a set of genes in the gut, butyrate promotes the growth of healthy cells, reduces inflammation, and halts the development of colorectal Cancer. Conversely, secondary bile acids, such as DCA, generated by bacteria from primary bile acids, can damage DNA, induce cellular stress, and release specific factors that contribute to the development of hepatocellular carcinomas and other complications. Furthermore, these secondary bile acids can further promote tumour growth by altering crucial signalling pathways, including the EGFR-MAPK and Beta-Catenin Pathways (Chen et al., 2023).

Moreover, the production of TMS by gut bacteria and its conversion to TMAO changes the entire body's metabolism. It is linked to inflammation, blood cholesterol, and several types of Cancer (Chen et al., 2023). By altering the immune system through AhR-activated pathways, bacteria that convert tryptophan to kynurenine facilitate the invasion of tumour cells into the immune system (Escriva et al., 2025). Inosine is one bacterial molecule that affects immune system cells, improving their ability to combat malignancies (Chen et al., 2023).

Overall, microbiome metabolites function as messenger molecules, altering the tumour environment by controlling metabolism, immunological responses, and gene activity in a manner that affects cancer biology in various ways. To create bacterial cancer therapeutics, it is crucial to understand how the metabolic activities of bacteria can impact Cancer (Escriva et al., 2025).

4. PROTECTIVE ROLES OF GUT MICROBIOTA IN CANCER

The gut microbiota plays a role in Cancer in two ways: it helps develop tumours or prevents tumour growth. Gaining insight into the tumour-inhibiting properties of certain gut bacteria, the impacts of microbiota-derived materials, and the value of probiotics all suggest viable ways to use the microbiome for fighting Cancer.

4.1 Tumour Suppressive Microbes and Their Mechanisms

Various gut microorganisms function as tumour suppressors, maintaining balance in the gut, modulating immune responses, and inhibiting cancer-promoting actions. Beneficial bacteria can outcompete harmful bacteria, maintain the skin cells' barrier, and produce molecules that reduce inflammation, all of which contribute to a healthy body and lower cancer risks (Hou et al., 2024). As an example, bacteria such as *Butyrivibrio fibrisolvens* and *Faecalibacterium prausnitzii*, which produce butyrate, are found in larger numbers in healthy individuals and may protect against colorectal Cancer by supporting the health of cells in the colon and stabilising the immune response (Kalyanaraman et al., 2024).

Microbes that lower the risks of tumour growth can also affect the host's immune system by increasing Tregs and suppressing pathways that cause chronic inflammation and cancer development (Hou et al., 2024). Traditionally, bacteria in the gut interact with both surface cells and immune cells below, helping to produce anti-inflammatory cytokines, including interleukin-10. Additionally, specific species of bacteria have been studied to determine how they regulate oncogenic signalling by inhibiting activities in the Wnt/β-catenin and various other pathways.

Research with gnotobiotic mice has proven that some bacteria help prevent Cancer. Letting bacteria that control tumour growth into the body can cut down the number of tumours, whereas less diversity among microbes or the absence of beneficial bacteria can increase tumour growth. They confirm that having the right mix of microbes in the digestive system is crucial for avoiding cancer (Kalyanaraman et al., 2024).

Table 1. Tumour-Suppressive Gut Microbes and Their Anticancer Actions

Microbe	Mechanism	Cancer type	Reference
Butyrivibrio fibrisolvens	Butyrate Production: supports colon cell health and stabilizes immune response	Colorectal Cancer	Kalyanaraman et al., 2024
Faecalibacterium prausnitzii	Butyrate Production: supports colon cell health and stabilizes immune response	Colorectal cancer	Kalyanaraman et al., 2024
Bacteroides fragilis (anti-inflammatory strain)	Boost Tregs; secrete IL-10; suppress inflammation	Various (Inflammation-driven cancers)	Hou et al., 2024
Salmonella enterica, Helicobacter pylori, and Pseudomonas aeruginosa	Inhibit oncogenic signals (e.g., Wnt/β-catenin)	Various	Hou et al., 2024
Beneficial microbial consortia (Mice)	Lower tumour count; preserve microbial diversity	Gastrointestinal cancers (in mouse models)	Kalyanaraman et al., 2024

4.2 Role of Short Chain-Fatty Acids and Other Metabolites

The most important microbial byproducts, mainly acetate, propionate, and butyrate, are short-chain fatty acids made by the fermentation of dietary fibres by gut anaerobes. It is now understood that gut microbiota utilises SCFAs to protect against Cancer by regulating energy in cells, influencing the immune system, and modulating gene expression, as well as combating inflammation (Hou et al., 2024; Kalyanaraman et al., 2024).

Butyrate especially helps stop tumours from growing in various ways. It encourages cell death in cancer cells and stops their division, using this approach to support the primary energy needs of healthy colon cells and protect the epithelial lining (Hou et al., 2024). Most significantly, butyrate inhibits histone deacetylase, allowing histones to be acetylated. This alters the function of genes involved in cell division and programmed cell death, also known as apoptosis. SCFAs also activate

G-protein receptors, such as GPR109A, which help reduce inflammation and maintain intestinal wall integrity (Luu et al., 2021).

Additionally, propionate and acetate contribute to these effects by modulating the function of immune cells and reducing inflammatory processes involved in carcinogenesis (Kalyanaraman et al., 2024; Luu et al., 2021). In addition, SCFAs contribute to tumour growth and metastasis by affecting angiogenesis and EMT, and this process is mediated by maintaining low levels of VEGF and TGF-β pathways (Hou et al., 2024). Documents have revealed that using SCFAs together with chemotherapy enhances the cancer-killing abilities while helping to reduce the toxic side effects (Luu et al., 2021).

These products are present in the gut and ultimately enter circulation, reaching and affecting the immune system in areas relevant to cancer treatment beyond the gut (Hou et al., 2024). Due to the connection between diet and bacteria, the specific SCFAs produced in the gut play a central role in preventing and treating Cancer.

4.3 Probiotics and Case Study: *Lactobacillus rhamnosus GG*

Probiotics are live bacteria that, when taken in adequate amounts, help the host's health. Modifying the gut Microbiota and immune responses has demonstrated promising new uses in cancer prevention and complementary therapy. Due to its exceptional safety record and diverse action methods, *Lactobacillus rhamnosus GG (LGG)* is one of the most researched and widely used probiotic strains. Through various pathways, including microbial homeostasis restoration, gut barrier integrity reinforcement, inflammatory regulation, and direct antiproliferative actions on cancer cells, LGG has anticancer benefits. According to preclinical studies, LGG can lower proinflammatory cytokines that are implicated in inflammation-associated gastrointestinal cancers, such as interleukin 6 (IL-6), interleukin 8 (IL-8), and tumour necrosis factor-alpha (TNF-alpha). Additionally, it has been discovered that LGG inhibits the activity of enzymes that promote tumour growth, like ornithine decarboxylase, which impacts polyamine metabolism essential for cancer cell growth (Owens et al., 2021).

Clinical studies on cancer patients, particularly those receiving chemotherapy or radiation therapy, have shown that taking LGG supplements lowers gastrointestinal side effects such as mucositis and diarrhoea, which enhances patient quality of life and treatment compliance. Furthermore, the administration of LGG has been associated with enhanced immunological markers, including a shift in the cytokine profile toward anti-tumour immunity and increased T-cell counts. Additionally, mechanistic studies demonstrate that cellular components and metabolites produced from LGG can activate the CD8+ T-cell response and promote dendritic cell maturation, which is necessary for efficient anticancer immunity (Owens et al., 2021). Furthermore, preclinical models employing LGG altered to create 3-hydroxybutyrate- a substance helpful in battling colon cancer cachexia- show that recent developments using genetically modified strains of LGG have improved its anticancer characteristics. LGG has systemic immune-modulatory effects beyond the gut, supporting its potential use in integrative oncology (Qiu et al., 2025).

5. GUT MICROBIOTA AS A TUMOUR PROMOTER

Despite the importance of the gut microbiota to the host's well-being, under certain conditions, it may stimulate tumour growth. To a large extent, this role is preceded by pathogenic bacteria, which stimulate carcinogenesis, activate chronic inflammation, and induce oxidative stress as a consequence of microbial dysbiosis, influencing tumour immune evasion and development. These pathogenic processes are crucial for elucidating the complex interplay between the microbiome and carcinogenesis, as they have important implications for warranted therapeutic processes.

5.1 Pathogenic Bacteria and Carcinogenesis

Specific pathogenic gut microbiota bacteria have been termed as direct determinants of carcinogenesis, as they produce DNA damage, modify cellular functions, and impact oncogenic signalling pathways. Notably, *Escherichia coli* strains that produce the genotoxin colibactin can induce DNA double-strand breaks in host cells, which are indicators of tumour development and genetic instability (Ivleva & Grivennikov, 2022). Similarly, the toxins produced by *Bacteroides fragilis*, especially enterotoxigenic strains, can trigger Ptc/-catenin signalling and inflammatory cascades, both of which contribute to the development of colorectal Cancer (CRC) (Chen et al., 2023). Expanded in CRC tissues, *Fusobacterium nucleatum* is implicated in generating a proinflammatory tumour microenvironment and the growth and invasion of cancer cells by activating immune invasion pathways (Zepeda-Rivera et al., 2024). These microorganisms incorporate carcinogenic processes, such as host genetic alteration, oncogenic signalling dysregulation, and immune remodelling environments, that promote tumour formation. The ubiquitous presence of bacteria in tumour tissue suggests that bacterial colonization directly affects carcinogenesis, which is the main reason they are central to the aetiology of gastrointestinal cancers (Ivleva & Grivennikov, 2022).

Table 2. Gut Bacteria producing Carcinogenic Pathogens Implicated in Carcinogenesis

Pathogenic bacterium	Mechanism of carcinogenesis	Associated Cancer	References
Escherichia coli (colibactin-producing strains)	Induces DNA double-strand breaks via genotoxin colibactin → genomic instability.	Colorectal Cancer (CRC)	Ivleva & Grivennikov, 2022
Bacteroides fragilis (enterotoxin strains)	Triggers beta-catenin signalling and proinflammatory cascades → tumour development	Colorectal Cancer (CRC)	Chen et al., 2023
Fusobacterium nucleatum	Promotes immune evasion and inflammation via activation of immune evasion pathways	Colorectal Cancer (CRC)	Zepeda-Rivera et al., 2024
Various tumour-associated bacteria	Modifies host genetic, oncogenic signalling, and immune environment	Gastrointestinal cancers	Ivleva & Grivennikov, 2022

5.2 Dysbiosis-Induced Chronic Inflammation and Oxidative Stress

Dysbiosis, where pathogenic microorganisms overprotect commensal species, leads to a chronic inflammatory condition and oxidative stress, both of which are stable markers of carcinogenesis. Dysbiosis of the gut microbiota is the cause of gut barrier integrity violation and the constant activation of immune cells that produce inflammatory mediators, including IL-6 and TNF-alpha, as well as reactive oxygen species, which induce DNA damage and mutagenesis. This inflammation disrupts the delicate balance between cell proliferation and apoptosis, thereby increasing the likelihood of tumour initiation and progression (Karam et al., 2025). In addition, epigenetic changes driven by ongoing oxidative stress due to dysbiosis compromise cancer-suppressing mechanisms, predisposing individuals to Cancer. The gut microbiota regulates oxidative balance by modulating redox signalling and immune pathways. Due to an unbalanced microbial population, the host environment may change in a way that promotes tumour growth. Tumour growth and malignancy are accelerated by a positive feedback loop created by chronic inflammation and oxidative stress (Mostafavi et al., 2024).

5.3 Influence on Immune Evasion and Tumour Progression

An influence of gut microbiota on the tumour immune microenvironment is of interest in modulating tumour immune evasion mechanisms that enable tumour cells to escape immune recognition and stimulate their further progression. Particular bacterial species, such as *Fusobacterium nucleatum*, have been observed to contribute to immune evasion by inhibiting anti-tumour T-cell responses and establishing an immunosuppressive tumour microenvironment through the recruitment of both regulatory T cells and myeloid-derived suppressor cells. Moreover, products of metabolism by intestinal microbes, known as microbial-associated molecular patterns (MAMPs), regulate cytokine and immune cell functions, and alter tumour-associated macrophage polarisation and the cytotoxic effect of lymphocytes. This dysbiosis further impaired antigen presentation, downregulating the signal required to mount an immune response, and promoting tolerance and refractoriness to therapies such as immune checkpoint blockade. Targeting gut microbiota-based approaches targeting faecal microbiota transplantation and administration of probiotics that aim to restore immune-dampened functions and reinforce immunotherapy response by manipulating the microbiota, and the profound impact of gut microbiota in tumour immune interactions. Such microbial modulations of host immunity contribute to tumour progression and therapeutic resistance (He et al., 2022).

6. GUT MICROBIOTA AND CANCER THERAPY

The gut microbiota, a complex community of organisms that colonise the human gastrointestinal tract, has recently become a significant modulator of the therapeutic effect in malignancy. It affects chemotherapy, immunotherapy, and radiotherapy, as well as the efficacy and toxicity of these treatments. Additionally, precise manipulation of the gut microbiota with probiotics, faecal microbiota transplantation (FMT), and antibiotics is also a promising prospect for enhancing therapeutic efficacy and reducing side effects. This section has explored the impact of gut microbiota on cancer treatment, the effects of radiotherapy on microbial composition, and the potential of microbiota-directed treatment.

6.1 Influence on Chemotherapy and Immunotherapy Outcomes

The gut microbiome plays a significant role in regulating the therapeutic efficacy and toxicity of chemotherapy and immunotherapy in oncology. Host-microbiota interactions are complex, involving immunomodulation, drug metabolism, or changes in the microbial community, which can affect the activity and toxicities of chemotherapeutic agents. Notably, some species of bacteria induce an antitumor immune response, thereby enhancing the efficacy of certain cytotoxic drugs, such as oxaliplatin and cyclophosphamide, through different mechanisms. Among these, myeloid cellular priming and T cell activation are particularly noteworthy. On the other hand, dysbiosis of the microbiota before chemotherapy with antibiotics was found to have harmful consequences for the therapy's functioning, which also confirms the importance of a well-balanced microbiome. Additionally, intestinal microorganisms can degrade chemotherapy agents themselves, alter their availability, and produce toxic metabolites, which can exacerbate side effects. For instance, microbial ß-glucuronidases can degrade irinotecan, leading to its side effect, mucositis (Chrysostomou et al., 2023).

Gut microbiota has also emerged as one of the strongest indicators of therapeutic outcome in immunotherapy, particularly with immune checkpoint inhibitors (ICIs). The investigations are associated with microbial diversity and distinct taxa, including Bifidobacterium, Akkermansia muciniphila, and Faecalibacterium, which may lead to better patient responses and progression-free survival. The reduced responses to ICIs in germ-free or antibiotic-treated mouse models can be converted back to responders by faecal microbial transplantation, which lends further causative strength. Mechanistically, intestinal microorganisms affect antitumor immunity by interacting with innate and adaptive immune cells, the tumour microenvironment and systemic immune activation. These findings have served as the starting point for numerous clinical trials investigating the modulation of microbiota to enhance the efficacy of immunotherapy (Kiousi et al., 2023).

6.2 Radiotherapy Effects on Gut Microbiota

Radiotherapy, one of the traditional cancer therapies, has a significant effect on the gut flora, which in turn affects how effective and harmful the radiation is. Low microbial diversity, the increase of pathogenic species (*Proteobacteria* and *Fusobacteria*), and the depletion of butyrate-producing bacteria (*Faecalibacterium* and *Bifidobacterium*) are all consequences of ionizing radiation-induced dysbiosis. This microvascular damage is linked to radiation gastrointestinal toxicities, including radiation diarrhoea and enteritis, which impair quality of life and treatment compliance. The adverse effects of radiation are further exacerbated by disruption of the gut microbiota, which mechanically results in local inflammation, epithelial barrier dysfunction, and systemic immune bottlenecking. Interestingly, the recently proposed concept of the gut-organ axis suggests that the gut microbiota is linked to extraintestinal organs. Thus, radiation-induced changes in the microbiota can lead to alterations in distal tissues, such as the brain and lungs, which may promote the development of neurocognitive dysfunctions and pulmonary complications. Recently, it has also been proposed that gut microbiota can modulate radiosensitivity and the abscopal effect, and microbial metabolites, particularly short-chain fatty acids (SCFAs), play a role in immune regulation during radiotherapy. Regardless of these developments, interactions between microbiota and radiotherapy represent a field of active research with significant implications for clinical practice (Li et al., 2022).

6.3 Microbiota-Targeted Interventions: Probiotics, FMT, and Antibiotics

Treatments targeting the gut microbiota can become appealing add-on therapies in oncology to enhance outcomes and reduce side effects. Probiotics are living microorganisms that have been demonstrated to have potential in mitigating the side effects of chemotherapy and radiotherapy, such as diarrhoea and mucositis, and in enhancing immune responses (Wierzbicka et al., 2024; Rodriguez-Arrastia et al., 2021). In practice, it is stated that taking probiotics during cancer treatment can reduce the risk of infections and positively influence the functioning of the gastrointestinal tract. However, the issues of which strains are most effective to use and which courses of treatment are most beneficial still require standardisation (Kiousi et al., 2023).

The procedure of faecal microbiota transplantation (FMT), containing the transfer of faecal microbial communities of a healthy donor to a patient, has become one of the most potent methods to recover microbial diversity and functionality in cancer patients, especially in those who are not responsive to immune checkpoint inhibitors (Chen et al., 2019). Previous clinical trials have demonstrated improved anti-tumour activity and control of immune parameters with FMT in combination with ICIs, supporting the notion that FMT can overcome therapeutic resistance (Chrysostomou et al., 2023). However, donor selection, safety and engraftment of microbiota longevity remain a problem (Li et al., 2022).

The use of antibiotics in cancer treatment is two-sided. Although antibiotics are necessary to fight infections, they can significantly alter the composition of gut microbes, reduce diversity, and potentially impact the outcome of both chemotherapy and immunotherapy. Antibiotics are recommended to be used carefully to achieve a balance between controlling infections and preserving microbiota. The new approaches include antibiotic selectivity or targeting inhibitors to specific microbe species, thereby reducing the harmful consequences (Chrysostomou et al., 2023). There is a possibility that incorporating comprehensive microbiota management into the cancer treatment process may maximise the effects of treatment (Otto-Dobos et al., 2024).

7. INFLAMMASOMES IN GUT MICROBIOTA

Inflammasomes, as significant intracellular multiprotein complexes, are now among the leading actors of the interconnection between gut microbiota, immune responses, and cancer development. Despite their key roles in microbial and danger signal sensing, triggering of inflammatory cascades, and modulation of cell death processes, their functions in tumorigenesis are multifaceted and context-dependent.

In this case, the section will cover what inflammasomes are composed of, their purpose, their tandem malfunctioning in Cancer, and their intricate interaction with the gut barrier and immune system.

7.1 Inflammasomes: Structure, Function, and Dual Role in tumorigenesis

Inflammasomes are cytosolic protein complexes comprising predominantly a sensor molecule, e.g. a Nod-like receptor (NLR), the adaptor protein apoptosis-associated speck-like protein with a caspase recruitment domain (ASC) and the effector enzyme procaspase-1. These proteins must be triggered by pathogen-associated molecular patterns (PAMPs) or damage-associated molecular patterns (DAMPs). After formation, they activate caspase-1, which triggers the maturation and release of proinflammatory cytokines interleukin-1 beta (IL-1β) and interleukin-18 (IL-18), as well as pyroptotic cell death. The best-described inflammasome is NLRP3, which has a tripartite domain architecture comprising a leucine-rich repeat (LRR) domain that binds ligands, an NACHT domain that oligomerizes, and an N-terminal pyrin domain that binds ASC (Shadab et al., 2023; Fu & Wu, 2023).

Inflammasomes have opposing roles in cancer biology. They can also promote tumour growth by generating a proinflammatory microenvironment favouring proliferation, angiogenesis, invasion, and immune evasion. For example, the activation of NLRP3 facilitates the production of IL-1, which activates cancer-associated fibroblasts and myeloid-derived suppressor cells that stimulate the growth and metastasis of breast and gastric cancers. Conversely, once pyroptosis, an inflammatory programmed cell death, is activated by inflammasomes, tumour suppression also occurs by killing cancerous cells. In addition, it is possible to employ inflammasome signalling to stimulate anti-tumour immunity by promoting the release of cytokines, activating the natural killer (NK) cells and cytotoxic T lymphocytes. The practical outcome depends on the type of tumour, stage, microenvironment and specific inflammasome components involved. These context-dependent two functions are sobering thoughts upon considering the use of inflammasomes as therapeutic targets (Shadab et al., 2023).

7.2 Interaction with Gut Barrier and Immune Responses

The first line of defence against invasion by microorganisms and the maintenance of homeostasis with commensal microbiota is represented by intestinal epithelial cells and the intestinal gut barrier, formed by tight junctions (Manshouri et al., 2024). The outcome of critical control of this barrier by inflammasomes is, on the one hand, the development of immune tolerance to commensal bacteria, and, on the other hand, the initiation of a cascade of inflammatory reactions to pathogens (Manshouri et al., 2024; Yang et al., 2023). In epithelial and myeloid cells, the inflammasome activation promotes the secretion of IL-18, which is required for epithelial repair and the maintenance of barrier integrity to avoid dysbiosis and tumorigenesis caused by inflammation (Deng et al., 2023).

In addition, inflammasomes can regulate gut immunity, affecting both innate and adaptive immune cells. They control the release of cytokines and chemokines, which recruit immune effectors, stimulate immune monitoring, and facilitate the elimination of transformed cells (Shadab et al., 2023). Nevertheless, the a rhamnosus GG or chronic stimulation of the inflammasome leads to harmful inflammation, tissue injury, and a pro-tumour microenvironment (Shadab et al., 2023; Deng et al., 2023). Bidirectional communication between inflammasomes and the gut microbiota thus plays a key role in balancing immune activation and tolerance (Manshouri et al., 2024; Yang et al., 2023). The dysregulation may cause gut barrier dissolution and the perpetuation of inflammatory bowel disease (IBD) and also predispose colorectal Cancer (Manshouri et al., 2024; Deng et al., 2023).

8. EMERGING CONCEPTS AND SPECIALIZED TOPICS

More recent findings in oncology have expanded the remit of the gut microbiota beyond its long-standing functions in tumorigenesis and alteration of therapy. The topics of future interest include the contribution of the gut microbiota in communicating with hormone-related malignancies through epigenetics and its necessity in cancer cachexia indicated through gut-organ axes. Such mini-reviews, targeting specific topics, shed light on the multifaceted molecular and systemic-level processes by which gut microbiota impact cancer development, progression, and associated comorbidities.

8.1 Hormones-Related Cancers and Epigenetics

Hormones and Cancer The interdependence of a large sub-group of cancers (breast, prostate, ovarian and endometrial cancers) on hormonal signalling to stimulate tumorigenesis has been exploited in recent findings that have used the ability of the gut microbiota to modulate hormone levels, metabolism and epigenetic regulation which impacts so substantially on hormone-related carcinogenesis (Soldado-Gordillo & Alvarez-Mercado, 2024; Farhat et al., 2023).

It was also shown that gut microbiota can impact the systemic and local access of hormones by involving enterohepatic circulation of steroid hormones, as well as the production of enzyme glucuronidase, which deconjugates hormone metabolites to reactivate oestrogens and androgens, thereby targeting hormone signalling pathways that are disrupted in Cancer. Dysbiosis can disrupt this balance and is associated with alterations in microbial composition and diversity, leading to aberrant hormone metabolism, increased levels of bioactive hormones, and an increased risk of hormone-dependent malignancies (Arnone et al., 2025).

In DNA methylation, histone changes, and non-coding RNA expression changes, contributions of gut microbial products to epigenetic changes in host cells have been discovered concerning tumorigenesis, in addition to hormone metabolism. The microbial metabolites short-chain fatty acids (SCFAs), folate, and others serve as substrates or cofactors for epigenetic enzymes, thereby regulating the epigenomic landscape that determines cell proliferation and differentiation. For example, a histone deacetylase inhibitor, butyrate, is produced by microbes and can re-activate silenced tumour suppressor genes in hormone-related cancers (Zhao et al., 2021). Remarkably, the tuning of microbial epigenetics is also associated with the immune checkpoint pathways and transductions of inflammation signals that intersect with hormone receptor activities and contribute to diverse therapeutic responses. Cross-talk gut microbiota-epigenetics holds promising possibilities to program personalized medicine to attack hormone-related cancers by modulating the microbiome composition and its metabolic capabilities to restore the perturbed hormonal and epigenome balance (Arnone et al., 2025; Zhao et al., 2021).

8.2 Cancer Cachexia and Gut Organ Axes

A subgroup of cancers includes breast, prostate, ovarian and endometrial cancers, in which the tumorigenesis process is dependent on hormonal signalling. This type of Cancer is now in the spotlight because it has become clear that the gut microbiota reigns supreme in regulating levels of hormones and metabolism, as well as epigenetic control, thus influencing gut microbiota-influenced carcinogenesis (Soldado-Gordillo & Álvarez-Mercado, 2024; Farhat et al., 2023).

Some further research indicates that gut microbiota could also influence systemic and local concentration of hormones via modulating enterohepatic circulation of steroid hormones. Moreover, gut microbiota synthesizes enzymes like glucuronidase that deconjugate hormone metabolites and activate oestrogen and androgens that normally suppress oestrogen and androgen signalling pathways abnormal in Cancer. Dysbiosis, a reduction in microbial composition and diversity, can change such a balance, resulting in abnormal hormone metabolism, elevated bioactive hormone levels, and the risk of developing hormone-dependent cancers (Arnone et al., 2025).

In addition to hormone metabolism, gut microbial product is also connected with the host cell epigenetic change, including changes in DNA methylation, histone and non-coding RNA expression, which is decisive in gene expression regarding cancer development. As epigenetic enzyme cofactors or substrates, microbial and gut ecosystem metabolites, including folate and short-chain fatty acids, change the epigenomic landscape and relieve the expression of genes related to cell division and proliferation. For example, the histone deacetylase inhibitor microbial SCFA butyrate can reinstate the tumour suppression genes' activity that is silent in hormone-driven malignancies. Crosstalk Gut microbiota-epigenetics holds positive potential crosstalk to design personalized medicine to target hormone-related malignancies by manipulating the microbiome constituents and metabolic capabilities to correct the perturbed hormonal and epigenomic balance (Zhao et al., 2021).

9. CHALLENGES AND FUTURE PERSPECTIVES

The emerging field of study between microbiota of the gut and Cancer holds enormous potential, and enormous challenge, to translating scientific discovery into the clinical practice of medicine. Following the realization that the microbiome plays a role in tumour initiation, response to therapy, and prognosis of patients, gaps in knowledge remain. These gaps must be filled to realize the potential of microbiome-modifying therapy and personalized medicine and translate these to medical practice. It is seen that the future will be guided by multidisciplinary platforms on next-generation technologies that will solve the challenges of today.

9.1 Research Gaps and Personalized Therapeutics

Although the gut microbiota-cancer association is becoming deciphered, important knowledge gaps still exist, especially when designing individualized therapies. The most significant task is to untangle the multifaceted, two-way relationships between the gut microbiome, host genetics, lifestyle, and environmental factors, which overall impact the development and response to treatment of cancers (Zalila-Kolsi et al., 2025). Composition and functional properties of gut microbiota vary inter-individually, meaning it is hard to identify universal microbiome-based interventions, and approaches need to be highly personalized. For example, although gut microbiota can modify the reactions to cancer treatments, notably immunotherapies, one of the primary objectives is determining which microbial targets are relevant to therapeutically manipulating them (Huang et al., 2023).

The existing approaches to modification based on microbiota, faecal microbiota transplantation (FMT), probiotics, and prebiotics are usually limited because of the natural diversity and dynamics of the microbiota. Hence, the following research step should be able to distinguish between profitable and unfavourable microbial targets capable of enhancing the effect of immunotherapy and expanding the use of microbiota precision medicine (Huang et al., 2023). An important feature is the combination of so-called omics technologies, including metagenomics and metabolomics, to better understand these complex interactions and to discover robust biomarkers to propose early detection and personalized therapeutic approaches. This will aid in filling the translational gap between the state-of-the-art research discoveries and their implementation into precision medicine in colorectal Cancer (CRC) (Zalila-Kolsi et al., 2025).

9.2 Clinical Integration and Technological Advances

The clinical application of the study of gut microbiota into the widespread practice of treating Cancer has some impediments, yet technological advances are bypassing these impediments. One of them is the standardization of the methodologies of microbiota study, including sample collection, processing, and analysis, to enable the comparability and reliability of studies between different research settings (Wei et al., 2021). Even though the scientific community is becoming increasingly interested in microbiota, its successful application in medical practice is just beginning. To illustrate, optimization of the microbiome so that it leads to clinical benefits and minimal adverse events is demanding. Individualized and integrated approaches must be used in future trials, and individual clinical and pathological histories must be considered to optimize the impact of microbiota-targeted treatments and minimize the administration of side effects (Wei et al., 2024).

New technologies, however, are rendering this integration very easy. With the introduction of metagenomics and Next-Generation Sequencing (NGS), the ecology of the gut microbiome has become a subject of study, and various aspects of the correlation between gut microbiota and CRC have been revealed that were not acknowledged before. Such high-throughput technologies provide the opportunity to explore the microbial community in detail, which can enhance diagnostic (e.g., detection of microbial DNA and RNA in peripheral blood), as well as prognosis (Wei et al., 2021). Additionally, predictive analytics performed by artificial intelligence (AI) is a splendid step towards treating each individual differently based on the data gained via the microbiome analysis (Hemmati et al., 2024).

Additionally, nanotechnology is rising as a potential instrument in regulating gut microbiota, with new options and mechanisms for specific interventions. The convergence of AI, genomics, and bioinformatics is further improving the future of personalized medicine, which enables the design of customized treatments depending on a person's genetic, environmental, and lifestyle factors, and the gut microbiome is emerging as a significant constituent. These technological breakthroughs will be essential in overcoming the complexities of the gut microbiome and towards a future where microbiota-based therapies are regularly being incorporated into the management of Cancer (Wei et al., 2024).

10. CONCLUSION

The gut microbiota and cancer interrelation are undoubtedly complex and exhibit a multifaceted effect on the initiation, development, and progression of a tumour, as well as the impact on the effectiveness of the therapy, which involves the movement of the gut microbiota. As a microbiome, a highly diverse community of microorganisms, the gut microbiota system sustains human metabolic and immune processes. However, impairment of this underpinning could significantly alter the process of cancer development. The above review has implied the twofold nature of the gut microbiome, which is simultaneously a great driver of tumour development and its possible defence mechanism (Sun et al., 2023).

On the one hand, the imbalance of microbial communities known as gut dysbiosis enables establishing an environment conducive to cancer development. The pathogenic bacteria can actively enhance the occurrence of carcinogenesis (by DNA damages and other alterations of the host cellular metabolism, and generation of permanent inflammation and oxidative stress. These molecular machineries of microbials, such as the activation of inflammasomes, favour genomic instability, immune evasion and facilitation of a pro-tumorigenic microenvironment that permits tumour growth. Such an effect is not only detected in the local gastrointestinal cancers but also extends to extraintestinal cancers as well as the systemic pathological conditions, such as cancer cachexia, signifying the wide-reaching place of microbiota-host relations (Zhou et al., 2021; Sun et al., 2023).

Conversely, the microbial portion of a gut harbouring a profile has even protective mechanisms that can stop the growth of tumours and enhance the effectiveness of treatment. Among them are effective microorganisms and their products, mostly short-chain fatty acids (SCFAs), including butyrate, with anti-inflammatory, anti-proliferative, and immunomodulatory activity, preserving the health of the recipient and directly inhibiting carcinogenesis. The probiotic intervention with *Lactobacillus rhamnosus GG* is a vivid example of the microbial modulation contribution in improving antitumor immunity, decreasing complications and adverse effects related to treatments, and improving the quality of life of patients (Zhou et al., 2021). The host dysbiosis is characterized by the microbiota/epigenetics destabilization, inducing a high level of regulation of gut microorganisms in Cancer (Sun et al., 2023).

Furthermore, the native microbial communities inhabiting the gut are influential in regulating the efficacy of the standard cancer treatment, such as chemotherapy, immunotherapy and radiotherapy, in addition to the frequency and extent of the side effects induced by these drugs and methods. Microbiome-directed interventions are emerging as valuable modalities to simplify therapeutic action, overcome drug resistance, and reduce adverse effects, either by treating the microbiome under probiotics, faecal microbiome transplantation (FMT), or minimal but considerate use of antibiotics. With such interventions, the changing nature of the microbiome is brought out as a possible treatment target that can be readily accessible in oncology (Zhou et al., 2021).

Despite the magnificent progress, the issue with transferring these sophisticated scientific discoveries into a standard clinical practice remains relevant. The key research gaps relate to thoroughly explaining the mechanisms of microbiota-host interactions, obtaining precise microbial biomarkers to diagnose and predict the disease before it is too late and designing personal prophylaxis and therapy depending on the patient's microbiome (Zhou et al., 2021). In the future, it is essential to pay attention to approaches to standardization, extensive clinical studies, and integration of new technological techniques of precision oncology such as next-generation sequencing, metagenomics, and artificial intelligence. The last hope is that the full potential of the gut microbiota may be used to prevent Cancer, enhance the efficacy, reduce the toxicity of treatments, and double the outcomes of the patients in the era of individualized healthcare. This continuous pursuit will change how Cancer is treated, as microbial consultation will involve the total diagnosis and treatment packages (Hemmati et al., 2024).

REFERENCES

Ağagündüz, D., Cocozza, E., Cemali, Ö., Bayazıt, A. D., Nanì, M. F., Cerqua, I., Morgillo, F., Saygılı, S. K., Berni Canani, R., Amero, P., & Capasso, R. (2023). Understanding the role of the gut microbiome in gastrointestinal cancer: A review. *Frontiers in Pharmacology, 14*, 1130562. DOI: 10.3389/fphar.2023.1130562 PMID: 36762108

Aghamajidi, A., & Maleki Vareki, S. (2022). The effect of the gut microbiota on systemic and anti-tumor immunity and response to systemic therapy against cancer. *Cancers (Basel), 14*(15), 3563. DOI: 10.3390/cancers14153563 PMID: 35892821

Alberti, G., Mazzola, M., Gagliardo, C., Pitruzzella, A., Fucarini, A., Giammanco, M., ... & Carini, F. (2021). Extracellular vesicles derived from gut microbiota in inflammatory bowel disease and colorectal cancer. *Biomedical Papers of the Medical Faculty of Palacky University in Olomouc, 165*(3).

Arnone, A. A., Ansley, K., Heeke, A. L., Howard-McNatt, M., & Cook, K. L. (2025). Gut microbiota interact with breast cancer therapeutics to modulate efficacy. *EMBO Molecular Medicine, 17*(2), 219–234. DOI: 10.1038/s44321-024-00185-0 PMID: 39820166

Chen, Z., Guan, D., Wang, Z., Li, X., Dong, S., Huang, J., & Zhou, W. (2023). Microbiota in cancer: Molecular mechanisms and therapeutic interventions. *MedComm, 4*(6), e417. DOI: 10.1002/mco2.417 PMID: 37937304

Chigurupati, M. (2025). Unraveling the Causal Effects of Risk Factors on Diabetes Mellitus Insights from Mendelian Randomization Studies. *North American Journal of Engineering Research, 6*(1).

Chrysostomou, D., Roberts, L. A., Marchesi, J. R., & Kinross, J. M. (2023). Gut microbiota modulation of efficacy and toxicity of cancer chemotherapy and immunotherapy. *Gastroenterology, 164*(2), 198–213. DOI: 10.1053/j.gastro.2022.10.018 PMID: 36309208

Deng, Z., Lu, L., Li, B., Shi, X., Jin, H., & Hu, W. (2023). The roles of inflammasomes in cancer. *Frontiers in Immunology, 14*, 1195572. DOI: 10.3389/fimmu.2023.1195572 PMID: 37497237

Eissa, M. (2024). The Gut Microbiome: A Potential Therapeutic Path in Complementary Medicine. *Journal of Research in Complementary Medicine, 1*(2), 55–55. DOI: 10.5455/JRCM.20240509063048

Escriva, P. P., Bernardino, C. C. T., & Letellier, E. (2025). De-coding the complex role of microbial metabolites in cancer. *Cell Reports*, *44*(3). PMID: 40023841

Farhat, E. K., Sher, E. K., Džidić-Krivić, A., Banjari, I., & Sher, F. (2023). Functional biotransformation of phytoestrogens by gut microbiota with impact on cancer treatment. *The Journal of Nutritional Biochemistry*, *118*, 109368. DOI: 10.1016/j.jnutbio.2023.109368 PMID: 37100304

Fu, J., & Wu, H. (2023). Structural mechanisms of NLRP3 inflammasome assembly and activation. *Annual Review of Immunology*, *41*(1), 301–316. DOI: 10.1146/annurev-immunol-081022-021207 PMID: 36750315

He, R., Qi, P., Shu, L., Ding, Y., Zeng, P., Wen, G., Xiong, Y., & Deng, H. (2025). Dysbiosis and extraintestinal cancers. *Journal of Experimental & Clinical Cancer Research : CR*, *44*(1), 44. DOI: 10.1186/s13046-025-03313-x PMID: 39915884

He, Y., Huang, J., Li, Q., Xia, W., Zhang, C., Liu, Z., Xiao, J., Yi, Z., Deng, H., Xiao, Z., Hu, J., Li, H., Zu, X., Quan, C., & Chen, J. (2022). Gut microbiota and tumor immune escape: A new perspective for improving tumor immunotherapy. *Cancers (Basel)*, *14*(21), 5317. DOI: 10.3390/cancers14215317 PMID: 36358736

Hemmati, M. A., Monemi, M., Asli, S., Mohammadi, S., Foroozanmehr, B., Haghmorad, D., Oksenych, V., & Eslami, M. (2024). Using new technologies to analyze gut microbiota and predict cancer risk. *Cells*, *13*(23), 1987. DOI: 10.3390/cells13231987 PMID: 39682735

Hou, M., Yu, Q. Q., Yang, L., Zhao, H., Jiang, P., Qin, L., & Zhang, Q. (2024). The role of short-chain fatty acid metabolism in the pathogenesis, diagnosis and treatment of cancer. *Frontiers in Oncology*, *14*, 1451045. DOI: 10.3389/fonc.2024.1451045 PMID: 39435279

Huang, G., Khan, R., Zheng, Y., Lee, P. C., Li, Q., & Khan, I. (2023). Exploring the role of gut microbiota in advancing personalized medicine. *Frontiers in Microbiology*, *14*, 1274925. DOI: 10.3389/fmicb.2023.1274925 PMID: 38098666

Ivleva, E. A., & Grivennikov, S. I. (2022). Microbiota-driven mechanisms at different stages of cancer development. *Neoplasia : an International Journal for Oncology Research*, *32*, 100829. DOI: 10.1016/j.neo.2022.100829 PMID: 35933824

Jang, W., Kim, S., Son, Y., Kim, S., Lee, S., Kim, H. J., Jo, H., Park, J., Lee, K., Lee, H., Rahmati, M., Woo, S., Hwang, J., Kang, J., Smith, L., & Yon, D. K. (2025). Global, regional, and national burden of pharyngeal cancer and projections to 2050 in 185 countries: A population-based systematic analysis of GLOBOCAN 2022. *Journal of Korean Medical Science*, *40*(30), e177. DOI: 10.3346/jkms.2025.40.e177 PMID: 40762594

Kalyanaraman, B., Cheng, G., & Hardy, M. (2024). The role of short-chain fatty acids in cancer prevention and cancer treatment. *Archives of Biochemistry and Biophysics*, *761*, 110172. DOI: 10.1016/j.abb.2024.110172 PMID: 39369836

Karam, F., El Deghel, Y., Iratni, R., Dakroub, A. H., & Eid, A. H. (2025). The gut microbiome and colorectal cancer: An integrative review of the underlying mechanisms. *Cell Biochemistry and Biophysics*, *83*(3), 1–14. DOI: 10.1007/s12013-025-01683-9 PMID: 39946032

Kim, J., & Lee, H. K. (2022). Potential role of the gut microbiome in colorectal cancer progression. *Frontiers in Immunology*, *12*, 807648. DOI: 10.3389/fimmu.2021.807648 PMID: 35069592

Kiousi, D. E., Kouroutzidou, A. Z., Neanidis, K., Karavanis, E., Matthaios, D., Pappa, A., & Galanis, A. (2023). The role of the gut microbiome in cancer immunotherapy: Current knowledge and future directions. *Cancers (Basel)*, *15*(7), 2101. DOI: 10.3390/cancers15072101 PMID: 37046762

Li, Z., Ke, X., Zuo, D., Wang, Z., Fang, F., & Li, B. (2022). New insights into the relationship between gut microbiota and radiotherapy for cancer. *Nutrients*, *15*(1), 48. DOI: 10.3390/nu15010048 PMID: 36615706

Li, Z., Xiong, W., Liang, Z., Wang, J., Zeng, Z., Kołat, D., Li, X., Zhou, D., Xu, X., & Zhao, L. (2024). Critical role of the gut microbiota in immune responses and cancer immunotherapy. *Journal of Hematology & Oncology*, *17*(1), 33. DOI: 10.1186/s13045-024-01541-w PMID: 38745196

Luu, M., Riester, Z., Baldrich, A., Reichardt, N., Yuille, S., Busetti, A., Klein, M., Wempe, A., Leister, H., Raifer, H., Picard, F., Muhammad, K., Ohl, K., Romero, R., Fischer, F., Bauer, C. A., Huber, M., Gress, T. M., Lauth, M., & Visekruna, A. (2021). Microbial short-chain fatty acids modulate CD8+ T cell responses and improve adoptive immunotherapy for cancer. *Nature Communications*, *12*(1), 4077. DOI: 10.1038/s41467-021-24331-1 PMID: 34210970

Manshouri, S., Seif, F., Kamali, M., Bahar, M. A., Mashayekh, A., & Molatefi, R. (2024). The interaction of inflammasomes and gut microbiota: Novel therapeutic insights. *Cell Communication and Signaling : CCS*, *22*(1), 209. DOI: 10.1186/s12964-024-01504-1 PMID: 38566180

Mostafavi Abdolmaleky, H., & Zhou, J. R. (2024). Gut microbiota dysbiosis, oxidative stress, inflammation, and epigenetic alterations in metabolic diseases. *Antioxidants*, *13*(8), 985. DOI: 10.3390/antiox13080985 PMID: 39199231

Olofsson, L. E., & Bäckhed, F. (2022). The metabolic role and therapeutic potential of the microbiome. *Endocrine Reviews*, *43*(5), 907–926. DOI: 10.1210/endrev/bnac004 PMID: 35094076

Otto-Dobos, L. D., Strehle, L. D., Loman, B. R., Seng, M. M., Sardesai, S. D., Williams, N. O., Gatti-Mays, M. E., Stover, D. G., Sudheendra, P. K., Wesolowski, R., Andridge, R. R., Bailey, M. T., & Pyter, L. M. (2024). Baseline gut microbiome alpha diversity predicts chemotherapy-induced gastrointestinal symptoms in patients with breast cancer. *NPJ Breast Cancer*, *10*(1), 99. DOI: 10.1038/s41523-024-00707-6 PMID: 39548124

Owens, J. A., Saeedi, B. J., Naudin, C. R., Hunter-Chang, S., Barbian, M. E., Eboka, R. U., Askew, L., Darby, T. M., Robinson, B. S., & Jones, R. M. (2021). Lactobacillus rhamnosus GG orchestrates an antitumor immune response. *Cellular and Molecular Gastroenterology and Hepatology*, *12*(4), 1311–1327. DOI: 10.1016/j.jcmgh.2021.06.001 PMID: 34111601

Qiu, X., Zou, Z., Lin, T., Guo, C., & Lin, D. (2025). Engineered Lactobacillus rhamnosus Producing 3-Hydroxybutyrate: A Dual-Action Therapeutic Strategy for Colon Cancer Cachexia. *Biotechnology and Bioengineering*, *122*(6), 1574–1589. DOI: 10.1002/bit.28972 PMID: 40055977

Rodriguez-Arrastia, M., Martinez-Ortigosa, A., Rueda-Ruzafa, L., Folch Ayora, A., & Ropero-Padilla, C. (2021). Probiotic supplements on oncology patients' treatment-related side effects: A systematic review of randomized controlled trials. *International Journal of Environmental Research and Public Health*, *18*(8), 4265. DOI: 10.3390/ijerph18084265 PMID: 33920572

Shadab, A., Mahjoor, M., Abbasi-Kolli, M., Afkhami, H., Moeinian, P., & Safdarian, A. R. (2023). Divergent functions of NLRP3 inflammasomes in cancer: A review. *Cell Communication and Signaling : CCS*, *21*(1), 232. DOI: 10.1186/s12964-023-01235-9 PMID: 37715239

Soldado-Gordillo, A., & Álvarez-Mercado, A. I. (2024). Epigenetics, Microbiota, and Breast Cancer: A Systematic Review. *Life (Chicago, Ill.)*, *14*(6), 705. DOI: 10.3390/life14060705 PMID: 38929688

Sun, J., Chen, F., & Wu, G. (2023). Potential effects of gut microbiota on host cancers: Focus on immunity, DNA damage, cellular pathways, and anticancer therapy. *The ISME Journal*, *17*(10), 1535–1551. DOI: 10.1038/s41396-023-01483-0 PMID: 37553473

Wei, L. Q., Cheong, I. H., Yang, G. H., Li, X. G., Kozlakidis, Z., Ding, L., Liu, N. N., & Wang, H. (2021). The application of high-throughput technologies for the study of microbiome and cancer. *Frontiers in Genetics*, *12*, 699793. DOI: 10.3389/fgene.2021.699793 PMID: 34394190

Wei, Y., Shen, F., Song, H., Zhao, R., Feng, W., Pan, Y., Li, X., Yu, H., Familiari, G., Relucenti, M., Aschner, M., Shi, H., Chen, R., Nie, G., & Chen, H. (2024). The challenge and opportunity of gut microbiota-targeted nanomedicine for colorectal cancer therapy. *iMeta*, *3*(4), e213. DOI: 10.1002/imt2.213 PMID: 39135695

Wong, C. C., & Yu, J. (2023). Gut microbiota in colorectal cancer development and therapy. *Nature Reviews. Clinical Oncology*, *20*(7), 429–452. DOI: 10.1038/s41571-023-00766-x PMID: 37169888

Yang, D., Wang, Z., Chen, Y., Guo, Q., & Dong, Y. (2023). Interactions between gut microbes and NLRP3 inflammasome in the gut-brain axis. *Computational and Structural Biotechnology Journal*, *21*, 2215–2227. DOI: 10.1016/j.csbj.2023.03.017 PMID: 37035548

Zalila-Kolsi, I., Dhieb, D., Osman, H. A., & Mekideche, H. (2025). The Gut microbiota and colorectal cancer: Understanding the link and exploring therapeutic interventions. *Biology (Basel)*, *14*(3), 251. DOI: 10.3390/biology14030251 PMID: 40136508

Zechner, E. L., & Kienesberger, S. (2024). Microbiota-derived small molecule genotoxins: Host interactions and ecological impact in the gut ecosystem. *Gut Microbes*, *16*(1), 2430423. DOI: 10.1080/19490976.2024.2430423 PMID: 39558480

Zepeda-Rivera, M., Minot, S. S., Bouzek, H., Wu, H., Blanco-Míguez, A., Manghi, P., Jones, D. S., LaCourse, K. D., Wu, Y., McMahon, E. F., Park, S.-N., Lim, Y. K., Kempchinsky, A. G., Willis, A. D., Cotton, S. L., Yost, S. C., Sicinska, E., Kook, J.-K., Dewhirst, F. E., & Johnston, C. D. (2024). A distinct Fusobacterium nucleatum clade dominates the colorectal cancer niche. *Nature*, *628*(8007), 424–432. DOI: 10.1038/s41586-024-07182-w PMID: 38509359

Zhao, Y., Wang, C., & Goel, A. (2021). Role of gut microbiota in epigenetic regulation of colorectal Cancer. *Biochimica et Biophysica Acta (BBA)-. Revisiones en Cáncer, 1875*(1), 188490. PMID: 33321173

Zhou, H., Yuan, Y., Wang, H., Xiang, W., Li, S., Zheng, H., Wen, Y., Ming, Y., Chen, L., & Zhou, J. (2021). Gut microbiota: A potential target for cancer interventions. *Cancer Management and Research, 13*, 8281–8296. DOI: 10.2147/CMAR.S328249 PMID: 34764691

Chapter 10
Function of Gut Microbiota in Longevity as a Futuristic Approach of Personalised Nutrition

Sumira Malik
https://orcid.org/0000-0001-5077-1493
Amity University, Ranchi, India

Rupjyoti Bharali
Biswanath College, India

Humayun Samir Ahmed Barbhuyan
https://orcid.org/0000-0002-4663-4768
St. John College, India

Jutishna Bora
Amity University, Ranchi, India

Smita Lata
Amity University, Ranchi, India

Ayush Madan
https://orcid.org/0000-0001-5089-1794
People's University, India

ABSTRACT

Microorganisms residing in the host gut collectively known as gut microbiota, plays a crucial role in the health of the host. The gut microbiota influences the immune system, cognitive abilty and other functions in an individual contributing towards the well-being of the individual. These gut colonizers eventually change throughout the life of an individual that are specific in nature. However, there is a set of conserved gut microbiota which is present in every individual. Longevity has been related to healthy aging referring to disease-free health in individuals which is further related to composition of gut microbiota. Life-style and dietary habits have been linked directly to impact the composition of these gut colonizers. An inclusive understanding of impact of gut microbiota interactions in longevity and on human body, are discussed in this chapter.

DOI: 10.4018/979-8-3373-4382-2.ch010

INTRODUCTION

The relationship between gut, physical and mental health has been long recognized in Ayurvedic ancient practice (Rajpurohit et al., 2024). The gastrointestinal tract of human beings is composed of diverse group of microorganisms which is collectively known as gut microbiota plays an important role in maintaining human health. Most of these microorganism population is mainly dominated by bacteria; however, it also includes fungi, viruses, and protozoa (Bull & Plummer, 2014). This complex companionship begins since birth by colonizing the gut of infant from microbes of different sources like environment, food and maternal. This is crucial for development of immune system (Hooper et al., 2010), neuro behavioural traits Hakansson & Molin, 2011; Levy et al., 2017) and metabolism in humans (Rothschild et al., 2018). The gut microbiota in an adult human body performs significant roles like synthesis of vitamins, food degradation, managing the intestinal barrier integrity (Lakshminarayanan et al., 2014; Sender et al., 2016). Disruption of this intestinal barrier causes dysbiosis leading to digestion related disorders, inflammation, and manifestation of various other metabolic diseases (Thevaranjan et al., 2017).

In this chapter we aim at summarizing the recent knowledge of the impact of intestinal microbiota composition on human body and longevity and, emphasizing on dietary habits and aging which determines the relationship between the host and the microbiota.

GUT MICROBIOTA

The term "microbiota" includes the living microorganisms which are found in definite environments such as oral, gut, skin etc. to carry out vital functions through mutual interactions that determines host physiology (Li *et al.,* 2014; Kim & Benayoun 2021). Thus, the term "gut microbiota (GM) refers to the distinct, diverse, and complex community of microorganisms that resides in the gastrointestinal (GI) tract of humans and are responsible for maintaining the overall health in humans. The microbiota in gut is dominated mainly by bacteria (members of Bacteroidetes, Firmicutes, Proteobacteria and Actinobacteria, Fusobacteria phyla precisely and, few from Verrucomicrobia) (Turnbaugh et al.,2006; Arumugam et al., 2011; Sirisinha 2016); however, it also includes fungi and virus.

Genera such as *Bacteroides* and *Prevotella* dominates the human gut belonging to phylum Bacteroidetes. In Firmicutes phylum, genera *Clostridium* dominates and other genera colonising the gut are *Bacillus*, *Enterococcus*, *Lactobacillus*, and *Ruminicoccus*. The genera included from other bacterial phyla are *Akkermansia muciniphila*, *Bifidobacterium* spp. and *Escherichia coli* belonging to phyla Verrucomicrobia, Actinobacteria and Proteobacteria respectively (Walker et al., 2011). In human gut, the most dominant genera of bacteria belong to the genera viz., *Bacteroides, Bifidobacterium, Clostridium, Eubacterium, Faecalibacterium, Peptidococcus, Peptidostreptococcus* and *Ruminococcus* (Cho & Blaser 2012; Yatsunenko et al., 2012; Cresci & Bawden, 2015). The composition of gut microbiota to maintain good health conditions relies on factors such as environment, diet, age and lifestyle (Simões et al., 2022).

GUT MICROBIOTA FUNCTIONS

The gut microbiota regulates many vital functions in a healthy host like xenobiotic and drug metabolism, nutrient metabolism, immunomodulation, maintains the integrity of the gut barrier and function and structure of gastrointestinal tract, and provides antimicrobial protection through their mutual interactions with the host gut mucosa (Jandhyala et al., 2015; Ribaldone et al., 2022). The gut bacteria can also synthesize essential vitamins, notably vitamin K and B group vitamins such as biotin, folate, and thiamine. In fact, for several B group vitamins (cobalamin, folate, niacin, pyridoxine), gut bacteria are estimated to contribute more than 25% of the daily recommended intake (Hossain et al., 2022).

IMPACT OF GUT MICROBIOTA ON HUMAN HEALTH

1) Gut microbiota in developing immune system

The immune responses of human immune system constantly interact with the microbiota to maintain a balanced environment in the human body. The innate immune response acts as a barrier to harmful bacteria and regulates the adaptive immune response which balances the immunity by maintaining the composition of healthy microbiota. However, the adaptive response varies depending on the microbiota species. Numerous immune cells reside in the gastrointestinal tract that interact continuously with the gut microbiota (Owaga et al.,2015).

The development of immune system is dependent on the development of healthy microbiota and any kind of disruption in the development of microbiota at the developmental phase of immune system will give rise to various immunological and autoimmune disorders in human body (Sekirov et al., 2010). Through the lymphoid tissues present in gut, the microbiota of gut takes part in the immune system maturation (Macpherson & Uhr 2004). It has also been shown in germ free animal models that presence of commensal microbiota is very essential for functional immune system and the absence of these microbiota leads to defects in lymphoid tissues of intestine thereby causing faults in immune response (Bauer et al., 1963).

Colonization of mucosal surfaces of host by microbiota starts immediately after birth in infants which is mainly contributed by maternal microbiota, greatly influences the development of immune system in the host body (Gensollen et al., 2016; Gomez et al., 2016). This early onset of interaction between host microbiota and immune system is very crucial exerting long term effects on host's health leading to development of immune-mediated diseases in case of subtle dysbiosis conditions at the neonatal phase (Zheng et al., 2020) *(Fig 2)*.

The intestinal immune system can distinguish the large changing diversity of commensal healthy microbiota and pathogenic microbiota thereby regulating immune tolerance to the former and immune responses towards the later (Mowat, 2018). Host microbiota and innate immune system are in constant communication wherein signals are sent by microbes and received by Toll-like receptors to generate immune responses against any infection (Chu & Mazmanian 2013). Similarly, the mutual relationship between host microbiota and adaptive immunity has been studied. The gut microbiota provides an adaptive mechanism of protection by playing a crucial role in inducing B-cell and T-cell responses against pathogens. Interaction between T-cells and gut microbiota in stable circumstances impacts the overall response of immune system (Heidari et al., 2024).

During stable conditions, gut microbiota and intestinal T cells interact harmoniously to influence the overall immune system response (Heidari et al., 2024). For instance, the composition of diverse microbiota in gut is influenced and sustained by the secretory immunoglobuin A produced by T-cell dependant pathway that aids in the development of anti-inflammatory Foxp3+ regulatory T cells (Kawamoto et al., 2014). Moreover, the secretory IgA antibodies prevent inflammation and disturbance of intestinal homeostasis by coating colitogenic bacteria (Palm et al., 2014).

The irregularities in the interaction between microbiota and immune system influenced by lifestyle, use of antibiotics, diet, and other environmental factors causes immune-mediated diseases *(Fig 1)*. `

Figure 1. Gut-brain axis bidirectional interactions and development of immune system and functions

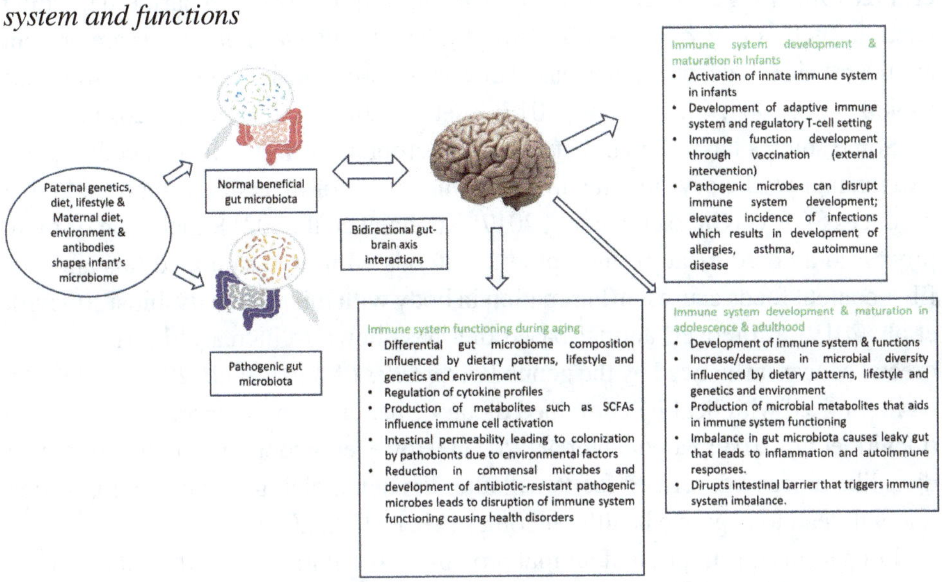

2) Interaction of gut microbiota with food and metabolism

Diet has a profound effect on composition of gut microbiota which regulates host metabolism and thereby responsible for the healthy or diseased state in individuals. Experimental studies have shown that an imbalance in the interaction between diet, gut microbiota and immune system affects the human body by causing chronic inflammatory diseases (Sirisinha, 2016). The interaction of diet and gut microbiota and its impact on health is multifaceted including lifestyle, environment and genetics (Soldán et al., 2024).

However, the recent studies have shown that diets like plant-based and mediterranean promotes diversity of healthy gut microbiota and their useful metabolites like short-chain fatty acids (SCFAs) thus improving the health by preventing diseases like cancer, cardiovascular disease, and other non-communicable diseases. Moreover, they lower the concentrations of trimethylamine-N-oxide (TMAO) which is responsible for negative health conditions. While western diet triggers the development of pathogenic bacteria that enhances the production of TMAO and lowers the production of SCFAs leading to development of chronic diseases causing mortality (reviewed in Soldán et al., 2024).

Studies have shown that healthy plant-based dietary patterns including wholesome foods like nuts, fruits and grains, minimises the risks of cancer, diabetes, kidney issues and cardiovascular diseases leading to death in individuals (Kim et al.,2019a; Kim et al.,2019b; Wang et al., 2022a; Wang et al., 2022b). The polysaccharide-degrading bacteria such as *Faecalibacterium prausnitzii* and *Eubacterium eligens* are present abundantly in wholesome plant-based diets possesses anti-inflammatory properties (Sokol et al., 2008; Chung et al., 2017; Li et al., 2021; Asnicar et al., 2021).

Some studies have shown that the gut microbiota is highly influenced in positive manner by dietary fiber leading to composition of diversified microbiota that produces SCFAs (Chassaing et al., 2017; Koponen et al., 2021). Inclusion of more processed and red meat, refined products, foods with high saturated fats and low fiber content foods causes inflammation in body with microbiota dysbiosis (Ocvirk et al., 2019). Moreover, animal-based diet has shown to increase the risk of colorectal cancer influenced by the genus *Bacteroides* (Alhinai et al., 2019) which can be minimised with healthy combined dietary fiber choices as reported in literature (Ocvirk et al., 2019; Koponen et al., 2021). However, adoption of unhealthy plant diets like processed, refined foods will alter the beneficial microbiota composition that will lead to negative health outcomes (Shen et al., 2024).

Long term consumption of animal proteins particularly from red meat and dairy produces N-nitroso compounds (endogenous) that are genotoxic in nature in gut of humans (Kuhnle et al., 2007). Moreover, proteins derived from animal-based diets has been reported to causes damage in genetic level by elevating the amount p-cresol in faeces mainly in colon by hindering progression in cell cycle (Moore et al., 1997; Andriamihaja et al., 2015). High intake of protein diets from animal sources without optimal amount of fiber upsurges the quantity of undigested proteins that is deposited in the colon which triggers the metabolic activity of microbes resulting in higher secretion of p-cresol thereby increasing the risk of cancer (Andriamihaja et al., 2015).

Gut microbiota responds differently to the variety of diets viz., plant-based, western-based or mediterranean-based and secretes metabolites accordingly through various pathways *(Fig3)* by interacting with the microenvironment of intestines thus regulating human health and longevity (Greer et al., 2011; Madsen et al., 2016). Exploring the capabilities of these metabolites secreted by gut microbes will help in deepening the knowledge of maintaining good health conditions and preventing life threating diseases in humans (Vernocchi et al., 2020).

Figure 2. Causes of variability in gut microbiota composition

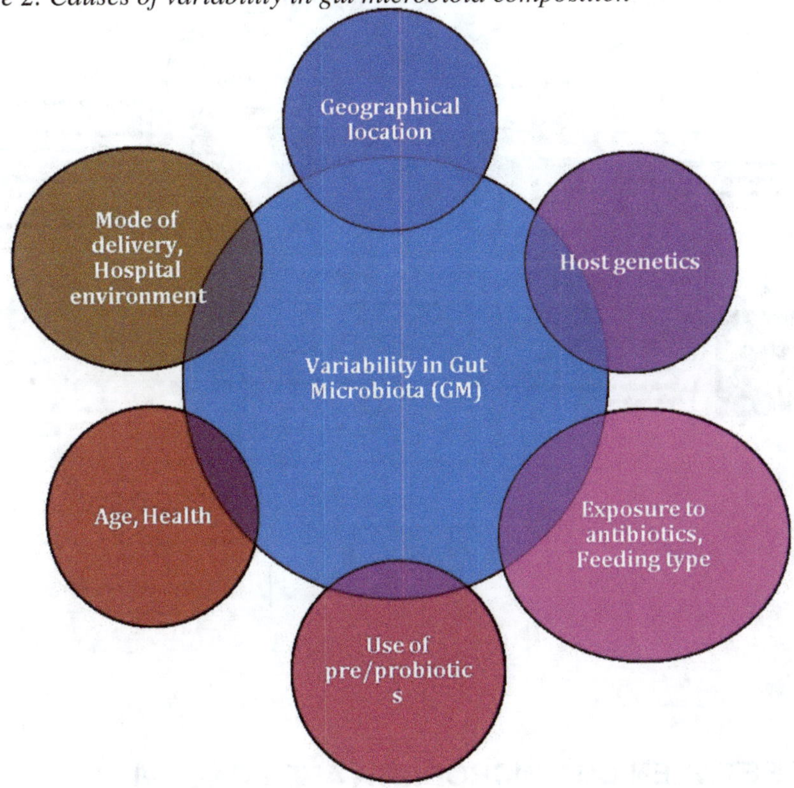

Figure 3. Effects of dietary patterns on healthy aging and longevity

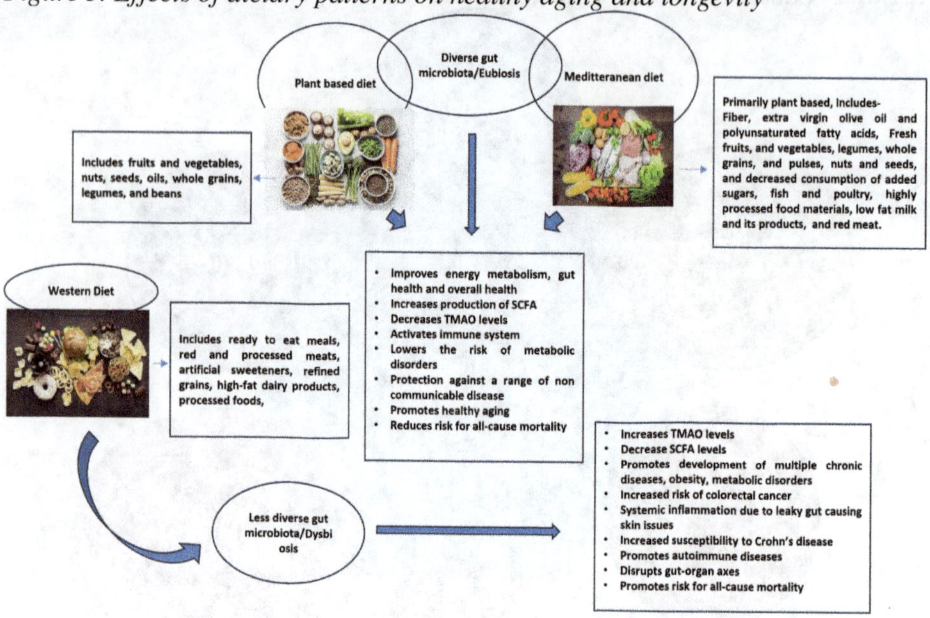

LINK BETWEEN GUT MICROBIOTA AND LONGEVITY

Several changes that are linked to age have been associated with gut microbiota which influences longevity (Clemente et al., 2012; Bana & Cabreiro 2019). Alteration in gut microbiome with aging leads to dysregulation in immune system responses as they are interconnected disrupting the balance between anti-inflammation and pro-inflammation process (Franceschi et al., 2000; Honda & Littman, 2012). Such changes during aging eventually leads towards development of various diseases and mortality (Ferrucci and Fabbri 2018). Through various gut-organ axes, gut microbiota regulates several functions in body providing perspectives to unlock different facets of aging and longevity *(Fig 4)*.

Earlier studies reported that there are certain core phyla of gut microbiome that maintains a state of equilibrium between them which is also influenced by other environmental factors are responsible for long healthy life (Yu et al., 2015; Jeffery et al., 2016; Odamaki et al., 2016; Odamaki et al., 2018; Tuikhar et al., 2019). The composition of micriobiota varies among different age groups which can be explained by the complex interactions between the environmental factors especially diet (Odamaki et al., 2016).

Percentage of taxa viz., *Akkermansia, Bifidobacterium, Butyricimonas, Christensenellaceae, Odoribacter, Parabacteroides*, and *Verrucomicrobia*, have been reported to be higher in oldest-old people and these taxa have been linked with anti-inflammatory activities promoting gut homeostasis, which is indicative of healthy aging and longevity (Yu et al., 2015; Biagi et al., 2016; Kim et al.2019; Tuikhar et al.,2019; Wu et al., 2019) *(Table 1)*. The host genetics alongwith environmental factors shapes the gut microbiome composition and function in healthy aging as evident from genome-based studies (Campbell et al., 2012; Dabrowska & Witkiewicz, 2016).

Based on some studies it has been found that in long-lived group of people some age dependent behaviours in terms of loss of appetite and digestion were not observed, moreover, they showed differences in their gut microbiota composition and functions such as increase in helath-beneficial taxa and thus increased levels of SCFA, vit B2 & K2 synthesis and good cellular metabolism indicating healthy aging and promoting longevity in those individuals (Kim et al., 2019; Wu et al., 2019). The flexible nature of gut microbiota which means it can be modified through dietary changes, active lifestyle, therapeutic interventions targeting microbiome such as probiotics and prebiotics, can promote longevity (Saad et al., 2013; Badal et al., 2020).

The taxa associated with healthy aging in long-lived group of people across studies shows inconsistency, and members of some taxa might be found in abundance in one cohort, while in others it shows less, and some members of the same taxa might dysregulate gut microbiome in any age group (Nagao-Kitamoto, 2017; Verdi et al., 2018; Tun et al., 2018; Wu et al., 2019).

Members of taxa that contributes towards maintenance of good health can be replaced with pathobionts due to several factors such as diet, lifestyle, sleep patterns and use of antibiotics over a period of time can decrease the diversity of commensals in gut and increase in pathobionts that are resistant to antibiotics (Ubeda et al., 2010; Dethlefsen and Relman, 2011; Jump et al., 2018; Haran et al., 2021; Larson et al., 2022).

The overall functional potential of gut microbiome is determined by metabolome and gut microbiota's metabolic pathways that changes during entire lifespan as evident in the abundance of genes that encode these pathways (Rampelli et al., 2013; Amedei & Morbidelli, 2019). Microbial metabolites from these pathways play a key role in shaping health and age-related variations through local or systemic mode of action (Nicholson et al., 2012), which is again dependent largely on dietary patterns, lifestyle patterns, genetics, and geography (Bressa et al., 2017; Allen et al., 2018; Henke et al., 2019).

Another fascinating functional trait of gut microbiome is their ability to alleviate any environmental toxins as evident in a study where supercentenarians and long-lived adults showed elevated ability of xenobiotic chemical degradation (Rampelli et al., 2020). In another study, it was observed that in the stools of young adults, the amount of cyclohexanecarboxylic acid, a toxin was higher than the long-lived adults which showed comparatively less amount of the toxin in the stool samples indicating metabolic degradation of the toxin (Tuikhar et al., 2019). However, there are more complex interactions and mechanisms that takes between host and the gut microbiome that broadly determines and impacts health, aging, and longevity (Bradley & Haran, 2024).

PROGRESS IN MICROBIOME RESEARCH IN CONTEXT OF LONGEVITY

Therapeutic interventions have emerged as potential strategy in impacting the overall gut health to promote healthy aging and thereby longevity by alleviating various age associated disorders.

Some of these emerging interventions are:

1) **Fecal microbiota transplantation:** The Fecal microbiota transplantation (FMT) has shown successful results in promotion of longevity specially in elderly people; in treatment of Crohn's disease, irritable bowel syndrome and other disorders (Kadyan et al., 2025). For instance, in a study, experimental mice showed improvements in disorders linked with age upon treating with FMT donated from long-lived cohort that promoted the count of beneficial microbes and their metabolites (Chen et al.,2020). FMT treatment enhances the production and concentration of SCFAs and using these as supplements has shown promising result in case of recovery from stroke (Lee et al., 2020; Zhang et al., 2020).

FMT is still developing and its success largely relies upon factors like selection of effective microbial strains from healthy donor, donor-recipient interactions and compatibility, planned ways for distribution (Ng et al., 2020). Development of FMT biobanks after thorough analysis from healthy donors from any age group will serve towards the goal of longevity (Kadyan et al., 2025). There are studies that shows capacity of FMT to enhance metabolic activity in the recipient by modifying the gut microbiota profile taken from the donor to reverse age related issues and increase the lifespan, however this needs further clinical trials involving large population (Shi et al., 2022). Barcena et al., (2019) in their study found an increase in gut microbes' composition and metabolic activities followed by a prolonged lifespan in progeroid mice upon FMT from wild-mice.

Another study by Parker et al., (2022), showed the variations in donor-recipient interaction during FMT, where faecal transplantation from older mice to younger mice disrupted the gut-barrier integrity and induced inflammation, while the age-related disorders in older mice were cured when FMT was from younger mice.

2) **Probiotics:** It includes wide range of beneficial and nutritional live microorganisms utilized to treat gut dysbiosis and maintaining the intestinal homeostasis by decreasing the count of pathobionts and increasing the number of healthy microbes and metabolites in gut (Sanders et al., 2011; Kim et al., 2019). With age, due to environmental exposure the composition of microbes in gut is altered causing pathogenic microbes to colonize intestine causing various disorders like colorectal cancer, crohn's disease, inflammatory bowel disease, antibiotic-associated diarrhea etc. (Kim et al., 2019).

Numerous studies have administered strains of beneficial probiotics in treatment of above-mentioned diseases and reported positive results. Some of the successful probiotic strains are *Lactobacillus acidophilus*, *Bifidobacterium animalis* subsp. *lactis* in inflammatory bowel disease (Blaabjerg et al., 2017); *Lactobacillus acidophilus*, *Bifidobacterium longum* and *Enterococcus faecalis* strains were also used as probiotics in treating colorectal cancer showing significant reduction in frequency of diarrhea in patients (Liong, 2008). VSL#3, a probiotic mixture and kind of medical food composed of eight bacterial strains viz., *L. acidophilus*, *L. casei*, *L. delbrueckii* subspecies *bulgaricus*, *L. plantarum*, and *Bifidobacterium breve*, *B. longum*, and *B. infantis* and *Streptococcus salivarius* subspecies *thermophilus* has shown anti-inflammatory effects and significant reduction in post-surgical recurrence of crohn's disease (Yang & Yu, 2018; Cheng et al., 2020).

Probiotics and its metabolites maintain the integrity of intestinal barrier by secreting mucus. For intstance, butyric acid a, metabolite of probiotics, in epithelium, elevates oxygen consumption and thereby enhances the HIF-responsive genes expression that are barrier-protective regulates the intestinal barrier integrity (Liu et al., 2020). Furthermore, probiotics are also known to minimise intestinal permeability, protecting the human gut from pathobionts (Monteagudo-Mera et al., 2019).

Identification, isolation, and selection of new beneficial probiotic strains has been made possible through various omics technologies including in vitro as well as in vivo experiments. Such information on an omics level on probiotics in context of human health would be very helpful in further development of probiotics research. Nevertheless, it is also very crucial to utilize probiotics in safe amounts or doses as it would exert negative health issues as evident from the report on overuse of Lactobacillus rhamnosus (probiotic) in patients showing inflammation in digestive organs caused infections (Boyle et al., 2006).

3) Prebiotics

Prebiotics are group of nutrients mainly from high fiber foods like resistant starches, galacto-/fructo-oligosaccharides, dietary fiber, that are degraded by the beneficial gut microbiota and utilized by them for their growth and activity. Prebiotics controls homeostasis in gut by improving intestinal barrier integrity and mucus secretion in aged people by maintaining the richness of saccharolytic bacteria and enzymes in gut (Arnold et al., 2021). Prebiotics focuses on production of SCFAs and controlling healthy composition of gut microbiota, also its effects on human health has been studied extensively mainly in conditions like IBD, mental health, obesity, immune system functioning through different pathways (Yoo et al., 2024).

4) Synbiotics

It is a mixture of probiotics and prebiotics and the term "symbiotic" was given by Glenn R. Gibson and Marcel Roberfroid in the year 1995 (Gibson & Roberfroid, 1995). It is basically a nutritional supplement that improves the useful effects of both pre and probiotics and administering these together yields desired effects on health (Kadyan et al.,2025). Such combination was designed to help the probiotic microorganisms to survive, grow in the gastrointestinal tract by dealing with challenges present therein (Hamasalim, 2016). The role of prebiotics in such combination is to supply nutrients and energy to probiotic microbial strains, to enhance the effect of synbiotics as a single product where the beneficial effects of both groups will be present (Markowiak & Slizewska, 2018).

Studies have reviewed synergistic traits of synbiotics for improving health conditions in elderly people, for e.g., in a clinical study, improved control on gut microbiome and overall gut health in older female patients was reported after administrating a synbiotic product viz., MPRO3 which is constituted of probiotic strains viz., *L. casei* HY2782, *L. plantarum* HY7712 and *B. animalis* spp. *lactis* HY8002, and prebiotics sourced from numerous dietary fibers (Lee et al., 2020).

5) Nutritional and dietary patterns

Diet especially plant based, plays the most projecting role among other interventions in controlling gut microbiome homeostasis as elucidated in the above sections. Dietary polyphenols are functional dietary component rich in antioxidants, shows anti-inflammatory activities, and are neuroprotective in function have the capacity to improve chronic health conditions such as neurodegenerative disorders (Kaydan et al., 2025).

The number of butyrate-producing bacteria can be increased in gut thereby reducing the occurrence of or improve the age-related modifications through procyanidin B2 and anthocyanin rich diets (Xiao et al., 2018; Li et al., 2019)

In a study it was found that combining certain strains of probiotics with diet rich in polyphenols, improved the inflammaging conditions in older and younger-old adults, moreover, the count of probiotic bacteria and SCFAs also increased in their gut (Meng et al., 2023). There are numerous herbs rich in antioxidants that can reverse aging by increasing the composition of beneficial gut microbes and minimising oxidative stress through several metabolic pathways (Peng et al., 2021). Ginseng, an antioxidant rich herb in its fermented form when supplemented with probiotics showed anti-aging properties in a study, by modulating the gut microbiome and triggering genes in antioxidant pathways (Xu et al., 2023). These studies reveal the importance of dietary patterns and nutrition in maintaining overall health and reducing the incidences of health disorders thereby promoting longevity.

Figure 4. Gut -organ axes regulating overall health and longevity

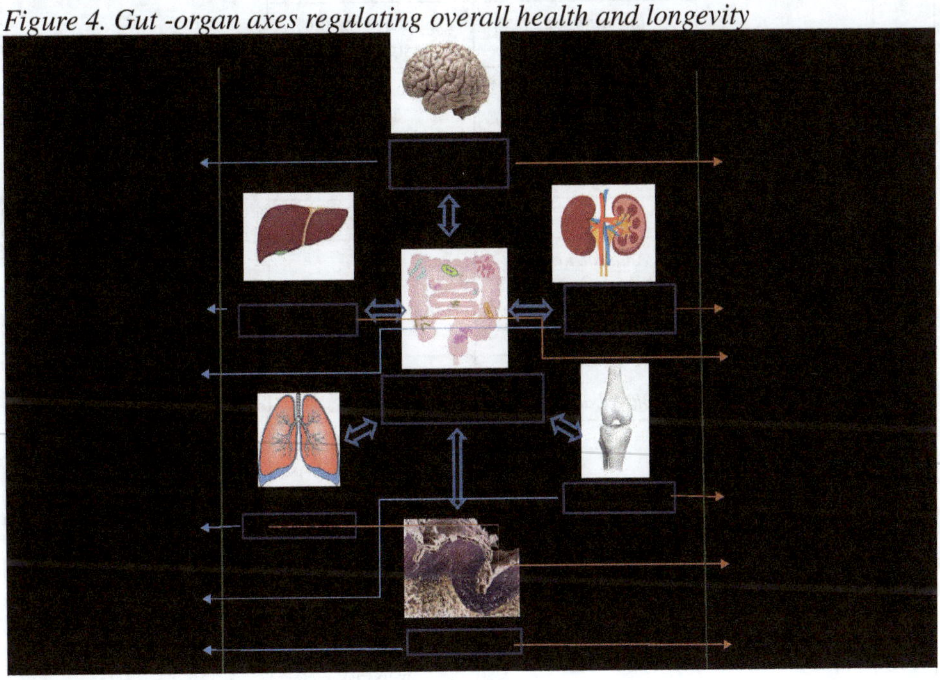

Table 1. Gut microbiota composition and functions in long-lived people.

S.no	Cohort	Beneficial gut microbiota	Functions	Reference
1	Long-lived adults	*Akkermansia muciniphila*	Anti-inflammatory activity	Chen et al., 2024
		Alistipes senegalensis	Reduces systemic inflammation	
		Alistipes shahii	Protective effects against some disorders	
		Eisenbergiella tayi	Protein N-glycosylation beneficial for longevity	
		Methanobrevibacter smithii	Maintains gut homeostasis	
2	Long-lived adults	*Bacteroides fragilis*	Regulates immune response	Wang et al., 2022
		Eubacterium ramulus	Supports colon health	
		Intestinimonas butyriciproducens	Enhance insulin signalling	
		Odoribacter splanchnicus	Anti-inflammatory activity	
		Ruthenibacterium lactatiformans	Commensal; probiotic	
3	Long-lived adults	*Anaerotruncus colihominis* et rel. (*Clostridium* cluster IV)	Modulates immune system	Den Besten et al., 2013; Biagi et al. 2016; Kong et al., 2016
		Bifidobacterium	Anti-inflammatory activity	
		Eubacterium limosum et rel. (*Clostridium* cluster XV)	Improves gut health by producing SCFAs; anti-inflammatory; maintains gut-barrier integrity	
		Akkermansia	Promotes intestinal integrity, minimises toxicity	
		Christensenellaceae	Lowers risk of cardiovascular disease and Type 2 diabetes	

continued on following page

Table 1. Continued

S.no	Cohort	Beneficial gut microbiota	Functions	Reference
4	Semi-Supercentenarians	*Akkermansia* and *Bifidobacterium*	Anti-inflammatory activity	Everard et al., 2013; Turoni et al., 2014
5	Semi-Supercentenarians	Christensenellaceae	Lowers risk of cardiovascular disease and Type 2 diabetes	Goodrich et al., 2014
6	Centenarians	*Akkermansia*	Maintains gut homeostasis; reduces inflammation, adiposity;	Kim et al., 2019
			Lowersrisk of cognitive and metabolic dysregulation	
		Christensenellaceae	Maintains gut homeostasis; reduces inflammation, adiposity;	
			Lowersrisk of cognitive and metabolic dysregulation	
		Clostridium	Butyrate (SCFAs) production; maintains gut barrier	
		Lactobacillus	Strengthens gut barrier; reduce inflammation	

continued on following page

Table 1. Continued

S.no	Cohort	Beneficial gut microbiota	Functions	Reference
		Akkermansia	Anti-inflammatory activity	
		Bifidobacterium	Maintains integrity of Intestinal barrier, impacts mental and immune health;	
			reduce inflammation	
		Butyricimonas	Produces SCFAs; suppress pathogens; anti-inflammatory	
		Christensenellaceae	Lowers risk of cardiovascular disease and Type 2 diabetes	
		Odoribacter	Anti-inflammatory activity	
7	Long-lived adults	Parabacteroides (few members)	Anti-inflammatory activity; Improves intestinal barrier	Yu et al., 2015; Biagi et al., 2016; Kim et al., 2019; Tuikhar et al., 2019; Wu et al, 2019;

CONCLUSION

Investigations on gut microbiome and its multifaceted interactions with host have paved way for exploring its role in overall health in all age group, healthy aging, and longevity. Inter-individual variations in gut microbiome composition and metabolic functions impacting health positively as well as in negative manner in different age group exists basically due to their exposure to different environments and dietary habits (Sepp et al., 2022). Numerous studies on the impact of integrated interventions on the gut microbiome like adoption of plant-based diet, exercise, maintaining sleep wake cycle, probiotics and prebiotic treatments have demonstrated potential benefits in health and longevity (Ngandu et al., 2015; Dedeyne et al., 2017; Zhonghui et al., 2024). However, it must be noted that even after various interventions, commensal taxa that are beneficial for health may not be able to reside in all individual's gut microbiome due to resistance as well as age-related factors. Further research on underlying crucial complex mechanisms will provide opportunities to develop distinguished health biomarkers (Sepp et al., 2022) and to decipher consequences of gut microbiome in overall health and longevity.

REFERENCES

Alhinai, E., Walton, G., & Commane, D. (2019). The role of the gut microbiota in colorectal cancer causation. *International Journal of Molecular Sciences*, *20*(21), 5295. DOI: 10.3390/ijms20215295 PMID: 31653078

Allen, J. M., Mailing, L. J., Niemiro, G. M., Moore, R., Cook, M. D., White, B. A., Holscher, H. D., & Woods, J. A. (2018). Exercise alters gut microbiota composition and function in lean and obese humans. *Medicine and Science in Sports and Exercise*, *50*(4), 747–757. DOI: 10.1249/MSS.0000000000001495 PMID: 29166320

Amedei, A., & Morbidelli, L. (2019). Circulating metabolites originating from gut microbiota control endothelial cell function. *Molecules (Basel, Switzerland)*, *24*(21), 3992. DOI: 10.3390/molecules24213992 PMID: 31694161

Arnold, J. W., Roach, J., Fabela, S., Moorfield, E., Ding, S., Blue, E., Dagher, S., Magness, S., Tamayo, R., Bruno-Barcena, J. M., & Azcarate-Peril, M. A. (2021). The pleiotropic effects of prebiotic galacto-oligosaccharides on the aging gut. *Microbiome*, *9*(1), 1–19. DOI: 10.1186/s40168-020-00980-0 PMID: 33388088

Arumugam, M., Raes, J., Pelletier, E., Le Paslier, D., Yamada, T., Mende, D. R., Fernandes, G. R., Tap, J., Bruls, T., Batto, J. M., Bertalan, M., Borruel, N., Casellas, F., Fernandez, L., Gautier, L., Hansen, T., Hattori, M., Hayashi, T., Kleerebezem, M., & Dore, J. (2011). Enterotypes of the human gut microbiome. *Nature*, *473*(7346), 174–180. DOI: 10.1038/nature09944 PMID: 21508958

Asnicar, F., Berry, S. E., Valdes, A. M., Nguyen, L. H., Piccinno, G., Drew, D. A., Leeming, E., Gibson, R., Le Roy, C., Khatib, H. A., Francis, L., Mazidi, M., Mompeo, O., Valles-Colomer, M., Tett, A., Beghini, F., Dubois, L., Bazzani, D., Thomas, A. M., & Spector, T. D. (2021). Microbiome connections with host metabolism and habitual diet from 1,098 deeply phenotyped individuals. *Nature Medicine*, *27*(2), 321–332. DOI: 10.1038/s41591-020-01183-8 PMID: 33432175

Badal, V. D., Vaccariello, E. D., Murray, E. R., Yu, K. E., Knight, R., Jeste, D. V., & Nguyen, T. T. (2020). The gut microbiome, aging, and longevity: A systematic review. *Nutrients*, *12*(12), 3759. DOI: 10.3390/nu12123759 PMID: 33297486

Bana, B., & Cabreiro, F. (2019). The microbiome and aging. *Annual Review of Genetics*, *53*(1), 239–261. DOI: 10.1146/annurev-genet-112618-043650 PMID: 31487470

Bárcena, C., Valdés-Mas, R., Mayoral, P., Garabaya, C., Durand, S., Rodríguez, F., Fernández-García, M. T., Salazar, N., Nogacka, A. M., Garatachea, N., Bossut, N., Aprahamian, F., Lucia, A., Kroemer, G., Freije, J. M. P., Quirós, P. M., & López-Otín, C. (2019). Healthspan and lifespan extension by fecal microbiota transplantation into progeroid mice. *Nature Medicine*, *25*(8), 1234–1242. DOI: 10.1038/s41591-019-0504-5 PMID: 31332389

Bauer, H., Horowitz, R. E., Levenson, S. M., & Popper, H. (1963). The response of the lymphatic tissue to the microbial flora: Studies on germfree mice. *American Journal of Pathology*, *42*(4), 471–483. PMID: 13966929

Biagi, E., Franceschi, C., Rampelli, S., Severgnini, M., Ostan, R., Turroni, S., Consolandi, C., Quercia, S., Scurti, M., Monti, D., Capri, M., Brigidi, P., & Candela, M. (2016). Gut microbiota and extreme longevity. *Current Biology*, *26*(11), 1480–1485. DOI: 10.1016/j.cub.2016.04.016 PMID: 27185560

Biagi, E., Franceschi, C., Rampelli, S., Severgnini, M., Ostan, R., Turroni, S., Consolandi, C., Quercia, S., Scurti, M., Monti, D., Capri, M., Brigidi, P., & Candela, M. (2016). Gut microbiota and extreme longevity. *Current Biology*, *26*(11), 1480–1485. DOI: 10.1016/j.cub.2016.04.016 PMID: 27185560

Bjerregård Madsen, J., Kaila, A., Vehviläinen-Julkunen, K., & Miettinen, M. (2016). Time allocation and temporal focus in nursing management: An integrative review. *Journal of Nursing Management*, *24*(8), 983–993. DOI: 10.1111/jonm.12411 PMID: 27411357

Blaabjerg, S., Artzi, D. M., & Aabenhus, R. (2017). Probiotics for the prevention of antibiotic-associated diarrhea in outpatients—A systematic review and meta-analysis. *Antibiotics (Basel, Switzerland)*, *6*(4), 21. DOI: 10.3390/antibiotics6040021 PMID: 29023420

Boyle, R. J., Robins-Browne, R. M., & Tang, M. L. (2006). Probiotic use in clinical practice: What are the risks? *The American Journal of Clinical Nutrition*, *83*(6), 1256–1264. DOI: 10.1093/ajcn/83.6.1256 PMID: 16762934

Bradley, E., & Haran, J. (2024). The human gut microbiome and aging. *Gut Microbes*, *16*(1), 2359677. DOI: 10.1080/19490976.2024.2359677 PMID: 38831607

Bressa, C., Bailén-Andrino, M., Pérez-Santiago, J., González-Soltero, R., Pérez, M., Montalvo-Lominchar, M. G., Maté-Muñoz, J. L., Domínguez, R., Moreno, D., & Larrosa, M. (2017). Differences in gut microbiota profile between women with active lifestyle and sedentary women. *PLoS One*, *12*(2), e0171352. DOI: 10.1371/journal.pone.0171352 PMID: 28187199

Bull, M. J., & Plummer, N. T. (2014). Part 1: The human gut microbiome in health and disease. *Integrative Medicine (Encinitas, Calif.)*, *13*(6), 17–22. PMID: 26770121

Campbell, J. H., Foster, C. M., Vishnivetskaya, T., Campbell, A. G., Yang, Z. K., Wymore, A., Palumbo, A. V., Chesler, E. J., & Podar, M. (2012). Host genetic and environmental effects on mouse intestinal microbiota. *The ISME Journal*, *6*(11), 2033–2044. DOI: 10.1038/ismej.2012.54 PMID: 22695862

Chassaing, B., Vijay-Kumar, M., & Gewirtz, A. T. (2017). How diet can impact gut microbiota to promote or endanger health. *Current Opinion in Gastroenterology*, *33*(6), 417–421. DOI: 10.1097/MOG.0000000000000401 PMID: 29019865

Chen, S., Zhang, Z., Liu, S., Chen, T., Lu, Z., Zhao, W., Mou, X., & Liu, S. (2024). Consistent signatures in the human gut microbiome of longevous populations. *Gut Microbes*, *16*(1), 2393756. DOI: 10.1080/19490976.2024.2393756 PMID: 39197040

Chen, Y., Zhang, S., Zeng, B., Zhao, J., Yang, M., Zhang, M., Li, Y., Ni, Q., Wu, D., & Li, Y. (2020). Transplant of microbiota from long-living people to mice reduces aging-related indices and transfers beneficial bacteria. *Aging (Albany NY)*, *12*(6), 4778–4793. DOI: 10.18632/aging.102872 PMID: 32176868

Cheng, F. S., Pan, D., Chang, B., Jiang, M., & Sang, L. X. (2020). Probiotic mixture VSL# 3: An overview of basic and clinical studies in chronic diseases. *World Journal of Clinical Cases*, *8*(8), 1361–1384. DOI: 10.12998/wjcc.v8.i8.1361 PMID: 32368530

Cho, I., & Blaser, M. J. (2012). The human microbiome at the interface of health and disease. *Nature Reviews. Genetics*, *13*(4), 260–270. DOI: 10.1038/nrg3182 PMID: 22411464

Chu, H., & Mazmanian, S. K. (2013). Innate immune recognition of the microbiota promotes host-microbial symbiosis. *Nature Immunology*, *14*(7), 668–675. DOI: 10.1038/ni.2635 PMID: 23778794

Chung, W. S. F., Meijerink, M., Zeuner, B., Holck, J., Louis, P., Meyer, A. S., Wells, J. M., Flint, H. J., & Duncan, S. H. (2017). Prebiotic potential of pectin and pectic oligosaccharides to promote anti-inflammatory commensal bacteria in the human colon. *FEMS Microbiology Ecology*, *93*(11), fix127. Advance online publication. DOI: 10.1093/femsec/fix127 PMID: 29029078

Clemente, J. C., Ursell, L. K., Parfrey, L. W., & Knight, R. (2012). The impact of the gut microbiota on human health: An integrative view. *Cell*, *148*(6), 1258–1270. DOI: 10.1016/j.cell.2012.01.035 PMID: 22424233

Cresci, G. A., & Bawden, E. (2015). Gut microbiome: What we do and don't know. *Nutrition in Clinical Practice*, *30*(6), 734–746. DOI: 10.1177/0884533615609899 PMID: 26449893

Dabrowska, K., & Witkiewicz, W. (2016). Correlations of host genetics and gut microbiome composition. *Frontiers in Microbiology*, *7*, 1357. DOI: 10.3389/fmicb.2016.01357 PMID: 27625642

Dedeyne, L., Deschodt, M., Verschueren, S., Tournoy, J., & Gielen, E. (2017). Effects of multi-domain interventions in (pre)frail elderly on frailty, functional, and cognitive status: A systematic review. *Clinical Interventions in Aging*, *12*, 873–896. DOI: 10.2147/CIA.S130794 PMID: 28579766

den Besten, G., van Eunen, K., Groen, A. K., Venema, K., Reijngoud, D.-J., & Bakker, B. M. (2013). The role of short-chain fatty acids in the interplay between diet, gut microbiota, and host energy metabolism. *Journal of Lipid Research*, *54*(9), 2325–2340. DOI: 10.1194/jlr.R036012 PMID: 23821742

Dethlefsen, L., & Relman, D. A. (2011). Incomplete recovery and individualized responses of the human distal gut microbiota to repeated antibiotic perturbation. *Proceedings of the National Academy of Sciences of the United States of America*, *108*(Suppl. 1), 4554–4561. DOI: 10.1073/pnas.1000087107 PMID: 20847294

Everard, A., Belzer, C., Geurts, L., Ouwerkerk, J. P., Druart, C., Bindels, L. B., Guiot, Y., Derrien, M., Muccioli, G. G., Delzenne, N. M., & Cani, P. D. (2013). Cross-talk between *Akkermansia muciniphila* and intestinal epithelium controls diet-induced obesity. *Proceedings of the National Academy of Sciences of the United States of America*, *110*(22), 9066–9071. DOI: 10.1073/pnas.1219451110 PMID: 23671105

Ferrucci, L., & Fabbri, E. (2018). Inflammageing: Chronic inflammation in ageing, cardiovascular disease, and frailty. *Nature Reviews. Cardiology*, *15*(9), 505–522. DOI: 10.1038/s41569-018-0064-2 PMID: 30065258

Franceschi, C., Bonafè, M., Valensin, S., Olivieri, F., De Luca, M., Ottaviani, E., & De Benedictis, G. (2000). Inflamm-aging: An evolutionary perspective on immunosenescence. *Annals of the New York Academy of Sciences*, *908*(1), 244–254. DOI: 10.1111/j.1749-6632.2000.tb06651.x PMID: 10911963

Gensollen, T., Iyer, S. S., Kasper, D. L., & Blumberg, R. S. (2016). How colonization by microbiota in early life shapes the immune system. *Science*, *352*(6285), 539–544. DOI: 10.1126/science.aad9378 PMID: 27126036

Gibson, G. R., & Roberfroid, M. B. (1995). Dietary modulation of the human colonic microbiota: Introducing the concept of prebiotics. *The Journal of Nutrition, 125*(6), 1401–1412. DOI: 10.1093/jn/125.6.1401 PMID: 7782892

Gomez de Agüero, M., Ganal-Vonarburg, S. C., Fuhrer, T., Rupp, S., Uchimura, Y., Li, H., Steinert, A., Heikenwalder, M., Hapfelmeier, S., Sauer, U., McCoy, K. D., & Macpherson, A. J. (2016). The maternal microbiota drives early postnatal innate immune development. *Science, 351*(6279), 1296–1302. DOI: 10.1126/science.aad2571 PMID: 26989247

Goodrich, J. K., Waters, J. L., Poole, A. C., Sutter, J. L., Koren, O., Blekhman, R., Beaumont, M., Van Treuren, W., Knight, R., Bell, J. T., Spector, T. D., Clark, A. G., & Ley, R. E. (2014). Human genetics shape the gut microbiome. *Cell, 159*(4), 789–799. DOI: 10.1016/j.cell.2014.09.053 PMID: 25417156

Greer, J. B., & O'Keefe, S. J. (2011). Microbial induction of immunity, inflammation, and cancer. *Frontiers in Physiology, 1*, 168. DOI: 10.3389/fphys.2010.00168 PMID: 21423403

Hamasalim, H. J. (2016). Synbiotic as feed additives relating to animal health and performance. *Advances in Microbiology, 6*(04), 288–302. DOI: 10.4236/aim.2016.64028

Haran, J. P., Zeamer, A., Ward, D. V., Dutta, P., Bucci, V., & McCormick, B. A. (2021). The nursing home older adult gut microbiome composition shows time-dependent dysbiosis and is influenced by medication exposures, age, environment, and frailty. *The Journals of Gerontology. Series A, Biological Sciences and Medical Sciences, 76*(11), 1930–1938. DOI: 10.1093/gerona/glab167 PMID: 34125200

Heidari, M., Maleki Vareki, S., Yaghobi, R., & Karimi, M. H. (2024). Microbiota activation and regulation of adaptive immunity. *Frontiers in Immunology, 15*, 1429436. DOI: 10.3389/fimmu.2024.1429436 PMID: 39445008

Henke, M. T., Kenny, D. J., Cassilly, C. D., Vlamakis, H., Xavier, R. J., & Clardy, J. (2019). *Ruminococcus gnavus*, a member of the human gut microbiome associated with Crohn's disease, produces an inflammatory polysaccharide. *Proceedings of the National Academy of Sciences of the United States of America, 116*(26), 12672–12677. DOI: 10.1073/pnas.1904099116 PMID: 31182571

Honda, K., & Littman, D. R. (2012). The microbiome in infectious disease and inflammation. *Annual Review of Immunology, 30*(1), 759–795. DOI: 10.1146/annurev-immunol-020711-074937 PMID: 22224764

Hooper, L. V., & Macpherson, A. J. (2010). Immune adaptations that maintain homeostasis with the intestinal microbiota. *Nature Reviews. Immunology, 10*(3), 159–169. DOI: 10.1038/nri2710 PMID: 20182457

Jeffery, I. B., Lynch, D. B., & O'Toole, P. W. (2016). Composition and temporal stability of the gut microbiota in older persons. *The ISME Journal, 10*(1), 170–182. DOI: 10.1038/ismej.2015.88 PMID: 26090993

Jump, R. L. P., Crnich, C. J., Mody, L., Bradley, S. F., Nicolle, L. E., & Yoshikawa, T. T. (2018). Infectious diseases in older adults of long-term care facilities: Update on approach to diagnosis and management. *Journal of the American Geriatrics Society, 66*(4), 789–803. DOI: 10.1111/jgs.15248 PMID: 29667186

Kawamoto, S., Maruya, M., Kato, L. M., Suda, W., Atarashi, K., Doi, Y., Tsutsui, Y., Qin, H., Honda, K., Okada, T., Hattori, M., & Fagarasan, S. (2014). $Foxp3^{+}$ T cells regulate immunoglobulin A selection and facilitate diversification of bacterial species responsible for immune homeostasis. *Immunity, 41*(1), 152–165. DOI: 10.1016/j.immuni.2014.05.016 PMID: 25017466

Kim, B.-S., Choi, C. W., Shin, H., Jin, S.-P., Bae, J.-S., Han, M., Seo, E. Y., Chun, J., & Chung, J. H. (2019). Comparison of the gut microbiota of centenarians in longevity villages of South Korea with those of other age groups. *Journal of Microbiology and Biotechnology, 29*(3), 429–440. DOI: 10.4014/jmb.1811.11023 PMID: 30661321

Kim, B.-S., Choi, C. W., Shin, H., Jin, S.-P., Bae, J.-S., Han, M., Seo, E. Y., Chun, J., & Chung, J. H. (2019). Comparison of the gut microbiota of centenarians in longevity villages of South Korea with those of other age groups. *Journal of Microbiology and Biotechnology, 29*(3), 429–440. DOI: 10.4014/jmb.1811.11023 PMID: 30661321

Kim, B.-S., Choi, C. W., Shin, H., Jin, S.-P., Bae, J.-S., Han, M., Seo, E. Y., Chun, J., & Chung, J. H. (2019). Comparison of the gut microbiota of centenarians in longevity villages of South Korea with those of other age groups. *Journal of Microbiology and Biotechnology, 29*(3), 429–440. DOI: 10.4014/jmb.1811.11023 PMID: 30661321

Kim, H., Caulfield, L. E., Garcia-Larsen, V., Steffen, L. M., Coresh, J., & Rebholz, C. M. (2019a). Plant-based diets are associated with a lower risk of incident cardiovascular disease, cardiovascular disease mortality, and all-cause mortality in a general population of middle-aged adults. *Journal of the American Heart Association, 8*(16), e012865. DOI: 10.1161/JAHA.119.012865 PMID: 31387433

Kim, H., Caulfield, L. E., Garcia-Larsen, V., Steffen, L. M., Grams, M. E., Coresh, J., & Rebholz, C. M. (2019b). Plant-based diets and incident CKD and kidney function. *Clinical Journal of the American Society of Nephrology; CJASN, 14*(5), 682–691. DOI: 10.2215/CJN.12391018 PMID: 31023928

Kim, S. K., Guevarra, R. B., Kim, Y. T., Kwon, J., Kim, H., Cho, J. H., Kim, H. B., & Lee, J. H. (2019). Role of probiotics in human gut microbiome-associated diseases. *Journal of Microbiology and Biotechnology, 29*(9), 1335–1340. DOI: 10.4014/jmb.1906.06064 PMID: 31434172

Kong, F., Hua, Y., Zeng, B., Ning, R., Li, Y., & Zhao, J. (2016). Gut microbiota signatures of longevity. *Current Biology, 26*(18), R832–R833. DOI: 10.1016/j.cub.2016.08.015 PMID: 27676296

Koponen, K. K., Salosensaari, A., Ruuskanen, M. O., Havulinna, A. S., Männistö, S., Jousilahti, P., Palmu, J., Salido, R., Sanders, K., Brennan, C., Humphrey, G. C., Sanders, J. G., Meric, G., Cheng, S., Inouye, M., Jain, M., Niiranen, T. J., Valsta, L. M., Knight, R., & Salomaa, V. V. (2021). Associations of healthy food choices with gut microbiota profiles. *The American Journal of Clinical Nutrition, 114*(2), 605–616. DOI: 10.1093/ajcn/nqab077 PMID: 34020448

Kuhnle, G. G. C., Story, G. W., Reda, T., Mani, A. R., Moore, K. P., Lunn, J. C., & Bingham, S. A. (2007). Diet-induced endogenous formation of nitroso compounds in the GI tract. *Free Radical Biology & Medicine, 43*(7), 1040–1047. DOI: 10.1016/j.freeradbiomed.2007.03.011 PMID: 17761300

Lakshminarayanan, B., Stanton, C., O'Toole, P. W., & Ross, R. P. (2014). Compositional dynamics of the human intestinal microbiota with aging: Implications for health. *The Journal of Nutrition, Health & Aging, 18*(9), 773–786. DOI: 10.1007/s12603-014-0549-6 PMID: 25389954

Larson, P. J., Zhou, W., Santiago, A., Driscoll, S., Fleming, E., Voigt, A. Y., Chun, O. K., Grady, J. J., Kuchel, G. A., Robison, J. T., & Oh, J. (2022). Associations of the skin, oral and gut microbiome with aging, frailty and infection risk reservoirs in older adults. *Nature Aging, 2*(10), 941–955. DOI: 10.1038/s43587-022-00287-9 PMID: 36398033

Lee, J., d'Aigle, J., Atadja, L., Quaicoe, V., Honarpisheh, P., Ganesh, B. P., Hassan, A., Graf, J., Petrosino, J., Putluri, N., Zhu, L., Durgan, D. J., Bryan, R. M.Jr, McCullough, L. D., & Venna, V. R. (2020). Gut microbiota–derived short-chain fatty acids promote poststroke recovery in aged mice. *Circulation Research, 127*(4), 453–465. DOI: 10.1161/CIRCRESAHA.119.316448 PMID: 32354259

Lee, S. H., You, H. S., Kang, H. G., Kang, S. S., & Hyun, S. H. (2020). Association between altered blood parameters and gut microbiota after synbiotic intake in healthy, elderly Korean women. *Nutrients, 12*(10), 3112. DOI: 10.3390/nu12103112 PMID: 33053824

Levy, M., Kolodziejczyk, A. A., Thaiss, C. A., & Elinav, E. (2017). Dysbiosis and the immune system. *Nature Reviews. Immunology*, *17*(4), 219–232. DOI: 10.1038/nri.2017.7 PMID: 28260787

Li, J., Wu, T., Li, N., Wang, X., Chen, G., & Lyu, X. (2019). Bilberry anthocyanin extract promotes intestinal barrier function and inhibits digestive enzyme activity by regulating the gut microbiota in aging rats. *Food & Function*, *10*(1), 333–343. DOI: 10.1039/C8FO01962B PMID: 30575836

Li, Y., Wang, D. D., Satija, A., Ivey, K. L., Li, J., Wilkinson, J. E., Wu, Y., Ding, E. L., Rimm, E. B., Hu, F. B., & Sun, Q. (2021). Plant-based diet index and metabolic risk in men: Exploring the role of the gut microbiome. *The Journal of Nutrition*, *151*(9), 2780–2789. DOI: 10.1093/jn/nxab175 PMID: 34114015

Liong, M. T. (2008). Roles of probiotics and prebiotics in colon cancer prevention: Postulated mechanisms and in-vivo evidence. *International Journal of Molecular Sciences*, *9*(5), 854–863. DOI: 10.3390/ijms9050854 PMID: 19325789

Liu, Q., Yu, Z., Tian, F., Zhao, J., Zhang, H., Zhai, Q., & Chen, W. (2020). Surface components and metabolites of probiotics for regulation of intestinal epithelial barrier. *Microbial Cell Factories*, *19*(1), 23. DOI: 10.1186/s12934-020-1289-4 PMID: 32024520

Macpherson, A. J., & Uhr, T. (2004). Induction of protective IgA by intestinal dendritic cells carrying commensal bacteria. *Science*, *303*(5664), 1662–1665. DOI: 10.1126/science.1091334 PMID: 15016999

Markowiak, P., & Śliżewska, K. (2018). The role of probiotics, prebiotics and synbiotics in animal nutrition. *Gut Pathogens*, *10*(1), 21. DOI: 10.1186/s13099-018-0250-0 PMID: 29930711

Meng, N., Zhou, Y., Zhang, Q., Yu, X., Li, H., Liu, Y., Liu, M., & Li, Q. (2023). Using inflammatory biological age to evaluate the preventing aging effect of a polyphenol-probiotic-enhanced dietary pattern in adults aged 50 years and older. *Journal of Agricultural and Food Chemistry*, *71*(16), 6314–6325. DOI: 10.1021/acs.jafc.2c07241 PMID: 37057839

Monteagudo-Mera, A., Rastall, R. A., Gibson, G. R., Charalampopoulos, D., & Chatzifragkou, A. (2019). Adhesion mechanisms mediated by probiotics and prebiotics and their potential impact on human health. *Applied Microbiology and Biotechnology*, *103*(16), 6463–6472. DOI: 10.1007/s00253-019-09978-7 PMID: 31267231

Moore, J. W., Millard, S., Babidge, W., Rowland, R., & Roediger, W. E. (1997). Hydrogen sulphide produces diminished fatty acid oxidation in the rat colon in vivo: Implications for ulcerative colitis. *ANZ Journal of Surgery*, *67*(4), 245–249. DOI: 10.1111/j.1445-2197.1997.tb01961.x PMID: 9152152

Mowat, A. M. (2018). To respond or not to respond: A personal perspective of intestinal tolerance. *Nature Reviews. Immunology*, *18*(6), 405–415. DOI: 10.1038/s41577-018-0002-x PMID: 29491358

Nagao-Kitamoto, H., & Kamada, N. (2017). Host-microbial cross-talk in inflammatory bowel disease. *Immune Network*, *17*(1), 1–12. DOI: 10.4110/in.2017.17.1.1 PMID: 28261015

Ng, S. C., Kamm, M. A., Yeoh, Y. K., Chan, P. K., Zuo, T., Tang, W., Sood, A., Andoh, A., Ohmiya, N., Zhou, Y., Ooi, C. J., Mahachai, V., Wu, C.-Y., Zhang, F., Sugano, K., & Chan, F. K. L. (2020). Scientific frontiers in faecal microbiota transplantation: Joint document of Asia-Pacific Association of Gastroenterology (APAGE) and Asia-Pacific Society for Digestive Endoscopy (APSDE). *Gut*, *69*(1), 83–91. DOI: 10.1136/gutjnl-2019-319407 PMID: 31611298

Ngandu, T., Lehtisalo, J., Solomon, A., Levälahti, E., Ahtiluoto, S., Antikainen, R., Bäckman, L., Hänninen, T., Jula, A., Laatikainen, T., Lindström, J., Mangialasche, F., Paajanen, T., Pajala, S., Peltonen, M., Rauramaa, R., Stigsdotter-Neely, A., Strandberg, T., Tuomilehto, J., & Kivipelto, M. (2015). A 2-year multidomain intervention of diet, exercise, cognitive training, and vascular risk monitoring versus control to prevent cognitive decline in at-risk elderly people (FINGER): A randomised controlled trial. *Lancet*, *385*(9984), 2255–2263. DOI: 10.1016/S0140-6736(15)60461-5 PMID: 25771249

Nicholson, J. K., Holmes, E., Kinross, J., Burcelin, R., Gibson, G., Jia, W., & Pettersson, S. (2012). Host–gut microbiota metabolic interactions. *Science*, *336*(6086), 1262–1267. DOI: 10.1126/science.1223813 PMID: 22674330

Ocvirk, S., Wilson, A. S., Appolonia, C. N., Thomas, T. K., & O'Keefe, S. J. D. (2019). Fiber, fat, and colorectal cancer: New insight into modifiable dietary risk factors. *Current Gastroenterology Reports*, *21*(11), 62. DOI: 10.1007/s11894-019-0725-2 PMID: 31792624

Odamaki, T., Bottacini, F., Kato, K., Mitsuyama, E., Yoshida, K., Horigome, A., Xiao, J., & van Sinderen, D. (2018). Genomic diversity and distribution of *Bifidobacterium longum* subsp. *longum* across the human lifespan. *Scientific Reports*, *8*(1), 85. DOI: 10.1038/s41598-017-18391-x PMID: 29311585

Odamaki, T., Kato, K., Sugahara, H., Hashikura, N., Takahashi, S., Xiao, J., Abe, F., & Osawa, R. (2016). Age-related changes in gut microbiota composition from newborn to centenarian: A cross-sectional study. *BMC Microbiology*, *16*(1), 90. DOI: 10.1186/s12866-016-0708-5 PMID: 27220822

Owaga, E., Hsieh, R. H., Mugendi, B., Masuku, S., Shih, C. K., & Chang, J. S. (2015). Th17 cells as potential probiotic therapeutic targets in inflammatory bowel diseases. *International Journal of Molecular Sciences*, *16*(9), 20841–20858. DOI: 10.3390/ijms160920841 PMID: 26340622

Palm, N. W., de Zoete, M. R., Cullen, T. W., Barry, N. A., Stefanowski, J., Hao, L., Degnan, P. H., Hu, J., Peter, I., Zhang, W., Ruggiero, E., Cho, J. H., Goodman, A. L., & Flavell, R. A. (2014). Immunoglobulin A coating identifies colitogenic bacteria in inflammatory bowel disease. *Cell*, *158*(5), 1000–1010. DOI: 10.1016/j.cell.2014.08.006 PMID: 25171403

Parker, A., Romano, S., Ansorge, R., Aboelnour, A., Le Gall, G., Savva, G. M., Pontifex, M. G., Telatin, A., Baker, D., Jones, E., Vauzour, D., Rudder, S., Blackshaw, L. A., Jeffery, G., & Carding, S. R. (2022). Fecal microbiota transfer between young and aged mice reverses hallmarks of the aging gut, eye, and brain. *Microbiome*, *10*(1), 1–25. DOI: 10.1186/s40168-022-01243-w PMID: 35501923

Peng, X., Hao, M., Zhao, Y., Cai, Y., Chen, X., Chen, H., Zhang, Y., Dong, L., Liu, X., Ding, C., Liu, W., Yang, M., & Luo, Y. (2021). Red ginseng has stronger anti-aging effects compared to ginseng possibly due to its regulation of oxidative stress and the gut microbiota. *Phytomedicine*, *93*, 153772. DOI: 10.1016/j.phymed.2021.153772 PMID: 34753028

Rampelli, S., Candela, M., Turroni, S., Biagi, E., Collino, S., Franceschi, C., O'Toole, P. W., & Brigidi, P. (2013). Functional metagenomic profiling of intestinal microbiome in extreme ageing. *Aging (Albany NY)*, *5*(12), 902–912. DOI: 10.18632/aging.100623 PMID: 24334635

Rampelli, S., Soverini, M., D'Amico, F., Barone, M., Tavella, T., Monti, D., Capri, M., Astolfi, A., Brigidi, P., Biagi, E., Franceschi, C., Turroni, S., & Candela, M. (2020). Shotgun metagenomics of gut microbiota in humans with up to extreme longevity and the increasing role of xenobiotic degradation. *mSystems*, *5*(2), e00124–e20. DOI: 10.1128/mSystems.00124-20 PMID: 32209716

Rothschild, D., Weissbrod, O., Barkan, E., Kurilshikov, A., Korem, T., Zeevi, D., Costea, P. I., Godneva, A., Kalka, I. N., Bar, N., Shilo, S., Lador, D., Vila, A. V., Zmora, N., Pevsner-Fischer, M., Israeli, D., Kosower, N., Malka, G., Wolf, B. C., & Segal, E. (2018). Environment dominates over host genetics in shaping human gut microbiota. *Nature*, *555*(7695), 210–215. DOI: 10.1038/nature25973 PMID: 29489753

Saad, N., Delattre, C., Urdaci, M., Schmitter, J. M., & Bressollier, P. (2013). An overview of the last advances in probiotic and prebiotic field. *Lebensmittel-Wissenschaft + Technologie*, *50*(1), 1–16. DOI: 10.1016/j.lwt.2012.05.014

Sanders, M. E., Heimbach, J. T., Pot, B., Tancredi, D. J., Lenoir-Wijnkoop, I., Lähteenmäki-Uutela, A., Gueimonde, M., & Bañares, S. (2011). Health claims substantiation for probiotic and prebiotic products. *Gut Microbes*, *2*(3), 127–133. DOI: 10.4161/gmic.2.3.16174 PMID: 21646865

Sekirov, I., Russell, S. L., Antunes, L. C. M., & Finlay, B. B. (2010). Gut microbiota in health and disease. *Physiological Reviews*, *90*(3), 859–904. DOI: 10.1152/physrev.00045.2009 PMID: 20664075

Sender, R., Fuchs, S., & Milo, R. (2016). Are we really vastly outnumbered? Revisiting the ratio of bacterial to host cells in humans. *Cell*, *164*(3), 337–340. DOI: 10.1016/j.cell.2016.01.013 PMID: 26824647

Sepp, E., Smidt, I., Rööp, T., Tšepetova, J., Kõljalg, S., Mikelsaar, M., Soidla, I., Ainsaar, M., Kolk, H., Vallas, M., Jaagura, M., & Mändar, R. (2022). Comparative analysis of gut microbiota in centenarians and young people: Impact of eating habits and childhood living environment. *Frontiers in Cellular and Infection Microbiology*, *12*, 851404. DOI: 10.3389/fcimb.2022.851404 PMID: 35372105

Shen, X., Tilves, C., Kim, H., Tanaka, T., Spira, A. P., Chia, C. W., Talegawkar, S. A., Ferrucci, L., & Mueller, N. T. (2024). Plant-based diets and the gut microbiome: Findings from the Baltimore Longitudinal Study of Aging. *The American Journal of Clinical Nutrition*, *119*(4), 628–638. DOI: 10.1016/j.ajcnut.2024.01.006 PMID: 38218318

Shi, X., Ma, T., Sakandar, H. A., Menghe, B., & Sun, Z. (2022). Gut microbiome and aging nexus and underlying mechanism. *Applied Microbiology and Biotechnology*, *106*(17), 5349–5358. DOI: 10.1007/s00253-022-12089-5 PMID: 35882675

Sirisinha, S. (2016). The potential impact of gut microbiota on your health: Current status and future challenges. *Asian Pacific Journal of Allergy and Immunology*, *34*(4), 249–264. DOI: 10.12932/AP0803 PMID: 28042926

Sokol, H., Pigneur, B., Watterlot, L., Lakhdari, O., Bermúdez-Humarán, L. G., Gratadoux, J. J., Blugeon, S., Bridonneau, C., Furet, J. P., Corthier, G., Grangette, C., Vasquez, N., Pochart, P., Trugnan, G., Thomas, G., Blottière, H. M., Doré, J., Marteau, P., Seksik, P., & Langella, P. (2008). *Faecalibacterium prausnitzii* is an anti-inflammatory commensal bacterium identified by gut microbiota analysis of Crohn disease patients. *Proceedings of the National Academy of Sciences of the United States of America*, *105*(43), 16731–16736. DOI: 10.1073/pnas.0804812105 PMID: 18936492

Soldán, M., Argalášová, Ľ., Hadvinová, L., Galileo, B., & Babjaková, J. (2024). The effect of dietary types on gut microbiota composition and development of non-communicable diseases: A narrative review. *Nutrients*, *16*(18), 3134. DOI: 10.3390/nu16183134 PMID: 39339734

Thevaranjan, N., Puchta, A., Schulz, C., Naidoo, A., Szamosi, J. C., Verschoor, C. P., Loukov, D., Schenck, L. P., Jury, J., Foley, K. P., Schertzer, J. D., Larche, M. J., Davidson, D. J., Verdu, E. F., Surette, M. G., & Bowdish, D. M. E. (2017). Age-associated microbial dysbiosis promotes intestinal permeability, systemic inflammation, and macrophage dysfunction. *Cell Host & Microbe*, *21*(4), 455–466. e4. DOI: 10.1016/j.chom.2017.03.002 PMID: 28407483

Tuikhar, N., Keisam, S., Labala, R. K., Ramakrishnan, P., Arunkumar, M. C., Ahmed, G., Biagi, E., & Jeyaram, K. (2019). Comparative analysis of the gut microbiota in centenarians and young adults shows a common signature across genotypically non-related populations. *Mechanisms of Ageing and Development*, *179*, 23–35. DOI: 10.1016/j.mad.2019.02.001 PMID: 30738080

Tuikhar, N., Keisam, S., Labala, R. K. I., Ramakrishnan, P., Arunkumar, M. C., Ahmed, G., Biagi, E., & Jeyaram, K. (2019). Comparative analysis of the gut microbiota in centenarians and young adults shows a common signature across genotypically non-related populations. *Mechanisms of Ageing and Development*, *179*, 23–35. DOI: 10.1016/j.mad.2019.02.001 PMID: 30738080

Tun, M. H., Tun, H. M., Mahoney, J. J., Konya, T. B., Guttman, D. S., Becker, A. B., Mandhane, P. J., Turvey, S. E., Subbarao, P., Sears, M. R., Brook, J. R., Lou, W., Takarao, T. K., Scott, J. A., & Kozyrskyj, A. L. (2018). Postnatal exposure to household disinfectants, infant gut microbiota and subsequent risk of overweight in children. *Canadian Medical Association Journal*, *190*(37), E1097–E1107. DOI: 10.1503/cmaj.170809 PMID: 30224442

Turnbaugh, P. J., Ley, R. E., Mahowald, M. A., Magrini, V., Mardis, E. R., & Gordon, J. I. (2006). An obesity-associated gut microbiome with increased capacity for energy harvest. *Nature, 444*(7122), 1027–1031. DOI: 10.1038/nature05414 PMID: 17183312

Ubeda, C., Taur, Y., Jenq, R. R., Equinda, M. J., Son, T., Samstein, M., Viale, A., Socci, N. D., van den Brink, M. R. M., Kamboj, M., & Pamer, E. G. (2010). Vancomycin-resistant *Enterococcus* domination of intestinal microbiota is enabled by antibiotic treatment in mice and precedes bloodstream invasion in humans. *The Journal of Clinical Investigation, 120*(12), 4332–4341. DOI: 10.1172/JCI43918 PMID: 21099116

Verdi, S., Jackson, M. A., Beaumont, M., Bowyer, R. C. E., Bell, J. T., Spector, T. D., & Steves, C. J. (2018). An investigation into physical frailty as a link between the gut microbiome and cognitive health. *Frontiers in Aging Neuroscience, 10*, 398. DOI: 10.3389/fnagi.2018.00398 PMID: 30564113

Vernocchi, P., Del Chierico, F., & Putignani, L. (2020). Gut microbiota metabolism and interaction with food components. *International Journal of Molecular Sciences, 21*(10), 3688. DOI: 10.3390/ijms21103688 PMID: 32456257

Walker, A. W., Ince, J., Duncan, S. H., Webster, L. M., Holtrop, G., Ze, X., Brown, D., Stares, M. D., Scott, P., Bergerat, A., Louis, P., McIntosh, F., Johnstone, A. M., Lobley, G. E., Parkhill, J., & Flint, H. J. (2011). Dominant and diet-responsive groups of bacteria within the human colonic microbiota. *The ISME Journal, 5*(2), 220–230. DOI: 10.1038/ismej.2010.118 PMID: 20686513

Wang, F., Baden, M. Y., Guasch-Ferré, M., Wittenbecher, C., Li, J., Li, Y., Sun, Q., Rimm, E. B., Manson, J. E., Willett, W. C., Hu, F. B., & Qi, L. (2022a). Plasma metabolite profiles related to plant-based diets and the risk of type 2 diabetes. *Diabetologia, 65*(7), 1119–1132. DOI: 10.1007/s00125-022-05692-8 PMID: 35391539

Wang, F., Ugai, T., Haruki, K., Wan, Y., Akimoto, N., Arima, K., Zhong, R., Twombly, T. S., Wu, K., Yin, K., Zhang, X., Giovannucci, E. L., Willett, W. C., & Ogino, S. (2022b). Healthy and unhealthy plant-based diets in relation to the incidence of colorectal cancer overall and by molecular subtypes. *Clinical and Translational Medicine, 12*(8), e893. DOI: 10.1002/ctm2.893 PMID: 35998061

Wang, J., Qie, J., Zhu, D., Zhang, X., Zhang, Q., Xu, Y., Wang, Y., Mi, K., Pei, Y., Liu, Y., Jia, G., & Liu, X. (2022). The landscape in the gut microbiome of long-lived families reveals new insights on longevity and aging – relevant neural and immune function. *Gut Microbes, 14*(1), e2107288. DOI: 10.1080/19490976.2022.2107288 PMID: 35939616

Wu, L., Zeng, T., Zinellu, A., Rubino, S., Kelvin, D. J., & Carru, C. (2019). A cross-sectional study of compositional and functional profiles of gut microbiota in Sardinian centenarians. *mSystems*, *4*(4), e00325–e19. DOI: 10.1128/mSystems.00325-19 PMID: 31289141

Xiao, Y., Dong, J., Yin, Z., Wu, Q., Zhou, Y., & Zhou, X. (2018). Procyanidin B2 protects against d-galactose-induced mimetic aging in mice: Metabolites and microbiome analysis. *Food and Chemical Toxicology*, *119*, 141–149. DOI: 10.1016/j.fct.2018.05.017 PMID: 29751077

Xu, H. Y., Li, Q. C., Zhou, W. J., Zhang, H. B., Chen, Z. X., Peng, N., Gong, S. Y., Liu, B., & Zeng, F. (2023). Anti-oxidative and anti-aging effects of probiotic fermented ginseng by modulating gut microbiota and metabolites in Caenorhabditis elegans. *Plant Foods for Human Nutrition (Dordrecht, Netherlands)*, *78*(2), 320–328. DOI: 10.1007/s11130-023-01055-9 PMID: 36947370

Yang, J., & Yu, J. (2018). The association of diet, gut microbiota and colorectal cancer: What we eat may imply what we get. *Protein & Cell*, *9*(5), 474–487. DOI: 10.1007/s13238-018-0543-6 PMID: 29713943

Yatsunenko, T., Rey, F. E., Manary, M. J., Trehan, I., Dominguez-Bello, M. G., Contreras, M., Magris, M., Hidalgo, G., Baldassano, R. N., Anokhin, A. P., Heath, A. C., Warner, B., Reeder, J., Kuczynski, J., Caporaso, J. G., Lozupone, C. A., Lauber, C., Clemente, J. C., Knights, D., & Gordon, J. I. (2012). Human gut microbiome viewed across age and geography. *Nature*, *486*(7402), 222–227. DOI: 10.1038/nature11053 PMID: 22699611

Yoo, S., Jung, S. C., Kwak, K., & Kim, J. S. (2024). The role of prebiotics in modulating gut microbiota: Implications for human health. *International Journal of Molecular Sciences*, *25*(9), 4834. DOI: 10.3390/ijms25094834 PMID: 38732060

Yu, X., Wu, X., Qiu, L., Wang, D., Gan, M., Chen, X., Wei, H., & Xu, F. (2015). Analysis of the intestinal microbial community structure of healthy and long-living elderly residents in Gaotian Village of Liuyang City. *Applied Microbiology and Biotechnology*, *99*(19), 9085–9095. DOI: 10.1007/s00253-015-6888-3 PMID: 26298698

Chapter 11
Ionizing Radiation–Induced Microbiota Dysbiosis:
From Intestinal Imbalance to Physiological Dysfunction

Saloua Mabsor-Zgandaoui
https://orcid.org/0009-0006-4601-9059

Biology and Health Laboratory, Department of Biology, Faculty of Sciences, Ibn Tofail University, Morocco

ABSTRACT

Ionizing radiation, whether environmental, diagnostic, or therapeutic, profoundly alters the gut microbiota, a key regulator of metabolism, nutrient absorption, and immunity. Radiation exposure disrupts microbial diversity, reduces beneficial taxa, and favors opportunistic species, impairing functions such as short-chain fatty acid production, vitamin synthesis, and bile acid metabolism. These disturbances weaken intestinal integrity and trigger systemic inflammation. In radiotherapy, especially for abdominal or pelvic cancers, dysbiosis is linked to gastrointestinal toxicity, inflammation, and reduced treatment tolerance. Radiation-induced microbial changes also affect gut–brain communication, influencing cognitive and emotional functions. Drawing from animal and human studies, this chapter explores how radiation reshapes microbial ecosystems and impacts host physiology. Understanding these mechanisms is vital for predicting radiation responses and developing microbiota-based strategies to protect intestinal and systemic health.

DOI: 10.4018/979-8-3373-4382-2.ch011

1. INTRODUCTION

The human gut is host to a complex microbial ecosystem composed of several billion microorganisms that play an essential role in digestion, metabolism and immune regulation. This dynamic balance, known as the gut microbiota, plays a central role in maintaining homeostasis. Any profound change in its composition or functioning could lead to significant disruptions, affecting not only intestinal health, but also distant physiological systems, such as the nervous system or energy metabolism (Dekaboruah et al. 2020).

Among the exogenous factors that can alter the gut microbiota, ionizing radiation (IR) occupies a special place. Whether environmental, medical or accidental, IR induces cell and tissue damage through direct and indirect pathways. Radiation triggers specific reactive oxygen species (ROS) and reactive nitrogen species (RNS) that cause oxidative damage which, unlike that generated in host cells, targets gut microbiota populations (Mabsor-Zgandaoui, Rachmoune, et al. 2025; Mabsor-Zgandaoui, Moussaif, et al. 2025).

In animals as well as in humans, shows that exposure to IR alters the composition and diversity of the gut microbiota. This often results in a decrease in beneficial bacteria, such as Lactobacillus, Bifidobacterium or certain species that produce short-chain fatty acids (SCFAs) and an expansion of opportunistic species, such as Proteobacteria. Such dysbiosis compromises vital functions such as fiber fermentation, vitamin and protective metabolite production, or even the integrity of the epithelial barrier. Over the long term, these disturbances promote inflammation, intestinal permeability alteration, and increased susceptibility to infection and systemic disease (Vancamelbeke and Vermeire 2017; Yang et al., 2025).

In clinical conditions, in patients who undergo abdominopelvic radiotherapy, such microbiota changes are associated with higher gastrointestinal toxicity, which is manifested by diarrhea, abdominal pain and sometimes with a tolerance to treatment. Moreover, certain recent findings imply that there is a relationship between RI-induced dysbiosis and damage at the intestinal-brain axis level, which may be responsible for cognitive or emotional disturbances arising under irradiation (Eaton et al. 2022).

It is therefore essential to understand the mechanisms by which IRs alter the gut microbiota, not only to appreciate the biological effects of these exposures, but also to design preventive or therapeutic interventions. The use of targeted strategies, such as probiotics, prebiotics, postbiotics or faecal microbiota transplants opens up new perspectives in the prevention or restoration of gut health in cases of radiation exposure (Cusumano et al. 2025; Cannizzaro et al. 2025; Gulliver et al. 2022).

This chapter aims to present in detail the impact of IR on the gut microbiota, explaining the mechanisms of action, alterations in composition and metabolic function, and their physiological and clinical implications. It draws on the latest findings in the literature and highlights emerging trends in radiation protection through microbiome modulation.

2. HISTORICAL PERSPECTIVE ON THE GUT MICROBIOTA: AN ECOLOGICAL BARRIER

The human gut microbiota is a complex community of bacteria, archaea, viruses, yeasts and fungi. It has an estimated cell density of nearly 10^4 bacterial cells and transforms individuals into true holobionts, comprising roughly half their cells being microbial in origin. They are all actively engaged in digestion, metabolism, and immunity, and their dysregulation. Dysbiosis, is now recognized to be a significant causative factor in a wide range of pathologies, from metabolic derangements to inflammatory or neurodevelopmental diseases (Sarah Maurel 2024).

2.1. Early observations (17th–19th centuries)

The scientific study of microbiota began in the 17th century, when Antoni van Leeuwenhoek first observed microorganisms, which he called 'animalcules,' in his own stool using his sophisticated microscope. However, it was not until the 19th century that their role in pathology began to be studied. In 1842, John Goodsir described *Sarcina ventriculi* in vomit, establishing the first link between a microbe and a digestive disease (Lewandowska-Pietruszka, Figlerowicz, and Mazur-Melewska 2022).

The 19th century marked a revolution: Pasteur and Koch formulated the germ theory, relegating the old miasma theory to the background. The cholera epidemic of 1854, studied by John Snow, provided decisive proof: the disease was transmitted by contaminated water. In 1883, Koch isolated *Vibrio cholerae*, confirming this mechanism and laying the foundations for his famous postulates linking a pathogen to a disease (Blevins and Bronze 2010).

2.2. Early 20th century: emergence of the beneficial role of microbiota

The turn of the 20th century saw the emergence of a new vision: microbes are not only pathogenic, some can be beneficial. Élie Metchnikov, working in Pasteur's laboratory, received the Nobel Prize (1908) for his work on phagocytosis. He also proposed that the consumption of yoghurt containing *Bacillus bulgaricus* explained the longevity of *Bulgarian peasants*, paving the way for probiotic therapy (Metchnikoff,

2004). Theodor Escherich described *Bacterium coli* commune, renamed *Escherichia coli*, and highlighted the importance of breast milk in protecting against childhood infections (Farré-Maduell and Casals-Pascual 2019). Henry Tissier discovered bifidobacteria in the stools of breastfed infants, suggesting their protective role and therapeutic potential against diarrhoea. The First World War further highlighted this protective role.

In 1917, *Alfred Nissle* isolated a strain of *E. coli* resistant to dysentery, which was developed as a probiotic and is still used today in the treatment of chronic inflammatory bowel disease (IBD) (Farré-Maduell and Casals-Pascual 2019).

2.3. Mid-20th Century: experimental models and ecological concepts

During the first half of the 20th century, a fundamental question emerged: is it possible to live without microbiota?

Experiments on animals stimulated under axenic conditions (sine germine) as early as the 1930s provided insightful answers: Axenic mice have an atrophied small intestine, a hypertrophied caecum, slowed transit, hypoplastic colonic mucosa and a 20% loss of cell populations. In terms of immunity, they show a significant decrease in IgA and increased susceptibility to infections. These observations demonstrate that the microbiota is not only essential for digestion, but also for neurological and immune development (Luczynski et al. 2016).

Within the same decades, Carl Woese's bacterial reclassification distinguishes bacteria, archaea and eukaryotes, rendering the notion of an 'intestinal flora' obsolete in favor of a 'microbiota'. At the same time, microbiologist René Dubos proposes the idea of the microbiota as an integrated ecosystem in its host, anticipating contemporary thinking (Fry 2024).

2.4. The Sequencing Revolution and Major Projects (21st Century)

The advent of high-throughput sequencing in the late 2000s ushered in a new era. Two major projects sparked this revolution:

The Human Microbiome Project (HMP) launched in 2007 by the NIH, and MetaHit (2008), project Indo-European. These initiatives allow the mapping of thousands of microbiome genomes. Many of the microorganisms are still described as OTU (Operational Taxonomic Units), but with this approach, systematic relationships between dysbiosis and chronic pathologies (obesity, diabetes, MICI, neurologic disorders) are revealed (Lewandowska-Pietruszka, Figlerowicz, and Mazur-Melewska 2022).

Today, balance of the microbiota (eubiose) is considered a health status essential to health. Its opposite, the dysbiosis, is a quantitative, qualitative, or functional disorder of this ecosystem with local (intestinal permeability, inflammation) and systemic (entero-cerebral axis, metabolism, immunity) consequences.

3. ANATOMY OF THE INTESTINE, MICROBIAL COMPOSITION AND ENVIRONMENTAL DISRUPTORS

3.1. Intestinal organogenesis

Research into the origin and formation of the digestive tract has long been marked by a debate between two theories: preformation, according to which the embryo is a miniature version of the adult, and epigenesis, which considers development to be a gradual process starting from an undifferentiated mass. Aristotle's observations on the development of the chick in the egg already supported epigenesis, but it was not until the 18th century, thanks to the work of Caspar Friedrich Wolff, that this theory was confirmed. Wolff demonstrated that organs, including the intestine, form gradually from cellular folds, thus introducing the concept of embryonic layers (endoderm, mesoderm and ectoderm), which are the origin of all tissues and organs (Van Speybroeck, De Waele, and Van De Vijver 2002).

In humans, prenatal development is divided into two main phases: the embryonic period (up to 8 weeks), characterised by the formation of organs, and the foetal period, during which growth and maturation take place. The major event is gastrulation, which forms the three embryonic layers and the body axes. The primitive digestive tract derives from the endoderm, formed by the folding of the embryo during the 4th week in humans (E7.5 to E9.5 in mice) (Sarah Maurel 2024).

The regionalisation of the digestive tract then occurs under the influence of molecular signal gradients, which guide the differentiation of segments into the oesophagus, stomach, small intestine and colon. At the same time, the intestinal epithelium, which is initially simple, evolves into a more complex organisation: pseudostratified then columnar, along a cranio-caudal axis. Between the 7th and 9th week of pregnancy, intestinal villi appear, increasing the absorption surface area. Later, between the 11th and 12th weeks, intestinal crypts emerge, which harbour Lgr5+ stem cells, ensuring the constant renewal of the epithelium (Sato et al. 2009; Wang et al., 2019).

Post-natal development involves regression of colique villosities and maturation of colon crypts. This structural organisation along the crypts-villi axis will be the basis for intestinal function in adults, allowing an equilibrium between regeneration, absorption, and defence. Recent progress in developmental biology, including the development of intestinal organoids from pluripotent stem cells (Sato et al. 2009), underlines the importance of this knowledge for modelling and understanding digestive pathologies.

3.2. Ontogenesis of the intestinal barrier and related functions

The intestinal barrier is a complex organism that develops during embryonic development and continues to mature after birth. It is composed of a set of physical, chemical, immune and ecological barriers that interact to maintain the balance between tolerance to microbial and food antigens and defence against pathogens.

Ontogenesis begins with the differentiation of the endoderm into a primitive intestinal tube, which gradually specialises into the different segments of the digestive tract. Epithelial cells differentiate into different specialised lineages, and the intestinal immune system (such as Peyer's patches and intraepithelial lymphocytes) develops. In new-borns, the intestinal barrier is still immature, which explains its increased permeability to antigens and a higher risk of enteric infections. With microbial colonisation and dietary diversification, the barrier strengthens and acquires its full functionality.

3.3. A physical-chemical barrier: the intestinal epithelium

The intestinal epithelium is the first line of defense against the luminal environment. It consists of a polarized single-cell layer, renewed every 4 to 5 days, which plays a key role in the selectivity of exchanges between the intestinal lumen and the internal environment (Vancamelbeke and Vermeire 2017).

3.3.1. The secretory lineage

The intestinal epithelium, which is constantly regenerating, relies on a differentiation process driven by cryptic stem cells. The secretory lineage is one of many lineages resulting from this differentiation: it occupies a strategic position in the body, as it plays an essential role in maintaining intestinal homeostasis and protecting the body from external aggressions. This lineage is composed mainly of four cell types: enteroendocrine cells, goblet cells, Paneth cells and tuft cells. Each of these has specific functions which, when combined, regulate the intestinal barrier, intercellular communication and the immune response (Vancamelbeke and Vermeire 2017).

Enteroendocrine cells represent less than 1% of the epithelial population, but they constitute the largest endocrine system in the body. They secrete a wide range of peptide hormones and biogenic amines, such as serotonin, glucagon-like peptide-1

(GLP-1), ghrelin and peptide YY. These regulate intestinal motility, enzyme secretion and nutrient absorption, and help control satiety and energy metabolism. Their function within the intestinal-brain axis is currently greatly appreciated, as they act as a bridge between signals derived from the microbiome and central regulation of physiological processes. Current research emphasizes the fact that enteroendocrine cells are sensitive to metabolites from the microbiome, such as short-chain fatty acids (SCFA), pointing to the involvement of the intestinal microbiome in hormonal regulation (Yang et al., 2025).

Goblet cells, on the other hand, are responsible for the synthesis and secretion of mucins, mainly MUC2, which form the protective mucus covering the intestinal epithelium. This mucus forms a viscous barrier that limits the adhesion and translocation of pathogenic bacteria to epithelial cells. It also provides an ecological support for commensal bacteria, which feed on glycoproteins in the mucus. In pathological conditions, such as chronic inflammatory bowel disease (IBD), a change in mucin secretion or destruction of the mucus leads to increased intestinal permeability and contributes to chronic inflammation (Gieryńska et al. 2022).

Paneth cells, located at the bottom of Lieberkühn crypts, are essential for innate intestinal immunity. They secrete antimicrobial peptides such as defensins, lysozyme and phospholipase A2, which limit the proliferation of pathogenic bacteria. They also contribute to microbiota homeostasis by promoting a balance between beneficial bacteria and potential pathogens. In addition, they provide trophic signals essential for the maintenance of intestinal stem cells, particularly via the Wnt pathway (Vancamelbeke and Vermeire 2017).

Tuft cells, although less studied, are emerging as important players in immune and chemosensory signaling. They are characterized by microvilli in bundles ('tufts') and are responsible for detecting parasitic and chemical signals in the intestinal lumen. These cells produce, in particular, interleukin-25 (IL-25), which triggers the type 2 immune response, essential for defense against helminths. In addition, they appear to interact closely with nerve fibers, promoting the integration of enteric-nervous signals. Their exact function in intestinal pathologies remains under study, but data point towards their implication in immune remodeling in the setting of chronic inflammation (Vancamelbeke and Vermeire 2017).

3.3.2. Intercellular junctions

Intestinal epithelial integrity is based on the cohesion of cells with each other, ensured by a complex network of intercellular junctions. These organelles are essential for preserving the intestinal barrier, selecting nutrients that pass through, and protecting against microbial translocation. The three main types of junctions are tight junctions, adherens junctions (zonula adherens and macula adherens/desmosomes) and gap junctions (Gieryńska et al. 2022).

Tight junctions are the first line of control for paracellular permeability. They are formed by transmembrane proteins such as claudin, occludin and JAM (junctional adhesion molecule), associated with the actin cytoskeleton by ZO (zonula occludens) adapter proteins. The system controls the selective transmission of ions and small molecules, but prevents the uncontrolled diffusion of macromolecules and bacteria. Disruptions to these junctions, which are generally induced by oxidative stress, pro-inflammatory cytokines (TNF-α, IFN-γ) or exposure to ionizing radiation, lead to intestinal hyperpermeability, known as "leaky gut" (Gieryńska et al. 2022).

Adherent junctions (zonula adherens) form an adhesion ring beneath tight junctions, consisting largely of cadherins (E-cadherin) and catenins. They are essential for the mechanical cohesion of epithelial cells and for the transmission of signals regulating cell polarity and differentiation. Macula adherens, or desmosomes, increase this cohesion by strongly immobilizing cells to each other using specific proteins such as desmoplakin and keratin. These structures give the intestinal epithelium its resistance to mechanical stress and shear flows induced by the passage of luminal contents (Yang et al., 2025).

Lastly, *gap junctions* provide for the direct passage of small molecules and ions between neighboring epithelial cells. They consist of connexins that aggregate to produce transmembrane channels. These junctions are essential for coordinating cellular response, such as transmission of calcium signals and coordination of epithelial secretion. They also have roles in tissue repair mechanisms and regulated apoptosis (Gieryńska et al. 2022).

Recent studies have highlighted the relevance of alterations in these junctions to the development of various intestinal pathologies, ranging from IBD to colorectal cancer. For instance, decreased expression of claudin-1 and occludin has been correlated with loss of barrier integrity and an increased risk of inflammation (Neurath, Artis, and Becker 2025).

3.4. An ecological barrier: the role of gut microbiota

The gut microbiota, composed of nearly 10^{14} microorganisms from the major phylogenic groups Firmicutes, Bacteroidetes, Actinobacteria and Proteobacteria, is an evolutionarily dynamic ecological barrier protecting the host from external attacks. Its diversity and balance are crucial for maintaining intestinal homeostasis. One of its main roles is to compete with pathogens for nutrients and epithelial adhesion sites. By colonising the mucosa at a rapid rate, commensal bacteria prevent the implantation of opportunistic microorganisms, a process known as colonisation resistance (Dekaboruah et al. 2020). Recent work has demonstrated that some strains of Lactobacillus and Bifidobacterium are able to generate antimicrobial peptides that are capable of inhibiting the direct growth of pathogenic enterobacteria, reinforcing such a barrier action (Vinayamohan et al. 2024).

The microbiota plays a key role in stimulating and regulating the intestinal immune system. It is involved in the development of regulatory T cells and in the formation of secretory immunoglobulin A (IgA), which limits the penetration of antigens and pathogens through the mucosa. Recent studies using axenic mouse models have shown that the absence of microbiota leads to profound immaturity of intestinal lymphoid structures and an impaired immune response to infections (León and Francino 2022).

The fundamental role of the microbiota has been established from studies conducted on germ-free (GF) mice or animals treated with antibiotics, confirming the idea that the development of the immune system coincides with the acquisition of a complex microbiota. GF mice have immature gut-associated lymphoid tissue (GALT), a decrease in the number of intestinal lymphocytes, decreased immunoglobulin (Ig) A production, and impaired antimicrobial peptides compared to colonized controls. Microbiota colonization restores many of these alterations, but some can only be restored if colonization occurs early in development (Salvo-Romero, Stokes, and Gareau 2020).

However, an imbalance in this community, or dysbiosis, can have harmful consequences. It often results in a decrease in beneficial butyrate-producing bacteria and an increase in pathobionts. It is associated with chronic inflammatory bowel disease (IBD), but also with metabolic diseases such as obesity and type 2 diabetes, as well as neurological disorders through the gut-brain axis. A number of studies suggested that alterations in the gut microbiota might cause the progression of neurodegenerative diseases such as Alzheimer's and Parkinson's disease by leading towards systemic inflammation and intestinal permeability (Ullah et al. 2023).

Thus, the gut microbiota is not only an ecological shield against pathogens; it is a true metabolic and immunomodulatory organ whose balance is essential to maintaining health. Recent advances in metagenomics and metabolomics confirm that restoring functional microbiota through approaches such as prebiotics, probiotics or faecal microbiota transplantation offers promising therapeutic prospects for many dysbiosis-related diseases (Dekaboruah et al. 2020).

4. THE EFFECT OF IONIZING RADIATION ON THE GUT MICROBIOME

Ionizing radiation consists of energy that is capable of removing electrons from atoms or molecules and thus ionizing them. IR is the result of decay from radionuclides and may either be electromagnetic waves (gamma (γ) or X-rays) or particles (alpha, beta, or neutrons) (Mabsor-Zgandaoui, Rachmoune, et al. 2025). Radiation-material interaction results in indirect and direct effects, ranging from free radical formation (mostly from water molecules) to the DNA molecule's alteration and eventual destruction (Mabsor-Zgandaoui, Moussaif, et al. 2025).

The intestinal tract has a high rate of cell renewal, a huge bacterial density, and exposure to physical and chemical stresses like bile, ROS/RNS, pH, bile acid, that strongly influence the microbial ecology. IR whether medical (repeated imaging, radiotherapy), environmental or from outer space, introduces oxidative stress and molecular damage that can affect both the host and microbes simultaneously (Fernandes et al. 2021). The cascading effects include: (a) high luminal oxidative stress, (b) barrier damage (tight junctions, mucus), (c) alterations in available nutrient substrates (fiber, mucins), (d) local/systemic inflammation that reconfigures ecological niches, and (e) changes in immobility/emptying and secretion that alter transit. IR triggers measurable dysbiosis decreased α-diversity, β-diversity reshaping, correlated with digestive toxicity and clinical outcomes (Wang et al., 2025).

Potential tissue damage after exposure depends on the radiation dose and the radiosensitivity of the tissues. The most radiosensitive cells are those that divide rapidly, are well nourished, and have high metabolic activity. However, above given thresholds, it is known that predictable acute effects will occur irrespective of the tissue (Figure 1).

Figure 1. Direct and Indirect effect of Ionizing radiation.

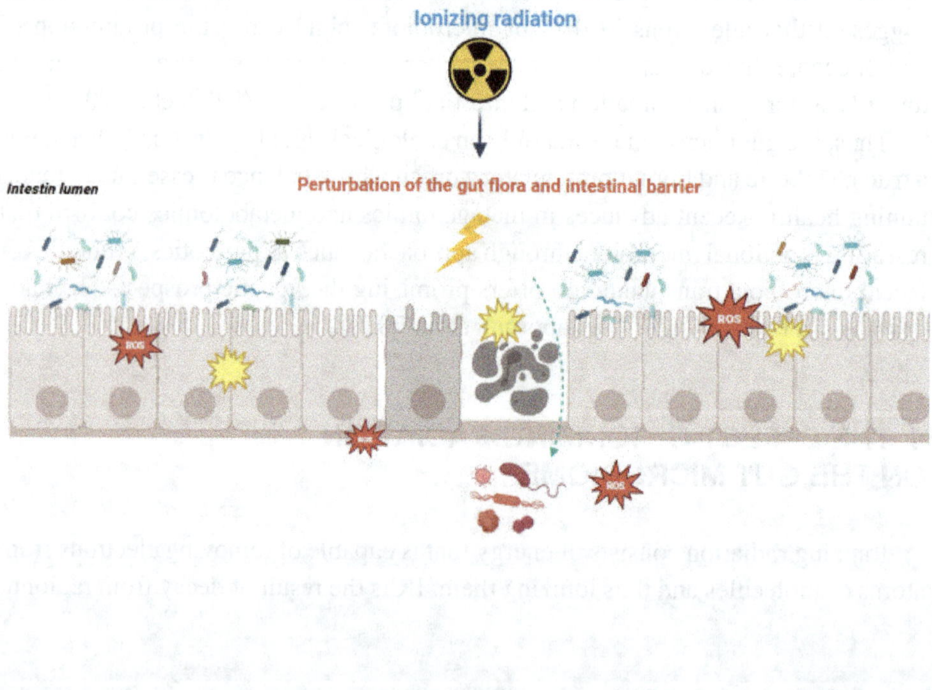

4.1. Mechanisms of action: from photons to the microbiotic phenotype

IR exerts its biological effects through two main mechanisms: direct damage and indirect damage. In the case of direct damage, the energy deposited by IR directly targets essential macromolecules in microbial cells, such as DNA, proteins and membrane lipids, causing irreversible structural alterations. Bacterial DNA can thus undergo single- and double-strand breaks, base modifications or cross-links, compromising the viability of microorganisms and their ability to reproduce (Mabsor-Zgandaoui, Rachmoune, et al. 2025).

Indirect damage is linked to the ionization of water and the cascade formation of ROS and nitrogen species (RNS), in particular the hydroxyl radical (OH-), superoxide anion (O2-) and peroxynitrite (ONOO–). These highly reactive molecules induce oxidative stress that damages DNA, proteins and lipids, thereby exacerbating the loss of functionality of intestinal microorganisms. The extent of this damage depends on the radiation dose, dose rate and oxygenation of the intestinal environment (Mabsor-Zgandaoui, Rachmoune, et al. 2025) (Figure 1).

However, radiosensitivity varies considerably from one bacterial species to another. This variability is influenced by cell wall structure, the presence of DNA repair systems such as RecA and the SOS response, and the ability of certain species to form protective biofilms. In addition, bacteria in the stationary phase or in a slowed metabolic state often show better tolerance to radiation stress than those in the exponential phase.

It is crucial to mention that IR has the potential to remodel the intestinal ecosystem by disturbing the ecological equilibrium. Certain aerotolerant species and *Proteobacteria*, i.e., *Escherichia coli* or *Enterobacter spp*., seem to benefit from the post-irradiation environment with its surplus of ROS, elevated nitrosated derivatives, and reduced competition with radiosensitive bacteria. This dynamic can lead to marked dysbiosis, where protective bacteria such as *Firmicutes* and *Bacteroidetes* decline in favor of opportunistic taxa that promote inflammation and metabolic complications (Fernandes et al. 2021).

Recent reviews (2023–2025) thus highlight a dual interaction of IR with the gut microbiota: on the one hand, a direct action through damage to the vital structures of microorganisms, and on the other hand, indirect effects mediated by changes in the host's intestinal environment, such as mucosal alteration and immune disruption. All of these mechanisms explain the complexity of microbial responses to radiation and the contribution of the microbiota to post-irradiation pathophysiology.

4.2. Host-mediated effects

The effects of IR on the gut microbiota are not restricted to direct damage to microorganisms. Much of the dysbiosis observed following irradiation is in fact, the result of changes in the gut ecosystem orchestrated by the host. These alterations involve epithelial damage, disruption of mucus and secretory cells, deregulation of microbial metabolism, and profound immune effects, which together redefine the available microbial niches and promote the emergence of opportunistic species (Shukla et al. 2016).

One of the first events triggered by irradiation is disruption of the integrity of the intestinal epithelium and its tight junctions. Key proteins such as occludin, claudins and zonula occludens-1 (ZO-1) are disorganised or fragmented after exposure, resulting in increased paracellular permeability, commonly referred to as "leaky gut". This loss of barrier function allows microbial components such as LPS and other pathogen-associated molecular patterns (PAMPs) to pass into the chorion. These signals activate inflammatory pathways, notably via TNF-α, IFN-γ and IL-1β, creating a pro-inflammatory microenvironment. The latter not only amplifies tissue damage, but also promotes the establishment of opportunistic pathobionts that take advantage of increased permeability and inflammation (Shukla et al. 2016).

Radiation also affects intestinal mucus and Paneth cells, two essential pillars of the physicochemical barrier. The expression and secretion of MUC2, a major mucus glycoprotein, are reduced, which diminishes the protective layer separating the luminal flora from the epithelium. Paneth cells see their antimicrobial granules (defensins, lysozyme) altered, which leads to a reduction in the trophic signals necessary for the maintenance of intestinal stem cells. Paneth cells see their antimicrobial granules altered, leading to a reduction in the trophic signals necessary for the maintenance of cryptic intestinal stem cells and a decrease in antimicrobial pressure on inflammophilic species. The cryptic niche then becomes more vulnerable, with compromised regeneration and colonization favored by opportunistic pathogenic bacteria (Neurath, Artis, and Becker 2025).

IR profoundly modulates the metabolism of microbial substrates. The decrease in butyrogenic bacteria, such as *Faecalibacterium prausnitzii* and *Roseburia*, results in a marked reduction in the production of SCFAs, particularly butyrate. However, this metabolite is the main source of energy for colonocytes and a major regulator of tight junction assembly via AMPK activation and occludin stabilization. The loss of butyrate creates a vicious circle: the weakening of the epithelial barrier increases the passage of PAMPs, which intensifies inflammation, which in turn further reduces butyrogenic populations.

Normal microbiota stimulates a delicate balance between regulatory T cells (Treg) and T helper 17 cells (Th17), as well as sustained IgA production and signaling via pattern recognition receptors (PRRs) such as TLR and NOD. After irradiation, this dialogue is disrupted: the Treg/Th17 balance is upset, IgA production drops, and PRR pathways are abnormally activated by the excessive passage of PAMPs. In addition, certain metabolites derived from tryptophan are reduced, weakening the IL-22/REG3 loops responsible for maintaining epithelial integrity and antimicrobial resistance. Taken together, these disruptions create a mucosal environment that is unfavorable to protective symbionts and conducive to the proliferation of inflammatory bacteria (Belkaid and Hand 2014).

Evidence has also demonstrated disruption of the gut microbial community during and after pelvic radiotherapy. Clinical and animal research conducted on patients who underwent pelvic irradiation showed a dynamic change in the composition of the gut microbiota, including changes in the abundance of specific taxa and microbial diversity. Disruption of the balance of the gut microbiome is also correlated with gastrointestinal diseases such as chronic IBD. In addition, radiation damage to the intestinal epithelial barrier increases the permeability of bacteria into the lumen and triggers immune responses.

4.3. Microbial composition modifications

4.3.1. Frequent taxonomic specificities

These ecological modifications following irradiation result in relatively robust taxonomic signatures, observed both in animal models and in critically ill patients who have already undergone radiotherapy treatments. The *Firmicutes* and *Bacteroidetes* phyla, which generally dominate the gut microbiota, are significantly reduced after irradiation, particularly butyrogenic genera such as *Faecalibacterium* and *Roseburia*. Similarly, beneficial bacteria such as *Lactobacillus* and *Bifidobacterium*, which strengthen the mucosal barrier and produce protective metabolites, are reduced. On the other hand, there is an expansion of opportunistic and aerotolerant species, such as those belonging to the phylum *Proteobacteria* (e.g. *Escherichia coli, Enterobacter*), but also other genera such as *Alistipes, Akkermansia* and certain species of *Verrucomicrobia*. These species take advantage of the inflammatory environment and post-irradiation oxidative stress. However, the severity of this dysbiosis depends on the context: dose, fractionation, irradiated area, but also the initial state of the microbiota and confounding factors such as diet or antibiotic therapy (Yang et al., 2025).

4.3.2. Dose, fractionation and location

The impact of IR on the gut microbiota is greatly influenced by the location of the irradiation field, the dose and the fractionation regimen. Pelvic and abdominal fields cause the most significant changes in the microbiota, as they directly irradiate the parts of the intestine that are richest in microbial biomass. Several observational studies and experimental series show that after pelvic irradiation, α diversity decreases rapidly during the first few weeks, reflecting an overall depletion of microbial richness that goes hand in hand with the onset of clinical symptoms (diarrhoea, abdominal pain, fatigue) (Yang et al., 2025).

Fractionation (small repeated doses as distinct from a single dose) influences the extent and dynamics of dysbiosis. Fractionated regimens (~1.8–2.0 Gy/fraction for a total of 45–50 Gy) in clinical radiotherapy induce 'progressive' dysbiosis: α diversity gradually decreases as the cumulative dose increases, and some β diversity remains affected in a high proportion of patients after treatment. Conversely, acute irradiation patterns (IRT or high-dose targeted irradiation) show instantaneous and abrupt collapses of the microbial community. Consequently, even if the loss of diversity is uniform, the kinetics (sudden vs. gradual) and persistence (complete recovery vs. incomplete restoration) depend on the fractionation and volume irradiated. This is why pelvic radiotherapy studies have reported correlations between cumulative dose and the severity of gastrointestinal symptoms, and between baseline microbial composition and the risk of acute toxicity: initial profiles dominated by proteobacteria and characterised by a low abundance of butyrogenic bacteria predispose to grade ≥ 2 diarrhoea during radiotherapy. Subsequent research conducted on cohorts of prostate cancer patients confirms that early faecal composition is a reliable predictor of acute gastrointestinal toxicity. Ultimately, the precise location is important, as the microbial composition itself is segmental and bacterial density is not uniform along the intestine. Pelvic niches, particularly the rectum and sigmoid colon, are compact and highly specialised. Ultimately, the precise is important, as the microbial composition itself is segmental and bacterial density is not uniform along the intestine (Eaton et al. 2022). Pelvic niches, particularly the rectum and sigmoid colon, are compact and highly specialized (Iacovacci et al., 2024; Wang et al., 2021).

4.3.3. Acute vs. chronic exposure

The temporal kinetics of microbial alterations depend on the mode of exposure. In murine models of acute irradiation (high-dose segmental irradiation or TBI), dysbiosis rapidly sets in: longitudinal studies show, within 24 to 72 hours, a marked regression in the metabolic pathways involved in the production of short-chain fatty acids (SCFAs), a disruption of epithelial tight junctions (claudins, occludin) and a depletion of the mucus layer. These initial events have two significant and connected effects: first, loss of functional metabolism (less butyrate, reduced colonocytic energy, AMPK and tight junction assembly compromised); second, structural change making the lamina propria accessible to PAMPs, supporting bacterial translocation and local systemic inflammatory response. Current research affirms that this impairment of SCFA metabolism and the mucin layer is not only premature but can be sustained even in the medium term, causing chronic sequelae in certain patients.

The experimental relationship between mucositis and dysbiosis has been studied: in a murine model of pelvic irradiation, it was demonstrated that mucositis precedes dysbiosis, i.e. tissue changes and inflammation are observed within the first 24 hours, while qualitative alterations in microbial composition are generally delayed and appear later. This sequence characterises the model in which IR first compromises the host (epithelium, mucus, junctions), and where microbial ecological disruption is secondary to this although downstream, dysbiosis causes and prolongs inflammation. This model has therapeutic implications: early maintenance of the epithelium and mucus layer intact (through antioxidants, mucoprotectors, targeted nutrition) could reduce secondary dysbiosis (Li et al. 2021).

In humans, fractionated exposures administered in radiotherapy trigger microbial alterations in 'stages': faecal chemistry varies with each degree of cumulative dose and, in a fraction of patients, the community does not recover to its baseline state after treatment cessation. Longitudinal cohort studies in pelvic oncology demonstrate a decline in α-diversity during the first week of RT and the persistence of differences in β-diversity in patients with chronic symptoms several months after treatment.

Certain studies have even demonstrated that the baseline composition (pre-RT) correlates with the risk of acute toxicity: patients with low levels of butyrogenic bacteria and a predominance of *Proteobacteria* were more likely to experience severe diarrhea during RT. These findings highlight the potential usefulness of pre-treatment microbacterial profile as a predictive biomarker and the potential for targeted preventive intervention measures before or during radiotherapy. Acute vs chronic is manifested in the way the impairment of microbiome functions (SCFA, bile acid conjugation, derivatives of tryptophan) manifests as first energy and immunomodulating losses (acute phase), then a stable reorganization of metabolic and immune networks (chronic phase) (Gulliver et al. 2022).

In the acute stage, butyrate decreases impaired the energy supply to colonocytes and reduced AMPK and pro-integrity of junction pathways activation; simultaneously, indole loss reduced AhR activation and IL-22/REG3 production, reducing antimicrobial defense. These functional changes explain why initial damage to the barrier predisposes to bacterial translocation and inflammation, and why, in some patients, this feedback loop becomes self-perpetuating and develops into chronic enteritis (Jameus et al. 2024).

4.3.4. Summary and clinical implications

The literature points to an integrative model: IR primarily affects the host (tight junctions, epithelium, mucus), inducing early mucositis that anticipates and predisposes to subsequent secondary dysbiosis; pelvic-abdominal localisation and fractionated regimens (small cumulative doses) provide the most clinically applicable profiles, with early decline in α diversity and persistent change in β diversity in some patients; acute exposures produce very rapid AGCC production and changes in mucosal layer thickness (24 to 72 hours), while fractionated regimens lead to progressive synchronous dysbiosis with accumulation of symptoms. They provide a rational basis for targeted prevention and treatment approaches: functional maintenance of the microbiota, timely defense of the barrier, and controlled trials of probiotics/FMT in high-risk patients identified on the basis of the pre-RT microbiome (Gulliver et al. 2022).

4.4. Functional changes: metabolites, metabolic pathways and barrier

4.4.1 SCFAs (acetate, propionate, butyrate)

The short-chain fatty acids (SCFAs) acetate, propionate and, in particular, butyrate is one of the metabolic pivots through which the microbiota maintains colonic physiology.

Butyrate provides direct energy to colonocytes, induces local oxidative respiration, activates AMPK and contributes to the tightening of tight junctions, reducing the permeability of the colonic mucosa. Butyrate directly provides energy to colonocytes, induces local oxidative respiration, activates AMPK and participates in tightening tight junctions, thereby reducing epithelial permeability. At the immunological level, butyrate is an inhibitor of histone deacetylases, inducing Treg and suppressing the amplification of pro-inflammatory responses; it also exerts antioxidant effects that counteract some of the oxidative stress induced by radiation (Cannizzaro et al. 2025).

These actions are responsible for the fact that the depletion of butyrogenic bacteria (*Faecalibacterium, Roseburia*) is directly linked to the weakening of the barrier and the worsening of the clinical effects of radiation. Several animal and human studies have noted a reduction in SCFAs immediately after irradiation, as well as downregulation of tight junction proteins and upregulation of bacterial translocation markers. Restoration of AGCC via increased fermentable fiber, administration of prebiotics or microencapsulated butyrate supplements improves barrier integrity and reduces endotoxinaemia in preclinical models, oral formulations of microencapsulated butyrate and translational trials in oncology patients are underway and show promising signs of reducing acute mucositis and treatment-related diarrhea.

In addition to butyrate, functional disruption of fermentation pathways has system-wide effects: acetate and propionate are involved in hepatic metabolism and inflammatory tone regulation, and their depletion is accompanied by an alteration in the faecal and plasma metabolomic profile observed after IR. Current metabolomic analyses confirm that the post-irradiation metabolic signature is characterized by a degradation of microbial fermentation products and an increase in oxidative markers, thus providing a more resilient functional readout than taxonomy alone (Sun et al. 2024; Cazzaniga et al. 2024).

4.4.2. Bile and vitamins

The microbiota is responsible for converting primary bile acids excreted by the host into secondary bile acids via microbial enzymatic processes (7α-dehydroxylation). Secondary bile acids act as ligands for nuclear and membrane receptors, modulating intestinal motility, epithelial permeability, and mucosal immunity (Guo et al. 2023).

Irradiation disrupts the taxonomic composition and enzymatic capacity of communities, leading to alteration of the bile pool (change in primary/secondary ratios) and deregulation of FXR/TGR5 signaling, which can result in motility disorders, increased inflammation and impaired epithelial repair. Recent studies highlight imbalances in bile metabolism after irradiation and demonstrate that modulation of bile acids (through analogues, supplements or microbial modulation) can mitigate some of the consequences (Guo et al. 2023).

Simultaneously, microbial pathways replacing vitamin biosynthesis (mainly B vitamins and vitamin K) are at risk of RI-induced diversity loss. Commensal bacteria contribute to the local availability of these cofactors, which are vital for nucleotide synthesis, redox maintenance and cell regeneration. These pathways have been shown to exhibit functional reductions based on irradiation by means of metabolomic and metagenomic analysis, signifying a plausible effect on tissue and local coagulation repair (vitamin K). Such findings call for targeted vitaminomic studies in irradiated subjects and consideration of applied nutritional intake or supplementation where indicated (Guo et al. 2023).

4.4.3. Tryptophan derivatives and AhR activation

The microbial metabolites of tryptophan, indoles and their derivatives, activate the aromatic hydrocarbon receptor (AhR) in epithelial and mucosal immune cells. AhR activation stimulates IL-22 production, induces the expression of antimicrobials such as REG3γ, and promotes epithelial regeneration. AhR activation stimulates IL-22 production, induces the expression of antimicrobials such as REG3γ, and promotes epithelial regeneration. Following irradiation, the depletion of indole-producing commensals reduces this protective pathway: the decrease in AhR activators results in lower IL-22/REG3 levels, less effective crypt repair, and greater susceptibility to microbial translocation. Current research, such as that on intestinal organoids and mouse models, shows that certain indole metabolites have radioprotective activity in vitro and in vivo, preserving crypt viability and reducing post-irradiation inflammation. These findings pave the way for the use of AhR ligands derived from the microbiota or dietary precursors (tryptophan-rich diets) as adjuvant therapies to limit IR-induced mucosal damage (Rueda et al. 2024).

5. THERAPEUTIC APPROACHES AND FUNCTIONAL MODULATION STRATEGIES

Understanding functional changes guides specific therapeutic approaches, ranging from simple nutritional treatment to sophisticated biological treatment. These treatments aim to (1) restore the integrity of the epithelial barrier, (2) maintain or restore the protective functions of the microbiome and (3) inhibit or slow the growth of pathobionts.

Fermentable fiber and nutrition. Increasing the intake of fermentable fiber (inulin, FOS, resistant starch) promotes butyrogens and replenishes SCFA reserves; Recent studies indicate that high-fiber diets may reduce the toxic gastrointestinal side effects of radiotherapy and could potentially improve antitumor response through immune-metabolic modulation. Clinical trials are underway to determine the value of specific nutritional support during RT.

Prebiotics, probiotics and synbiotics. Recent meta-analyses and trials show that probiotic formulations reduce the frequency and severity of chemotherapy/radiotherapy-induced diarrhea in certain clinical settings. Efficacy depends heavily on the strain, timing of administration and the patient's immune status. Butyrate-promoting probiotics or consortia comprising SCFA producers appear very promising for limiting mucositis. Synbiotics (prebiotics + probiotics) may have an effect. Synbiotics (prebiotic + probiotic) may have a synergistic effect by feeding the administered strains. However, large-scale randomised trials and safety studies are needed, particularly in immunocompromised patients. Postbiotics and butyrate supplements.

Direct administration of butyrate (topically, orally microencapsulated, or as an enema) has been shown in preclinical and small clinical trials to have positive effects on mucosal integrity and reduction of symptoms of radical proctitis. Postbiotics (isolated microbial metabolites), such as SCFAs or indole derivatives, promote direct delivery of the missing function without full restoration of the microbial community, which may be advantageous in controlled therapeutic windows. Controlled-release formulations of indole-3-aldehyde and butyrate are under development. Pharmacological modulation of bile acids and AhR. FXR/TGR5 modulating drugs or bile acid analogs can be employed to restore functional derangements following irradiation; preclinical models show that modulation of these pathways impacts tissue repair and inflammation. Selective AhR agonists or tryptophan-enriched amino acid precursors (or indole supplements) also partially restore the IL-22/REG3 pathway and improve mucosal resistance to injury in animal models, but the complexity of AhR actions, which depend on context and ligands, requires caution in extrapolation (Xie et al. 2024).

Faecal microbiota transplantation (FMT). FMT rapidly restores microbial diversity and function in models where dysbiosis is established. Case series and pilot trials report symptom relief in patients with refractory chronic radicular enteritis after FMT, with partial restoration of SCFA pathways and clinical relief. Standardization (donor selection, preparation, route of administration) and safety assessment remain challenges for widespread use (Lagier and Raoult 2016).

Strategic antibiotics and 'guided ecology'. Experimental studies suggest that targeted antibiotic therapy (e.g., oral vancomycin) may sometimes enhance the antitumor effect of RT by influencing the immunosuppressive microbiome, but it is also responsible for a loss of butyrogens and a risk of complications (dysbiosis, C. difficile). The 'guided ecology' strategy consists of considering the selective and temporary use of antibiotics, followed by guided microbial reconstitution, but this requires careful clinical assessment (Cusumano et al. 2025).

Antioxidants and mucoprotectants. Antioxidant drugs and mucus stabilizers can inhibit the first wave of epithelial lesions and therefore blunt the cascade to dysbiosis. Preclinical experiments and some pilot clinical trials support the idea of barrier protection provided that therapy is initiated early.

6. CONCLUSION

IR has profound and diverse effects on the gut microbiome, altering its composition, reducing beneficial taxa and enriching opportunistic species. Microbial alterations impair crucial functions such as SCFA production, bile acid processing, and vitamin synthesis, ultimately compromising epithelial barrier integrity and promoting inflammation. Clinically, radiation-induced dysbiosis is strongly associated with gastrointestinal toxicity, systemic immunosuppression, and potentially disturbances in the gut-brain axis. Existing data highlight that baseline microbial profiles may even predict patient response to radiotherapy, highlighting the potential of the microbiome as a mediator and biomarker of radiation effects. Reversing these disruptions through the use of microbiota-focused approaches, ranging from dietary adjustments to pre/probiotics, second-generation postbiotics, and faecal microbiota transplantation, offers promising avenues for inhibiting radiation-induced damage. Future work on the dynamics of the microbiome in the context of host response will be essential to the mission of personalized radiation protection and achieving optimal therapeutic outcomes.

REFERENCES

Belkaid, Y., & Hand, T. W. (2014). Role of the microbiota in immunity and inflammation. *Cell, 157*(1), 121–141. DOI: 10.1016/j.cell.2014.03.011 PMID: 24679531

Blevins, S. M., & Bronze, M. S. (2010). Robert Koch and the "golden age" of bacteriology. *International Journal of Infectious Diseases, 14*(9), e744–e751. DOI: 10.1016/j.ijid.2009.12.003 PMID: 20413340

Cannizzaro, R., Maiero, S., Pelizzo, P., Gulotta, M., Facchin, S., Tessarolo, G., Zucchetto, A., Matrone, F., Realdon, S., & Bortolus, R. (2025). Microencapsulated sodium butyrate in the prevention of acute radiotherapy proctitis: Single-center prospective study. *Journal of Clinical Medicine, 14*(13), 4783. Advance online publication. DOI: 10.3390/jcm14134783 PMID: 40649157

Cazzaniga, M., Cardinali, M., Di Pierro, F., Zonzini, G. B., Palazzi, C. M., Gregoretti, A., Zerbinati, N., Guasti, L., & Bertuccioli, A. (2024). The potential role of probiotics, especially butyrate producers, in the management of gastrointestinal mucositis induced by oncologic chemo-radiotherapy. *International Journal of Molecular Sciences, 25*(4), 2306. Advance online publication. DOI: 10.3390/ijms25042306 PMID: 38396981

Cusumano, G., Angeles Flores, G., Venanzoni, R., & Angelini, P. (2025). The impact of antibiotic therapy on intestinal microbiota: Dysbiosis, antibiotic resistance, and restoration strategies. *Antibiotics (Basel, Switzerland), 14*(4), 371. Advance online publication. DOI: 10.3390/antibiotics14040371 PMID: 40298495

Dekaboruah, E., Suryavanshi, M. V., Chettri, D., & Verma, A. K. (2020). Human microbiome: An academic update on human body site-specific surveillance and its possible role. *Archives of Microbiology, 202*(8), 2147–2167. DOI: 10.1007/s00203-020-01931-x PMID: 32524177

Eaton, S. E., Kaczmarek, J., Mahmood, D., McDiarmid, A. M., Norarfan, A. N., Scott, E. G., Then, C. K., Tsui, H. Y., & Kiltie, A. E. (2022). Exploiting dietary fibre and the gut microbiota in pelvic radiotherapy patients. *British Journal of Cancer, 127*(9), 1535–1546. DOI: 10.1038/s41416-022-01980-7 PMID: 36175620

Farré-Maduell, E., & Casals-Pascual, C. (2019). The origins of gut microbiome research in Europe: From Escherich to Nissle. *Human Microbiome Journal, 14*, 100065. Advance online publication. DOI: 10.1016/j.humic.2019.100065

Fernandes, A., Oliveira, A., Soares, R., & Barata, P. (2021). The effects of ionizing radiation on gut microbiota: A systematic review. *Nutrients, 13*(9), 3025. Advance online publication. DOI: 10.3390/nu13093025 PMID: 34578902

Fry, M. (2024). The discovery of archaea: From observed anomaly to consequential restructuring of the phylogenetic tree. *History and Philosophy of the Life Sciences*, *46*(2), 16. Advance online publication. DOI: 10.1007/s40656-024-00616-8 PMID: 38530473

Gieryńska, M., Szulc-Dąbrowska, L., Struzik, J., Mielcarska, M. B., & Gregorczyk-Zboroch, K. P. (2022). Integrity of the intestinal barrier: The involvement of epithelial cells and microbiota—A mutual relationship. *Animals (Basel)*, *12*(2), 145. Advance online publication. DOI: 10.3390/ani12020145 PMID: 35049768

Gulliver, E. L., Young, R. B., Chonwerawong, M., D'Adamo, G. L., Thomason, T., Widdop, J. T., Rutten, E. L., Rossetto Marcelino, V., Bryant, R. V., Costello, S. P., O'Brien, C. L., Hold, G. L., Giles, E. M., & Forster, S. C. (2022). Review article: The future of microbiome-based therapeutics. *Alimentary Pharmacology & Therapeutics*, *56*(2), 192–208. DOI: 10.1111/apt.17049 PMID: 35611465

Guo, L., Da, F., Gao, Q., Miao, X., Guo, J., Zhang, W., Li, J., Wang, J., & Liu, J. (2023). Irradiation-induced intestinal injury is associated with disorders of bile acids metabolism. *International Journal of Radiation Oncology, Biology, Physics*, *115*(2), 490–500. DOI: 10.1016/j.ijrobp.2022.08.007 PMID: 35948117

Iacovacci, J., Serafini, M. S., Avuzzi, B., Badenchini, F., Cicchetti, A., Devecchi, A., Dispinzieri, M., Doldi, V., Giandini, T., Gioscio, E., Mancinelli, E., Noris Chiorda, B., Orlandi, E., Palorini, F., Possenti, L., Reis Ferreira, M., Villa, S., Zaffaroni, N., De Cecco, L., & Rancati, T. (2024). Intestinal microbiota composition is predictive of radiotherapy-induced acute gastrointestinal toxicity in prostate cancer patients. *EBioMedicine*, *106*, 105246. Advance online publication. DOI: 10.1016/j.ebiom.2024.105246 PMID: 39029427

Jameus, A., Dougherty, J., Narendrula, R., Levert, D., Valiquette, M., Pirkkanen, J., Lalonde, C., Bonin, P., Gagnon, J. D., Appanna, V. D., Tharmalingam, S., & Thome, C. (2024). Acute impacts of ionizing radiation exposure on the gastrointestinal tract and gut microbiome in mice. *International Journal of Molecular Sciences*, *25*(6), 3339. Advance online publication. DOI: 10.3390/ijms25063339 PMID: 38542312

Lagier, J.-C., & Raoult, D. (2016). Greffe de microbiote fécal et infections. *Medecine Sciences*, *32*(11), 1015–1020. DOI: 10.1051/medsci/20163211015 PMID: 28008840

León, E. D., & Francino, M. P. (2022). Roles of secretory immunoglobulin A in host–microbiota interactions in the gut ecosystem. *Frontiers in Microbiology*, *13*, 880484. Advance online publication. DOI: 10.3389/fmicb.2022.880484 PMID: 35722300

Lewandowska-Pietruszka, Z., Figlerowicz, M., & Mazur-Melewska, K. (2022). The history of the intestinal microbiota and the gut–brain axis. *Pathogens (Basel, Switzerland), 11*(12), 1540. Advance online publication. DOI: 10.3390/pathogens11121540 PMID: 36558874

Li, K., Epperly, M. W., Acosta Barreto, G., Greenberger, J. S., & Methé, B. A. (2021). Longitudinal fecal microbiome study of total body irradiated mice treated with radiation mitigators identifies bacterial associations with survival. *Frontiers in Cellular and Infection Microbiology, 11*, 715396. Advance online publication. DOI: 10.3389/fcimb.2021.715396 PMID: 34621689

Luczynski, P., Neufeld, K. A. M. V., Oriach, C. S., Clarke, G., Dinan, T. G., & Cryan, J. F. (2016). Growing up in a bubble: Using germ-free animals to assess the influence of the gut microbiota on brain and behavior. *The International Journal of Neuropsychopharmacology, 19*(8), pyw020. Advance online publication. DOI: 10.1093/ijnp/pyw020 PMID: 26912607

Mabsor-Zgandaoui, S., Moussaif, A., El Hessni, A., Mesfioui, A., El Mzibri, M., Iddar, A., & Moutaouakkil, A. (2025). Ionising and ultraviolet radiation induce the secretion of melanin in *Tetrahymena pyriformis. The International Journal of Environmental Studies, 82*(1), 1–14. DOI: 10.1080/00207233.2024.2412455

Mabsor-Zgandaoui, S., Rachmoune, K., El Hessni, A., El Mzibri, M., Iddar, A., & Moutaouakkil, A. (2025). Effect of hydrogen peroxide pre-treatment on enhancing the cellular resistance of *Tetrahymena pyriformis* exposed to ionizing radiation. *Toxicological and Environmental Chemistry, 107*(2), 294–309. DOI: 10.1080/02772248.2025.2460804

Maurel, S. (2024). *Rôle de l'implantation du microbiote intestinal sur la susceptibilité au syndrome de l'intestin irritable à l'âge adulte* (Doctoral dissertation). Université Paris-Saclay.

Metchnikoff, I. I. (2004). *The prolongation of life: Optimistic studies (Reprint of* (1907 ed.). Springer.

Neurath, M. F., Artis, D., & Becker, C. (2025). The intestinal barrier: A pivotal role in health, inflammation, and cancer. *The Lancet. Gastroenterology & Hepatology, 10*(6), 573–592. Advance online publication. DOI: 10.1016/S2468-1253(24)00390-X PMID: 40086468

Rueda, G. H., Causada-Calo, N., Borojevic, R., Nardelli, A., Pinto-Sanchez, M. I., Constante, M., Libertucci, J., Mohan, V., Langella, P., Loonen, L. M. P., Wells, J. M., Collins, S. M., Sokol, H., Verdu, E. F., & Bercik, P. (2024). Oral tryptophan activates duodenal aryl hydrocarbon receptor in healthy subjects: A crossover randomized controlled trial. *American Journal of Physiology. Gastrointestinal and Liver Physiology, 326*(6), G687–G696. DOI: 10.1152/ajpgi.00306.2023 PMID: 38591144

Salvo-Romero, E., Stokes, P., & Gareau, M. G. (2020). Microbiota–immune interactions: From gut to brain. *LymphoSign Journal, 7*(1), 1–23. DOI: 10.14785/lymphosign-2019-0018

Sato, T., Vries, R. G., Snippert, H. J., van de Wetering, M., Barker, N., Stange, D. E., van Es, J. H., Abo, A., Kujala, P., Peters, P. J., & Clevers, H. (2009). Single Lgr5 stem cells build crypt-villus structures in vitro without a mesenchymal niche. *Nature, 459*(7244), 262–265. DOI: 10.1038/nature07935 PMID: 19329995

Shukla, P. K., Gangwar, R., Manda, B., Meena, A. S., Yadav, N., Szabo, E., Balogh, A., Lee, S. C., Tigyi, G., & Rao, R. K. (2016). Rapid disruption of intestinal epithelial tight junction and barrier dysfunction by ionizing radiation in mouse colon in vivo: Protection by N-acetyl-L-cysteine. *American Journal of Physiology. Gastrointestinal and Liver Physiology, 310*(9), G705–G715. DOI: 10.1152/ajpgi.00314.2015 PMID: 26822914

Speybroeck, L. V., De Waele, D., & Van de Vijver, G. (2002). Theories in early embryology: Close connections between epigenesis, preformationism, and self-organization. *Annals of the New York Academy of Sciences, 981*(1), 7–49. DOI: 10.1111/j.1749-6632.2002.tb04910.x PMID: 12547672

Sun, J., Chen, S., Zang, D., Sun, H., Sun, Y., & Chen, J. (2024). Butyrate as a promising therapeutic target in cancer: From pathogenesis to clinic [Review]. *International Journal of Oncology, 64*(4), 44. Advance online publication. DOI: 10.3892/ijo.2024.5632 PMID: 38426581

Ullah, H., Arbab, S., Tian, Y., Liu, C. Q., Chen, Y., Qijie, L., Khan, M. I. U., Hassan, I. U., & Li, K. (2023). The gut microbiota–brain axis in neurological disorder. *Frontiers in Neuroscience, 17*, 1225875. Advance online publication. DOI: 10.3389/fnins.2023.1225875 PMID: 37600019

Vancamelbeke, M., & Vermeire, S. (2017). The intestinal barrier: A fundamental role in health and disease. *Expert Review of Gastroenterology & Hepatology, 11*(9), 821–834. DOI: 10.1080/17474124.2017.1343143 PMID: 28650209

Vinayamohan, P., Joseph, D., Viju, L. S., Baskaran, S. A., & Venkitanarayanan, K. (2024). Efficacy of probiotics in reducing pathogenic potential of infectious agents. *Fermentation (Basel, Switzerland), 10*(12), 599. Advance online publication. DOI: 10.3390/fermentation10120599

Wang, L., Wang, X., Zhang, G., Ma, Y., Zhang, Q., Li, Z., Ran, J., Hou, X., Geng, Y., Yang, Z., Feng, S., Li, C., & Zhao, X. (2021). The impact of pelvic radiotherapy on the gut microbiome and its role in radiation-induced diarrhoea: A systematic review. *Radiation Oncology (London, England), 16*(1), 187. Advance online publication. DOI: 10.1186/s13014-021-01899-y PMID: 34563216

Wang, Q., Xu, G., Yan, O., Wang, S., & Wang, X. (2025). Radiation-induced injury and the gut microbiota: Insights from a microbial perspective. *Therapeutic Advances in Gastroenterology, 18*, 17562848251347347. Advance online publication. DOI: 10.1177/17562848251347347 PMID: 40535532

Wang, S., Walton, K. D., & Gumucio, D. L. (2019). Signals and forces shaping organogenesis of the small intestine. In *Current Topics in Developmental Biology* (Vol. 132, pp. 31–65). Academic Press., DOI: 10.1016/bs.ctdb.2018.12.001

Xie, L. W., Cai, S., Lu, H. Y., Tang, F. L., Zhu, R. Q., Tian, Y., & Li, M. (2024). Microbiota-derived I3A protects the intestine against radiation injury by activating AhR/IL-10/Wnt signaling and enhancing the abundance of probiotics. *Gut Microbes, 16*(1), 2347722. Advance online publication. DOI: 10.1080/19490976.2024.2347722 PMID: 38706205

Yang, K., Li, G., Li, Q., Wang, W., Zhao, X., Shao, N., Qiu, H., Liu, J., Xu, L., & Zhao, J. (2025). Distribution of gut microbiota across intestinal segments and their impact on human physiological and pathological processes. *Cell & Bioscience, 15*(1), 47. Advance online publication. DOI: 10.1186/s13578-025-01385-y PMID: 40241220

Yang, S., Liu, H., & Liu, Y. (2025). Advances in intestinal epithelium and gut microbiota interaction. *Frontiers in Microbiology, 16*, 1499202. Advance online publication. DOI: 10.3389/fmicb.2025.1499202 PMID: 40104591

Chapter 12
Wearable and Digital Health Technologies in Microbiome Monitoring

Radhika Kande
Independent Researcher, USA

P. Selvakumar
https://orcid.org/0000-0002-3650-4548
Department of Science and Humanities, Nehru Institute of Technology, Coimbatore, India

T. C. Manjunath
https://orcid.org/0000-0003-2545-9160
Rajarajeswari College of Engineering, Bengaluru, India

Anupama Manish Mohabansi
https://orcid.org/0009-0006-1939-8989
G.H. Raisoni College of Engineering and Management, India

T. Saminathan
SRM Institute of Science and Technology, India

ABSTRACT

In recent years, the field of microbiome research has undergone a profound transformation, driven by advances in sequencing technologies, computational biology, and the growing recognition of the microbiome's critical role in human health. The human microbiome—the collective genome of trillions of microorganisms inhabiting the body—has been implicated in a wide range of physiological processes, from digestion and immune function to mental health and metabolic regulation.

DOI: 10.4018/979-8-3373-4382-2.ch012

Understanding the dynamic interactions between these microbial communities and their host has opened up new frontiers in personalized medicine and preventive health. One of the most exciting and rapidly developing areas in this domain is the integration of microbiome monitoring with wearable and digital health technologies, which promises to revolutionize how we track, understand, and ultimately manipulate our microbial ecosystems in real-time.

INTRODUCTION

In recent years, the field of microbiome research has undergone a profound transformation, driven by advances in sequencing technologies, computational biology, and the growing recognition of the microbiome's critical role in human health. The human microbiome—the collective genome of trillions of microorganisms inhabiting the body—has been implicated in a wide range of physiological processes, from digestion and immune function to mental health and metabolic regulation. Understanding the dynamic interactions between these microbial communities and their host has opened up new frontiers in personalized medicine and preventive health. One of the most exciting and rapidly developing areas in this domain is the integration of microbiome monitoring with wearable and digital health technologies, which promises to revolutionize how we track, understand, and ultimately manipulate our microbial ecosystems in real-time. Historically, microbiome studies relied on invasive sampling methods such as stool collection, biopsies, or swabs, which, while effective for snapshot analyses, provided limited insight into the temporal dynamics and environmental influences affecting microbial populations. These traditional methods, often coupled with expensive and time-consuming laboratory processing, restricted microbiome research primarily to specialized settings and isolated time points. However, the advent of wearable biosensors and digital health platforms has begun to shift this paradigm by enabling continuous, non-invasive, and real-time monitoring of microbial-related biomarkers and physiological parameters. This transition aligns with a broader trend in healthcare toward decentralization and patient empowerment, leveraging the convergence of biotechnology, microelectronics, and data science.

Wearable devices tailored for microbiome monitoring utilize a range of innovative technologies, including biosensors capable of detecting microbial metabolites, volatile organic compounds (VOCs), and other biochemical signals indicative of microbiome activity or dysbiosis. For example, breath analyzers embedded in wearables can measure specific VOCs produced by gut microbes, offering indirect but informative markers of microbial metabolism linked to digestive health, inflammation, or disease states. Similarly, skin patches embedded with microfluidic channels and biochemical sensors can capture sweat metabolites or other secretions, providing clues about the skin microbiome's composition and health status. These devices are often paired with smartphones or dedicated digital platforms that collect, analyze, and visualize data, enabling users and healthcare providers to monitor trends, receive alerts, and make data-driven decisions(ACS Appl. Interfaces, 2020). The integration of machine learning and artificial intelligence (AI) algorithms within digital health platforms further enhances microbiome monitoring by facilitating pattern recognition, predictive analytics, and personalized recommendations. By analyzing large datasets generated from wearable sensors alongside other health metrics—such as diet, exercise, sleep patterns, and environmental exposures—AI models can identify correlations and causal links between microbiome fluctuations and health outcomes. This holistic approach supports the emergence of precision microbiome medicine, where interventions such as dietary modifications, probiotics, prebiotics, or targeted therapeutics can be tailored to an individual's unique microbial profile and lifestyle factors. Moreover, the continuous data streams provided by wearables allow for dynamic tracking of treatment efficacy and early detection of microbiome perturbations that may signal disease onset or progression.

Commercial interest and research investment in this area have surged, leading to a diverse ecosystem of startups, academic labs, and healthcare providers developing microbiome-monitoring wearables and digital tools. Companies are exploring devices that combine microbiome data with other biosignals—such as heart rate variability, glucose levels, and physical activity—to create integrated health insights. For instance, smart toilets equipped with sensors to analyze stool consistency, microbiome composition, and other biomarkers are emerging as potential home-based diagnostic tools. Meanwhile, advances in miniaturized sequencing technologies and point-of-care testing are anticipated to further enhance the resolution and accessibility of microbiome data, possibly enabling direct microbial profiling in real time. Despite these promising developments, several challenges remain in realizing the full potential of wearable microbiome monitoring. Technological limitations include the sensitivity, specificity, and stability of biosensors in complex biological matrices, as well as issues related to data accuracy and reproducibility(Aggarwal et al., 2023). The interpretation of microbiome data is complicated by high inter-individual variability, transient microbial shifts, and the influence of confounding factors such as diet, medication, and environment. Additionally, ethical and privacy concerns arise with the continuous collection of personal biological data, necessitating robust frameworks for data security, informed consent, and equitable access. Regulatory pathways for approval and clinical validation of microbiome-based diagnostics and interventions are still evolving, requiring multidisciplinary collaboration between scientists, clinicians, technologists, and policymakers.

Looking forward, the future of microbiome monitoring in wearable and digital health technologies is poised to be shaped by several key trends. First, advancements in multi-omics integration—combining genomics, metabolomics, proteomics, and microbiomics data—will deepen insights into host-microbiome interactions and enable more precise phenotyping of health states. Second, the proliferation of interoperable digital health ecosystems will facilitate data sharing and longitudinal tracking across populations, enhancing epidemiological studies and public health initiatives. Third, user-centric design and behavioral science will be critical to ensure adherence, engagement, and meaningful health outcomes, particularly as microbiome monitoring transitions from research settings into everyday wellness and clinical care. Finally, personalized microbiome interventions may evolve from static treatments to adaptive, feedback-driven therapies that dynamically respond to microbial changes captured by wearables, ushering in an era of truly personalized, real-time microbial management. In conclusion, the convergence of microbiome science with wearable and digital health technologies represents a transformative revolution in health monitoring and management(Artif. Intell. Med., 2024a). By enabling continuous, non-invasive, and personalized tracking of microbial ecosystems, these innovations hold the promise to not only deepen our understanding of the microbiome's role in health and disease but also to empower individuals and clinicians with actionable insights. As the technology matures and integration challenges are addressed, microbiome monitoring is expected to become a cornerstone of precision health, contributing to more effective prevention, diagnosis, and treatment strategies tailored to the unique microbial and physiological makeup of each individual. The microbiome revolution is thus not only reshaping biomedical research but also redefining the future of healthcare delivery in the digital age.

UNDERSTANDING THE MICROBIOME: IMPORTANCE FOR HUMAN HEALTH

The human microbiome—the vast and diverse collection of microorganisms, including bacteria, viruses, fungi, and archaea, that inhabit various ecological niches of the human body—has emerged as a pivotal factor influencing health, disease, and overall well-being. Comprising trillions of microbial cells that outnumber human cells by an estimated ratio of about 1.3:1, and encoding a genetic repertoire far surpassing that of the human genome, the microbiome constitutes a dynamic, integral component of our biology. This microbial community, established early in life and shaped by genetics, diet, environment, and lifestyle, performs a multitude of essential functions that are indispensable for normal physiological processes. Understanding the microbiome's importance is critical for unraveling the complex interactions between host and microbes that dictate health outcomes, and it is rapidly transforming the fields of medicine, nutrition, immunology, and even mental health. One of the most fundamental roles of the microbiome is its contribution to digestion and metabolism. In the gut, where microbial density and diversity are highest, commensal bacteria facilitate the breakdown of complex polysaccharides, fibers, and other dietary components that are otherwise indigestible by human enzymes(Artif. Intell. Med., 2024b). This microbial fermentation results in the production of short-chain fatty acids (SCFAs) such as acetate, propionate, and butyrate, which serve as vital energy sources for colonocytes and exert anti-inflammatory effects. SCFAs also play a role in regulating lipid and glucose metabolism, thus influencing energy homeostasis and metabolic health. Disruptions in microbial composition—commonly referred to as dysbiosis—have been linked to metabolic disorders such as obesity, type 2 diabetes, and non-alcoholic fatty liver disease, highlighting the microbiome's key role in metabolic regulation and disease susceptibility.

Beyond metabolism, the microbiome is indispensable for the development and function of the immune system. Microbial colonization from birth educates the immune system to distinguish between harmful pathogens and benign or beneficial microbes, thus fostering immune tolerance and preventing inappropriate inflammatory responses. Commensal microbes stimulate the production of regulatory T cells and influence the balance between pro- and anti-inflammatory cytokines, shaping immune responses throughout life. This microbial-immune crosstalk is crucial for maintaining mucosal barrier integrity and defending against infections. Conversely, perturbations in the microbiome have been associated with autoimmune diseases, allergies, asthma, and inflammatory bowel diseases (IBD), indicating that microbiome composition and diversity are integral to immune homeostasis and the prevention of immune-mediated pathologies(Deng et al., 2023). The microbiome's influence extends to the central nervous system via the gut-brain axis, a bidirectional communication pathway linking the gastrointestinal tract and the brain through neural, hormonal, and immune signaling. Emerging research has demonstrated that gut microbes can affect brain function and behavior by producing neurotransmitters, modulating systemic inflammation, and impacting the hypothalamic-pituitary-adrenal (HPA) axis. Alterations in gut microbiota composition have been implicated in neurodevelopmental disorders such as autism spectrum disorder (ASD), as well as neuropsychiatric conditions including depression, anxiety, and Parkinson's disease. This expanding understanding of the microbiome's role in mental health suggests potential novel therapeutic avenues targeting the gut microbiota for neurological and psychiatric disorders.

The skin microbiome, another critical microbial ecosystem, serves as the first line of defense against environmental insults and pathogens. Comprising a complex consortium of bacteria, fungi, and viruses adapted to the unique microenvironments of the skin, these microbes contribute to the maintenance of skin barrier function, pH balance, and antimicrobial defense. Dysbiosis of the skin microbiome has been linked to common dermatological conditions such as acne, eczema, psoriasis, and atopic dermatitis. Similarly, the oral microbiome, residing in the mouth's diverse niches, plays an essential role in maintaining oral health by preventing colonization by pathogenic species and supporting immune responses. Imbalances in oral microbial communities are associated not only with dental diseases such as caries and periodontitis but also with systemic conditions like cardiovascular disease, diabetes, and adverse pregnancy outcomes(Diabetes Technol. Ther., 2024). The human microbiome also participates in the detoxification of xenobiotics, including environmental chemicals, drugs, and carcinogens, thereby influencing drug metabolism and efficacy. Microbial enzymes can modify pharmaceutical compounds, impacting bioavailability, therapeutic effects, and side effect profiles. This interplay underscores the importance of microbiome composition in personalized medicine, where understanding an individual's microbial makeup could optimize drug dosing and minimize adverse reactions.

In addition to these functional roles, the microbiome acts as a crucial modulator of human evolution and adaptation. The co-evolution of humans with their microbiota has shaped immune defenses, dietary capabilities, and even reproductive fitness. Variations in microbiome composition across different populations and geographic regions reflect adaptations to diverse diets, environments, and cultural practices, emphasizing the microbiome's role in human diversity and resilience. The loss of microbial diversity in modern, industrialized societies due to lifestyle changes, antibiotic use, and urbanization has been hypothesized to contribute to the rising incidence of chronic inflammatory and metabolic diseases, a phenomenon described as the "disappearing microbiota" hypothesis. Given the microbiome's extensive influence on health, its study has spurred the development of novel diagnostic, preventive, and therapeutic strategies. Microbiome profiling through high-throughput sequencing technologies allows the identification of microbial signatures associated with specific diseases, enabling earlier diagnosis and risk stratification. Therapeutically, interventions such as probiotics, prebiotics, synbiotics, fecal microbiota transplantation (FMT), and diet modifications aim to restore microbial balance and improve health outcomes. While many of these approaches show promise, challenges remain in understanding the complexity of microbe-host interactions and the personalized nature of microbiome-based therapies.

Ethical, legal, and social implications of microbiome research also warrant consideration, especially as microbiome data becomes integrated into clinical and consumer health platforms. Issues related to data privacy, informed consent, and equitable access to microbiome-based interventions are critical to address to ensure that the benefits of microbiome science are realized in a fair and responsible manner. In conclusion, the microbiome represents a fundamental dimension of human biology with profound implications for health and disease. Its importance spans numerous physiological systems and disease processes, underscoring the need for comprehensive research and thoughtful clinical translation. As our understanding deepens, the microbiome is poised to become a cornerstone of personalized medicine, preventive healthcare, and innovative therapeutic development. Embracing the complexity and dynamism of the human microbiome offers unprecedented opportunities to enhance human health, resilience, and longevity in the 21st century and beyond(Diagnostics, 2019). Wearable technologies designed to track microbiome health represent a groundbreaking frontier in personalized medicine and health monitoring, leveraging the convergence of biotechnology, miniaturized sensors, microfluidics, and digital platforms to provide continuous, real-time insights into the dynamic microbial ecosystems that inhabit the human body. Traditionally, understanding the human microbiome—complex communities of bacteria, fungi, viruses, and other microorganisms—relied on periodic, often invasive sampling methods such as stool collection, skin swabs, or mucosal biopsies followed by laboratory analysis. These approaches, while invaluable for advancing microbiome science, offer only snapshots of microbial composition and activity, lacking the temporal resolution necessary to capture rapid microbial fluctuations and their interactions with environmental and lifestyle factors. Wearable technologies, by contrast, hold the promise of transforming microbiome research and clinical care by enabling non-invasive, longitudinal, and personalized monitoring of microbial-related biomarkers directly from the body or through indirect proxies, thereby opening new avenues for health management, disease prevention, and therapeutic optimization.

At the core of wearable microbiome tracking devices are advanced biosensors capable of detecting a broad spectrum of biochemical signals associated with microbial activity, such as metabolites, volatile organic compounds (VOCs), proteins, and nucleic acids. These sensors integrate with miniaturized electronic circuits, microfluidic systems, and wireless communication modules to continuously collect, process, and transmit data to paired digital devices such as smartphones, tablets, or cloud-based platforms. Among the most extensively explored modalities are breath analyzers, skin patches, ingestible capsules, and smart textiles, each targeting specific microbiome niches and health indicators. Breath-based wearables leverage the detection of VOCs generated by gut and respiratory tract microbes. The human breath contains hundreds of VOCs, some of which are metabolites or signaling molecules produced by microbiota, including short-chain fatty acids, alcohols, ketones, and sulfur-containing compounds. Sensors such as metal oxide semiconductor sensors, gas chromatography–mass spectrometry (GC-MS) miniaturized components, and infrared spectroscopy integrated into handheld or wearable breathalyzers can quantify these compounds, enabling the indirect assessment of gut microbial metabolism and health status. For example, elevated hydrogen or methane in breath tests can indicate small intestinal bacterial overgrowth (SIBO) or dysbiosis, while specific VOC signatures have been associated with gastrointestinal diseases such as irritable bowel syndrome (IBS), inflammatory bowel disease (IBD), and colorectal cancer(Duan et al., 2025). Breath-based wearables offer the advantages of being non-invasive, user-friendly, and capable of real-time monitoring, which can facilitate early detection of dysbiosis and personalized dietary or therapeutic interventions. Additionally, these patches may incorporate stimuli-responsive elements that release therapeutics or modulate local environments based on detected microbial signals, merging diagnostics with targeted treatments in a closed-loop system. Ingestible electronic capsules represent a cutting-edge class of wearables designed for direct gastrointestinal microbiome monitoring(Front. Anal. Sci., 2024).

Figure 1. Recent advances in smart wearable sensors for continuous human health monitoring

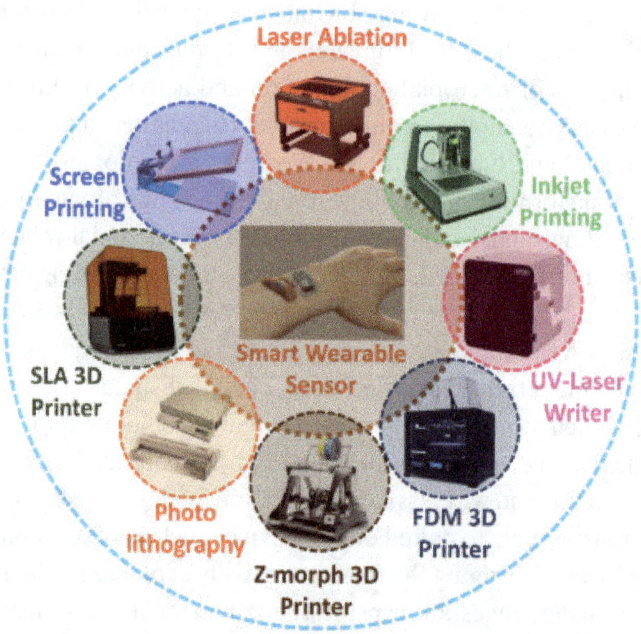

Smart textiles and wearable garments incorporating microbiome-sensing technologies are emerging as promising tools for continuous health monitoring in daily life. By embedding biosensors into fabrics, these textiles can non-invasively sample skin secretions and detect microbial biomarkers associated with health or disease states. For example, antimicrobial resistance genes or pathogen-specific metabolites could be identified, supporting early infection detection or management of chronic skin conditions. The combination of comfort, unobtrusiveness, and connectivity positions smart textiles for applications in sports medicine, occupational health, and personalized skincare. The data collected by microbiome-tracking wearables are typically processed through sophisticated digital health platforms that employ machine learning, artificial intelligence (AI), and big data analytics to interpret complex microbial and physiological signals(Front. Physiol., 2024). These platforms integrate microbiome data with other health metrics—such as diet, physical activity, sleep, medication use, and environmental exposures—to generate personalized health insights, predictive models, and actionable recommendations. For instance, AI algorithms can detect early signs of microbiome imbalance, suggest dietary adjustments, or recommend probiotic supplementation tailored to the user's unique microbial profile and lifestyle. Furthermore, remote monitoring capabilities enable healthcare providers to track patient status continuously, adjust treatments dynamically, and improve clinical outcomes, thereby advancing the paradigm of precision medicine.

Despite the significant promise, several challenges and limitations accompany wearable microbiome technologies. Sensor sensitivity and specificity remain critical technical hurdles, as the biochemical milieu in sweat, breath, or gut fluids is complex, dynamic, and subject to interference by environmental and physiological factors. Calibration, standardization, and validation of sensor outputs against gold-standard laboratory methods are essential to ensure reliable and clinically meaningful data. Privacy and data security issues also arise due to the sensitive nature of microbiome and health information, necessitating robust cybersecurity measures and ethical frameworks for data use and sharing. Moreover, user adherence, device ergonomics, and cost-effectiveness are practical considerations that influence the adoption and scalability of these technologies. The future of wearable microbiome monitoring is poised to benefit from advances in sensor miniaturization, materials science, synthetic biology, and multi-omics integration(Frontiers in Digital Health, 2025). Emerging nanomaterials and flexible electronics will enhance sensor performance and comfort, while engineered microbial biosensors capable of producing detectable signals in response to specific stimuli may revolutionize in situ microbial sensing. Integration of genomic, transcriptomic, proteomic, and metabolomic data streams will provide holistic insights into host-microbe interactions and disease mechanisms. Additionally, the development of interoperable health ecosystems and standardized data frameworks will facilitate large-scale studies, population health management, and equitable access to microbiome-based healthcare innovations.

WEARABLE BIOSENSORS: REAL-TIME MICROBIOME TRACKING

Wearable biosensors represent a cutting-edge innovation at the intersection of biotechnology, electronics, and data science, designed to provide continuous, real-time monitoring of biological parameters relevant to the human microbiome. The advent of these miniaturized, highly sensitive devices marks a significant advancement from traditional microbiome sampling methods, which are typically invasive, discrete, and limited to laboratory analysis. Wearable biosensors enable dynamic monitoring of microbial-related biomarkers directly from the body or its secretions, facilitating an unprecedented understanding of microbiome fluctuations and their impact on health(Frontiers in Bioeng. Biotechnol., 2025). By leveraging advances in materials science, microfabrication, microfluidics, and molecular detection, wearable biosensors offer promising tools for precision health, early disease detection, and personalized therapeutics that respond to the complex and temporal nature of the microbiome. At the core of wearable biosensors designed for microbiome tracking is the ability to detect and quantify specific biochemical signatures associated with microbial activity, including metabolites, volatile organic compounds (VOCs), enzymes, nucleic acids, and immunological markers. These sensors typically employ a variety of detection modalities such as electrochemical, optical, piezoelectric, and magnetic sensing, each with distinct advantages in sensitivity, selectivity, and integration potential. Electrochemical sensors, for instance, utilize biochemical reactions to generate electrical signals proportional to the concentration of target analytes such as short-chain fatty acids (SCFAs), lactic acid, or ammonia produced by microbes. Optical biosensors rely on fluorescence, absorbance, or surface plasmon resonance to detect changes in light properties upon binding microbial molecules or cells. Piezoelectric sensors measure mass changes or mechanical vibrations caused by molecular interactions on their surface, while magnetic sensors can track magnetically labeled microbial components or metabolites.

One prominent application of wearable biosensors for microbiome monitoring is in breath analysis. Breath contains a rich array of VOCs derived from both host metabolism and microbial fermentation processes, particularly those of the gut and respiratory microbiomes. Miniaturized gas sensors embedded into wearable breathalyzers employ metal oxide semiconductors, carbon nanotubes, or graphene-based materials to selectively detect microbial VOCs such as hydrogen, methane, ethanol, and sulfur compounds. Real-time detection of these gases provides insights into gastrointestinal disorders like small intestinal bacterial overgrowth (SIBO), inflammatory bowel disease (IBD), and colorectal cancer, where microbial metabolism is disrupted(Harindranath & Desai, 2025). Breath biosensors offer the advantages of non-invasiveness, rapid response times, and potential for continuous or frequent measurements outside clinical settings. Skin-based wearable biosensors form another important category, designed to monitor the skin microbiome and its metabolic products via sampling of sweat, sebum, or interstitial fluid. Flexible, epidermal sensors incorporating microfluidic channels and electrochemical or optical detection elements can quantify microbial metabolites such as lactic acid, urea, and antimicrobial peptides, which reflect the health of the skin's microbial ecosystem. These devices enable monitoring of skin conditions like acne, eczema, psoriasis, and infections, by detecting inflammatory markers or dysbiosis-associated molecules. Advances in stretchable electronics and biocompatible materials have enhanced the comfort, durability, and accuracy of these biosensors, allowing long-term monitoring in everyday environments.

Ingestible biosensors represent a frontier in real-time gastrointestinal microbiome tracking. These swallowable devices navigate through the digestive tract, collecting localized data on microbial metabolites, pH, temperature, and mechanical activity. Recent innovations have led to capsules equipped with biosensing elements capable of detecting microbial enzymes or nucleic acids in situ, although these technologies are still emerging. The wireless transmission of data from these capsules to external receivers provides spatially resolved, temporal microbiome profiles inaccessible through conventional stool analysis. This direct gut monitoring is vital for diagnosing localized dysbiosis, infections, and inflammatory conditions, as well as assessing responses to diet or therapeutics with high precision. Wearable biosensors generate vast quantities of complex data, necessitating integration with sophisticated digital health platforms for interpretation, visualization, and actionable feedback. Machine learning and artificial intelligence (AI) algorithms play a crucial role in deciphering patterns from multi-dimensional biosensor data, correlating microbial signatures with health outcomes, lifestyle factors, and environmental exposures(Hubballi et al., 2025). Such digital ecosystems enable personalized health insights, early warnings of microbial imbalance, and dynamic adjustment of interventions such as diet, probiotics, or medications. Remote monitoring and telemedicine applications also benefit from wearable biosensors, facilitating continuous patient supervision and data-driven clinical decision-making without the need for frequent hospital visits. The integration of biosensor data with electronic health records and clinical workflows must be handled with care to maximize benefits and minimize risks(Jagannath et al., 2024). Equitable access to these advanced technologies also warrants attention to prevent disparities in healthcare.

Future directions for wearable biosensors in microbiome tracking are highly promising. Emerging nanomaterials such as graphene, transition metal dichalcogenides, and quantum dots offer enhanced sensitivity and multiplexing capabilities. Synthetic biology approaches may enable living biosensors—engineered microbes or cells embedded within wearables that respond to microbial signals with measurable outputs. Multi-modal sensing platforms combining chemical, physical, and biological signals will provide richer, more accurate microbiome profiles. Advances in wireless power transfer and energy harvesting may support longer device lifespans and reduce the need for recharging. Integration with other omics data—genomics, metabolomics, proteomics—will facilitate comprehensive systems biology approaches to health monitoring(Kim et al., 2020). The fusion of biosensor innovation with microbiome science is thus reshaping the landscape of biomedical research and healthcare delivery for the future. One of the foremost considerations in designing microbiome-friendly wearables is the choice of materials that come into direct or indirect contact with the skin or mucosal surfaces(Kotte, Attaluri & Selvakumar, 2025). Another critical aspect in microbiome-friendly wearable design is the minimization of contamination and cross-talk between the device and microbiota(Liu et al., 2022). Since these devices often aim to monitor subtle changes in microbial populations or their metabolic products, any introduction of foreign microbes or chemicals from the device itself can confound results and impair longitudinal tracking.

User comfort and adherence are paramount to the success of microbiome-friendly wearables. Devices must be lightweight, flexible, and discreet to encourage prolonged wear, which is essential for capturing dynamic microbiome data over time. Materials must not provoke allergic reactions or dermatitis, conditions known to alter the skin microbiome and confound measurements. Design features such as adjustable straps, breathable fabrics, and skin-like elasticity enhance wearability. The devices should also be easy to apply, remove, and clean without requiring complex maintenance, as improper handling could introduce external microbes or damage sensors(Maheswaran et al., 2025). In summary, the design of microbiome-friendly wearables demands a sophisticated synthesis of material innovation, sensor technology, biological understanding, and user-centric principles to achieve accurate, reliable, and non-disruptive monitoring of the human microbiome(MDPI, 2023). These devices not only capture crucial data for advancing microbiome science but also empower individuals to engage proactively with their microbial health, potentially transforming preventive medicine and personalized therapeutics. Overcoming challenges related to biocompatibility, sensor specificity, contamination control, and user experience will be key to realizing the full potential of microbiome-friendly wearables. As this field evolves, it promises to redefine how we measure, interpret, and influence the microbiome—ushering in a new era of holistic health monitoring that embraces the intimate partnership between humans and their microbial inhabitants.

CONTINUOUS MONITORING: WEARABLE DEVICES FOR MICROBIOME HEALTH

Continuous monitoring of microbiome health via wearable devices represents a revolutionary shift in how we understand and manage the intricate microbial ecosystems that reside within and on the human body. Unlike traditional microbiome assessments, which rely on infrequent sampling and laboratory analysis, continuous monitoring enables dynamic, real-time tracking of microbial fluctuations and their interactions with host physiology, lifestyle factors, and environmental influences. This shift toward persistent observation is crucial because the microbiome is highly dynamic, responding rapidly to dietary changes, stress, medication, infections, and other stimuli. Capturing these temporal variations in microbial communities and their metabolic outputs through wearable technologies opens unprecedented opportunities for early disease detection, personalized health management, and preventive care, transforming microbiome science from a static snapshot to a living narrative of health. Wearable devices designed for continuous microbiome monitoring encompass a diverse range of sensor technologies and form factors, each tailored to specific microbial niches such as the gut, skin, oral cavity, and respiratory tract. These devices employ advanced biosensors capable of detecting key microbial metabolites, volatile organic compounds (VOCs), enzymatic activities, and molecular markers that serve as proxies for microbial composition and function. Breath analyzers, for example, continuously sample exhaled air to detect microbial VOCs like hydrogen, methane, and short-chain fatty acids, providing non-invasive insight into gut microbial fermentation and dysbiosis. Skin patches embedded with electrochemical or optical sensors monitor sweat and sebum composition, capturing metabolites and immune markers that reflect the skin microbiome's status. Ingestible capsules equipped with miniaturized sensors traverse the gastrointestinal tract, collecting spatially resolved data on microbial metabolites, pH, and temperature throughout the gut(MDPI, 2024). Smart textiles integrated with biosensors represent an emerging modality capable of long-term skin microbiome monitoring in a comfortable and unobtrusive manner.

The technology underlying continuous microbiome wearables integrates state-of-the-art sensor materials, microfluidics, low-power electronics, wireless communication, and data analytics. Biosensors leverage electrochemical detection, fluorescence, surface plasmon resonance, and gas sensing to achieve high sensitivity and selectivity for microbial biomarkers. Microfluidic systems enable controlled sample collection, filtration, and reaction within the device, enhancing signal specificity by minimizing interference from complex bodily fluids. Low-power circuit design and energy harvesting methods extend device operation, enabling prolonged wear without frequent charging. Wireless protocols such as Bluetooth Low Energy (BLE) or Near-Field Communication (NFC) facilitate seamless data transmission to smartphones or cloud platforms, where sophisticated algorithms analyze the data to identify patterns and anomalies. Continuous data streams from microbiome wearables integrate into digital health ecosystems that combine microbiome information with other physiological and behavioral metrics such as heart rate, sleep, diet, activity, and medication adherence. Artificial intelligence (AI) and machine learning models process these multidimensional datasets to provide actionable health insights(Micromachines, 2022). For instance, sudden shifts in microbial metabolites detected by a wearable breath sensor may signal early onset of gastrointestinal inflammation or infection, prompting timely medical intervention. Personalized feedback loops can suggest dietary modifications, probiotic supplementation, or lifestyle changes to restore microbial balance. Moreover, clinicians can remotely monitor patients with chronic diseases such as inflammatory bowel disease (IBD), metabolic syndrome, or skin disorders, enabling adaptive, data-driven care tailored to individual microbiome dynamics.

The continuous nature of monitoring overcomes limitations of traditional microbiome assessment, which often misses transient or episodic microbial changes linked to disease flare-ups, treatment responses, or environmental exposures. By capturing longitudinal data, wearables help delineate causal relationships between microbiome alterations and health outcomes. This temporal resolution facilitates the development of predictive models that anticipate disease progression or relapse before clinical symptoms manifest, enabling proactive healthcare strategies. Additionally, continuous microbiome monitoring empowers users with real-time awareness of their microbial health, fostering engagement in preventive behaviors and adherence to therapeutic regimens. Despite these advantages, continuous microbiome monitoring via wearables faces several challenges. Sensor accuracy and specificity are critical, given the complexity of biological matrices such as sweat, breath, or gut fluids, which contain numerous potential interferents(Nat. Electron., 2021). Ensuring reliable biomarker detection amidst variable physiological conditions and external contaminants requires robust sensor design, calibration, and signal processing. Biocompatibility and user comfort are essential to support long-term wear without causing irritation or microbiome disruption. Data privacy and security concerns must be addressed rigorously, given the sensitive nature of microbiome data, which can reveal personal health information. Regulatory pathways for approval of microbiome wearables as medical devices are still evolving, requiring evidence of safety, efficacy, and clinical utility.

Future directions in continuous microbiome monitoring envision further miniaturization and integration of multifunctional sensors capable of multiplexed detection of genetic, metabolic, proteomic, and immunological markers. Advances in synthetic biology may yield living biosensors that respond dynamically to microbial changes with enhanced sensitivity and specificity. Wearable devices are expected to become increasingly seamless, integrated into everyday clothing or accessories, enabling ubiquitous microbiome health tracking. The convergence of microbiome data with other omics layers and environmental sensing will support holistic models of health and disease, facilitating truly personalized and preventive medicine. In conclusion, wearable devices for continuous monitoring of microbiome health offer a transformative approach to understanding and managing human microbial ecosystems in real time(Nature Biomed. Eng., 2022). At their core, microbiome tracking mobile apps serve as interactive platforms that aggregate data from various sources, including user inputs, wearable biosensors, laboratory microbiome test results, dietary logs, physical activity trackers, and environmental sensors. Users typically begin by submitting baseline information—such as health history, symptoms, and dietary habits—and may upload microbiome sequencing reports obtained from direct-to-consumer or clinical testing services. Some apps integrate directly with wearable biosensors that monitor microbial metabolites through sweat, breath, or skin emissions, providing continuous or periodic real-time data streams(Nature Electronics, 2021). By harmonizing these multidimensional datasets, the apps create personalized microbiome profiles that reflect microbial diversity, abundance of key taxa, metabolic activity, and potential dysbiosis indicators. Sophisticated algorithms and machine learning models embedded within these mobile apps analyze the incoming data to detect trends, deviations, and correlations with health metrics. For instance, fluctuations in gut microbial diversity may be linked to digestive symptoms such as bloating or irregular bowel movements, while skin microbiome imbalances might correlate with acne or eczema flare-ups. Mobile apps often provide visualizations such as heatmaps, charts, and microbiome "fingerprints" to help users intuitively grasp their microbiome status and changes over time. They may also feature personalized recommendations for diet adjustments, probiotic or prebiotic supplementation, stress management, and lifestyle modifications aimed at fostering a balanced and resilient microbiome. These suggestions are frequently updated based on ongoing data collection and emerging scientific evidence, creating a dynamic, adaptive wellness plan.

Another key advantage of microbiome-focused mobile apps is their ability to facilitate longitudinal tracking and behavioral modification. By encouraging users to log food intake, medication use, sleep patterns, exercise, and symptoms, these apps build a comprehensive contextual dataset that helps identify specific factors influencing microbiome health. Real-time feedback and reminders promote adherence to recommended regimens, empowering users to take proactive steps to optimize their microbial ecosystems. Social and community features embedded within some apps create supportive environments for sharing experiences, challenges, and successes, enhancing motivation and engagement. Gamification elements, such as achievement badges or progress tracking, further incentivize sustained user interaction. Mobile apps also serve as valuable platforms for clinical research and patient management. Aggregated, anonymized data from app users can be leveraged for large-scale microbiome studies, enabling researchers to explore population-level patterns and novel biomarkers of disease or health resilience(Nature Rev. Mater., 2022). Clinicians may use these apps to monitor patient microbiome status remotely, tailoring treatments and tracking responses in chronic conditions such as inflammatory bowel disease, metabolic syndrome, or dermatological disorders. Integration with electronic health records (EHRs) and telemedicine services facilitates seamless communication between patients and healthcare providers, enhancing coordinated care.

The development of microbiome tracking mobile apps involves several technological and design challenges. Ensuring data accuracy and validity is paramount, as self-reported information and sensor-derived data are prone to variability and errors. Calibration of biosensors and standardization of microbiome data across different sequencing platforms require ongoing efforts to maintain comparability and reliability. Privacy and security considerations are critical, given the sensitive nature of microbiome data, which can potentially reveal information about diet, lifestyle, and disease risk. Developers must comply with stringent data protection regulations such as GDPR and HIPAA, employing encryption, anonymization, and secure data storage solutions to protect user information. User-friendly interfaces that accommodate diverse populations—including those with limited technical literacy—are essential to maximize accessibility and usability. Furthermore, microbiome science itself is still evolving, and translating complex scientific findings into actionable, evidence-based recommendations poses inherent difficulties. Mobile apps must carefully balance providing helpful guidance with avoiding overpromising or misinterpretation of microbiome data(NPJ Digit. Med., 2020). Collaboration between microbiologists, clinicians, bioinformaticians, and software developers is essential to ensure that app content is accurate, clinically relevant, and regularly updated to reflect advances in the field. Transparent communication about the limitations of microbiome testing and the probabilistic nature of health predictions fosters user trust and realistic expectations.

Looking ahead, the future of microbiome tracking mobile apps is poised to benefit from advances in artificial intelligence, sensor technology, and integrative health platforms. Enhanced AI-driven analytics will enable deeper insights into causal relationships between microbiome dynamics and health outcomes, facilitating predictive modeling and personalized intervention strategies. Integration with emerging wearable biosensors capable of multiplexed, real-time detection of microbial metabolites and immune markers will enrich data streams and improve monitoring granularity(Talanta, 2022a). Interoperability standards will promote seamless data exchange across apps, devices, and healthcare systems, supporting holistic health management. Additionally, augmented reality (AR) and virtual coaching interfaces may offer immersive, engaging user experiences that further motivate lifestyle changes supportive of microbiome health. In conclusion, mobile apps for tracking microbiome health and wellness represent a transformative tool in the democratization of microbiome science and personalized healthcare. By harnessing the power of data integration, real-time monitoring, and AI-driven insights, these apps empower users to actively engage with their microbial health, make informed decisions, and adopt behaviors that promote microbial diversity and stability. As technology, science, and user engagement strategies continue to evolve, mobile microbiome apps will play an increasingly central role in preventive medicine, chronic disease management, and health optimization—ushering in a new era where microbiome health is an integral part of everyday wellness.

DIGITAL PLATFORMS: ANALYZING MICROBIOME DATA

The advent of high-throughput sequencing technologies and multi-omics approaches has resulted in an explosion of microbiome data, necessitating sophisticated digital platforms for efficient, accurate, and scalable analysis. Digital platforms dedicated to microbiome data analysis serve as comprehensive ecosystems that integrate raw data processing, bioinformatics pipelines, statistical analysis, visualization tools, and interpretative frameworks to transform vast volumes of complex microbial information into actionable insights. These platforms are foundational to advancing microbiome research and translating microbiome science into clinical, commercial, and personalized health applications. Their design and functionality must address unique challenges inherent to microbiome data, including high dimensionality, compositionality, biological variability, and the need for multi-modal integration, all while maintaining accessibility for users ranging from expert bioinformaticians to clinicians and citizen scientists. At the core of microbiome digital platforms lies the capacity to handle raw sequencing data from various technologies, such as 16S rRNA gene sequencing, whole metagenome shotgun sequencing (WMS), metatranscriptomics, metabolomics, and proteomics(Saha et al., 2022). These diverse datasets require specialized preprocessing steps including quality control, adapter trimming, error correction, and assembly. State-of-the-art platforms incorporate automated workflows that streamline these procedures using established tools like QIIME2, DADA2, MetaPhlAn, HUMAnN, and others. The integration of containerized environments and cloud computing infrastructure has significantly enhanced the scalability and reproducibility of these pipelines, enabling the analysis of large cohorts or longitudinal studies that generate terabytes of data. Cloud-based platforms such as Qiita, MicrobiomeAnalyst, and MG-RAST provide users with user-friendly interfaces and powerful backend resources, democratizing access to advanced bioinformatics without the need for extensive computational infrastructure.

Beyond raw data processing, digital platforms excel in performing taxonomic and functional profiling, which are fundamental to understanding microbiome composition and metabolic potential. Taxonomic classification algorithms leverage reference databases like SILVA, Greengenes, and GTDB to assign microbial identities at various taxonomic levels, from phyla to strain. Functional profiling uses gene annotation tools and pathway databases such as KEGG, MetaCyc, and UniProt to infer microbial metabolic capabilities and interaction networks. The combined taxonomic and functional profiles enable researchers and clinicians to explore correlations between microbiome features and health or disease states. Advanced platforms implement differential abundance testing, diversity metrics calculation (alpha and beta diversity), and network analysis to reveal community structure and dynamics. Interactive visualizations—such as heatmaps, ordination plots, phylogenetic trees, and metabolic maps—facilitate data interpretation and hypothesis generation, empowering users to explore patterns intuitively(Sakthivel et al., 2025). One of the most transformative aspects of digital microbiome platforms is their capacity to integrate multi-omics and clinical data, thereby offering holistic views of microbiome-host interactions. Integrative analysis modules allow the simultaneous examination of microbial genomics, transcriptomics, metabolomics, proteomics, and immunological markers alongside patient metadata such as demographics, clinical parameters, medication use, diet, and lifestyle factors. Machine learning and artificial intelligence algorithms embedded within these platforms enable predictive modeling, biomarker discovery, and stratification of disease phenotypes based on complex microbiome signatures. For example, classifiers built on microbiome data can distinguish between healthy individuals and those with inflammatory bowel disease, colorectal cancer, or metabolic syndrome with remarkable accuracy. Longitudinal data integration supports the tracking of microbiome dynamics in response to interventions such as antibiotics, probiotics, or dietary changes, informing personalized treatment plans and adaptive clinical management.

Despite their power, microbiome digital platforms face significant analytical and interpretative challenges. Microbiome data are inherently compositional, meaning that relative abundance values are constrained and interdependent, which can lead to spurious correlations if not properly handled. Platforms must incorporate compositional data analysis methods, such as centered log-ratio transformations and advanced statistical models, to address these issues. Biological variability stemming from sample collection, DNA extraction, sequencing depth, and batch effects requires normalization and robust experimental design, which platforms must facilitate through quality assurance modules. Moreover, the heterogeneity of microbial communities across body sites, individuals, and populations complicates the establishment of universal reference baselines, necessitating the development of context-specific databases and classifiers(Sci. Rep., 2022). Data standardization efforts, including the use of standardized ontologies (e.g., MIxS) and reporting guidelines, are essential to improve comparability and meta-analyses across studies and platforms. Data privacy and security constitute another critical dimension for microbiome digital platforms, especially those handling human microbiome data linked to personal health information. Platforms must implement stringent encryption protocols, secure user authentication, and compliance with data protection regulations such as the GDPR and HIPAA. Ethical considerations around data ownership, informed consent, and responsible data sharing require transparent governance frameworks to maintain user trust and foster collaborative research. Open data initiatives and community-driven platforms play vital roles in accelerating scientific discovery by enabling data sharing and benchmarking while balancing privacy concerns.

Looking forward, digital platforms for microbiome data analysis are poised to become increasingly intelligent, integrative, and user-centric. The incorporation of artificial intelligence advances, such as deep learning models, will enhance pattern recognition and enable the discovery of subtle microbial signatures linked to health outcomes. Real-time analytics and edge computing integration may facilitate on-device microbiome monitoring and feedback, closing the loop between data collection and health intervention. Platforms will increasingly support interoperability with electronic health records (EHRs), mobile health applications, and wearable biosensors, fostering comprehensive digital health ecosystems. The rise of federated learning approaches promises collaborative data analysis across institutions without compromising data privacy. Additionally, user interfaces will become more intuitive and accessible, catering to a broad spectrum of users including clinicians, researchers, and laypersons, thereby democratizing microbiome science and its applications. In conclusion, digital platforms for analyzing microbiome data are indispensable enablers of the microbiome revolution, providing the computational backbone required to decode complex microbial ecosystems and translate these insights into meaningful health and wellness applications. By integrating advanced bioinformatics, multi-omics data fusion, machine learning, and secure data management, these platforms empower a diverse user base to harness the power of the microbiome. As the field progresses, ongoing innovation in platform design, algorithm development, and data governance will be essential to overcome current challenges and fully realize the potential of microbiome-informed precision medicine, ultimately transforming how we monitor, understand, and modulate the human microbiome for improved health outcomes.

TELEMEDICINE AND REMOTE MONITORING: MICROBIOME HEALTH

Telemedicine and remote monitoring technologies have become increasingly vital in modern healthcare, particularly in the realm of microbiome health, where dynamic, personalized, and longitudinal data are essential for understanding and managing the complex microbial ecosystems influencing human wellness(Science Transl. Med., 2018). The integration of telemedicine platforms with remote microbiome monitoring enables continuous, real-time assessment of an individual's microbiome status, facilitating timely interventions, improved patient engagement, and more personalized treatment plans without the constraints of traditional clinical settings. This transformation is especially significant for chronic and multifactorial conditions linked to microbiome imbalances, such as inflammatory bowel disease (IBD), irritable bowel syndrome (IBS), metabolic disorders, skin diseases, and even mental health conditions. By leveraging digital communication, wearable biosensors, home sampling kits, and data analytics, telemedicine and remote monitoring foster a proactive, patient-centered approach that bridges the gap between patients and healthcare providers, enabling seamless, data-driven microbiome health management. Remote microbiome monitoring encompasses a variety of technological innovations designed to collect and transmit microbiome-related data from patients' homes or everyday environments to healthcare providers for analysis and interpretation. Wearable biosensors capable of detecting microbial metabolites, volatile organic compounds (VOCs), or immune markers in sweat, breath, or skin secretions provide continuous, non-invasive data streams that reflect microbial activity and host responses. Ingestible capsules embedded with sensors offer spatially resolved sampling along the gastrointestinal tract, while home microbiome testing kits allow patients to self-collect samples such as stool, saliva, or skin swabs that are mailed to laboratories or analyzed on-site with portable devices. These technologies generate rich datasets capturing microbial composition, function, and dynamics in real time or near-real time, enabling clinicians to monitor disease activity, treatment efficacy, and lifestyle impacts remotely. Integration with mobile health applications ensures seamless data transfer, real-time alerts, and personalized feedback to patients, enhancing adherence and engagement.

Despite these advantages, implementing telemedicine and remote microbiome monitoring involves significant challenges. Ensuring the accuracy, reliability, and standardization of biosensors and home sampling devices is critical to generate clinically actionable data. Variability in sample collection, environmental contamination, and device calibration can affect data quality, necessitating rigorous validation and quality control protocols. Data privacy and security concerns are paramount, given the sensitive nature of microbiome information, which may reveal personal health risks, lifestyle habits, or disease states. Telemedicine platforms must comply with regulatory frameworks such as HIPAA and GDPR, employing encryption, secure data storage, and transparent consent processes. Additionally, disparities in digital literacy, access to technology, and internet connectivity can limit the equitable adoption of telemedicine and remote monitoring, underscoring the need for inclusive design and support strategies. Integration and interoperability remain key technical challenges, as microbiome data streams must be harmonized with electronic health records (EHRs), laboratory information systems, and other digital health tools to create comprehensive patient profiles(Sempionatto et al., 2019). Advanced data analytics, including machine learning and artificial intelligence, are essential to interpret complex microbiome datasets in clinical contexts, identify meaningful patterns, and generate predictive models for personalized interventions. Telemedicine platforms must evolve to incorporate these capabilities and support clinicians in decision-making without increasing cognitive workload or workflow disruptions.

Looking forward, the future of telemedicine and remote microbiome monitoring promises further innovation and expansion. Emerging wearable biosensors with multiplexed detection of microbial, metabolic, and immunological markers will provide deeper insights into host-microbe interactions in real time. Miniaturized, non-invasive devices capable of continuous gut microbiome surveillance could revolutionize management of gastrointestinal diseases. Integration of microbiome monitoring with other physiological sensors—tracking heart rate, glucose levels, sleep, and stress—will enable holistic digital phenotyping and multi-dimensional health assessments. Telemedicine platforms will increasingly leverage AI-driven virtual health assistants and personalized coaching to support behavior change and optimize microbiome health. Regulatory advances and standardized protocols will facilitate clinical validation and reimbursement, promoting wider adoption in routine care. In conclusion, telemedicine and remote monitoring represent transformative approaches to managing microbiome health, combining cutting-edge sensor technology, digital communication, and data analytics to enable personalized, continuous, and accessible care. These innovations empower patients and clinicians to collaboratively monitor and modulate the microbiome, improving disease management, preventive care, and overall wellness. Overcoming technological, regulatory, and social challenges through multidisciplinary collaboration will be essential to fully realize the potential of telemedicine and remote microbiome monitoring in shaping the future of precision health and microbiome-informed medicine.

PERSONALIZED MEDICINE: MICROBIOME-BASED TREATMENT

Personalized medicine, an approach that tailors healthcare interventions to individual genetic, environmental, and lifestyle factors, has witnessed a transformative evolution with the integration of microbiome science. The human microbiome—a complex, dynamic community of microorganisms inhabiting various body sites—plays a pivotal role in health and disease, influencing metabolism, immunity, and even neurological function. This understanding has catalyzed the development of microbiome-based personalized medicine, where interventions are customized based on an individual's unique microbial composition and functional characteristics. By leveraging high-resolution microbiome profiling, multi-omics integration, and advanced computational tools, clinicians and researchers are moving beyond one-size-fits-all treatments toward precision therapeutics that optimize efficacy, minimize adverse effects, and promote long-term health through targeted modulation of the microbiome. The promise of microbiome-based personalized medicine lies in its ability to address the heterogeneity of human disease by recognizing that microbial community structures and functions vary significantly between individuals and populations. Diseases such as inflammatory bowel disease (IBD), colorectal cancer, obesity, diabetes, allergies, and neuropsychiatric disorders have been linked to specific alterations in microbiome composition—often termed dysbiosis—which differ widely among patients. Traditional treatment paradigms frequently fail to account for this microbial variability, resulting in inconsistent therapeutic outcomes. In contrast, personalized microbiome interventions seek to restore or enhance beneficial microbial functions tailored to the patient's distinct microbial ecosystem, thereby improving treatment precision and patient response.

One of the foundational tools enabling microbiome-based personalized medicine is comprehensive microbial profiling through next-generation sequencing (NGS) technologies. Techniques such as 16S rRNA gene sequencing, whole-genome shotgun metagenomics, metatranscriptomics, metabolomics, and proteomics provide detailed taxonomic and functional insights into an individual's microbiome. This information facilitates the identification of microbial biomarkers predictive of disease susceptibility, progression, or therapeutic response. For example, in oncology, the composition of the gut microbiome has been shown to influence the efficacy and toxicity of immune checkpoint inhibitors, with certain bacterial taxa correlating with enhanced response rates. Personalized treatment plans can incorporate microbiome profiling to select or modify immunotherapy regimens, potentially improving clinical outcomes. Personalized microbiome interventions encompass a broad spectrum of strategies, including targeted probiotics and prebiotics, fecal microbiota transplantation (FMT), dietary modifications, antibiotics, and small molecule therapeutics designed to modulate specific microbial pathways. Targeted probiotics involve the administration of live microorganisms selected or engineered to restore missing or depleted beneficial species or functions. These probiotics may be tailored to the patient's microbiome profile, addressing specific deficits or imbalances. Similarly, prebiotics—non-digestible dietary fibers or compounds—can be personalized to stimulate the growth of beneficial microbes identified as underrepresented in a given individual. Dietary interventions personalized to microbiome data have also demonstrated efficacy in managing metabolic disorders and inflammatory conditions by promoting favorable microbial shifts.

FMT represents a more radical and potent microbiome-based therapeutic modality, wherein fecal material from a healthy donor is transferred to a patient to restore microbial diversity and function. While FMT has proven highly effective in treating recurrent Clostridioides difficile infection, its application in other diseases remains experimental, and personalized approaches are emerging to optimize donor selection and recipient matching based on microbiome compatibility and functional criteria. Advances in synthetic microbiota consortia—engineered communities of well-characterized microbial strains—promise safer, more controlled alternatives to conventional FMT, allowing precise manipulation of microbiome composition and metabolic outputs. In addition to microbial community modulation, microbiome-based personalized medicine explores host-microbe interactions at molecular and cellular levels, enabling the development of small molecule drugs and biologics that target microbial metabolites, enzymes, or signaling pathways. For instance, certain microbial metabolites such as short-chain fatty acids (SCFAs) and bile acids have profound effects on host immunity and metabolism; manipulating these pathways through personalized interventions can ameliorate inflammatory or metabolic disorders. Furthermore, pharmacomicrobiomics—the study of how the microbiome affects drug metabolism and response—highlights the potential for microbiome-informed dosing and drug selection to enhance therapeutic safety and efficacy.

Looking ahead, the future of microbiome-based personalized medicine is promising and poised for rapid advancement. Integration of multi-omics data—combining microbiome profiles with host genomics, transcriptomics, metabolomics, and environmental factors—will enable more comprehensive and accurate models of health and disease. Advances in artificial intelligence and systems biology will facilitate predictive analytics to tailor interventions dynamically and optimize treatment regimens. The development of precision probiotics, next-generation synbiotics (combinations of probiotics and prebiotics), and designer microbial therapeutics will expand the armamentarium of personalized treatments. Furthermore, longitudinal monitoring through wearable sensors and digital health platforms will allow real-time assessment of microbiome dynamics, supporting adaptive interventions and preventive care. In conclusion, microbiome-based personalized medicine represents a paradigm shift in healthcare, harnessing the complexity and individuality of the human microbiome to inform precise, effective, and patient-centered treatments. By integrating advanced sequencing technologies, bioinformatics, targeted therapeutics, and digital health tools, this approach promises to revolutionize the management of a broad range of diseases and promote long-term health through tailored microbiome modulation. Continued interdisciplinary research, technological innovation, and ethical stewardship will be essential to translate the full potential of microbiome-informed personalized medicine into clinical practice, ultimately improving outcomes and quality of life for diverse patient populations.

DISEASE PREVENTION: MICROBIOME MONITORING AND INSIGHTS

The burgeoning field of microbiome research has unveiled the intricate and critical role that the diverse communities of microorganisms inhabiting the human body play in maintaining health and preventing disease. One of the most impactful applications of microbiome monitoring in disease prevention lies in the early detection and management of chronic inflammatory conditions such as inflammatory bowel disease (IBD), rheumatoid arthritis, and allergies. For example, subtle changes in gut microbial diversity or the relative abundance of key species such as Faecalibacterium prausnitzii or Bacteroides fragilis have been correlated with disease onset and severity. By monitoring these microbial indicators over time, clinicians can identify patients at elevated risk and implement preemptive interventions including dietary modulation, probiotics, or targeted antimicrobials to restore microbial balance and avert disease progression. Similarly, microbiome insights have advanced preventive strategies in metabolic syndrome and type 2 diabetes, where specific microbial metabolites like short-chain fatty acids (SCFAs) influence insulin sensitivity and systemic inflammation(Wang et al., 2022). Personalized microbiome profiling can guide nutritional and lifestyle recommendations that favor beneficial microbial functions, thereby reducing the risk of metabolic disease. In infectious disease prevention, microbiome monitoring plays a vital role in understanding colonization resistance—the natural ability of the resident microbiota to inhibit pathogenic invasion. Disruptions caused by antibiotics or environmental factors often compromise this resistance, increasing susceptibility to infections such as Clostridioides difficile colitis, urinary tract infections, or respiratory tract infections. Continuous monitoring enables identification of vulnerability windows and supports timely interventions such as probiotic administration or fecal microbiota transplantation (FMT) to restore protective microbial communities. In hospital settings, microbiome-based surveillance can aid in infection control and antimicrobial stewardship by tracking microbial dynamics and resistance gene prevalence, ultimately reducing healthcare-associated infections. Furthermore, ethical and privacy concerns surrounding microbiome data—given its potential to reveal sensitive information about an individual's health, lifestyle, and genetic predispositions—require robust regulatory frameworks and transparent consent processes(Zheng et al., 2021). Accessibility and equity also present barriers to widespread adoption of microbiome monitoring in disease prevention. Disparities in healthcare infrastructure, digital literacy, and affordability may limit the reach of these advanced technologies, underscoring the need for inclusive design and policy interventions to ensure equitable benefits. Education and engagement initiatives are vital to enhance public understanding of microbiome health and encourage proactive participation in monitoring programs.

CONCLUSION

Looking forward, the integration of microbiome monitoring into precision public health frameworks offers exciting prospects for population-level disease prevention and health promotion. Combining microbiome data with environmental, socioeconomic, and behavioral determinants through big data analytics can inform targeted interventions and resource allocation to high-risk communities. Advances in synthetic biology and microbiome engineering may enable the development of designer microbial consortia that confer protective effects, functioning as living therapeutics to bolster host defenses and resilience. Additionally, longitudinal microbiome biobanks linked to electronic health records (EHRs) will facilitate longitudinal epidemiological studies, enabling early detection of emerging health threats and evaluation of preventive strategies at scale. In conclusion, microbiome monitoring and insights herald a new frontier in disease prevention, shifting the healthcare paradigm toward proactive, personalized, and holistic management of health. By harnessing advanced molecular technologies, digital health innovations, and computational analytics, this approach enables early detection of disease risk, informed preventive interventions, and sustained microbial homeostasis conducive to wellness. Addressing current scientific, technological, ethical, and social challenges through multidisciplinary collaboration will be essential to fully realize the preventive potential of microbiome science. Ultimately, integrating microbiome monitoring into routine healthcare promises to reduce disease burden, improve quality of life, and foster resilient health ecosystems at both individual and population levels. Disease prevention through microbiome monitoring and insights represents a transformative approach that leverages the dynamic interactions between host and microbiota to anticipate, mitigate, and preempt the onset of illness. This paradigm shift—from reactive treatment to proactive health management—is grounded in the recognition that disruptions or imbalances in the microbiome, often termed dysbiosis, are implicated in a wide spectrum of diseases ranging from infectious and inflammatory conditions to metabolic, neurological, and autoimmune disorders. Continuous microbiome monitoring, combined with sophisticated data analysis, offers unprecedented opportunities to detect early warning signs of disease, understand risk factors, personalize preventive strategies, and promote resilient microbial ecosystems conducive to long-term health. Microbiome monitoring for disease prevention employs advanced molecular and digital technologies that enable the detailed characterization and longitudinal tracking of microbial communities across various body sites such as the gut, skin, oral cavity, respiratory tract, and urogenital system. High-throughput sequencing technologies—including 16S rRNA gene sequencing and shotgun metagenomics—allow comprehensive profiling of microbial taxonomy and functional potential. When integrated with metatranscriptomics, metabolomics, and proteomics, these technologies provide multi-dimensional snapshots of microbiome activity, revealing metabolic pathways and signaling networks relevant to health and disease processes. Importantly, the temporal dimension afforded by continuous or periodic sampling enables the detection of microbiome shifts that precede clinical symptoms, serving as predictive biomarkers of disease risk or impending flare-ups.

REFERENCES

Aggarwal, V.. (2023). Electrochemical (Bio)Sensing Devices for Human Microbiome Related Biomarkers. *Sensors (Basel)*, *23*(2), 837. DOI: 10.3390/s23020837 PMID: 36679633

ACS Appl. Interfaces. (2020). *Skin-like thermal mapping devices*. DOI: 10.1021/acsami.0c04747

Artif. Intell. Med. (2024a). *Intelligent wearable assisted digital healthcare industry 5.0*. DOI: 10.1016/j.artmed.2024.103000

Artif. Intell. Med. (2024b). *Remote patient monitoring using AI: current state, applications, and challenges*. DOI: 10.1016/j.artmed.2023.102049

Deng, Z., Guo, L., Chen, X., & Wu, W. (2023). Smart Wearable Systems for Health Monitoring. *Sensors (Basel)*, *23*(5), 2479. DOI: 10.3390/s23052479 PMID: 36904682

Diabetes Technol. Ther. (2024). *Noninvasive real-time glucose monitoring in the near future*. DOI: 10.1089/dia.2024.0005

Diagnostics. (2019). *RF and microwave techniques for non-invasive glucose monitoring*. DOI: 10.3390/diagnostics9010008

Duan, L., Zhao, J., & Wang, X.. (2025). Wearable Electrochemical Biosensors for Advanced Healthcare Monitoring. *Advancement of Science*, *202411433*(2), 2411433. Advance online publication. DOI: 10.1002/advs.202411433 PMID: 39588557

Front. Anal. Sci. (2024). *Future directions: What lies ahead for smart biochemical wearables*. DOI: 10.3389/frans.2024.1509815

Front. Physiol. (2024). *Integrated framework of load monitoring: smartphone + wearables + point of care*. [DOI pending]

Frontiers in Bioeng. Biotechnol. (2025). *Wearable sensors–based assistive technologies for patient health monitoring*. DOI: 10.3389/fbioe.2025.1437877

Frontiers in Digital Health. (2025). *Returning individual wearable sensor results to participants*. DOI: 10.3389/fdgth.2025.1569452

Harindranath, S., & Desai, D. (2025). Wearable technology in inflammatory bowel disease: Current state and future direction. *Expert Review of Medical Devices*, *22*(2), 121–126. DOI: 10.1080/17434440.2025.2453561 PMID: 39798078

Hubballi, R. B., Selvakumar, P., Seenivasan, R., & Basava Aradhya, S. G., Dinesh, N., & Seelam, P. K. (2025). Overview of Current AI Technologies in Education. In L. Kyei-Blankson & E. Ntuli (Eds.), *Transformative AI Practices for Personalized Learning Strategies* (pp. 1–26). IGI Global. DOI: 10.4018/979-8-3693-8744-3.ch001

Jagannath, B., Lin, K.-C., Pali, M., Sankhala, D., Muthukumar, S., & Prasad, S. (2024). A sweat-based wearable enabling technology for real-time monitoring of IL-1β and CRP as potential markers for inflammatory bowel disease. *Inflammatory Bowel Diseases*. Advance online publication. DOI: 10.1093/ibd/izaa191 PMID: 32720974

Kim, Y. C.. (2020). An integrated wearable microneedle array for the continuous monitoring of multiple biomarkers in interstitial fluid. *Nature Biomedical Engineering*, *6*(11), 1214–1222. DOI: 10.1038/s41551-022-00887-1 PMID: 35534575

Kotte, K. R., Attaluri, V., & Selvakumar, P. (2025). Revolutionising Retail Banking with AI and Virtual Technologies AI-Driven Financial Training. In Nair, A. J., Manohar, S., Limbu, Y. B., & Huhmann, B. A. (Eds.), *Intersecting Natural Language Processing and FinTech Innovations in Service Marketing* (pp. 421–440). IGI Global., DOI: 10.4018/979-8-3693-9944-6.ch020

Liu, Y., Tang, Y., Cheng, Y., Huang, W., & Xiang, L. (2022). Electrochemical Biosensors Based on Saliva Electrolytes for Rapid Detection and Diagnosis. *Journal of Materials Chemistry. B*, *11*(1), 33–45. DOI: 10.1039/D2TB02031A PMID: 36484271

Maheswaran, K., Selvakumar, P., Shaikh, M., Shashank, G., Gupta, S., & Manjunath, T. C. (2025). The Evolution of Smart Urban Mobility With Emerging Technologies. In Ponnusamy, S., Assaf, M., Youssef, B., Jeon, G., & Kalyanaraman, S. (Eds.), *Leveraging VANETs and Blockchain Technology for Urban Mobility* (pp. 1–28). IGI Global., DOI: 10.4018/979-8-3373-0265-2.ch001

MDPI. (2024). Recent advances in wearable healthcare devices: From material to application. *Biosensors (Basel)*, *11*(4), 358. DOI: 10.3390/bios11040358 PMID: 38671780

Micromachines. (2022). Flexible wearable sensors for sports: kinematics to physiologies. DOI: 10.3390/mi13010058

Nat. Electron. (2021). Wearable devices for COVID-19 detection. DOI: 10.1038/s41928-020-00505-5

Nature Biomedical Engineering. (2022). Integrated wearable microneedle array for biomarker monitoring. DOI: 10.1038/s41551-022-00916-z

Nature Electronics. (2021). Smart lens COVID-19 detection. DOI: 10.1038/s41928-020-00504-6

Nature Reviews Materials. (2022). End-to-end design of wearable sensors. DOI: 10.1038/s41578-022-00460-x

NPJ Digital Medicine. (2020). Wireless monitoring of CSF shunts. DOI: 10.1038/s41746-020-00408-x

Plasmonic Sensor for Hydrogen Sulfide in Saliva: Multisensor Platform and Bag Format. *Talanta*, 245, 123449. DOI: 10.1016/j.talanta.2022.123449

Saha, T.. (2022). Non-invasive monitoring of interstitial fluid lactate through an epidermal iontophoretic device. *Talanta, 254*, 124122. DOI: 10.1016/j.talanta.2022.124122 PMID: 36459870

Sakthivel, M., Jaganathan, A., Mohanraj, M., & Selvakumar, P. Mohit, & Manjunath, T. (2025). Brand Loyalty through AI and Personalisation: AI-Generated Content for Financial Marketing. In A. J. Nair, S. Manohar, Y. B. Limbu, & B. A. Huhmann (Eds.), *Intersecting Natural Language Processing and FinTech Innovations in Service Marketing* (pp. 77–96). IGI Global. DOI: 10.4018/979-8-3693-9944-6.ch006

Science Translational Medicine. (2018). Epidermal electronics for shunt monitoring. DOI: 10.1126/scitranslmed.aau2423

Scientific Reports. (2022). Reshaping healthcare with wearable biosensors. DOI: 10.1038/s41598-022-26951-z

Sempionatto, J. R., Lin, M., & Yin, L.. (2019). Pacifier Biosensor: Toward Noninvasive Saliva Biomarker Monitoring. *Analytical Chemistry*, *91*(23), 13883–13891. DOI: 10.1021/acs.analchem.9b03379 PMID: 31573188

Shajari, S., Kuruvinashetti, K., Komeili, A., & Sundararaj, U.MDPI. (2023). The emergence of AI-based wearable sensors for digital health. *Sensors (Basel)*, *23*(23), 9498. DOI: 10.3390/s23239498 PMID: 38067871

Wang, Y., Nie, Y., Wang, P., Li, Y., Ma, Q., & Yu, D. (2022). A novel bacterial imprinted polymers-electrochemiluminescent sensor for Lactobacillus salivarius detection. *Sensors and Actuators. B, Chemical*, *358*, 131467. DOI: 10.1016/j.snb.2022.131467

Zheng, P., Zhang, F., Wang, K., Zhang, W., Li, Y., Sun, Y., Sun, X., Li, C., Dong, B., Wang, L., & Xu, L. (2021). Smart Biosensors and Intelligent Devices for Salivary Biomarker Detection. *Trends in Analytical Chemistry*, *140*, 116281. DOI: 10.1016/j.trac.2021.116281

Chapter 13

AI-Based Microbiome: Biomarkers for Nutritional Health

Naresh Kumar Sripada
https://orcid.org/0000-0002-0724-1750
SR University, India

Sirikonda Shwetha
https://orcid.org/0000-0002-2738-680X
Sumathi Reddy Institute of Technology for Women, India

P. Selvakumar
https://orcid.org/0000-0002-3650-4548
Department of Science and Humanities, Nehru Institute of Technology, Coimbatore, India

T. C. Manjunath
https://orcid.org/0000-0003-2545-9160
Rajarajeswari College of Engineering, Bengaluru, India

S. Lokesh
https://orcid.org/0000-0003-1915-6294
SRM Institute of Science and Technology, India

Sumit Kushwaha
Chandigarh University, India

ABSTRACT

The rapid advancement in microbiome science, combined with the emergence of powerful artificial intelligence (AI) analytics, is transforming the future of personalized nutrition by unlocking novel biomarkers that reflect human health, dietary responses, and disease susceptibilities. The human gut microbiome, consisting of trillions of microorganisms including bacteria, archaea, fungi, and viruses, is now recognized as a dynamic metabolic organ that influences digestion, immune regulation, metabolic homeostasis, and even neural signaling pathways through the gut–brain axis. Yet, its complexity poses significant challenges in deciphering how specific dietary components modulate microbial networks and how these networks, in turn, shape individual nutritional needs. Traditional nutritional guidelines have

DOI: 10.4018/979-8-3373-4382-2.ch013

been developed for the average person, assuming uniform responses to food; however, mounting evidence shows that metabolic reactions to the same diet can vary dramatically across individuals due to microbiome composition.

UNLOCKING THE MICROBIOME: AI-DRIVEN BIOMARKERS FOR PERSONALIZED NUTRITION

The rapid advancement in microbiome science, combined with the emergence of powerful artificial intelligence (AI) analytics, is transforming the future of personalized nutrition by unlocking novel biomarkers that reflect human health, dietary responses, and disease susceptibilities. The human gut microbiome, consisting of trillions of microorganisms including bacteria, archaea, fungi, and viruses, is now recognized as a dynamic metabolic organ that influences digestion, immune regulation, metabolic homeostasis, and even neural signaling pathways through the gut–brain axis. Yet, its complexity poses significant challenges in deciphering how specific dietary components modulate microbial networks and how these networks, in turn, shape individual nutritional needs. Traditional nutritional guidelines have been developed for the average person, assuming uniform responses to food; however, mounting evidence shows that metabolic reactions to the same diet can vary dramatically across individuals due to microbiome composition, gene–environment interactions, lifestyle patterns, and underlying health conditions. This interindividual variability underscores the necessity of shifting from a universal diet model to a precision nutrition paradigm. (Albayati et al., 2023)Here, AI-driven microbiome biomarker discovery emerges as a key enabler, supporting the identification of subtle yet clinically relevant microbial signatures, functional pathways, and metabolic outputs that conventional statistical methods fail to detect.

Machine learning and deep learning techniques are increasingly being applied to vast metagenomics, metabolomics, and clinical datasets to reveal causal associations between microbial taxa, metabolic products, and personalized dietary outcomes. These models integrate multi-omics features—including genetic variants, microbial species abundance, metatranscriptomic gene expressions, short-chain fatty acid profiles, and dietary logs—to predict individualized responses such as postprandial glucose spikes, lipid fluctuations, inflammation markers, nutrient absorption efficiency, and appetite regulation. The success of AI-powered prediction models, such as those used in personalized glycemic control programs, demonstrates how algorithmic approaches can outperform fixed nutritional labels in optimizing metabolic health based on microbiome-informed biomarker panels. Additionally, AI-derived biomarkers are accelerating early disease detection and risk assessment by identifying microbial dysbiosis patterns associated with obesity, metabolic syndrome, type 2 diabetes, inflammatory bowel disease, allergies, and even neurological conditions. These advances shift the focus from treating disease to actively managing health through precision dietary strategies targeted to restore microbial balance.(Aljamaan et al., 2024)Beyond predictive modeling, AI is facilitating hypothesis generation through unsupervised learning, network analysis, and causal inference frameworks that reveal previously undiscovered microbial interactions. For instance, machine learning-driven clustering can group individuals into microbiome-based subtypes that correlate with dietary behavior, metabolic responses, and potential intervention strategies. Reinforcement learning further supports adaptive nutrition guidance by continuously refining personalized recommendations based on real-world feedback.

GUT INSTINCT: AI-BASED MICROBIOME BIOMARKERS FOR NUTRITIONAL HEALTH

The emergence of artificial intelligence (AI) as a critical analytical framework in microbiome research is transforming our understanding of nutritional health and enabling the development of highly personalized, biomarker-driven dietary strategies. The gut microbiome—comprising trillions of microorganisms including commensal, symbiotic, and opportunistic species—functions as an essential regulator of human physiology by contributing to nutrient metabolism, immune maturation, intestinal barrier integrity, and neuromodulation via the gut–brain axis. (Bano & Siddiqui, 2024)Nutrition, in turn, is one of the most powerful modulators of the microbial ecosystem, shaping community structure, gene expression, and metabolite production that influence host metabolic pathways. However, population-level nutritional recommendations traditionally overlook interindividual variation in dietary responses, despite growing evidence that identical meals can produce vastly different metabolic consequences in different individuals due to distinct microbial profiles. AI-based microbiome biomarker discovery aims to bridge this gap by capturing complex, nonlinear interactions among microbiome composition, dietary inputs, host genetics, and clinical outcomes, ultimately enabling precision nutrition that optimizes health based on the biological uniqueness of each person.At the core of this advancement are machine learning and deep learning approaches that integrate high-dimensional metagenomic, metatranscriptomic, and metabolomic data to uncover relationships that would remain invisible through traditional statistics. Algorithms such as random forests, support vector machines, and neural networks identify microbial signatures—specific taxa patterns, functional genes, metabolic networks, or gut metabolite profiles—that serve as predictive biomarkers of nutritional responses and disease risk. One of the most notable applications is the prediction of individualized glycemic control, demonstrating that microbiome-informed AI models outperform calorie counting or macronutrient labels in forecasting postprandial glucose levels and guiding dietary recommendations for metabolic health.(Cardon et al., 2023).

In addition to predictive capabilities, AI supports mechanistic discovery in microbiome-nutrition interactions by revealing causal pathways that can be translated into targeted dietary therapies. Unsupervised learning methods identify microbiome community states and ecological subtypes that classify individuals by their metabolic potential, enabling stratification of nutritional strategies based on microbial functionality rather than phenotype alone. (Chen & Esmaeilzadeh, 2024) Network-based AI techniques map inter-species relationships, metabolic dependencies, and keystone microbial players that can serve as intervention points for dietary modulation. Reinforcement learning approaches further enable adaptive nutrition systems that refine dietary guidance through continuous feedback from real-world biomarker changes. Meanwhile, explainable AI (XAI) frameworks are gaining importance for improving interpretability, enhancing clinical trust, and ensuring that biomarker-driven decisions can be validated by host–microbiome biology rather than treated as "black-box" outputs.

THE MICROBIOME ADVANTAGE: AI-POWERED BIOMARKERS FOR HEALTHIER EATING

The integration of microbiome science with artificial intelligence (AI) is redefining the foundations of health-driven nutrition by uncovering precise biological markers that guide personalized eating strategies. The gut microbiome, widely recognized as a key determinant of human physiological balance, influences digestion, immune regulation, endocrine signaling, cognitive function, and long-term metabolic resilience. Yet, its inherent complexity—characterized by trillions of microbial cells organized into dynamic ecosystems—has historically limited our ability to translate microbiome knowledge into practical dietary guidance. Conventional nutrition relies on generalized recommendations designed for a hypothetical average human, but individual dietary responses vary strikingly due to differences in microbial composition, functional gene expression, lifestyle, and host genetics. As a result, foods perceived universally as "healthy," such as certain fruits or whole grains, may trigger glucose spikes, immune irritation, or inefficient nutrient absorption in some individuals while delivering metabolic benefits to others. This mismatch between universal dietary guidelines and biological individuality has created an urgent need for more targeted nutritional decision-making. (de Marcellis-Warin et al., 2022) AI-powered microbiome biomarker discovery offers a pathway to overcome these challenges, enabling the identification of microbial signals and metabolic fingerprints that accurately reflect a person's nutritional needs, tolerances, and disease risk profiles.AI brings unprecedented analytical capability to microbiome research by deciphering high-dimensional omics datasets that integrate metagenomics, metabolomics, proteomics, transcriptomics, and clinical monitoring data.

For example, AI can forecast postprandial glycemic responses by analyzing microbial taxa abundances together with behavioral and anthropometric data, allowing personalized carbohydrate recommendations that stabilize blood sugar and support metabolic health. Similarly, biomarkers associated with lipid metabolism, gut inflammation, satiety hormone regulation, and vitamin biosynthesis are increasingly integrated into predictive systems for optimized nutrition. Tools such as feature selection algorithms and explainable AI methods help clarify which microbial traits—such as short-chain fatty acid production capacity, mucin-degrading activity, or bile acid conversion efficiency—serve as critical levers for healthier eating practices. These models are empowering the shift from descriptive microbiome profiling to actionable insight, where the function of the microbial community matters as much as its composition.Importantly(Dudley et al., 2014), AI-driven biomarker systems translate microbiome insights into tailored dietary interventions that enhance overall health outcomes. Personalized nutrition platforms now combine microbiome sequencing with real-time data from wearable sensors—tracking glucose levels, physical activity, sleep quality, and stress markers—to deliver dynamic food recommendations backed by biological signal monitoring. These programs offer individualized guidance on prebiotic fiber intake to encourage the growth of beneficial bacteria, probiotic supplementation to restore missing functions, and nutrient-dense food choices optimized for a person's metabolic and microbial context.

MICROBIOME MEETS MACHINE LEARNING: REVOLUTIONIZING NUTRITIONAL HEALTH

The convergence of microbiome science and machine learning is driving a transformative shift in nutritional health, offering unprecedented insights into how diet interacts with human biology on an individualized level. The gut microbiome—a complex and dynamic community of trillions of microorganisms living in symbiotic relationship with the human host—plays a pivotal role in shaping nutrient metabolism, immune function, cognitive processes, and disease risk. Historically, nutritional guidance has relied on broad population-level recommendations designed to meet the general needs of most people; however, individual responses to food vary dramatically based on differences in microbial composition, metabolic capacity, and host–environment interactions.(Fui-Hoon Nah et al., 2023) As a result, dietary interventions that benefit one person may be ineffective or even harmful for another. Machine learning, with its capacity to analyze high-dimensional datasets and uncover nonlinear patterns invisible to traditional statistical approaches, provides a powerful framework for predicting individualized nutritional responses and identifying biomarkers that reflect the unique interplay between diet, microbiome function, and health outcomes. This emerging field supports a paradigm shift from generic nutritional prescriptions toward precision nutrition rooted in personalized biology.Machine learning enables deep interrogation of multi-omics data including metagenomics, metabolomics, metatranscriptomics, and clinical phenotypes to reveal functionally relevant microbial characteristics.

The integration of machine learning with real-time digital health monitoring is further amplifying personalization in nutritional care. Wearable biosensors, mobile health apps, and automated diet logging systems generate continuous streams of data on physiological states, physical activity, sleep patterns, and emotional stress—all factors that influence microbiome composition and dietary response. (Hoofnagle et al., 2019)Machine learning systems update nutritional recommendations dynamically as lifestyle and microbial conditions evolve, providing adaptive dietary support. For consumers participating in microbiome-based nutrition programs, these technologies translate complex biological insights into simple, actionable guidance—identifying which foods optimize microbial function and which may trigger metabolic dysregulation. In health care settings, machine learning–assisted microbiome assessments support early detection of diet-linked disorders such as obesity, type 2 diabetes, inflammatory bowel disease, and colorectal cancer, enabling dietary interventions that mitigate progression. Furthermore, growing research highlights connections between diet, microbiome-produced neuroactive metabolites, and cognitive health, suggesting that personalized nutrition may become an integral strategy for managing mental well-being and neurodegenerative disease risk.Beyond individual outcomes, machine learning is reshaping scientific understanding of diet–microbiome–host interactions. Unsupervised learning and clustering methods identify microbiome community phenotypes and classify individuals by metabolic response patterns, revealing stratified nutritional needs within populations. Causal inference models uncover mechanistic drivers behind biomarker signals, helping distinguish correlation from biological impact.

AI-DRIVEN INSIGHTS: MICROBIOME BIOMARKERS FOR PRECISION NUTRITION

Artificial intelligence (AI) has emerged as a transformative force in advancing precision nutrition by enabling the discovery, interpretation, and application of microbiome biomarkers that reflect personalized health needs and dietary responses. (Iriart, 2019)The human gut microbiome—rich in metabolic capabilities and uniquely tailored within each individual—maintains a symbiotic relationship with its host, influencing nutrient digestion, immune regulation, inflammation balance, and central nervous system signaling. However, the complexity and variability of microbial ecosystems have long impeded efforts to translate microbiome knowledge into personalized dietary recommendations. Traditional nutritional models rely on population-wide assumptions that overlook profound differences in metabolic outcomes among individuals consuming the same foods. AI-driven microbiome biomarker analytics bridge this gap by assimilating multi-omics data and detecting intricate patterns that reveal how specific microbial features govern nutritional responses, disease risk, and physiological resilience. Through machine learning, deep learning, and network-based computational methods, microbiome characteristics are transformed into quantifiable biomarkers that inform dietary decisions tailored to individual biology—marking a paradigm shift away from one-size-fits-all nutrition and toward a model centered on biological precision.AI's value in precision nutrition lies in its ability to analyze massive datasets that integrate microbiome composition, gene expression, metabolite production, and real-world lifestyle metrics. Machine learning models identify microbial indicators of metabolic efficiency—such as the abundance of short-chain fatty acid (SCFA)-producing bacteria, bile acid-transforming species, or fiber-fermenting guilds—and link them to clinical markers including postprandial glucose responses, lipid fluctuations, inflammatory signaling profiles, and satiety hormone levels.

These biomarkers move beyond traditional metrics like calorie counts or macronutrient ratios by providing a more direct window into how the body processes food at a biochemical level. Deep neural networks can predict how an individual will respond to the glycemic load of specific meals based on microbial signatures, enabling dietary personalization that supports diabetes prevention, weight management, and metabolic control. Natural language processing tools contribute by extracting insights from scientific literature and harmonizing classifications of microbial functions, ensuring that emerging microbiome research continuously informs AI models. Collectively, these computational advances shift microbiome biomarkers from observational associations to actionable predictive tools(Ivanov et al., 2024).The integration of AI-driven microbiome biomarkers into clinical and consumer nutrition platforms is growing rapidly. Personalized nutrition programs now pair microbiome sequencing with biosensor data from continuous glucose monitors, wearable devices tracking sleep and physical activity, and mobile diet-tracking applications.

THE FUTURE OF NUTRITION: AI-BASED MICROBIOME BIOMARKERS

The future of nutrition is rapidly evolving toward a precision-driven model powered by artificial intelligence (AI) and microbiome biomarker discovery, fundamentally transforming how individuals understand and manage their health through diet. Nutrition science—once constrained by broad generalizations and standardized food guidelines—is becoming increasingly personalized as researchers uncover the profound role of the gut microbiome in shaping metabolic Machine learning models can identify microbial biomarkers associated with critical nutrition-related processes such as fiber fermentation capacity, short-chain fatty acid production, bile acid transformation, oxidative stress regulation, and fat and carbohydrate metabolism. Deep learning systems further integrate metabolomic and transcriptomic indicators to predict physiological outcomes including postprandial glycemic responses, immune activation, neurotransmitter balance, and microbiome-driven nutrient bioavailability. (Jenkins et al., 2020)These biomarkers reflect real biological mechanisms—not superficial dietary metrics—making them an invaluable foundation for precise dietary recommendations. Over time, AI systems will refine their predictions using longitudinal data, recognizing how microbiome responses change across life stages from childhood growth to aging-related metabolic decline. In this future, nutritional guidance will become increasingly anticipatory rather than corrective, alerting individuals when diet quality diverges from optimal microbial function and preventing health decline before it emerges clinically.

The practical implementation of AI-driven microbiome biomarkers is already reshaping the food and healthcare ecosystem, with rapid expansion expected in the coming decade. Personalized nutrition programs that combine microbiome sequencing with wearable health sensors are helping individuals monitor dietary impacts in real time. Digital dieticians guided by reinforcement learning models will dynamically adapt meal plans based on microbial response patterns, continuously optimizing metabolic performance, sleep quality, cognitive function, and emotional resilience.(Le et al., 2023) Clinical dietetics will incorporate biomarker-based strategies to support treatment pathways for conditions such as obesity, type 2 diabetes, metabolic syndrome, inflammatory bowel disease, non-alcoholic fatty liver disease, and allergies—allowing dietary therapy to be customized with medical precision. Additionally, mental health interventions may increasingly rely on biomarkers related to the gut–brain axis, targeting microbial pathways that influence anxiety, mood stability, and neuroinflammation. These developments signal a shift toward nutrition that enhances total human performance—not only physically, but also cognitively and psychologically.AI-enabled biomarker science will also transform food production and product innovation. The food and agriculture industries are beginning to design precision-engineered functional foods and microbial therapeutics that target specific biomarker-defined needs, such as enhancing SCFA production, modulating inflammatory microbial species, or improving micronutrient biosynthesis.

MICROBIOME BIOMARKERS AND AI: A NEW ERA IN NUTRITIONAL HEALTH

The convergence of microbiome science and artificial intelligence (AI) is catalyzing a paradigm shift in nutritional health, enabling a transition from generalized dietary recommendations to truly individualized nutrition strategies rooted in biological specificity. The human gut microbiome—comprising trillions of microorganisms, including bacteria, archaea, fungi, and viruses—plays a fundamental role in digestion, immune regulation, metabolic homeostasis, and even cognitive function through the gut–brain axis. Variations in microbial composition and function have been strongly linked to diverse health outcomes, including obesity, diabetes, cardiovascular disease, inflammatory bowel disease, and malnutrition. However, the sheer complexity, dynamic nature, and inter-individual variability of gut microbial ecosystems have long hindered the ability of clinicians and nutritionists to translate microbiome data into actionable dietary insights. (Li, 2023)AI-driven analytics and machine learning (ML) algorithms are now addressing these limitations by uncovering hidden patterns within high-dimensional multi-omic datasets—such as metagenomics, metabolomics, transcriptomics, and dietary exposure data—to identify robust microbial biomarkers capable of predicting diet responsiveness and personalized nutrition needs.

Figure 1. Gut microbiome and nutrition-related predictors of response

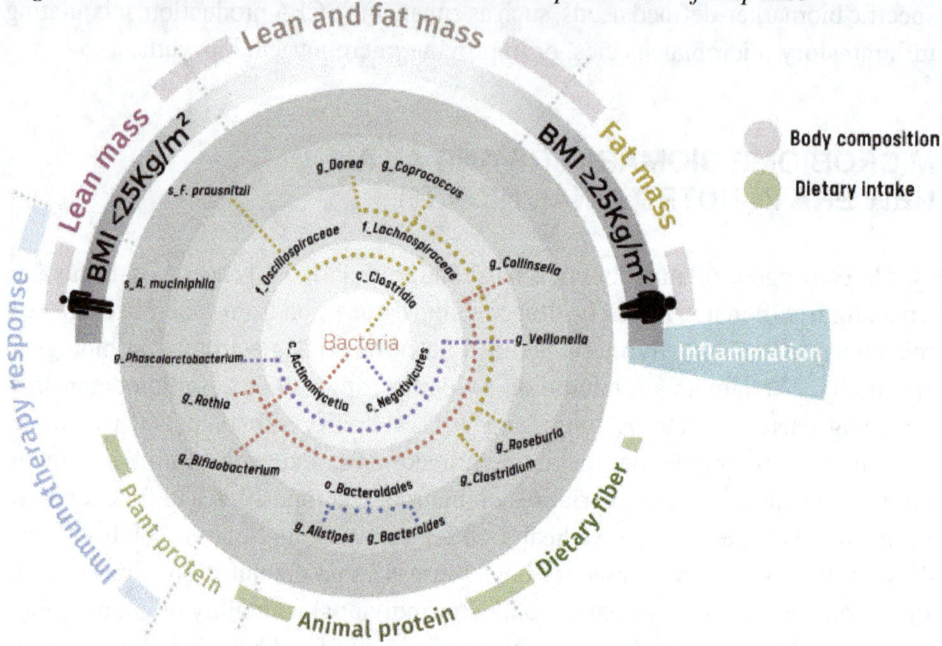

AI-enabled microbiome biomarkers are reshaping nutritional assessment by providing quantitative indicators of gut microbial function and related metabolic outcomes. Unlike traditional nutritional evaluation, which often depends on self-reported recalls, generalized nutrient guidelines, or static clinical measures, microbiome-based biomarkers offer real-time biological snapshots that reflect an individual's physiological response to food intake. Machine learning systems can integrate clinical parameters—like glucose response curves, lipid profiles, inflammatory cytokines, and gastrointestinal symptom patterns—with microbiome sequencing results to generate predictive models for personalized diet plans. For example, pioneering studies have demonstrated that postprandial glycemic responses vary widely between individuals consuming identical meals, with gut microbial signatures emerging as significant predictors of glucose metabolism. (Manjunath et al., 2026)AI models trained on population-scale microbiome datasets have accurately forecasted personalized glycemic reactions and informed optimized dietary recommendations that substantially improve blood sugar control. This personalized glycemic modulation approach exemplifies how AI-derived biomarkers can drive nutritional precision by accounting for host-microbiome interactions, dietary habits, lifestyle factors, and genetic predispositions.

AI-POWERED MICROBIOME ANALYSIS: UNLOCKING NUTRITIONAL SECRETS

AI-powered microbiome analysis represents a transformative advancement in nutritional science, revealing previously hidden biological mechanisms that govern individual dietary responses, digestive health, and metabolic regulation. The gut microbiome is now recognized as a dynamic system essential for nutrient absorption, energy metabolism, immune modulation, and neurochemical communication through the gut–brain axis. However, the extraordinary diversity and functional complexity of microbial communities—differing significantly between individuals based on genetics, diet, environment, age, and lifestyle—have historically impeded attempts to define consistent nutritional guidance grounded in personalized biology. (Pawar et al., 2026)Artificial intelligence is rapidly overcoming these barriers by applying machine learning (ML), deep learning (DL), and high-dimensional data mining techniques to multi-omics data such as metagenomics, transcriptomics, metabolomics, proteomics, and dietary intake patterns. These computational tools identify predictive microbial signatures, metabolic pathways, and functional biomarkers that elucidate how specific foods interact with the microbiome to influence health outcomes. In doing so, AI reveals nutritional secrets embedded within the gut ecosystem, paving the way for precision nutrition strategies tailored to each individual's microbial profile rather than relying on generalized dietary recommendations.

One of the most profound contributions of AI in microbiome science is its ability to decode the functional consequences of microbial composition beyond traditional taxonomic analysis. Conventional sequencing approaches often focus on cataloging microbial species present in the gut, yet microbial function—such as short-chain fatty acid (SCFA) generation, bile acid metabolism, or dietary fiber breakdown—is more closely tied to metabolic health and disease prevention. AI-driven functional profiling interprets complex gene expression and metabolite production patterns, producing actionable insights on how dietary choices affect host physiology in real time.(Seshanna et al., 2026) For instance, predictive AI models can analyze how different individuals metabolize carbohydrates, fats, and proteins, identifying whether a person is more prone to high glycemic responses, lipid dysregulation, or inflammatory reactions after specific meals. Integrating this data with continuous glucose monitoring, food-tracking apps, and wearable health sensors allows for dynamic nutritional recommendations that adapt to evolving microbiome states and lifestyle behaviors. Thus, AI converts microbiome data from static snapshots into powerful predictive tools that inform proactive dietary interventions.

FROM GUT TO TABLE: AI-BASED MICROBIOME BIOMARKERS FOR PERSONALIZED DIETS

The emerging synergy between microbiome research and artificial intelligence (AI) is fundamentally transforming how diets are designed, evaluated, and personalized. For decades, nutrition science has operated within a framework of generalized dietary recommendations, often failing to account for the immense inter-individual variability in metabolic responses to foods. Today, AI-based microbiome biomarkers are enabling an unprecedented shift: dietary personalization grounded in the biological realities of each person's gut microbial ecosystem. The human gut microbiome — comprising trillions of microorganisms with millions of unique genes — plays a central role in digestion, nutrient assimilation, immune function, metabolic regulation, and neuromodulation.(Selvakumar et al., 2026) Microbial diversity, ecological balance, and functional pathways profoundly influence how different individuals metabolize carbohydrates, fats, proteins, vitamins, and phytochemicals. Yet, due to its complexity and dynamic nature, the microbiome has remained a largely hidden contributor to dietary outcomes. AI now acts as the critical bridge "from gut to table," decoding the intricate relationships between microbial signatures and nutritional needs to support precision diets uniquely tailored to each individual's health goals and biological profile.AI-driven microbiome biomarkers function by extracting meaningful indicators from high-dimensional multi-omic datasets including metagenomics, metatranscriptomics, metabolomics, proteomics, and digital dietary tracking. Traditional dietary assessments rely on subjective food diaries or universal health metrics, which inadequately reflect actual metabolic responses. In contrast, AI algorithms can integrate microbial species abundance, functional gene pathways, metabolite outputs, glucose and lipid responses, inflammatory markers, and lifestyle inputs to generate predictive models that map how specific foods will affect a particular person. This approach has revealed striking insights: two individuals consuming identical meals can exhibit completely different glycemic or lipid responses due to differences in microbial metabolic potential. (Tsasis & Bains, 2008) AI-powered biomarker systems quantify these patterns to provide personalized diet recommendations that optimize blood sugar stability, reduce systemic inflammation, and enhance digestive efficiency. As a result, food choices become biologically informed — transitioning nutrition planning from guesswork to precision strategy.

Weight management and metabolic disease prevention are among the areas where AI-based microbiome biomarkers are demonstrating the most notable impact. Gut microbes help determine caloric energy harvest from foods, regulate hunger hormones such as ghrelin and leptin, and influence insulin sensitivity and fat storage. Machine learning models trained on population-scale microbiome datasets can identify microbial features associated with favorable metabolic adaptations, such as higher proportions of short-chain fatty acid (SCFA)-producing bacteria including *Roseburia* and *Butyricicoccus*, or the presence of *Akkermansia muciniphila*, linked to improved gut barrier integrity and metabolic resilience. By measuring these biomarkers, AI tools can recommend diets that selectively support the growth and activity of beneficial microbes — such as fiber-rich functional foods, resistant starches, polyphenols, and fermented products — and limit foods that promote dysbiosis. This targeted approach enables individuals to achieve sustainable metabolic health unlike uniform calorie-restriction models, marking a distinct evolution beyond traditional dieting paradigms.AI-powered microbiome biomarker analysis is also revolutionizing dietary management for digestive disorders and food sensitivities. Conditions such as irritable bowel syndrome (IBS), lactose malabsorption, fructose intolerance, small intestinal bacterial overgrowth (SIBO), and inflammatory bowel disease (IBD) involve unique microbial imbalances and immune triggers. Historically, individuals have navigated these conditions through trial-and-error elimination diets, which are time-consuming and often health, (Ulita et al., 2024)AI-based microbiome biomarkers are uncovering nutrition's influence on psychological well-being through the gut–brain axis. Microbial metabolites such as tryptophan derivatives and SCFAs affect neurotransmitter synthesis, neuroinflammation, and stress signaling. AI-enabled analyses identify biomarker profiles associated with anxiety, depression, or cognitive fatigue, enabling nutrition strategies that support neurochemical balance and emotional resilience. Functional foods enriched with prebiotics, omega-3 fatty acids, fermented components, or anti-inflammatory phytochemicals can be prescribed in alignment with microbiome data to enhance mental performance through microbiota-mediated pathways. This expansion into nutritional psychiatry underscores the holistic potential of AI-powered biomarker-driven diet personalization.

MICROBIOME-BASED BIOMARKERS: AI-DRIVEN SOLUTIONS FOR NUTRITIONAL HEALTH

Microbiome-based biomarkers powered by artificial intelligence (AI) are revolutionizing the landscape of nutritional health, shifting the paradigm from generalized dietary guidance to personalized, biologically informed interventions. The human gut microbiome — a vast and dynamic community of trillions of microorganisms — plays a central role in nutrient metabolism, immune function, inflammation regulation, and gut-brain communication. Inter-individual variation in microbial composition and metabolic potential influences how people respond to identical foods, including glycemic tolerance, lipid processing, and satiety signaling. Traditional nutrition science has long relied on population averages and standardized dietary guidelines that often fail to reflect the metabolic uniqueness of individuals. AI-driven microbiome biomarker discovery is overcoming these limitations by analyzing complex, high-dimensional biological data to identify measurable microbial and metabolic signatures that serve as reliable predictors of nutritional responses and health outcomes. These advancements pave the way for precision nutrition — an approach that aligns dietary strategies with the unique microbiological and metabolic profile of each person.

The identification of robust microbiome-based biomarkers requires the integration of multi-omic datasets including metagenomics, metatranscriptomics, metabolomics, proteomics, and digital dietary logs. Such datasets capture the breadth of microbial structure and function, yet their immense complexity renders traditional analytics insufficient. AI and machine learning (ML) algorithms excel in this realm by detecting nonlinear relationships, hidden clusters, and predictive molecular patterns that human analysis cannot easily perceive. By combining microbial abundance data with host phenotypes such as blood glucose levels, lipid panels, inflammatory cytokines, and anthropometric indicators, AI models generate personalized risk profiles and dietary response predictions. (Wang et al., 2024)For example, predictive tools leveraging microbiome biomarkers can estimate individualized postprandial glycemic reaction to specific foods, enabling precision carbohydrate management and reducing the risk of insulin resistance and type 2 diabetes. Similarly, microbial metabolite biomarkers such as short-chain fatty acid (SCFA) production provide insight into metabolic resilience, digestive performance, and colonocyte energy supply — informing dietary recommendations that promote microbial-mediated metabolic benefits.Metabolic disease prevention is a particularly compelling application of AI-enabled microbiome-based biomarker innovation. Dysbiosis — microbial imbalance characterized by reduced diversity and functional instability — has been strongly linked to obesity, cardiovascular disease, non-alcoholic fatty liver disease, and chronic inflammation. AI models trained on large clinical microbiome datasets can identify biomarker signatures predictive of metabolic dysfunction long before disease symptoms emerge. This facilitates early dietary intervention, such as increasing prebiotic fibers and polyphenol-rich foods that support beneficial taxa like *Akkermansia muciniphila* and *Bifidobacterium* species, while reducing consumption of pro-inflammatory or dysbiosis-triggering foods. By targeting microbial mechanisms of disease at the dietary level, AI-powered microbiome biomarkers support preventive nutrition strategies validated by biological response rather than general advice.

AI-DRIVEN MICROBIOME RESEARCH: NEW FRONTIERS IN NUTRITIONAL SCIENCE

AI-driven microbiome research is creating unprecedented opportunities in nutritional science, transforming our understanding of how food interacts with the human body at the molecular, microbial, and systemic levels. The gut microbiome — a highly diverse ecosystem enriched with bacteria, archaea, fungi, and viruses — acts as a crucial mediator between dietary intake and physiological outcomes, influencing digestion, nutrient metabolism, immune homeostasis, and neuroendocrine signaling. For decades, nutrition science relied heavily on population-level recommendations, simplifying dietary guidance into universal rules that often failed to work for every individual. (Wei et al., 2024)Yet, growing evidence reveals extreme variability in dietary responses among individuals, even when consuming identical meals. This variability stems largely from differences in gut microbial composition, gene expression, and metabolic byproducts, making the microbiome a key determinant of personalized nutrition needs. AI has emerged as a groundbreaking tool capable of decoding this complexity by integrating high-dimensional biological data and uncovering mechanistic insights that traditional methods cannot easily identify. Through advanced predictive modeling, machine learning (ML), and deep learning (DL), AI-powered analytics are accelerating biomarker discovery, optimizing dietary strategies, and enabling precision nutrition interventions that align with each individual's unique microbial ecosystem.

One of the most transformative impacts of AI in microbiome research lies in its ability to analyze multi-omic datasets — including metagenomics, metatranscriptomics, metabolomics, proteomics, and phenotypic clinical variables — to map how specific microbial functions regulate nutrient processing. These AI approaches go beyond identifying which microbes are present in the gut, focusing instead on how microbial pathways convert dietary substrates into metabolites that influence systemic health. For example, short-chain fatty acids (SCFAs) such as butyrate, acetate, and propionate play essential roles in maintaining gut lining integrity, regulating inflammation, and modulating energy metabolism. (Wysocki et al., 2023) AI-driven models can evaluate the abundance of SCFA-producing functional genes and predict whether dietary fiber intake will yield positive metabolic improvements in a given individual, assisting in personalized dietary recommendations. Similarly, AI algorithms trained on continuous glucose monitoring and microbiome sequencing data have revealed that individualized postprandial glycemic responses can be accurately predicted from microbial biomarkers — enabling precision carbohydrate management to prevent metabolic diseases like type 2 diabetes. These predictive capabilities redefine nutritional assessment by leveraging real biological response patterns rather than generalized nutritional metrics.AI-driven microbiome science is also accelerating progress in combating obesity, metabolic syndrome, fatty liver disease, and cardiovascular disorders. Dysbiosis — an imbalance in gut microbial diversity and function — is strongly correlated with systemic inflammation, insulin resistance, and dysregulated lipid metabolism. AI can detect early dysbiosis markers and stratify individuals based on the likelihood of developing metabolic complications, allowing targeted dietary interventions long before disease onset. Machine learning models identify which foods selectively enhance beneficial microbial taxa such as *Bifidobacterium* and *Akkermansia muciniphila*, known for improving metabolic resilience, gut permeability, and immune function.(Xu et al., 2024) AI-guided nutrition thus supports disease prevention through precise dietary adjustments that restore ecological balance and enhance metabolic stability.Beyond metabolism, AI-assisted microbiome research is reshaping our understanding of gastrointestinal disorders and allergies. Chronic gut-related conditions such as irritable bowel syndrome (IBS), inflammatory bowel disease (IBD), celiac disease, and food sensitivities are characterized by abnormal microbial interactions and impaired nutrient processing. Traditional diagnostic methods rely heavily on symptom tracking and invasive procedures, leading to delayed diagnoses and burdensome treatment pathways. AI models trained on microbiome biomarkers can identify subtle microbial disturbances, inflammation pathways, and dietary trigger patterns that help clinicians design personalized dietary regimens rooted in microbial function. This enables patients to achieve symptom relief more efficiently while preserving nutritional diversity, improving their quality of life.

THE MICROBIOME-BRAIN CONNECTION: AI-BASED BIOMARKERS FOR NUTRITIONAL PSYCHIATRY

The human gut microbiome has emerged as a vital regulator of brain function and emotional well-being, reshaping scientific understanding of the intricate communication network known as the gut-brain axis. This axis integrates neural, endocrine, immune, and metabolic pathways, enabling bidirectional signaling between intestinal microbes and the central nervous system through mechanisms such as microbial metabolite production, vagus nerve activation, and modulation of systemic inflammation. Increasing evidence indicates that disruptions in gut microbial composition—dysbiosis—can contribute to neuropsychiatric conditions including depression, anxiety disorders, autism spectrum disorder, and cognitive decline. Nutritional psychiatry, an emerging discipline at this intersection of diet, mental health, and microbiome science, aims to leverage food-based interventions to improve psychological outcomes. However, the complexity of microbial ecosystems, combined with vast individual variability in diet, genetics, and lifestyle, presents substantial barriers to establishing standardized dietary recommendations for mental health management. Artificial intelligence (AI) and machine learning have therefore become indispensable tools, capable of transforming microbiome data into actionable biomarkers that enable precision-based nutritional psychiatry. The surge in microbiome research has generated multi-omic datasets—including metagenomics, metabolomics, transcriptomics, and proteomics—that are too complex and high-dimensional for traditional statistical methods. (Yim et al., 2024)AI approaches efficiently extract meaningful patterns from this biological complexity by integrating diverse datasets and uncovering nonlinear relationships between gut microbes, dietary exposures, and neurobehavioral outcomes. Deep learning and unsupervised clustering methods help classify microbial signatures associated with specific psychiatric phenotypes, while supervised machine learning models enable predictions of treatment responsiveness or disease progression based on microbiome-derived biomarker profiles. For instance, alterations in short-chain fatty acid (SCFA)–producing bacteria, tryptophan-metabolizing taxa, and immune-triggering pathobionts have been linked to neurotransmitter imbalances and heightened systemic inflammation—key pathways involved in depression and anxiety. AI systems can identify these subtle microbial shifts long before clinical symptoms fully manifest, enabling early diagnosis and targeted dietary interventions before psychological conditions progress to chronic stages.

Dietary modulation is one of the most effective and accessible strategies for restoring microbiome balance and enhancing mental health. AI-based biomarker discovery is driving innovation in personalized nutrition programs that incorporate brain-relevant microbiome targets. By analyzing an individual's microbial composition, metabolic outputs, and diet-related behavioral data, AI algorithms can recommend tailored nutritional plans—increasing intake of prebiotic fibers to boost SCFA production, incorporating fermented foods to enhance microbial diversity, or guiding strategic supplementation of psychobiotics such as *Lactobacillus* and *Bifidobacterium* strains shown to modulate stress responses. These individualized interventions can be continuously optimized through adaptive learning systems that monitor real-time physiological feedback via wearable sensors and stool-based diagnostics, refining diet recommendations to maximize psychological benefits. Mobile applications that integrate AI-driven microbiome analytics are also improving adherence and accessibility, making precision nutritional psychiatry a practical reality for patients and clinicians.Another transformative aspect of AI in this field is its role in mapping the causal architecture of the gut-brain axis. While correlations between microbiome composition and psychiatric symptoms are well documented, establishing causality has remained challenging due to the complex and dynamic nature of microbial ecosystems. Reinforcement learning, causal inference modeling, and mechanistic AI frameworks are now being used to simulate metabolic interactions and neuroimmune pathways, revealing how specific microbial metabolites—such as serotonin precursors, gamma-aminobutyric acid (GABA), or kynurenine pathway products—shape mood regulation and cognitive function. These insights enable precise biomarker validation, supporting the development of next-generation diagnostic tools and psychobiotic therapeutic strategies. Clinical trials increasingly incorporate AI-guided microbiome assessments to stratify participants, predict outcomes, and identify novel response phenotypes, accelerating translation from bench to bedside. Despite rapid advancements, several ethical, technical, and clinical challenges must be addressed before AI-enabled nutritional psychiatry becomes mainstream. (Yuan et al., 2005)A lack of standardized protocols in microbiome sampling, sequencing methods, and metadata reporting complicates cross-study integration and model reproducibility. Many clinical studies rely on small and geographically homogenous cohorts, limiting generalizability and equity in biomarker-based recommendations. AI systems must therefore incorporate diverse population datasets while adopting transparent, explainable decision-making frameworks that allow clinicians to understand how microbiome features influence outcomes. Privacy concerns also arise with the integration of microbiome data—considered a unique biological identifier—into digital health platforms. Effective governance policies and strong data security measures are essential to maintaining public trust and safeguarding sensitive information. Furthermore, clinical validation of AI-based biomarkers requires long-term, interdisciplinary collaboration among gastroenterologists, psychiatrists, dietitians, bioinformaticians, and behavioral scientists.

AI-BASED MICROBIOME BIOMARKERS FOR CHRONIC DISEASE PREVENTION

The human gut microbiome has emerged as a central determinant of long-term health, influencing physiological systems ranging from immune regulation and metabolism to endocrine function and cellular homeostasis. In recent years, a growing body of research has linked microbial dysbiosis—an imbalance in gut microbial communities—to the onset and progression of major chronic diseases including type 2 diabetes, cardiovascular disease, obesity, inflammatory bowel disease, neurodegenerative disorders, and certain cancers. As noncommunicable diseases (NCDs) continue to rise globally—now accounting for over 70% of worldwide mortality—innovative strategies for early detection and prevention have become a critical public health priority. Artificial intelligence (AI) has emerged as a powerful tool in this field, capable of transforming complex microbiome data into clinically meaningful biomarkers that support precision prevention approaches. By integrating multi-omic datasets, behavioral information, and environmental exposures,

AI enables the identification of early microbial signatures associated with disease risk, well before conventional diagnostic markers become apparent. (Zhang et al., 2024)This positions AI-driven microbiome biomarkers at the forefront of future preventive healthcare, shifting the model from treatment of established disease to proactive maintenance of metabolic and immunological equilibrium.Microbiome datasets are inherently high-dimensional, capturing thousands of microbial taxa and their functional contributions through genomic sequencing, metabolomic profiling, and transcriptomic analysis. Traditional analytical methods struggle to uncover the nonlinear, interconnected relationships between microbial structure, metabolic outputs, and host health outcomes. Machine learning and deep learning techniques excel in this environment, enabling sophisticated pattern recognition and biomarker discovery. For example, random forests, support vector machines, and neural networks have demonstrated the ability to classify individuals at risk of developing type 2 diabetes by identifying subtle changes in bacterial species involved in insulin sensitivity, bile acid metabolism, and short-chain fatty acid (SCFA) synthesis. In cardiovascular disease research, AI models have detected microbial signatures associated with increased trimethylamine-N-oxide (TMAO) production—a gut-derived metabolite linked to atherosclerosis—allowing prediction of cardiovascular events beyond traditional risk factors like LDL cholesterol. Similarly, AI-enabled analysis of microbial diversity, pathobiont abundance, and inflammation-related metabolites helps identify individuals predisposed to obesity and metabolic syndrome, enabling early intervention with targeted nutritional or lifestyle programs.

The integration of AI-driven microbiome biomarkers into preventive nutrition strategies presents a significant opportunity to reduce chronic disease risk through personalized dietary guidance. Diet is one of the most influential determinants of microbiome composition, and individualized nutrition can restore microbial balance to support metabolic health. AI systems analyze not only microbiome data but also dietary intake, health history, and lifestyle patterns collected through mobile applications, wearables, and digital health records. By modeling how specific dietary components influence microbial activity, these algorithms generate customized dietary recommendations designed to promote the growth of beneficial bacteria, enhance SCFA production, modulate inflammatory responses, and optimize metabolic function. Clinical studies have demonstrated that personalized dietary interventions guided by microbiome analysis can improve glycemic control, reduce systemic inflammation, and support healthy weight management more effectively than generalized nutrition advice. Over time, continuous data collection contributes to adaptive learning models that refine recommendations, delivering a dynamic preventive health approach that evolves with the individual's microbiome.Beyond metabolic conditions, AI-based microbiome biomarkers are also advancing prevention in immune-related and neurodegenerative diseases. Inflammatory bowel disease (IBD) research has shown that early detection of microbial imbalances through AI models—particularly reduced microbial diversity and loss of anti-inflammatory taxa—can support preventive treatment strategies to delay or reduce disease flare-ups in high-risk individuals such as those with a family history. In neurodegenerative disease research, alterations in gut microbial metabolites affecting blood–brain barrier integrity, neuroinflammation, and oxidative stress are being used as predictive indicators for conditions such as Parkinson's and Alzheimer's disease. AI-powered causal modeling helps clarify mechanisms underlying these associations, supporting biomarker validation that could ultimately allow clinicians to deploy dietary and lifestyle interventions that preserve neurological function decades before symptom onset. Similar approaches are being explored in oncology, where AI-assisted microbiome profiling can help identify microbial signatures linked to colorectal cancer risk and inform preventive screening strategies.

NUTRIGENOMICS MEETS AI: MICROBIOME BIOMARKERS FOR PERSONALIZED NUTRITION

The convergence of nutrigenomics, microbiome science, and artificial intelligence (AI) is driving a paradigm shift in how nutrition is understood and delivered, enabling a transition from population-based guidelines to truly individualized dietary strategies. Nutrigenomics explores how nutrients influence gene expression and how genetic variation shapes dietary responses, while the human microbiome represents a dynamic ecosystem of trillions of microorganisms influencing digestion, metabolism, immune regulation, and overall health. The intersection of these fields reveals that genes and microbes engage in complex, bidirectional interactions that determine how individuals process foods, extract nutrients, produce bioactive metabolites, and maintain metabolic homeostasis. However, the sheer complexity and heterogeneity within both the human genome and the microbiome make it difficult to predict dietary responses using conventional analytical approaches. AI has emerged as a powerful computational solution capable of integrating genomic, microbial, environmental, and behavioral data to identify predictive biomarkers that inform personalized nutrition interventions tailored to the biological needs of each individual.Microbiome-based biomarkers provide key insights into the metabolic capabilities of gut microorganisms, revealing how dietary components are transformed into molecules that either support or impair health. For instance, differences in the abundance of bacteria associated with short-chain fatty acid (SCFA) production, bile acid modification, and amino acid fermentation influence a person's risk of obesity, insulin resistance, chronic inflammation, and gastrointestinal disorders. Meanwhile, genetic variability within host nutrient transporters, metabolic enzymes, and taste receptors determines how the body absorbs and utilizes nutrients, shaping individual nutritional requirements. AI models—ranging from random forests and gradient boosting machines to neural networks and reinforcement learning—are instrumental in mapping these multilayered relationships and extracting reliable predictive signatures from the extensive datasets generated by multi-omic sequencing. By integrating host genetics with microbiome profiles and dietary intake patterns, AI helps identify biomarker combinations that can accurately determine which foods optimize metabolic function, stabilize blood glucose responses, reduce inflammation, and promote long-term health.

One of the most important applications of AI-driven nutrigenomics is the prediction of postprandial glycemic responses (PPGR), a highly individualized metabolic outcome strongly associated with diabetes risk. Research has demonstrated that PPGR varies significantly even when individuals consume identical foods, driven largely by microbiome composition and metabolic activity. AI-based models trained on genomic and microbial biomarkers, together with lifestyle data such as physical activity and sleep, can forecast an individual's glycemic reaction to specific meals. These models support the creation of tailored dietary plans that sustain glucose balance and reduce risk of type 2 diabetes more effectively than generalized nutrition recommendations. Similarly, AI-enabled discovery of microbiome biomarkers linked to lipid metabolism, fiber fermentation efficiency, and dietary fat tolerance supports precision interventions that reduce cardiovascular disease risk and improve gut health outcomes.As personalized nutrition tools become more accessible through digital platforms, smartphone apps, and at-home gut testing, AI continuously enhances the user experience by adapting recommendations based on real-time feedback. Wearable devices measuring glucose variability, dietary adherence, mood, sleep, and physical activity feed new data into learning models, enabling dynamic updates to dietary guidance. (Raj et al., 2026a)The addition of explainable AI frameworks ensures users understand the rationale behind personalized recommendations, building trust and promoting sustained behavioral change. Furthermore, AI-based microbiome biomarker tracking enables early detection of diet-induced dysbiosis and guides corrective interventions such as targeted probiotics, prebiotic fibers, and fermented foods to restore microbial equilibrium. This adaptive and preventive approach is central to future healthcare, where lifestyle and diet serve as primary tools for reducing chronic disease burden.

AI-POWERED MICROBIOME DIAGNOSTICS: A NEW TOOL FOR NUTRITIONAL HEALTH

Artificial intelligence (AI)–powered microbiome diagnostics are revolutionizing the field of nutritional health by enabling earlier identification of metabolic imbalances, individualized dietary interventions, and a proactive approach to disease prevention at scale. The human gut contains a highly diverse and dynamic community of microorganisms that directly influence nutrient metabolism, immune function, intestinal barrier integrity, and endocrine signaling. Disruptions to this ecosystem, known as dysbiosis, have been linked to a spectrum of nutrition-related chronic conditions including obesity, type 2 diabetes, cardiovascular disease, irritable bowel syndrome (IBS), inflammatory bowel disease (IBD), and food intolerances. Traditional clinical diagnostics often detect disease only after significant physiological deterioration has occurred, but AI-enhanced microbiome analytics can uncover invisible biological changes long before symptoms develop. By transforming high-dimensional sequencing data into actionable biomarker insights, AI supports a shift in nutritional health from reactive treatment to predictive, personalized prevention. Microbiome diagnostics generate multi-omic datasets through metagenomic sequencing, metabolomic profiling, proteomic measurements, and transcriptomic analysis. These datasets capture the taxonomic composition of the gut, the functions encoded within microbial genes, and the bioactive metabolites produced through nutrient breakdown. The complexity and interdependency of these data exceed the capabilities of traditional statistical tools, making AI indispensable in extracting clinically relevant patterns. Machine learning models such as support vector machines, random forests, and neural networks have proven capable of diagnosing early metabolic dysfunction based on subtle microbial shifts including reduced production of short-chain fatty acids (SCFAs), elevated levels of pro-inflammatory metabolites, and altered pathways in lipid and bile acid metabolism. (Raj et al., 2026b) Meanwhile, deep learning techniques enable prediction of host dietary responses by modeling nonlinear relationships between microbiome structure, food intake behavior, and metabolic biomarkers such as glycemic variability, cholesterol levels, and inflammatory markers.

AI-powered microbiome diagnostics have been particularly transformative in personalized nutrition. Unlike conventional dietary guidelines that assume universal nutrient responses, these systems reveal that dietary impacts differ dramatically between individuals due to unique microbial and genomic profiles. AI tools analyze stool samples alongside lifestyle metrics, genetics, anthropometrics, and continuous glucose monitoring data to generate individualized nutrition recommendations designed to optimize metabolic health. For example, personalized diet platforms leveraging microbiome biomarkers can accurately forecast postprandial glycemic responses (PPGR) to specific foods—critical for diabetes prevention—allowing customized meal planning that minimizes glucose spikes. Similar approaches are applied to dietary fiber tolerance, lipid metabolism efficiency, and the selection of probiotics or prebiotics most beneficial to an individual's microbial composition. As users provide ongoing dietary and health feedback through mobile applications and wearable devices, AI models dynamically adjust recommendations, creating a closed-loop system for nutritional optimization.In clinical practice, AI-driven microbiome diagnostics are supporting earlier detection of gastrointestinal and systemic conditions. For instance, machine learning classifiers trained on microbial diversity indices, pathogen abundance, and mucosal immune markers can identify individuals at risk for IBD flare-ups, enabling preventive nutritional strategies that reduce disease severity. AI-based colorectal cancer screening methods integrate microbial biomarkers such as *Fusobacterium nucleatum* abundance to detect cancer risk with high sensitivity, offering a minimally invasive complement to colonoscopy. In pediatric nutritional health, microbiome biomarkers assist in monitoring early immune system development, predicting risks such as food allergies and malnutrition, and guiding personalized infant feeding practices that foster lifelong metabolic resilience. Additionally, AI models are being explored for the detection of micronutrient deficiencies—linking microbial metabolic signatures with vitamin synthesis and absorption pathways—introducing new avenues for nutrition-focused diagnostics in both clinical and public health contexts.Commercial adoption of AI-enabled microbiome testing is expanding rapidly as home-based stool collection kits and mobile health platforms make diagnostics more accessible to the general population. Companies are developing user-friendly interfaces that transform complex biomarker results into clear nutritional guidance, empowering individuals to take ownership of their health. However, the accuracy and reliability of consumer microbiome tests vary significantly across platforms, reflecting broader challenges in data standardization. Differences in sequencing techniques, machine learning model training, and reference databases can produce inconsistent interpretations. To ensure clinical trustworthiness, regulatory bodies and scientific organizations are working to establish validated standards for microbiome diagnostics, including reproducibility benchmarks, transparent reporting practices, and clinical validation requirements.

THE MICROBIOME AND AI: A POWERFUL PARTNERSHIP FOR NUTRITIONAL DISCOVERY

The fusion of microbiome science and artificial intelligence (AI) is transforming the field of nutritional discovery, enabling researchers and clinicians to unravel how diet shapes health at a level of complexity that was once impossible to decode. The human gut microbiome—comprising trillions of bacteria, fungi, viruses, and archaea—plays a fundamental role in digestion, metabolic regulation, immune system activation, and the biosynthesis of vitamins and neuroactive compounds. Variation in microbiome composition helps explain why individuals respond differently to the same foods, why certain diets produce dramatic health improvements in some but not others, and how nutritional imbalances contribute to chronic disease risk. However, microbiome ecosystems are extraordinarily dynamic, with microbial genes outnumbering human genes by orders of magnitude and interacting through biochemical networks that are still only partially understood. AI offers the computational power and analytical sophistication required to interpret these complex systems, accelerating nutritional discovery by uncovering new biomarkers, metabolic pathways, and personalized dietary strategies that support long-term health. Multi-omic technologies—such as metagenomics, metabolomics, proteomics, and transcriptomics—have generated vast datasets revealing the enormous functional diversity of the gut microbiome. Yet high dimensionality, nonlinear interactions, and environmental influences make these data difficult to analyze using traditional tools. Machine learning and deep learning techniques excel in pattern recognition, enabling the identification of microbial features linked to specific nutritional outcomes such as glycemic response, lipid metabolism efficiency, inflammatory load, and intestinal barrier health. AI-powered analysis helps classify microbial communities into health-relevant phenotypes, detect dysbiosis patterns associated with early disease risk, and map how dietary inputs are transformed into metabolic outputs. By integrating dietary records, wearable sensor data, genomics, and physiological biomarkers, AI systems can predict individualized responses to specific nutrients—from carbohydrate tolerance to fat absorption dynamics—paving the way for precision nutrition solutions grounded in microbial and metabolic individuality.

A key area in which the microbiome-AI partnership is driving discovery is the understanding of how microbial metabolites shape metabolic and neurological pathways. Short-chain fatty acids (SCFAs), bile acid derivatives, neurotransmitter precursors, and immune-modulating molecules produced by gut microbes act as signaling agents across the gut–brain, gut–liver, and gut–immune axes. AI models can quantify the influence of specific dietary changes on these biochemical pathways and identify the microbial drivers responsible for beneficial or detrimental metabolic states. For example, reinforcement learning approaches simulate how iterative changes in fiber or polyphenol intake optimize SCFA production, which in turn enhances insulin sensitivity and reduces inflammation. Similarly, causal inference modeling allows researchers to examine how microbial tryptophan metabolism affects serotonin availability and mood regulation, supporting nutritional psychiatry interventions that target mental well-being through gut health.AI is also accelerating the discovery of novel dietary compounds and microbiome-modulating interventions. By analyzing thousands of foods, phytochemicals, and microbial growth responses, AI tools can identify previously unrecognized prebiotics or food ingredients that nurture beneficial bacterial strains. These discoveries support the design of functional foods and personalized probiotic therapies tailored to an individual's gut ecology. Furthermore, AI-enabled predictive modeling helps refine clinical trials by identifying microbial biomarkers linked to treatment responsiveness, reducing trial duration and improving translational outcomes. Startups and research organizations are leveraging these capabilities to develop dynamic nutrition platforms that continuously evolve recommendations based on real-time microbiome monitoring through stool analysis, breath tests, or ingestible biosensors.The microbiome-AI partnership is not only advancing clinical and consumer nutrition but also contributing to global public health and sustainability. Large-scale AI-powered analyses of microbiome data across populations enable researchers to identify dietary patterns that promote microbial diversity and resilience—key indicators of long-term disease prevention. Such insights support the development of dietary guidelines that better reflect cultural diversity, geographical variability, and genetic differences. Additionally, microbiome-based agricultural research—supported by machine learning—is helping identify plant-based nutrition sources and food production methods that improve gut health while reducing environmental footprint, aligning nutritional discovery with planetary well-being.

CONCLUSION

The convergence of microbiome science, artificial intelligence (AI), and sustainable food innovation is ushering in a transformative shift in how societies understand the interrelations between diet, health, and environmental conservation. The escalating global challenges of food insecurity, dietary-related chronic diseases, and ecological degradation demand nutritional strategies that are not only personalized and health-promoting but also resource-efficient and climate-conscious. Within this landscape, AI-based microbiome biomarkers are emerging as powerful instruments for decoding the complex interactions between human gut microbial ecosystems and food systems of the future. The gut microbiome—an expansive community of bacteria, fungi, viruses, and archaea—plays a central role in nutrient metabolism, immune regulation, appetite control, mental health, and long-term disease risk. Yet, the microbiome varies profoundly among individuals due to genetics, lifestyle, geography, environmental exposures, and most critically, dietary inputs. Traditional nutritional guidelines—which adopt a one-size-fits-all perspective—struggle to address this biological heterogeneity. AI-driven approaches help overcome this limitation by extracting meaningful biomarkers from multi-omics datasets, including metagenomics, metabolomics, transcriptomics, and dietary data streams, thereby enabling predictive and dynamic models of personalized dietary response.Future foods—encompassing plant-based alternatives, cultured proteins, precision-fermented ingredients, algae-derived nutrients, and climate-resilient crops—represent a cornerstone of sustainable food systems. However, the physiological impacts of these novel foods cannot be fully understood through conventional nutrient composition analysis. The microbiome acts as a functional mediator between innovative food sources and human health outcomes. AI-based biomarker discovery enables rapid, high-fidelity evaluation of microbial responses to emerging food technologies, identifying beneficial changes such as improved short-chain fatty acid production, increased vitamin biosynthesis, enhanced fiber fermentation, and favorable modulation of immune-linked microbial pathways. Moreover, AI systems can detect detrimental microbial shifts resulting from excessive food additives, antinutrients, or imbalanced macronutrient formulations, facilitating iterative product reformulation to optimize gut-friendly design. Thus, microbiome analytics not only supports personalized diet recommendations but also accelerates the research, development, and regulatory assessment of sustainable foods.

From a planetary health perspective, AI-powered microbiome insights contribute to a paradigm where dietary patterns are shaped to reduce environmental burdens while maximizing human well-being. Diets that promote microbial diversity—particularly those rich in dietary fibers, resistant starches, polyphenols, and minimally processed plant ingredients—are often aligned with environmentally sustainable agricultural practices and lower greenhouse gas emissions. AI models incorporating microbiome biomarkers can quantify the health impacts of transitioning to sustainable diets, such as flexitarian, plant-forward, or culturally adapted regenerative food systems. This positions microbiome-aware nutrition policy as a strategic lever for achieving Sustainable Development Goals (SDGs) related to climate action, good health, responsible consumption, and food system resiliency. Additionally, precision nutrition guided by AI-enabled biomarkers can reduce overconsumption and food waste by tailoring portion sizes and nutrient composition to individual metabolic needs, reducing the ecological cost of dietary inefficiencies.The integration of microbiome biomarker discovery with digital health platforms—wearable sensors, mobile diet tracking, smart kitchen ecosystems, and cloud analytics—creates a continuous feedback loop between dietary behaviors and real-time biological response. These technologies empower consumers to understand how sustainable food choices influence their microbiome and overall health, making personalized nutrition accessible beyond clinical or research settings. At the same time, advancements in explainable AI ensure that prediction models retain transparency, enabling clinicians, nutritionists, and consumers to interpret microbiome-linked dietary recommendations with confidence. Blockchain-based traceability and AI-enabled safety monitoring can further reinforce trust in future foods by validating their microbial impacts across diverse demographic groups.Despite immense promise, challenges persist in data standardization, cross-population generalizability, ethical handling of microbiome-related health data, and regulatory frameworks for AI-assisted food labeling and personalized nutrition services. The microbiome's complexity means that biomarkers must be validated across time, environments, and cultural dietary practices to avoid biased or inequitable dietary guidance. Additionally, the commercialization of microbiome testing raises concerns around data privacy, informed consent, and affordability. Robust international governance, open science collaborations, and multidisciplinary workforce development—spanning food science, computational biology, microbiology, behavioral science, and sustainability research—are crucial for translating AI-microbiome insights into globally applicable nutritional solutions.

REFERENCES

Albayati, H., Alistarbadi, N., & Rho, J. J. (2023). Assessing engagement decisions in NFT metaverse based on the theory of planned behavior (TPB). *Telematics and Informatics Reports*, *10*, 100045. DOI: 10.1016/j.teler.2023.100045

Aljamaan, F., Temsah, M.-H., Altamimi, I., Al-Eyadhy, A., Jamal, A., Alhasan, K., Mesallam, T. A., Farahat, M., & Malki, K. H. (2024). Reference hallucination score for medical artificial intelligence chatbots: Development and usability study. *JMIR Medical Informatics*, *12*(1), e54345. DOI: 10.2196/54345 PMID: 39083799

Bano, N., & Siddiqui, S. (2024). Consumers' intention towards the use of smart technologies in tourism and hospitality (T&H) industry: A deeper insight into the integration of TAM, TPB and trust. *Journal of Hospitality and Tourism Insights*, *7*(3), 1412–1434. DOI: 10.1108/JHTI-06-2022-0267

Cardon, P., Fleischmann, C., Aritz, J., Logemann, M., & Heidewald, J. (2023). The challenges and opportunities of AI-assisted writing: Developing AI literacy for the AI age. *Business and Professional Communication Quarterly*, *86*(3), 257–295. DOI: 10.1177/23294906231176517

Chen, Y., & Esmaeilzadeh, P. (2024). Generative AI in medical practice: In-depth exploration of privacy and security challenges. *Journal of Medical Internet Research*, *26*, e53008. DOI: 10.2196/53008 PMID: 38457208

de Marcellis-Warin, N., Marty, F., Thelisson, E., & Warin, T. (2022). Artificial intelligence and consumer manipulations: From consumer's counter algorithms to firm's self-regulation tools. *AI and Ethics*, *2*(2), 259–268. DOI: 10.1007/s43681-022-00149-5

Dudley, R., Dodgson, G., Sarll, G., Halhead, R., Bolas, H., & McCarthy-Jones, S. (2014). The effect of arousal on auditory threat detection and the relationship to auditory hallucinations. *Journal of Behavior Therapy and Experimental Psychiatry*, *45*(3), 311–318. DOI: 10.1016/j.jbtep.2014.02.002 PMID: 24632145

Fui-Hoon Nah, F., Zheng, R., Cai, J., Siau, K., & Chen, L. (2023). Generative AI and ChatGPT: Applications, challenges, and AI-human collaboration. *Journal of Information Technology Case and Application Research*, *25*(3), 277–304. DOI: 10.1080/15228053.2023.2233814

Hoofnagle, C. J., Van Der Sloot, B., & Borgesius, F. Z. (2019). The European union general data protection regulation: What it is and what it means. *Information & Communications Technology Law*, *28*(1), 65–98. DOI: 10.1080/13600834.2019.1573501

Iriart, J. A. B. (2019). Precision medicine/personalized medicine: A critical analysis of movements in the transformation of biomedicine in the early 21st century. *Cadernos de Saude Publica, 35*, e00153118. DOI: 10.1590/0102-311x00153118 PMID: 30916181

Ivanov, S., Soliman, M., Tuomi, A., Alkathiri, N. A., & Al-Alawi, A. N. (2024). Drivers of generative AI adoption in higher education through the lens of the theory of planned behaviour. *Technology in Society*, *77*, 102521. DOI: 10.1016/j.techsoc.2024.102521

Jenkins, E. L., Ilicic, J., Barklamb, A. M., & McCaffrey, T. A. (2020). Assessing the credibility and authenticity of social media content for applications in health communication: Scoping review. *Journal of Medical Internet Research, 22*(7), e17296. DOI: 10.2196/17296 PMID: 32706675

Le, H. D., Wolinska, J. M., Baertschiger, R. M., & Himidan, S. A. (2023). Complication is inevitable, but suffering is optional—Psychological aspects of dealing with complications in surgery. *European Journal of Pediatric Surgery*, *33*(03), 181–190. DOI: 10.1055/s-0043-1767830 PMID: 36948212

Li, J. (2023). Information avoidance in the age of COVID-19: A meta-analysis. *Information Processing & Management*, *60*(1), 103163. DOI: 10.1016/j.ipm.2022.103163 PMID: 36405670

Manjunath, M., Ogwu, M. C., Udayakumar, S., Kuchipudi, J. D., Rengarajan, C., Selvakumar, P., & Manjunath, T. C. (2026). Chromatography in Food Contaminant Analysis: Principles, Advances, and Applications for Food Safety. In Ogwu, M., & Izah, S. (Eds.), *Detection, Identification, and Monitoring of Food Contaminants* (pp. 207–238). IGI Global Scientific Publishing., DOI: 10.4018/979-8-3373-3982-5.ch007

Pawar, P., Anute, N., Tripathi, S., Ahluwalia, G. K., Kalshetti, P., & Selvakumar, P. (2026). AI and Its Importance in the Development of Luxury Consumption. In Vale, V. (Ed.), *Multidisciplinary Approach to Luxury Consumption and AI* (pp. 1–34). IGI Global Scientific Publishing., DOI: 10.4018/979-8-3693-8422-0.ch001

Raj, R., Bhope, A., Kodmalwar, P. A., Sudindra, V. R., Sharma, A., Selvakumar, P., & Manjunath, T. C. (2026). Exchange Rates and Trade Dynamics. In Canguende-Valentim, C., Madaleno, M., Victorino, S., & Jungo, J. (Eds.), *Monetary Dynamics and Socio-Economic Development in Emerging Economies* (pp. 195–220). IGI Global Scientific Publishing., DOI: 10.4018/979-8-3693-9765-7.ch007

Raj, R., Lavanya, K., Chavan, S., Gokila, S., Hubballi, R. B., Selvakumar, P., & Manjunath, T. (2026). Econometric Models to Explain the Economic Growth of a Country or Region. In Reyes Ruiz, G. (Ed.), *Impacts of Military Spending on Economic Growth* (pp. 43–72). IGI Global Scientific Publishing., DOI: 10.4018/979-8-3373-3456-1.ch002

Selvakumar, P., & Haashni, S. SudhaAnanthi, G., & Manjunath, T. C. (2026). Cybernetic Systems Thinking: Foundations for Organizational Adaptability. In L. Tsvasman (Ed.), Cybernetic Leadership for Sustainable Innovation (pp. 99-124). IGI Global Scientific Publishing. DOI: 10.4018/979-8-3373-2484-5.ch004

Seshanna, S. V., Gopalakrishnan, G., Anute, N., Deepthi Reddy, K., Sharma, M., Selvakumar, P., & Manjunath, T. C. (2026). Digital Transformation and Cybersecurity. In Saeed, S., & Tahir, S. (Eds.), *User-Centric Cybersecurity Implications for Sustainable Digital Transformation* (pp. 1–30). IGI Global Scientific Publishing., DOI: 10.4018/979-8-3373-3171-3.ch001

Tsasis, P., & Bains, J. (2008). Management of complex chronic disease: Facing the challenges in the Canadian health-care system. *Health Services Management Research*, *21*(4), 228–235. DOI: 10.1258/hsmr.2008.008001 PMID: 18957400

Ulita, N., Kartanegara, A. T., Salsabila, J., Saleh, A., & Queen, Z. (2024). Empathy map gen z towards healthy food: A foodpreneur design strategy. [ATT]. *Aptisi Transactions on Technopreneurship*, *6*(2), 242–253. DOI: 10.34306/att.v6i2.404

Wang, C., Wang, H., & Li, Y.. (2024). Factors influencing university students' behavioral intention to use generative artificial intelligence: Integrating the theory of planned behavior and AI literacy. *International Journal of Human-Computer Interaction*, •••, 1–23. DOI: 10.1080/10447318.2024.2383033

Wei, C., Nawi, H. M., & Naeem, S. B. (2024). The uses and gratifications (U&G) model for understanding fake news sharing behavior on social media. *Journal of Academic Librarianship*, *50*(5), 102938. DOI: 10.1016/j.acalib.2024.102938

Wysocki, O., Davies, J. K., Vigo, M., Armstrong, A. C., Landers, D., Lee, R., & Freitas, A. (2023). Assessing the communication gap between AI models and healthcare professionals: Explainability, utility and trust in AI-driven clinical decision-making. *Artificial Intelligence*, *316*, 103839. DOI: 10.1016/j.artint.2022.103839

Xu, Y., Wang, M., Bao, L., Cheng, Z., & Li, X. (2024). A cross-sectional study based on the comprehensive model of information seeking: Which factors influence health information-seeking behavior in patients with periodontitis. *BMC Oral Health*, *24*(1), 1307. DOI: 10.1186/s12903-024-05068-x PMID: 39468496

Yim, D., Khuntia, J., Parameswaran, V., & Meyers, A. (2024). Preliminary evidence of the use of generative AI in health care clinical services: Systematic narrative review. *JMIR Medical Informatics*, *12*(1), e52073. DOI: 10.2196/52073 PMID: 38506918

Yuan, K.-H., Bentler, P. M., & Zhang, W. (2005). The effect of skewness and kurtosis on mean and covariance structure analysis: The univariate case and its multivariate implication. *Sociological Methods & Research*, *34*(2), 240–258. DOI: 10.1177/0049124105280200

Zhang, N., Xu, Y., Lu, Q., Zhu, L., An, R., Zhou, X., Wang, Y., Ma, Y., Deng, H., Guo, H., Wang, L., Sun, J., Bo, H., & Wang, X. (2024). Exploring the behavioral intentions of PICC-related thrombosis prevention in breast cancer patients undergoing chemotherapy: A qualitative study based on theory of planned behavior. *Supportive Care in Cancer*, *32*(10), 1–13. DOI: 10.1007/s00520-024-08827-2 PMID: 39235516

Chapter 14
Future Perspectives and Ethical Considerations in Microbiome-Based Nutrition

K. Gayathri
https://orcid.org/0009-0007-3786-2009
Department of Microbiology, Sacred Heart College, Tirupattur, India

K. Kesavardhini
https://orcid.org/0009-0005-8235-042X
Department of Microbiology, Sacred Heart College, Tirupattur, India

P. Saranraj
https://orcid.org/0000-0002-5052-6532
Department of Microbiology, Sacred Heart College, Tirupattur, India

B. Lokeshwari
https://orcid.org/0009-0005-6612-5134
Department of Microbiology, Sacred Heart College, Tirupattur, India

M. Manigandan
https://orcid.org/0000-0002-8115-2713
Department of Microbiology, Sacred Heart College, Tirupattur, India

A. Mubarak Ali
https://orcid.org/0009-0009-6367-7864
Department of Microbiology, Sacred Heart College, Tirupattur, India

ABSTRACT

The microbiome-based nutrition is a revolutionary change in nutritional science since it identifies the gut microbiome as the key node between diet and human health. The conventional dietary advice has been mostly based on the population-wide guidelines, but there is increasing evidence to show that how individuals respond to food is highly dependent on the composition and the capacity of the gut microbial communities. Human gut microbiome, which contains trillions of microorganisms, is a dynamic and metabolic and immunological organ that regulates nutrient usage, energy, inflammatory response, and host physiology by generating bioactive

DOI: 10.4018/979-8-3373-4382-2.ch014

metabolites, including short-chain fatty acid, vitamins, and signaling molecules. Recent developments in the high-throughput sequencing, multi-omics technologies, bioinformatics and artificial intelligence have sped up the comprehension of diet-microbiome-host interactions and made the possibility of precision and personalized nutrition strategies possible.

1. INTRODUCTION

The microbiome-based nutrition is a new and fast-moving subsector of the nutritional science that is changing the conventional understanding of the role of diet in human health. During decades, the nutritional recommendations were mostly grounded on generalized population-level recommendations, in which the nutritional needs of the host were considered in terms of both macronutrient and micronutrient needs. But increasingly scientific evidence points towards the fact that physiological effects of food cannot be completely comprehended without considering the complex and dynamic community of microorganisms that inhabits the human gastrointestinal tract. The gut microbiome, which is also known as this community, is composed of trillions of bacteria, archaea, fungi, viruses and protozoa that interact in an extremely interactive ecosystem. The gut microbiome is effectively an extra organ, which is involved in the key processes of the digestive system, metabolism, immunology, and endocrine interactions, and the general state of health (Asher et al., 2015).

The human intestinal microbiome plays one of the most vital roles in the metabolism of complex nutritional substances that cannot be digested by the enzymes of the human intestines. Gut microbes metabolize dietary fibers, resistant starch and oligosaccharides into bioactive products, such as short-chain fatty acids (SCFAs), vitamins (including vitamin K and some B vitamins), bile acid derivatives, and a broad array of signaling molecules. The effects of these microbial metabolites on host physiology are extensive, including the regulation of intestinal barrier, the control of inflammatory pathways, the impact of lipids and glucose metabolism, and the immune tolerance. As a result of this, gut microbiome is an influential mediator between diet and health, defining the way in which nutrients are processed and how dieting patterns are changed into physiological results (Bharti et al., 2020).

Individual differences in the composition and functional aspects of the microbiome have also highlighted the shortcomings of general dietary guidelines. That is because the gut microbial communities of individuals who eat the same foods can significantly differ in their metabolic and immunological responses. The genomics, age, early life exposures, use of antibiotics, lifestyle, geographical location, and cultural dietary practices are among the factors that influence the structure and functionality of the microbiome. This heterogeneity has prompted a growing interest in microbiome-informed/microbiome-based nutrition, which aims to personalize dietary recommendations based on the unique microbial composition of an individual as opposed to depending on the generalized nutritional recommendations (Shapira et al., 2020).

The high-throughput sequencing technologies and computational biology have advanced rapidly and have played a significant role in accelerating this area. Among the techniques that have allowed the global characterization of microbial diversity, functional gene content, and metabolic activity, are 16S rRNA gene sequencing, whole-genome shotgun metagenomics, metatranscriptomics, metaproteomics, and metabolomics. These tools combined with bioinformatics, artificial intelligence, and systems biology methods enable researchers to chart intricate dietmicrobiomehost interactions in unmatched detail and accuracy. These integrative studies have shown that dietary compounds have active roles in the formation of a microbial community and their metabolic productivity that affect host physiology well beyond elementary nutrient uptake (Dong et al., 2021).

Owing to these findings, microbiome-based dietary interventions are proving to be an effective means of prevention and control of a plethora of chronic disorders. Due to the gut-brain axis, dysbiosis, characterized by the state of an imbalance in microbial composition or activity, has been identified as the cause of obesity, type 2 diabetes, cardiovascular diseases, inflammatory bowel disease, allergies, autoimmune diseases, and even neuropsychiatric diseases. Dietary strategies to control the microbiome, including diets high in microbial accessible carbohydrates, prebiotics, probiotics, synbiotics, and even functional foods, are non-invasive and possibly sustainable ways of restoring microbial balance. The strategies promote long-term dietary patterns that result in microbial resilience and ecosystem stability unlike traditional drug therapies (Chopra et al., 2022).

In addition to disease treatment, the microbiome-based nutrition has significant potential in improving the healthspan and well-being. New studies indicate that functional capacity, microbial diversity and healthy aging are strongly correlated to immune competence and age-associated disease resistance. Diets favorably supporting the diversity of the microflora, especially rich in plant-based foods and dietary fibres, have been linked to a lower degree of systemic inflammation and a higher metabolic state. Microbiome-based nutrition by adopting nutritional practices that match the ecological needs of beneficial gut microbes can help to promote better life and longer lifespan (Meena et al., 2022).

Even considering its enormous potential, microbiome science is a difficult field to translate into practical and clinically actionable nutritional advice. Microbiome of the gut is extremely dynamic and sensitive to temporary fluctuations in the diet, stress, disease and drugs used. Transient changes and microbial responses based on their context makes it difficult to interpret microbiome data and reduces reproducibility across studies. Moreover, it is scientifically challenging in defining the cause-effect relationships between certain microbial taxa, food ingredients and health effects because of the interactive and dynamic environment of the microbial ecosystem (Karnwal et al., 2023).

Alongside scientific and technical issues, the microbiome-based nutrition attracts some significant ethical, social, and regulatory concerns. Microbiome data is highly personal and could give sensitive information regarding risk of diseases, lifestyle, and environmental exposure. Concerns about information privacy, possession, informed consent, and security storage are thus key to responsible research and practice. The growing commoditization of microbiome assay kits and individualized nutrition platforms has also become a cause of concerns with regard to inflated health assertions, scientifically unsound and inconsistent regulatory regulation (Tanwar et al., 2023).

Another important problem is equity and accessibility. Pharmacogenomic microbiome-based nutrition can be highly dependent on novel sequencing technologies, web-based interfaces, and technical skills, which are economically and technologically out of reach of broad groups of the global population. Such innovations may cause further health disparities in the hands of the privileged groups unless the policies are inclusive and designed with the aim of the common good and health. The ethical application of microbiome-based nutrition should then be based on such values as cost-effectiveness, cultural competence, and international applicability, especially in low- and middle-income communities (Ding et al., 2024).

2. EMERGING TRENDS IN MICROBIOME-BASED NUTRITION

There is an accelerated growth of microbiome-based nutrition which is propelled by advancements in technology, increasing biological knowledge, and a general rise in understanding of the microbiome as a significant health determinant. The new trends are focusing on personalization, innovation of functional foods, on targeted manipulation of the microbiome and integration into clinical and preventive healthcare systems. All these changes are transforming the conceptualization and practice of nutrition whether in the research or practice (Liu et al., 2024).

2.1 Precision and Personalized Nutrition

A transition to precision and personalized nutrition is one of the most notable new trends in microbiome-based nutrition. Contrary to the traditional dietary recommendations, which are based on a one-size-fits-all strategy, precision nutrition acknowledges that reactions to food may vary greatly and be highly dependent on the composition of the gut microbiome, the host genetics, metabolic condition, lifestyle, and the environmental exposures. Individualized dietary prescriptions on the basis of microbiome profiling are intended to maximize the efficiency of metabolism, enhance glycemic variability, control lipid metabolism, and decrease the threat of chronic illnesses (Longo et al., 2016).

Research studies have shown that the postprandial glucose responses, lipid metabolism, and inflammatory markers of people who eat the same foods can differ significantly, and it is mainly because of the gut microbial composition and activity. When the profile of the microbiome of a person is analyzed, in addition to clinical and lifestyle data, specific dietary interventions can also be adapted to ensure the activation of beneficial microbial pathways and inhibition of harmful ones. These interventions are especially applicable in the treatment of such metabolic disorders like obesity, type 2 diabetes and cardiovascular diseases (Reinke et al., 2019).

Precision nutrition is likely to develop with the help of machine learning and artificial intelligence (AI). The computational tools can combine big data multi-omics, such as metagenomics, metabolomics, host genomics, dietary intake, and clinical parameters. The accuracy of dietary response predictions can be enhanced by relying on AI-driven predictive models which can detect complex patterns and interactions that cannot be identified by the conventional statistical approaches. With further development of these models, the precision nutrition will probably be more predictive, dynamic, and clinically implementable (Świątkiewicz et al., 2021).

2.2 Functional Foods and Next-Generation Probiotics

The other significant movement in microbiome-based nutrition is the creation of functional items and the next generation probiotics that target to selectively regulate gut microbial communities. Conventional probiotics, which are usually Lactobacillus and Bifidobacterium strains, have proven to have health benefits but in most cases poor colonization ability as well as strain specificity. The next generations of strategies are going to be beyond these traditional formulations and more precise and functional microbial interventions (Lanzaro et al., 2023).

The next-generation probiotics include commensal anaerobic bacteria, e.g. *Akkermansia muciniphila* and *Faecalibacterium prausnitzii*, which are strongly linked to metabolic wellbeing, immune control, and intestinal barrier strength. Genetically engineered probiotic strains are also under investigation due to their capacity to provide therapeutic molecules, digest harmful metabolites or control certain metabolic pathways in the gut ecosystem. Multi-strain microbial consortia are also receiving a growing level of interest due to their ability to provide an ecosystem with balance more efficiently than single-strain probiotics (Goyal et al., 2023).

Another emerging field of innovation is functional foods that are fortified with prebiotics, synbiotics, postbiotics, and microbiota-accessible carbohydrates (MACs).

Prebiotic selectively stimulate the growth of good microbes, whereas postbiotic are non-viability microbial products or metabolites that do not require live organisms and still have health benefits. Such functional ingredients can be added to ordinary food, and the microbiome modulation becomes more affordable and sustainable. It is anticipated that such foods will be in the centre of promoting gut health and preventing diet-related illnesses at the population level (Tahara et al., 2013).

2.3 Microbiome Editing and Therapeutic Nutrition

Microbiome editing is a novel movement that goes past the passive dietary control to a more focused and controlled control of microbial communities. Novel strategies involve using bacteriophages to selectively kill pathogenic bacteria, bacteriocins to kill certain populations of microbes, or using CRISPR-based technologies to modify the genes of microbes or to regulate the behavior of microbes in the gut ecosystem. The strategies promise more precise and fewer off-target effects compared to broad-spectrum antibiotics in correcting dysbiosis (Shen et al., 2024).

Therapeutic nutrition is also being used together with microbiome editing tools in order to improve treatment efficacy. Diet may be utilized to develop a desirable ecological niche favoring the existence and operation of useful microorganisms unveiled by specific interventions. Using dietary fibers and certain nutrients as an example, it is possible to employ strategic applications of these factors to enhance the integration of helpful strains after microbiome editing or fecal microbiota transplantation. These combined strategies have potential in the management of complicated conditions, such as metabolic syndrome, inflammatory bowel disease, neurodegenerative and neuropsychiatric disorders associated with the gut-brain axis. Through the combination of nutritional interventions and those aimed at microbiome modification, potentially more long-lasting and customized treatment effects can be obtained (Gaur et al., 2022).

2.4 Integration with Preventive and Clinical Nutrition

One important trend of future in microbiome-based nutrition is its incorporation into preventive and clinical health systems. Given the weight of evidence illustrating a role for the microbiome in disease risk and prognosis, microbiome-informed dietary approaches should become an essential aspect of clinical nutrition and public health initiatives. Microbiome-based dietary plans could potentially aid in early detection of the disease, risk stratification and personalized prevention. In the clinical setting, microbiome-directed nutrition may enhance traditional pharmacological interventions by improving drug response, reducing side effects, and targeting drug-nutrient-microbe interactions. For instance, some gut bacteria mediate drug metabolism and bioavailability; thus, dietary-based manipulation of these microbial populations may improve the efficacy of drug therapy (González et al., 2025). From a preventive medicine perspective, the use of population-level microbiome information could theoretically be used to drive food-based dietary guideline recommendations designed to limit the onset and impact of chronic diseases. From a public health perspective, including microbiome science in nutrition policy may play part of the transition of healthcare systems toward prevention rather than remedy. Microbiome-based nutrition could aid in decreasing health costs, increasing optimal long-term health and support for sustainable healthcare through the promotion of dietary patterns that favor microbial diversity and resilience (Nadeem et al., 2017).

3. TECHNOLOGICAL AND SCIENTIFIC CHALLENGES

Nevertheless, although there are impressive developments in microbiome research and increasing interest in the idea of microbiome-based nutrition, there are still a number of technological and scientific obstacles that hamper the successful implementation of this concept in practical nutrition. The gut microbiome is a very difficult, dynamic, and context-specific ecosystem, and its relations with diet and host physiology is a very daunting challenge to comprehend. These issues need to be tackled in order to guarantee the reliability, reproducibility, and clinical validity of microbiome-informed nutritional interventions (Gorthy et al., 2024). Among the major issues, inter-individual variations in microbiome composition and functionality can be highlighted. The gut microbial profiles of no two people are the same, even in populations or individuals that are genetically related or adhering to a similar diet. This difference is due to many factors such as the genetics, age, sex, exposure to microbes during early periods of life, the birthing process, history of breastfeeding, antibiotic exposure, lifestyle, stress, geography and cultural food habits. Consequently, the effects of interventions based on dietary benefits may be inconsequential or even negative in another person. This heterogeneity makes it difficult to come up with generalizable dietary guidelines, and requires large and heterogeneous datasets to represent significant patterns of people (Ahmed et al., 2025).

Temporal instability and plasticity of the microbiome is closely related to inter-individual variability. The gut microbiome is not an environment that remains constant over time; it varies with time with short-term changes in diet, disease, drugs, traveling, and psychological stress. Although such flexibility enables the microbiome to react to environmental stimuli, it also creates research and clinical translation challenges. A single point in time might not be representative of the long-term microbial condition of an individual, providing inconsistent interpretations and low predictive ability. There is a need to use longitudinal studies to resolve microbiome dynamics hence this has been expensive thus logistically difficult (Rao et al., 2023). The other significant scientific weakness is that microbial genes and pathways lack complete functional annotation. Despite the fact that a significant number of millions of microbial genes are identified with metagenomic sequencing, a large fraction of them have not had an opportunity to be functionally characterized. This gap in knowledge limits the capacity to associate certain microbial functions with the contents of the diet and health outcomes. Moreover, gene presence may not directly mean that the gene is expressed or active, which is why such complementary techniques as metatranscriptomics, metaproteomics, and metabolomics are required. The combination of these datasets to produce a functional knowledge on the activity of microorganisms is still computationally demanding and necessitates sophisticated analytical models (Rawat et al., 2023).

Another important barrier is to create causal relationships between diet, changes in microbiome, and health outcomes. Most of the microbiome studies are observational and it is hard to determine causality as opposed to effect. As an illustration, although there are microbial profiles that are related to a disease state, it is not always clear whether such alterations are related to the development of the disease or that they are just an indication of the underlying pathological processes (Guan et al., 2023). Causality could be addressed in controlled dietary intervention studies and mechanistic experiments involving gnotobiotic animal models, yet there is a difficult issue of extrapolating the results of these models to human populations because of species-specific differences in microbiome composition and host physiology. Variations in the methodology among studies also make the field complex. Microbiome data has a significant potential of variation due to differences in sample collection methods, storage conditions, DNA extraction protocols, sequencing platforms, and bioinformatics pipelines. These discrepancies make cross-study comparisons and meta-analyses difficult, reducing the external validity of the results. Microbiome-based nutritional guidelines need therefore to be standardized and based on best practices to enhance reproducibility and trust in microbiome-based nutritional recommendations (Thanoon et al., 2023).

There are also other problems with data analysis and interpretation, which are connected with the enormous amounts and complexity of microbiome datasets. The sequencing of genome data in high-throughput measurements produces large volumes of data that involve the use of advanced computational instruments and statistical skills. Results and interpretations may be affected by biases that are brought about during the data processing like normalization process and taxonomic classification algorithms (Shariff et al., 2023). In addition, the microbiome data used along with diet, host genomics, metabolomics, and clinical measures is one of the key issues of analysis especially in the presence of no standardized models of multi-omics analysis. The other technological drawback is related to the correct determination of the diet that is paramount in associating diet with the change of microbiomes. The conventional dietary assessment procedures including food frequency questionnaires and self-reported dietary recalls are susceptible to recall bias and error. These constraints decrease the accuracy of diet-microbiome association research and make predictive models weaker. New digital tools, wearable, and metabolomic biomarkers resemble good options, but they are not standardized and accessible yet (Khan et al., 2023).

Inadequate biomarkers to determine whether microbiome is healthy also complicate microbiome-based nutrition. The diversity of microbes is commonly referred to as an indicator of health, yet the increased diversity is not always positive, and the circumstances are important. It is still a challenge to recognise trustworthy functional and metabolic indicators that are sufficient in showing the state of health. In the absence of proper benchmarks, it is inherently unclear how microbiome data can be converted into practical dietary recommendations. Practical challenges are also related to scalability and implementation in clinical contexts. Most microbiome analyses are based on expensive analytical facilities, unique human resources, and financial resources at present. Such requirements reduce the chances of their use in standard clinical practice and population health. It is critical to develop a set of diagnostic tools that are cost-effective, fast, and standardized and make microbiome-based nutrition accessible outside the laboratory (Gayap et al., 2024).

Lastly, technological issues are overlaped with ethical and regulatory uncertainty. Lack of specific regulatory principles of microbiome-based nutritional interventions may delay the clinical translation and confuse the researchers, clinicians, and industry stakeholders. It is important to assure public trust, avoid premature or misleading applications and assure scientific rigor, safety, and transparency. To conclude, microbiome-based nutrition has a great potential, but its successful implementation as a reliable and effective method is limited by serious technological and scientific issues. The diversity among individuals, the instability of the situation over time, the incomplete functional knowledge, the inabilities to form causative links, and the absence of the methodological norms are all evidence of the complexity of the given field. These difficulties will need interdisciplinary efforts, longitudinal, long-term studies, standardized methods, advanced computational, and strong regulatory measures to overcome them. To make the development of microbiome research clinically relevant and ethically responsible nutritional solutions, it is necessary to address these barriers (Alheeti et al., 2024).

4. MID- TO LONG-TERM PERSPECTIVES

4.1 Routine Use of Microbiome Profiling in Clinical Nutrition

In the coming 5-15 years, microbiome profiling is likely to become a research-based instrument, which will be used as a routine in the process of clinical nutritional evaluation. With the decrease in the cost of sequencing technologies, their increased speed and standardization, clinicians might soon regularly include gut microbiome data with the more common biomarkers, including anthropometry, biochemical indices, and dietary intake histories. This integration will be specifically helpful in the treatment of the metabolic disorders (obesity, type 2 diabetes, and metabolic syndrome), malnutrition, inflammatory bowel diseases, and the diet-responsive disorders such as irritable bowel syndrome (Hassan et al., 2024). Nonetheless, the general clinical acceptance of microbiome profiling will rely on creation of strong clinical evidence that indicates clinical usefulness i.e., that microbiome-informed nutritional diseases result in better health conditions than traditional dietary recommendations. Moreover, successful implementation will entail the formulation of reimbursement systems, inclusion of microbiome tests in clinical practice, and specialized training that will provide the dietitians, clinicians and healthcare providers with the competence to insure responsible and effective interpretation of microbiome data (Ansari et al., 2025).

4.2 Microbiome-Guided Therapeutics and Precision Synbiotics

The maturation of microbiome-directed therapeutics is a significant long-term development of microbiome-based nutrition. It is assumed that future interventions will be based on more specific, tailored interventions like designer probiotics, rationally designed microbial consortia, precision prebiotics, synbiotics, and bacteriophage based interventions. These applications will be specific to address discrete functional deficits of the gut microbiome, including dysfunctional short-chain fatty acid biosynthesis, disordered bile acid metabolism, or excess pro-inflammatory signaling. Such therapeutics can have synergistic effect when used together with individualized dietary interventions and improve metabolic regulation and prevention of diseases. However, they will need strict regulation during their translation into the routine use, in this case, in terms of Good Manufacturing Practices (GMP), strain characterization, genetic stability, safety profiling, and long-term ecological impact in the gut. The global agreement on regulatory routes and the content and efficacy of the regulatory standards will be essential to guarantee the safety, effectiveness and confidence in the population towards these emerging microbiome based nutritional therapeutics (Rajpoot and Tiwari, 2025).

4.3 AI and Automated Nutrition Advice at Scale

The artificial intelligence will have a transformative role in the provision of microbiome-based nutrition in large-scale. Over time, AI-based platforms can constantly compare longitudinal data of the microbiome with dietary intake, lifestyle, clinical parameters, and outputs of wearable sensors to offer adaptive, real-time nutritional advice. These systems might be dynamically regulated by dietary recommendations as the microbiome of an individual changes in response to diet, medication, stress or illness. Nonetheless, the application of AI-based nutritional guidance creates profound issues pertaining to data privacy, algorithmic accountability, and regulation. To ensure that these systems are accepted by the users and approved by the regulators, it will be necessary to ensure that such systems are mindful of individual autonomy, do not discriminate, and offer explainable suggestions. In addition, the strong validation in various populations and their association with the healthcare system instead of a stand-alone consumer application will be needed to avoid abuses and over-dependence on automated decision-making in nutrition and health management (Wang et al., 2025).

4.4 Population-Level and Public Health Applications

In addition to personalized care, microbiome data can also be used to grow both population-based nutrition and population health interventions. Massive microbiome surveillance may be used to establish microbial trends by community in relation to diet, environmental exposures or vulnerability to disease and therefore inform region-specific nutritional prescriptions and intervention. As an illustration, microbiome knowledge can be used to guide fortification policies, dietary diversification policies, or non-communicable disease policies. Nevertheless, there is a need to be careful when translating microbiome science into a public health practice (Zhou et al., 2025). Categorization of populations on the basis of microbiome signatures has the potential to cause stigmatizing or simplistic interpretation, especially when microbial disparities are analyzed without proper attention to socioeconomic, cultural and ecological factors. Public health practice that is ethical should thus focus on inclusiveness, cultural sensitivity and environmental sustainability making sure that microbiome informed policies do not overtake but rather enhance existing principles of nutrition related to the subject of public health (Obayya et al., 2023).

4.5 Global Health and Equity Challenges

One of the most significant issues of microbiome-based nutrition development in the long term is the strong unbalance in the world research representation. The available databases on microbiomes are mainly of high-income nations, and hence, the implications of the results to different populations with varying diets, lifestyles, and exposure to the environment are constrained. Microbiome-based nutrition can adversely strengthen global health inequities unless there is a conscious effort to involve low- and middle-income countries (LMICs). It will be necessary to develop research capacity, infrastructure and local expertise within LMICs to produce context-relevant information and interventions (Anjum et al., 2024). Besides, the adoption of precision nutrition under resource-constrained conditions also introduces practical questions of cost, accessibility, technological feasibility, and cultural relevance. These challenges will be overcome by new low-cost microbiome assessment devices, community-participatory research paradigm, and policies that uphold equity, which will mean that the advantages of microbiome-derived nutrition will be experienced by the entire world, not just the wealthy segments (Murph et al., 2024).

5. ETHICAL CONSIDERATIONS

Nutrition through microbiomes presents a multifaceted ethical dilemma that is both outside the scope of traditional nutritional science due to the biological sensitivity of microbiome information, and is further complicated by the fact that more sophisticated analytics (including artificial intelligence) are needed as well as the growing commercialization of personalized health solutions. In contrast to the usual dietary recommendations, microbiome-based ones are based on biological samples which can provide insights about the risk of a disease and about lifestyle and perhaps characteristic features which can be identified. Ethical considerations thus cut across informed consent, privacy, equity, governance, commercial interests and cultural sensitivity. It is crucial that the solution to these problems should be provided before they arise so that the microbiome-based nutrition can become an acceptable, fair, and socially responsible discipline instead of a field based on the power of technology or the need of the market (Casadevall et al., 2023).

5.1 Informed Consent and Comprehension

An informed consent is a basic ethical standard in microbiome-based nutrition, but it poses special problems because the scientific complexity and dynamism of microbiome studies make it challenging to implement. Test outcomes of microbiomes are commonly not a diagnosis but a probability, and their predictive ability on various health outcomes is not well known. Ethical consent practices should then clarify what microbiome testing is and is not able to tell, such as the constraints of the existing science (Zhang, 2023). The participants need to be aware of how their information can be utilized beyond instant dietary counseling, including further study, algorithm schooling, or product creation. Plain-language summaries, visual aids as well as the decision-support tools are essential in seeing to it that true understanding is acquired as opposed to formal consent. Informed consent should also cover the possible risks, uncertainty in the long term, reversibility of interventions as well as the necessity of follow up monitoring, particularly when the evidence is still being worked out in the case of interventions that require live or engineered microbes (Tiwari et al., 2018).

5.2 Privacy, Data Governance, and Re-identifiability

Microbiome data lie in a mediating position between genetic, clinical and lifestyle data in terms of ethical concerns. Even though the microbiome profiles cannot be compared to the human genomes sequences, they may be used as quasi-identifiers when supplemented with other metadata like diet, locality, or health conditions. Some of these risks are re-identification, secondary use, inference of disease susceptibility and commercial profiling without express consent (Su et al., 2021). Effective policies to promote ethical governance thus involves sound policies to protect data such as de-identification, encryption, controlled-access databases and straightforward policies on data-retention. Developing technical solutions like federated learning and privacy-preserving analytics are a potentially viable solution because they allow the models to develop without sharing data centrally. Clear governance systems should also establish access to microbiome information by whom, to what end, and under what circumstances and be held accountable with AI-driven analytics becoming more an inherent part of nutrition and healthcare decision-making (Wani et al., 2022).

5.3 Direct-to-Consumer Testing and Commercialization

The fast development of direct to consumer (DTC) microbiome testing services is a different ethical dilemma. Several DTC systems offer individualized nutritional advice through the analysis of microbiomes without adequate clinical support or expert advice. This brings into question false health claims, misconception among consumers and the possible harm of improper use of diet or other forms of supplements. Moreover, consumers might lack the information about the methods of their biological samples and data storage, reuse, or sale. Commercialization of evidence-based research needs to be ethical and conveyed through clear communication on strength of evidence, recommendation limitations and policy of data use. The regulatory standards and consumer protection policies are necessary to allow claims to be supported by evidence and consumers not to be deceived by the marketing narratives that surpass the scientific wisdom. The global moves towards consensus guidelines are one of the steps toward solving such challenges (Shabbir et al., 2024).

5.4 Responsibility and Accountability for AI-Driven Recommendations

With the growth of artificial intelligence as the foundation of microbiome-based nutrition platforms, the responsibility and accountability issues are of utmost importance. In case AI-based dietary recommendations cause negative results, it is not always clear who should take the blame the software developer, the medical professional, or the commercial force allowing the service. To make AI systems ethically used, it is necessary to report on model design, training data, performance measures, and known limitations. Risks can be addressed with the help of human-in-the-loop models, when clinicians or certified professionals still have control over AI suggestions. There should also be post-market monitoring and reporting and correcting error mechanisms. The regulatory precedents that have been observed due to other uses of clinical AI highlight the need to ensure that validation is done rigorously, constant monitoring is undertaken and accountability is well defined in terms of ensuring the safety of the users (Singh et al., 2022).

5.5 Cultural, Dietary, and Ecological Considerations

Food is heavily both culturally rooted within cultural identity, and within social practices and the local ecosystem. Any microbiome-based nutritional counseling that ignores cultural patterns of food consumption runs the risk of low compliance, lack of ethical sensitivity and unanticipated social outcomes. The ethics of nutrition approach should therefore be culturally sensitive and flexible to local ones instead of introducing homogenized or western-centric ones. Furthermore, the mass-scale changes in diet or the use of engineered microbes can have ecological consequences such as food systems, biodiversity, and environmental sustainability. The development and introduction of microbiome-based nutrition should incorporate and integrate environmental risk assessment and ecological ethics to make sure it is consistent with larger priorities of sustainability and planetary health (Weir, 2023).

6. REGULATORY, LEGAL, AND POLICY LANDSCAPE

The quick development of microbiome-based nutrition has surpassed most of the current regulatory and legal frameworks leaving researchers, clinicians, industry and consumers uncertain. In contrast to conventional nutritional interventions, microbiome-based interventions typically require biological measurements, sophisticated computational models, and live biomimicking products, and each of them can be classified under a different regulatory framework. It is necessary to create transparent, compatible and evidence-based regulatory channels to promote safety, effectiveness, transparency and trust by the people and at the same time promote innovation (Bai et al., 2023).

6.1 Regulation of Tests, Algorithms, and Therapeutics

There are several regulatory areas of microbiome-based nutrition products, such as diagnostic tests, software decision-support tools, and live biotherapeutic products. Tests involving the use of microbiome that can be used to produce dietary recommendations can be considered in vitro diagnostics but AI-based algorithms that can analyze the results of microbiome tests may be subject to regulation as a medical device, especially when such information can be used to impact clinical decision-making (Ratiner et al., 2023). Simultaneously, engineered biotherapeutic products like defined microbial consortia, engineered probiotics and bacteriophages are frequently regulated as biologics or live biotherapeutic products. The United States and European Union regulatory bodies have started to provide specifications regarding AI in healthcare as well as microbiome-based therapeutics, including risk-based classification principles, transparency, and lifecycle management. One of the key policy concerns is harmonization of regulatory classification, evidentiary requirements and post-market surveillance among these product types as hybrid products are becoming more of a combination of diagnostics, algorithms and therapeutics. The recent regulatory assent of AI tools to be utilized in clinical practice indicates that, under strict validation and continuous monitoring, more complicated digital and biological technologies may be incorporated into health care interventions, which will be the precedent in future application of microbiome-associated technologies (Iacomino et al., 2024).

6.2 Intellectual Property and Strain Commercialization

The intellectual property (IP) implications are particularly complicated with microbiome-based nutrition where the innovation can be based on naturally occurring microbial strains, engineered organisms, and proprietary data analytics. Although patent protection might encourage investment and innovation, excessive IP protection can lower availability, prevent independent validation and restrict scientific cooperation. The protection of commercial interests should be weighed with the aim of the policymakers on the protection of the public health and the research transparency (Shang et al., 2024). Ambiguities and court battles regarding patentability of microbial strains, genetic modifications and functional claims should be prevented by having clear guidelines to assess such matters. Also, the policies of data sharing, biobanking, and the accessibility of microbial samples may improve the reproducibility and transparency, as well as protecting the rights of participants. Moral IP systems must also consider benefit-sharing, especially where microbial resources or data are provided by a particular population or region, and commercialization must not be used as a tool to take advantage of the providers or to hurt the trust of the population (Whelan et al., 2024).

Table 1 summarizes the major scientific and technological limitations associated with microbiome-based nutrition. Although this approach holds great promise for personalized dietary interventions, several challenges—including biological variability, lack of causal evidence, and methodological constraints—currently restrict its reliable clinical application.

Table 1. Scientific and Technological Limitations in Microbiome-Based Nutrition

Limitation / Challenge	**Detailed Description and Implications**
Lack of proven causality	Most microbiome–nutrition studies are correlational rather than causal. Although specific microbial taxa or metabolites are associated with health outcomes, it remains unclear whether these microbes drive the condition or simply reflect underlying physiological changes. This limits the translation of findings into definitive dietary prescriptions.
Inter-individual variability	The gut microbiome differs markedly among individuals due to genetics, age, early-life exposure, antibiotic usage, lifestyle, geography, and cultural diet. Consequently, identical dietary interventions may produce diverse or even opposing responses, complicating standardization of recommendations.
Temporal instability of the microbiome	The microbiome is highly dynamic and can change rapidly in response to short-term dietary shifts, stress, illness, or medication. Single-time-point sampling may not represent long-term microbial states, reducing predictive reliability and reproducibility of results.
Incomplete functional annotation	A substantial proportion of microbial genes identified through metagenomics lack known functions. This restricts accurate interpretation of diet–microbiome–host interactions and limits mechanistic understanding of microbial contributions to health.
Methodological inconsistencies	Variations in sample collection, DNA extraction methods, sequencing platforms, and bioinformatic pipelines introduce technical bias. These inconsistencies hinder cross-study comparisons, meta-analyses, and formulation of universally accepted guidelines.
Limitations of AI and ML models	AI-driven nutrition models depend heavily on large, diverse, and high-quality datasets. Training on biased or limited datasets can result in overfitting, reduced generalizability, and inaccurate dietary predictions for underrepresented populations.

continued on following page

Table 1. Continued

Limitation / Challenge	Detailed Description and Implications
Inadequate biomarkers of "microbiome health"	There is no universally accepted definition of a "healthy microbiome." Measures such as microbial diversity do not always correlate with positive health outcomes, making it difficult to define clear clinical benchmarks.
Challenges in dietary assessment	Self-reported dietary data (food frequency questionnaires, recalls) are prone to recall bias and inaccuracies, weakening diet–microbiome association studies and limiting the accuracy of predictive nutritional models.

7. LIMITATIONS AND RISKS

Although the idea of microbiome-based nutrition could hold a great potential, it is important to note that the area has a gross number of limitations and unclear gaps that have yet to be mitigated properly. A lot of the existing information is on the associative studies but not on the proven causal relationships. Although specific microbial taxa, metabolic pathways and health outcomes are often associated with correlation, it is difficult to determine causality because host-microbe-diet interactions are intricate. Interindividual variability, temporal instability of the microbiome, confounding effects of genetics, environment and lifestyle make it difficult to interpret. Consequently, there is an implicit uncertainty in translating microbiome signatures to dependable dietary data or therapeutic intervention, which highlights the significance of carefully planned mechanistic experiments and interventional trials over a longer period (Abeltino et al., 2024).

Another drawback of interpreting microbiomes data using artificial intelligence and machine-learning models to create individualized nutrition recommendations. These models are very sensitive to the quality, size and diversity of datasets upon which they are trained. In cases where the training data are small, or biased, which is common when biased on certain groups of people or diet, models will overfit, learning noisy, but non-biological signals. This type of bias may cause incorrect predictions and lower performance when used on new or diverse populations and, in a way, increase health disparities. To mitigate this risk, it is necessary to have models developed in a transparent way, with external validation on different populations, and updating the algorithms with new information as it becomes accessible (Nazir et al., 2024).

It is also uncertain the ecological impact of the introduction of engineered microbes or live biotherapeutic products at a large scale. Although these interventions are expected to act in the controlled conditions of the human gut, their ecological behaviour in the long term is not completely comprehended. Designed or intentionally enriched microbial strains could last longer than desired, intermix incompletely with native microbiota, or can be transferred between or to the environment. These opportunities bring up the issues of interference with microbial ecology and horizontal gene transfer. This is why continuous monitoring, post-market surveillance, and ecological risk assessment are the necessary aspects of responsible implementation of microbiome-based interventions (Porcari et al., 2024).

The quick commercialization of microbiome nutrition is a massive threat to abuse and overestimate of the benefits. Business interests could drive the early release of products and services and market them to promote the bottom line at the expense of health rather than the positive results of scientific studies. This may give a blow to the populace, may confuse consumers, and even hurt them with unsuitable diet or treatment suggestions. In the absence of robust regulatory controls, professional ethics, and evidence-based care, the profession will be effectively controlled by a culture of hype instead of science. It is important to identify and discuss these limitations and uncertainties to make sure that microbiome-based nutrition develops as a valid, safe and beneficial part of the contemporary nutrition science (Metwaly et al., 2025).

This image 1: summarizes the microbiome-based nutrition by highlighting the central role of the gut microbiome in linking diet, health, and personalized nutrition. It illustrates how advanced tools such as sequencing, multi-omics, and artificial intelligence enable targeted dietary interventions, including functional foods, probiotics, and microbiome editing. The figure also emphasizes the balance between potential benefits—such as disease prevention and healthy aging—and key challenges, including individual variability and ethical concerns. Overall, the image conveys the need to integrate scientific innovation with responsible governance for effective microbiome-based nutrition.

Figure 1. Integrating Microbiome Science into Precision and Ethical Nutrition

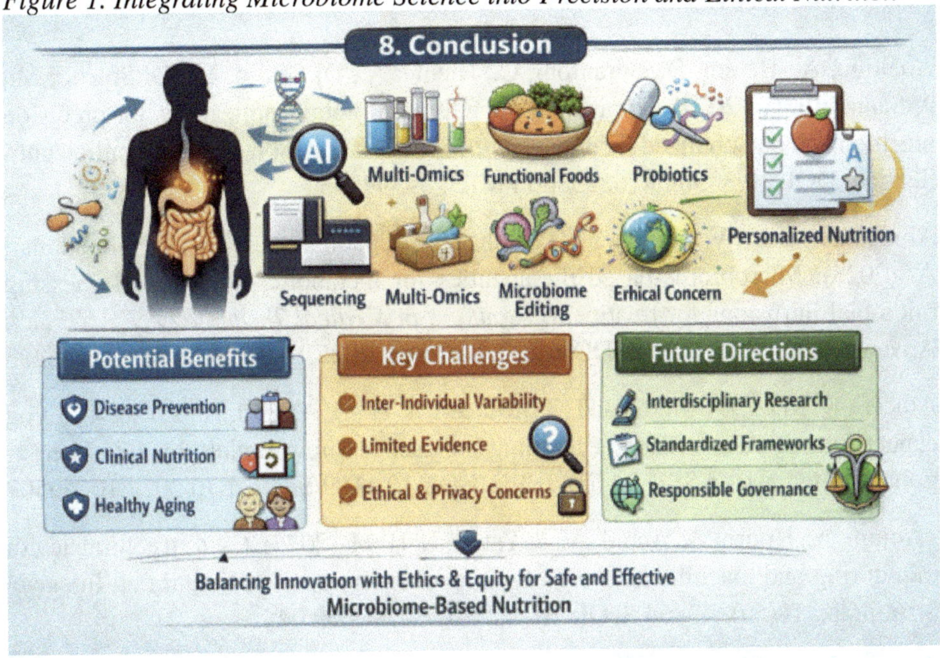

8. CONCLUSION

The microbiome-based nutrition is a paradigm change in the world of nutritional science because it focuses on the gut microbiome as one of the main intermediaries between food and the human body. The development of sequencing technologies, multi-omics, and artificial intelligence have facilitated more detailed insights into diet–microbiome–host interactions, which have led to accuracy and personalized nutrition. The future of disease prevention, clinical nutrition and healthy aging lie in the emerging interventions such as functional foods, second-generation probiotics, microbiome editing, and AI-based dietary advice. But such issues as inter-individual variability, time-varying stability of the microbiome, paucity of causal data, inconsistencies in methodology, and ethical issues of data privacy, equity, and commercialization still limit broad use in clinical practice. To ensure that microbiome-based nutrition is turned into safe, effective, and equitable health solutions, it will be necessary to address these limitations with respect to interdisciplinary research, standardized frameworks, and responsible governance.

9. REFERENCES

Abeltino, A., Hatem, D., Serantoni, C., Riente, A., Di Giulio, M., Di Spirito, M., & Santarelli, G. (2024). Unraveling the gut microbiota: Implications for precision nutrition and personalized medicine. *Nutrients*, *16*(22), 3806. Advance online publication. DOI: 10.3390/nu16223806 PMID: 39599593

Ahmed, N., Gaur, V., Kamle, M., Chauhan, A., Chauhan, R., Kumar, P., & Kumar, A. (2025). Microbiome-based therapeutics for metabolic disorders: Harnessing microbial intrusions for treatment. *Frontiers in Medical Technology*, *7*, 1695329. Advance online publication. DOI: 10.3389/fmedt.2025.1695329 PMID: 41246285

Alheeti, K. M. A., Al-Shouka, T. T., Majeed, S. H., & Ahmed, A. A. (2024). Lung cancer detection using machine learning and deep learning models. In 2024 International Conference on SSD (p. 63). IEEE. DOI: 10.1109/SSD61670.2024.10549507

) Anjum, A., Hrairi, M., Aabid, A., & Yatim, N. H. M. (2024). Civil structural health monitoring and machine learning: A comprehensive review. Frattura ed Integrità Strutturale, 18(69), 43–64. DOI: 10.3221/IGF-ESIS.69.04

Ansari, M. M., Kumar, S., Chola, C., Heyat, M. B. B., Akhtar, F., Hayat, M. A. B., & Yuan, Y. (2025). A novel machine and deep learning–based ensemble techniques for automatic lung cancer detection. *BioMed Research International*, *2025*(1), 6666688. Advance online publication. DOI: 10.1155/bmri/6666688

Asher, G., & Sassone-Corsi, P. (2015). Time for food: The intimate interplay between nutrition, metabolism, and the circadian clock. *Cell*, *161*(1), 84–95. DOI: 10.1016/j.cell.2015.03.015 PMID: 25815987

Bai, X., Huang, Z., Duraj-Thatte, A., Ebert, M., Zhang, F., Burgermeister, E., & Kong, J. (2023). Engineering the gut microbiome. *Nature Reviews Bioengineering*, *1*(9), 665–680. DOI: 10.1038/s44222-023-00072-2

Bharti, S. K., Pathak, V., Alam, T., Arya, A., Basak, G., & Awasthi, M. G. (2020). Materiality of edible film packaging in muscle foods: A worthwhile conception. *Journal of Packaging Technology and Research*, *4*(2), 117–132. DOI: 10.1007/s41783-020-00087-9

Casadevall, G., Duran, C., & Osuna, S. (2023). AlphaFold2 and deep learning for elucidating enzyme conformational flexibility and its application for design. *JACS Au*, *3*(6), 1554–1566. DOI: 10.1021/jacsau.3c00188 PMID: 37388680

Chopra, G., Kaushik, S., & Kain, P. (2022). Nutrient sensing via gut in *Drosophila melanogaster. International Journal of Molecular Sciences*, *23*(5), 2694. Advance online publication. DOI: 10.3390/ijms23052694 PMID: 35269834

Ding, L., Weger, B. D., Liu, J. Y., Zhou, L., Lim, Y., Wang, D., & Sassone-Corsi, P. (2024). Maternal high fat diet induces circadian clock-independent endocrine alterations impacting the metabolism of the offspring. *iScience*, *27*(5), 110343. Advance online publication. DOI: 10.1016/j.isci.2024.110343 PMID: 39045103

Dong, Y., Wei, Z., & Xue, C. (2021). Recent advances in carrageenan-based delivery systems for bioactive ingredients: A review. *Trends in Food Science & Technology*, *112*, 348–362. DOI: 10.1016/j.tifs.2021.04.012

Gaur, V. K., Gupta, S., Sharma, P., Gupta, P., Varjani, S., Srivastava, J. K., & Rodriguez-Couto, S. (2022). Metabolic cascade for remediation of plastic waste: A case study on microplastic degradation. *Current Pollution Reports*, *8*(1), 30–42. DOI: 10.1007/s40726-021-00210-7

Gayap, H. T., & Akhloufi, M. A. (2024). Deep machine learning for medical diagnosis, application to lung cancer detection: A review. *BioMedInformatics*, *4*(1), 236–257. DOI: 10.3390/biomedinformatics4010015

González-Hernández, A., Escamilla, A., Pérez-Ruiz, E., Rios, A., Frecha, C., Vaca-Paniagua, F., & Tenorio, J. (2025). From genes to personalized cancer care: A systematic review of toxicity-associated genetic variants in solid tumor treatments. *bioRxiv*. DOI: 10.1101/2025.10.21.25338446

Gorthy, S., Sargar, P., Hugar, C., Li, J., & Habyarimana, E. (2024). Summary of the potential and exploitation of omics and biotechnological breakthroughs in sorghum. In *Sorghum science and biotechnology* (p. 405). Springer., DOI: 10.1007/978-981-97-4347-6_17

Goyal, V. K., Rani, D., Arora, R., Mehrotra, S., Deng, C., & Wang, Y. (2023). Unlocking the potential of nano-enabled precision agriculture for efficient and sustainable farming. *Plants*, *12*(21), 3744. Advance online publication. DOI: 10.3390/plants12213744 PMID: 37960100

Guan, P., Yu, K., Wei, W., Tan, Y., & Wu, J. (2023). Big data analytics on lung cancer diagnosis framework with deep learning. *IEEE/ACM Transactions on Computational Biology and Bioinformatics*, *21*(2), 757–770. DOI: 10.1109/TCBB.2023.3281638 PMID: 37256795

Hassan, A., Khan, H., Ali, A., Din, I. U., Sajid, A., Husain, M., & Amin, R. (2024). An enhanced lung cancer identification and classification based on advanced deep learning and convolutional neural network. [BBE]. *Bulletin of Business and Economics, 13*(1), 136–150. DOI: 10.61506/01.00308

Iacomino, G., Rufián-Henares, J. Á., & Lauria, F. (2024). Editorial: Personalized nutrition and gut microbiota: Current and future directions. *Frontiers in Nutrition, 11*, 1375157. Advance online publication. DOI: 10.3389/fnut.2024.1375157 PMID: 38487630

Karnwal, A., Dohroo, A., & Malik, T. (2023). Unveiling the potential of bioinoculants and nanoparticles in sustainable agriculture for enhanced plant growth and food security. *BioMed Research International, 2023*(1), 6911851. Advance online publication. DOI: 10.1155/2023/6911851 PMID: 38075309

Khan, R. H., Miah, J., Nipun, S. A. A., Islam, M., Amin, M. S., & Taluckder, M. S. (2023). Enhancing lung cancer diagnosis with machine learning methods and systematic review synthesis. In 2021 7th International Conference on Electrical, Electronics and Information Engineering (ICEEIE) (p. 1). IEEE. DOI: 10.1109/ICEEIE59078.2023.10334739

Lanzaro, F., Barlabà, A., De Nigris, D., Di Domenico, F., Verde, V. L., Del Giudice, E. M., & Staiano, A. (2023). Pediatric diabetic nephropathy: Novel insights from microRNAs. *Journal of Clinical Medicine, 12*(4), 1447. Advance online publication. DOI: 10.3390/jcm12041447 PMID: 36835983

Liu, B., Zhou, H., Tan, L., Siu, K. T. H., & Guan, X. (2024). Exploring treatment options in cancer: Tumor treatment strategies. *Signal Transduction and Targeted Therapy, 9*(1), 175. Advance online publication. DOI: 10.1038/s41392-024-01856-7 PMID: 39013849

Longo, V. D., & Panda, S. (2016). Fasting, circadian rhythms, and time-restricted feeding in healthy lifespan. *Cell Metabolism, 23*(6), 1048–1059. DOI: 10.1016/j.cmet.2016.06.001 PMID: 27304506

Meena, K., Visarada, K., & Meena, D. K. (2022). *Sorghum bicolor* (L.) Moench a multifarious crop—Fodder to therapeutic potential and biotechnological applications: A future food for the millennium. *Future Foods : a Dedicated Journal for Sustainability in Food Science, 6*, 100188. Advance online publication. DOI: 10.1016/j.fufo.2022.100188

Metwaly, A., Kriaa, A., Hassani, Z., Carraturo, F., Druart, C., Arnauts, K., & de Vos, W. M. (2025). A consensus statement on establishing causality, therapeutic applications and the use of preclinical models in microbiome research. *Nature Reviews. Gastroenterology & Hepatology*, *22*(5), 343–357. DOI: 10.1038/s41575-025-01041-3 PMID: 40033063

Murph, A., Marston, C., Bramley, D., Trevelyan, C., & Allington, G. (2024). Dynamic token contextualization for adaptive knowledge synthesis in large language models. *OSF Preprints*. DOI: 10.31219/osf.io/8dsa7

Nadeem, M. A., Nawaz, M. A., Shahid, M. Q., Doğan, Y., Cömertpay, G., Yıldız, M., & Baloch, F. S. (2017). DNA molecular markers in plant breeding: Current status and recent advancements in genomic selection and genome editing. *Biotechnology, Biotechnological Equipment*, *32*(2), 261–285. DOI: 10.1080/13102818.2017.1400401

Nazir, A., Hussain, F. H. N., & Raza, A. (2024). Advancing microbiota therapeutics: The role of synthetic biology in engineering microbial communities for precision medicine. *Frontiers in Bioengineering and Biotechnology*, *12*, 1511149. Advance online publication. DOI: 10.3389/fbioe.2024.1511149 PMID: 39698189

Obayya, M., Arasi, M. A., Alruwais, N., Alsini, R., Mohamed, A., & Yaseen, I. (2023). Biomedical image analysis for colon and lung cancer detection using tuna swarm algorithm with deep learning model. *IEEE Access : Practical Innovations, Open Solutions*, *11*, 94705–94720. DOI: 10.1109/ACCESS.2023.3309711

Porcari, S., Mullish, B. H., Asnicar, F., Ng, S. C., Zhao, L., Hansen, R., & Segal, E. (2024). International consensus statement on microbiome testing in clinical practice. *The Lancet. Gastroenterology & Hepatology*, *10*(2), 154–163. DOI: 10.1016/S2468-1253(24)00311-X PMID: 39647502

Rajpoot, A., & Tiwari, S. (2025). Predictive modeling of structural performance using machine learning: A comprehensive review. *Deleted Journal*, *3*(1), 25–40. DOI: 10.47392/IRJAEH.2025.0005

Rao, B., & Arshad, M. Y. (2023). Early detection of lung cancer using machine learning technique. In *2022 International Conference on Computer Communication and Informatics (ICCCI)* (p. 1). IEEE. DOI: 10.1109/ICCCI56745.2023.10128389

Ratiner, K., Ciocan, D., Abdeen, S. K., & Elinav, E. (2023). Utilization of the microbiome in personalized medicine. *Nature Reviews. Microbiology*, *22*(4), 291–305. DOI: 10.1038/s41579-023-00998-9 PMID: 38110694

Rawat, D., Sharma, S., & Bhadula, S. (2023). Deep learning techniques in digital clinical diagnostic system for lung cancer. In 2022 8th International Conference on Advanced Computing and Communication Systems (ICACCS) (p. 1232). IEEE. DOI: 10.1109/ICACCS57279.2023.10113055

Reinke, H., & Asher, G. (2019). Crosstalk between metabolism and circadian clocks. *Nature Reviews. Molecular Cell Biology*, *20*(4), 227–241. DOI: 10.1038/s41580-018-0096-9 PMID: 30635659

Shabbir, K., Noureldin, M., & Sim, S. (2024). Data-driven model for seismic assessment, design, and retrofit of structures using explainable artificial intelligence. *Computer-Aided Civil and Infrastructure Engineering*. Advance online publication. DOI: 10.1111/mice.13338

Shang, Z., Pai, L., & Patil, S. (2024). Unveiling the dynamics of gut microbial interactions: A review of dietary impact and precision nutrition in gastrointestinal health. *Frontiers in Nutrition*, *11*, 1395664. Advance online publication. DOI: 10.3389/fnut.2024.1395664 PMID: 38873568

Shapira, S. N., & Christofk, H. R. (2020). Metabolic regulation of tissue stem cells. *Trends in Cell Biology*, *30*(7), 566–576. DOI: 10.1016/j.tcb.2020.04.004 PMID: 32359707

) Shariff, V., Paritala, C., & Ankala, K. (2023). An analysis on advances in lung cancer diagnosis with medical imaging and deep learning techniques: Challenges and opportunities.

Shen, H., Zhang, C., Li, S., Liang, Y., Lee, L. T., Aggarwal, N., & Lu, T. K. (2024). Prodrug-conjugated tumor-seeking commensals for targeted cancer therapy. *Nature Communications*, *15*(1), 4343. Advance online publication. DOI: 10.1038/s41467-024-48661-y PMID: 38773197

Singh, A., Rajput, V. D., Rawat, S., Sharma, R., Singh, A. K., Kumar, P., & Minkina, T. (2022). Geoinformatics and nanotechnological approaches for coping up abiotic and biotic stress in crop plants. In *Nanotechnology in plant growth promotion and protection* (p. 337). Wiley., DOI: 10.1002/9781119808565.ch17

Su, C., Hsu, Y., Thangudu, S., Chen, W., Huang, Y., Yu, C., & Wu, M. (2021). Application of multiparametric MR imaging to predict the diversification of renal function in miR29a-mediated diabetic nephropathy. *Scientific Reports*, *11*(1), 81519. Advance online publication. DOI: 10.1038/s41598-021-81519-7 PMID: 33479331

Świątkiewicz, I., Woźniak, A., & Taub, P. R. (2021). Time-restricted eating and metabolic syndrome: Current status and future perspectives. *Nutrients*, *13*(1), 221. Advance online publication. DOI: 10.3390/nu13010221 PMID: 33466692

Tahara, Y., & Shibata, S. (2013). Chronobiology and nutrition. *Neuroscience*, *253*, 78–88. DOI: 10.1016/j.neuroscience.2013.08.049 PMID: 24007937

Tanwar, R., Panghal, A., Chaudhary, G., Kumari, A., & Chhikara, N. (2023). Nutritional, phytochemical and functional potential of sorghum: A review. *Food Chemistry Advances*, *3*, 100501. Advance online publication. DOI: 10.1016/j.focha.2023.100501

Thanoon, M. A., Zulkifley, M. A., Zainuri, M. A. A. M., & Abdani, S. R. (2023). A review of deep learning techniques for lung cancer screening and diagnosis based on CT images. *Diagnostics (Basel)*, *13*(16), 2617. Advance online publication. DOI: 10.3390/diagnostics13162617 PMID: 37627876

Tiwari, S., Yadav, S. K., Sahu, V. K., & Tripathi, M. K. (2018). Current status and future prospects of marker assisted breeding for genetic improvement of minor millets. *International Journal of Current Microbiology and Applied Sciences*, *7*(12), 2587–2601. DOI: 10.20546/ijcmas.2018.712.293

Wang, J., Haq, A. U., Afzal, N., Khan, S., Alsolai, H., Alanazi, S. M., & Alshammari, W. M. (2025). Developing an innovative lung cancer detection model for accurate diagnosis in AI healthcare systems. *Scientific Reports*, *15*(1), 22945. Advance online publication. DOI: 10.1038/s41598-025-03960-2 PMID: 40592932

Wani, S. H., Choudhary, M., Barmukh, R., Bagaria, P. K., Samantara, K., Razzaq, A., & Kumar, A. (2022). Molecular mechanisms, genetic mapping, and genome editing for insect pest resistance in field crops. *Theoretical and Applied Genetics*, *135*(12), 3875–3901. DOI: 10.1007/s00122-022-04060-9 PMID: 35267056

Weir, T. L. (2023). Grand challenges: Actualizing the potential of the gut microbiome to address global nutrition challenges. *Frontiers in Microbiomes*, *2*, 1146827. Advance online publication. DOI: 10.3389/frmbi.2023.1146827

Whelan, K., Alexander, M., Gaïani, C., Lunken, G., Holmes, A., Staudacher, H. M., & Whelan, K. (2024). Design and reporting of prebiotic and probiotic clinical trials in the context of diet and the gut microbiome. *Nature Microbiology*, *9*(11), 2785–2796. DOI: 10.1038/s41564-024-01831-6 PMID: 39478082

Zhang, S. (2023). Artificial intelligence and applications in structural and material engineering. Highlights in Science. *Engineering and Technology*, *75*, 240–248. DOI: 10.54097/9qknfc57

Zhou, M., Huang, Z., Ma, Z., Chen, J., Lin, S., Yang, X., & Xu, X. (2025). The next frontier in antibody-drug conjugates: Challenges and opportunities in cancer and autoimmune therapy. *Cancer Drug Resistance (Alhambra, Calif.)*, *8*(1), 34–52. DOI: 10.20517/cdr.2025.49 PMID: 40843358

Compilation of References

Abbasi, A., Rad, A. H., Ghasempour, Z., Sabahi, S., Kafil, H. S., Hasannezhad, P., Rahbar Saadat, Y., & Shahbazi, N. (2022). The biological activities of postbiotics in gastrointestinal disorders. *Critical Reviews in Food Science and Nutrition*, *62*(22), 5983–6004. DOI: 10.1080/10408398.2021.1895061

Abdalkareem Jasim, S., Jade Catalan Opulencia, M., Alexis Ramírez-Coronel, A., & Markov, A. (2022). The emerging role of microbiota-derived short-chain fatty acids in immunometabolism. *International Immunopharmacology*, *110*, 108983. DOI: 10.1016/j.intimp.2022.108983

Abdulsalam, M., Hamisu, A. A., Ahmad, A. M., Wakili, F. B., Annu, F. S., & Garba, M. M. (2024). Microbiome dynamics and strategic management strategies: Exploring synergies between integrative medicine modalities and microbial balance. *Biological Sciences*, *4*(3), 725–735. DOI: 10.55006/biolsciences.2024.4307

Abeltino, A., Hatem, D., Serantoni, C., Riente, A., De Giulio, M. M., De Spirito, M., De Maio, F., & Maulucci, G. (2024). Unraveling the Gut Microbiota: Implications for Precision Nutrition and Personalized Medicine. *Nutrients*, *16*(22), 3806. DOI: 10.3390/nu16223806

Abondio, P., Sazzini, M., Garagnani, P., Boattini, A., Monti, D., Franceschi, C., Luiselli, D., & Giuliani, C. (2019). The Genetic Variability of APOE in Different Human Populations and Its Implications for Longevity. *Genes*, *10*(3), 222. DOI: 10.3390/genes10030222

Abusleme, L., Hoare, A., Hong, B.-Y., & Diaz, P. I. (2021). Microbial signatures of health, gingivitis, and periodontitis. *Periodontology 2000*, *86*(1), 57–78. DOI: 10.1111/prd.12362 PMID: 33690899

ACS Appl. Interfaces. (2020). *Skin-like thermal mapping devices*. DOI: 10.1021/acsami.0c04747

Adamska, A., Nowak, M., Piłaciński, S., Pilacinski, B., Adamska, B., Malewski, W., & Krętowski, A. (2016). Small intestinal bacterial overgrowth in adult patients with type 1 diabetes: Its prevalence and relationship with metabolic control and the presence of chronic complications of the disease. *Polish Archives of Internal Medicine*, *126*(9), 628–634. DOI: 10.20452/pamw.3501 PMID: 27535109

Ağagündüz, D., Cocozza, E., Cemali, Ö., Bayazıt, A. D., Nanì, M. F., Cerqua, I., Morgillo, F., Saygılı, S. K., Berni Canani, R., Amero, P., & Capasso, R. (2023). Understanding the role of the gut microbiome in gastrointestinal cancer: A review. *Frontiers in Pharmacology*, *14*, 1130562. DOI: 10.3389/fphar.2023.1130562 PMID: 36762108

Aggarwal, V.. (2023). Electrochemical (Bio)Sensing Devices for Human Microbiome Related Biomarkers. *Sensors (Basel)*, *23*(2), 837. DOI: 10.3390/s23020837 PMID: 36679633

Aghamajidi, A., & Maleki Vareki, S. (2022). The effect of the gut microbiota on systemic and anti-tumor immunity and response to systemic therapy against cancer. *Cancers (Basel)*, *14*(15), 3563. DOI: 10.3390/cancers14153563 PMID: 35892821

Aghebati-Maleki, L., Hasannezhad, P., Abbasi, A., & Khani, N. (2021). Antibacterial, antiviral, antioxidant, and anticancer activities of postbiotics: A review of mechanisms and therapeutic perspectives. *Biointerface Research in Applied Chemistry*, *12*(2), 2629–2645. DOI: 10.33263/BRIAC122.26292645

Aguilar-Toalá, J. E., Garcia-Varela, R., Garcia, H. S., Mata-Haro, V., González-Córdova, A. F., Vallejo-Cordoba, B., & Hernández-Mendoza, A. (2018). Postbiotics: An evolving term within the functional foods field. *Trends in Food Science & Technology*, *75*, 105–114. DOI: 10.1016/j.tifs.2018.03.009

Agus, A., Planchais, J., & Sokol, H. (2018). Gut Microbiota Regulation of Tryptophan Metabolism in Health and Disease. *Cell Host & Microbe*, *23*(6), 716–724. DOI: 10.1016/j.chom.2018.05.003 PMID: 29902437

Ahmed, N., Gaur, V., Kamle, M., Chauhan, A., Chauhan, R., Kumar, P., & Kumar, A. (2025). Microbiome-based therapeutics for metabolic disorders: Harnessing microbial intrusions for treatment. *Frontiers in Medical Technology*, *7*, 1695329. Advance online publication. DOI: 10.3389/fmedt.2025.1695329 PMID: 41246285

Akour, A. (2020). Probiotics and COVID-19: Is there any link? *Letters in Applied Microbiology*, *71*(3), 229–234. DOI: 10.1111/lam.13334

Al Assal, K., Prifti, E., Belda, E., Sala, P. C., Clément, K., Dao, M.-C., Doré, J., Levenez, F., Taddei, C. R., Fonseca, D. C., Rocha, I. M., Balmant, B. D., Thomas, A. M., Santo, M. A., Dias-Neto, E., Setubal, J. C., Zucker, J.-D., Belarmino, G., Torrinhas, R. S., & Waitzberg, D. L. (2020). Gut Microbiota Profile of Obese Diabetic Women Submitted to Roux-en-Y Gastric Bypass and Its Association with Food Intake and Postoperative Diabetes Remission. *Nutrients*, *12*(2), 278. DOI: 10.3390/nu12020278 PMID: 31973130

Alagiakrishnan, K., & Halverson, T. (2021). Microbial therapeutics in neurocognitive and psychiatric disorders. *Journal of Clinical Medicine Research*, *13*(9), 439–459. DOI: 10.14740/jocmr4575

Alam, M. T., Amos, G. C. A., Murphy, A. R. J., Murch, S., Wellington, E. M. H., & Arasaradnam, R. P. (2020). Microbial imbalance in inflammatory bowel disease patients at different taxonomic levels. *Gut Pathogens*, *12*(1), 1. DOI: 10.1186/s13099-019-0341-6 PMID: 31911822

Albayati, H., Alistarbadi, N., & Rho, J. J. (2023). Assessing engagement decisions in NFT metaverse based on the theory of planned behavior (TPB). *Telematics and Informatics Reports*, *10*, 100045. DOI: 10.1016/j.teler.2023.100045

Alberti, G., Mazzola, M., Gagliardo, C., Pitruzzella, A., Fucarini, A., Giammanco, M., ... & Carini, F. (2021). Extracellular vesicles derived from gut microbiota in inflammatory bowel disease and colorectal cancer. *Biomedical Papers of the Medical Faculty of Palacky University in Olomouc, 165*(3).

Alheeti, K. M. A., Al-Shouka, T. T., Majeed, S. H., & Ahmed, A. A. (2024). Lung cancer detection using machine learning and deep learning models. In 2024 International Conference on SSD (p. 63). IEEE. DOI: 10.1109/SSD61670.2024.10549507

Alhinai, E., Walton, G., & Commane, D. (2019). The role of the gut microbiota in colorectal cancer causation. *International Journal of Molecular Sciences*, *20*(21), 5295. DOI: 10.3390/ijms20215295 PMID: 31653078

Aljamaan, F., Temsah, M.-H., Altamimi, I., Al-Eyadhy, A., Jamal, A., Alhasan, K., Mesallam, T. A., Farahat, M., & Malki, K. H. (2024). Reference hallucination score for medical artificial intelligence chatbots: Development and usability study. *JMIR Medical Informatics*, *12*(1), e54345. DOI: 10.2196/54345 PMID: 39083799

Allali, I., Bakri, Y., Amzazi, S., & Ghazal, H. (2021). Gut-Lung axis in COVID-19. *Interdisciplinary Perspectives on Infectious Diseases*, *2021*(1), 6655380. DOI: 10.1155/2021/6655380

Allen, J. M., Mailing, L. J., Niemiro, G. M., Moore, R., Cook, M. D., White, B. A., Holscher, H. D., & Woods, J. A. (2018). Exercise alters gut microbiota composition and function in lean and obese humans. *Medicine and Science in Sports and Exercise*, *50*(4), 747–757. DOI: 10.1249/MSS.0000000000001495 PMID: 29166320

Allison, J., Kaliszewska, A., Uceda, S., Reiriz, M., & Arias, N. (2021). Targeting DNA Methylation in the Adult Brain through Diet. *Nutrients*, *13*(11), 3979. DOI: 10.3390/nu13113979 PMID: 34836233

Almeida-Santos, A. C., Novais, C., Peixe, L., & Freitas, A. R. (2021). Enterococcus spp. as a producer and target of bacteriocins: A double-edged sword in the antimicrobial resistance crisis context. *Antibiotics (Basel, Switzerland)*, *10*(10), 1215. DOI: 10.3390/antibiotics10101215 PMID: 34680796

Almonacid, D. E., Kraal, L., Ossandon, F. J., Budovskaya, Y. V., Cardenas, J. P., Bik, E. M., Goddard, A. D., Richman, J., & Apte, Z. S. (2017). 16S rRNA gene sequencing and healthy reference ranges for 28 clinically relevant microbial taxa from the human gut microbiome. *PLoS One*, *12*(5), e0176555. DOI: 10.1371/journal.pone.0176555 PMID: 28467461

Alpino, G. C. Á., Pereira-Sol, G. A., Dias, M. M., Aguiar, A. S., & Peluzio, M. C. G. (2024). Beneficial effects of butyrate on brain functions: A view of epigenetic. *Critical Reviews in Food Science and Nutrition*, *64*(12), 3961–3970. DOI: 10.1080/10408398.2022.2137776 PMID: 36287024

Al-Rashidi, H. E. (2022). Gut microbiota and immunity relevance in eubiosis and dysbiosis. *Saudi Journal of Biological Sciences*, *29*(3), 1628–1643. DOI: 10.1016/j.sjbs.2021.10.068 PMID: 35280528

Altay, O.. (2019). Systems biology perspective for studying the gut microbiota interactions. *Frontiers in Physiology*, *10*, 1177. DOI: 10.3389/fphys.2019.01177

Amar, J., Burcelin, R., Ruidavets, J. B., Cani, P. D., Fauvel, J., Alessi, M. C., Chamontin, B., & Ferrières, J. (2008). Energy intake is associated with endotoxemia in apparently healthy men. *The American Journal of Clinical Nutrition*, *87*(5), 1219–1223. DOI: 10.1093/ajcn/87.5.1219 PMID: 18469242

Amar, J., Chabo, C., Waget, A., Klopp, P., Vachoux, C., Bermúdez-Humarán, L. G., Smirnova, N., Bergé, M., Sulpice, T., Lahtinen, S., Ouwehand, A., Langella, P., Rautonen, N., Sansonetti, P. J., & Burcelin, R. (2011). Intestinal mucosal adherence and translocation of commensal bacteria at the early onset of type 2 diabetes: Molecular mechanisms and probiotic treatment. *EMBO Molecular Medicine*, *3*(9), 559–572. DOI: 10.1002/emmm.201100159 PMID: 21735552

Ambrogi, V., Bottacini, F., Cao, L., Kuipers, B., Schoterman, M., & van Sinderen, D. (2023). Galacto-oligosaccharides as infant prebiotics: Production, application, bioactive activities and future perspectives. *Critical Reviews in Food Science and Nutrition, 63*(6), 753–766. DOI: 10.1080/10408398.2021.1953437

Amedei, A., & Morbidelli, L. (2019). Circulating metabolites originating from gut microbiota control endothelial cell function. *Molecules (Basel, Switzerland), 24*(21), 3992. DOI: 10.3390/molecules24213992 PMID: 31694161

Ames, N., Storsley, J., & Thandapilly, S. J. (2018). In Beta, T., & Camire, M. E. (Eds.), *Functionality of beta-glucan from oat and barley and its relation with human health. Cereal Grain-based Functional Foods: Carbohydrate and Phytochemical Components* (pp. 147–166). The Royal Society of Chemistry., DOI: 10.1039/9781788012799-00147

Anas, M., Khattak, W. A., Fahad, S., Alrawiq, N., Alrawiq, H. S., Abdelsalam, N. R., Jaremko, M., & Quraishi, U. M. (2025). Mitigating heavy metal pollution in agriculture: A multi-omics and nanotechnology approach to safeguard global wheat production. *Journal of Hazardous Materials Advances, 17*, 100584. https://doi.org/https://doi.org/10.1016/j.hazadv.2024.100584. DOI: 10.1016/j.hazadv.2024.100584

An, B. C., Ahn, J. Y., Kwon, D., Kwak, S. H., Heo, J. Y., Kim, S., Ryu, Y., & Chung, M. J. (2023). Anti-cancer roles of probiotic-derived P8 protein in colorectal cancer cell line DLD-1. *International Journal of Molecular Sciences, 24*(12), 9857. DOI: 10.3390/ijms24129857

Anjana, a., & Tiwari, S. K. (2022). Bacteriocin-producing probiotic lactic acid bacteria in controlling dysbiosis of the gut microbiota. *Frontiers in Cellular and Infection Microbiology, 12*, 851140.

Ansaldo, E., Farley, T. K., & Belkaid, Y. (2021). Control of immunity by the microbiota. *Annual Review of Immunology, 39*(1), 449–479. DOI: 10.1146/annurev-immunol-093019-112348

Ansari, M. M., Kumar, S., Chola, C., Heyat, M. B. B., Akhtar, F., Hayat, M. A. B., & Yuan, Y. (2025). A novel machine and deep learning–based ensemble techniques for automatic lung cancer detection. *BioMed Research International, 2025*(1), 6666688. Advance online publication. DOI: 10.1155/bmri/6666688

Anwar, F., Altayb, H. N., Al-Abbasi, F. A., Al-Malki, A. L., Kamal, M. A., & Kumar, V. (2021). Antiviral effects of probiotic metabolites on COVID-19. *Journal of Biomolecular Structure & Dynamics, 39*(11), 4175–4184. DOI: 10.1080/07391102.2020.1775123

Anwer, E. K., Ajagbe, M., Sherif, M., Musaibah, A. S., Mahmoud, S., ElBanbi, A., & Abdelnaser, A. (2025). Gut microbiota secondary metabolites: Key roles in GI tract cancers and infectious diseases. *Biomedicines*, *13*(1), 100. DOI: 10.3390/biomedicines13010100 PMID: 39857684

Anyanwu, R. C., & Jukes, D. J. (1990). Food safety control systems for developing countries. *Food Control*, *1*(1), 17–26. DOI: 10.1016/0956-7135(90)90116-T

Arneth, B. M. (2018). Gut–brain axis biochemical signalling from the gastrointestinal tract to the central nervous system: Gut dysbiosis and altered brain function. *Postgraduate Medical Journal*, *94*(1114), 446–452. DOI: 10.1136/postgradmedj-2017-135424 PMID: 30026389

Arnold, J. W., Roach, J., Fabela, S., Moorfield, E., Ding, S., Blue, E., Dagher, S., Magness, S., Tamayo, R., Bruno-Barcena, J. M., & Azcarate-Peril, M. A. (2021). The pleiotropic effects of prebiotic galacto-oligosaccharides on the aging gut. *Microbiome*, *9*(1), 1–19. DOI: 10.1186/s40168-020-00980-0 PMID: 33388088

Arnone, A. A., Ansley, K., Heeke, A. L., Howard-McNatt, M., & Cook, K. L. (2025). Gut microbiota interact with breast cancer therapeutics to modulate efficacy. *EMBO Molecular Medicine*, *17*(2), 219–234. DOI: 10.1038/s44321-024-00185-0 PMID: 39820166

Aronsson, L., Huang, Y., Parini, P., Korach-André, M., Håkansson, J., Gustafsson, J. Å., Pettersson, S., Arulampalam, V., & Rafter, J. (2010). Decreased fat storage by Lactobacillus paracasei is associated with increased levels of angiopoietin-like 4 protein (ANGPTL4). *PLoS One*, *5*(9), e13087. DOI: 10.1371/journal.pone.0013087 PMID: 20927337

Arora, M., & Baldi, A. (2017). Comparative study of regulatory framework for probiotics: Current status and future recommendations. *Applied Clinical Research, Clinical Trials and Regulatory Affairs*, *4*(2), 140–156. DOI: 10.2174/2213476X04666170620100145

Arora, T., & Bäckhed, F. (2016). The gut microbiota and metabolic disease: Current understanding and future perspectives. *Journal of Internal Medicine*, *280*(4), 339–349. DOI: 10.1111/joim.12508 PMID: 27071815

Artif. Intell. Med. (2024a). *Intelligent wearable assisted digital healthcare industry 5.0*. DOI: 10.1016/j.artmed.2024.103000

Artif. Intell. Med. (2024b). *Remote patient monitoring using AI: current state, applications, and challenges*. DOI: 10.1016/j.artmed.2023.102049

Arumugam, M., Raes, J., Pelletier, E., Le Paslier, D., Yamada, T., Mende, D. R., Fernandes, G. R., Tap, J., Bruls, T., Batto, J. M., Bertalan, M., Borruel, N., Casellas, F., Fernandez, L., Gautier, L., Hansen, T., Hattori, M., Hayashi, T., Kleerebezem, M., & Dore, J. (2011). Enterotypes of the human gut microbiome. *Nature*, *473*(7346), 174–180. DOI: 10.1038/nature09944 PMID: 21508958

Asher, G., & Sassone-Corsi, P. (2015). Time for food: The intimate interplay between nutrition, metabolism, and the circadian clock. *Cell*, *161*(1), 84–95. DOI: 10.1016/j.cell.2015.03.015 PMID: 25815987

Asif, R., Liu, R., de Souza, R. J., Azab, S., Chong, M., Anand, S. S., & Deng, W. Q. (2025). A Scoping Review of Epigenetic Signatures of Diet and Diet-related Metabolites: Insights from Epigenome-Wide Association Studies and Their Implications for Cardiometabolic Health and Diseases. *The Yale Journal of Biology and Medicine*, *98*(2), 203–225. DOI: 10.59249/BDGN2070 PMID: 40589935

Asnicar, F., Berry, S. E., Valdes, A. M., Nguyen, L. H., Piccinno, G., Drew, D. A., Leeming, E., Gibson, R., Le Roy, C., Khatib, H. A., Francis, L., Mazidi, M., Mompeo, O., Valles-Colomer, M., Tett, A., Beghini, F., Dubois, L., Bazzani, D., Thomas, A. M., & Segata, N. (2021). Microbiome connections with host metabolism and habitual diet from 1,098 deeply phenotyped individuals. *Nature Medicine*, *27*(2), 321–332. DOI: 10.1038/s41591-020-01183-8 PMID: 33432175

Averina, O. V., Zorkina, Y. A., Yunes, R. A., Kovtun, A. S., Ushakova, V. M., Morozova, A. Y., Kostyuk, G. P., Danilenko, V. N., & Chekhonin, V. P. (2020). Bacterial metabolites of human gut microbiota correlating with depression. *International Journal of Molecular Sciences*, *21*(23), 9234. DOI: 10.3390/ijms21239234 PMID: 33287416

Ayesha, I. E., Monson, N. R., Klair, N., Patel, U., Saxena, A., Patel, D., & Ayesha, I. E. (2023). Probiotics and their role in the management of type 2 diabetes mellitus (Short-term versus long-term effect): A systematic review and meta-analysis. *Cureus*, *15*(10). Advance online publication. DOI: 10.7759/cureus.46741

Babu, M., & Snyder, M. (2023). Multi-Omics Profiling for Health. *Molecular & Cellular Proteomics*, *22*(6), 100561. DOI: 10.1016/j.mcpro.2023.100561 PMID: 37119971

Badal, V. D., Vaccariello, E. D., Murray, E. R., Yu, K. E., Knight, R., Jeste, D. V., & Nguyen, T. T. (2020). The gut microbiome, aging, and longevity: A systematic review. *Nutrients*, *12*(12), 3759. DOI: 10.3390/nu12123759 PMID: 33297486

Bai, X., Huang, Z., Duraj-Thatte, A., Ebert, M., Zhang, F., Burgermeister, E., & Kong, J. (2023). Engineering the gut microbiome. *Nature Reviews Bioengineering*, *1*(9), 665–680. DOI: 10.1038/s44222-023-00072-2

Balaguer, F., Enrique, M., Llopis, S., Barrena, M., Navarro, V., Álvarez, B., Chenoll, E., Ramón, D., Tortajada, M., & Martorell, P. (2022). Lipoteichoic acid from Bifidobacterium animalis subsp. lactis BPL1: A novel postbiotic that reduces fat deposition via IGF-1 pathway. *Microbial Biotechnology*, *15*(3), 805–816. DOI: 10.1111/1751-7915.13769

Bana, B., & Cabreiro, F. (2019). The microbiome and aging. *Annual Review of Genetics*, *53*(1), 239–261. DOI: 10.1146/annurev-genet-112618-043650 PMID: 31487470

Banan, A., Fields, J. Z., Decker, H., Zhang, Y., & Keshavarzian, A. (2000). Nitric oxide and its metabolites mediate ethanol-induced microtubule disruption and intestinal barrier dysfunction. *The Journal of Pharmacology and Experimental Therapeutics*, *294*(3), 997–1008. DOI: 10.1016/S0022-3565(24)39164-5

Bandyopadhyay, B., & Mandal, N. C. (2014). Probiotics, prebiotics and synbiotics-in health improvement by modulating gut microbiota: The concept revisited. *International Journal of Current Microbiology and Applied Sciences*, *3*(3), 410–420.

Bano, N., & Siddiqui, S. (2024). Consumers' intention towards the use of smart technologies in tourism and hospitality (T&H) industry: A deeper insight into the integration of TAM, TPB and trust. *Journal of Hospitality and Tourism Insights*, *7*(3), 1412–1434. DOI: 10.1108/JHTI-06-2022-0267

Bárcena, C., Valdés-Mas, R., Mayoral, P., Garabaya, C., Durand, S., Rodríguez, F., Fernández-García, M. T., Salazar, N., Nogacka, A. M., Garatachea, N., Bossut, N., Aprahamian, F., Lucia, A., Kroemer, G., Freije, J. M. P., Quirós, P. M., & López-Otín, C. (2019). Healthspan and lifespan extension by fecal microbiota transplantation into progeroid mice. *Nature Medicine*, *25*(8), 1234–1242. DOI: 10.1038/s41591-019-0504-5 PMID: 31332389

Barone, M., D'Amico, F., Brigidi, P., & Turroni, S. (2022). Gut microbiome–micronutrient interaction: The key to controlling the bioavailability of minerals and vitamins? *BioFactors (Oxford, England)*, *48*(2), 307–314. DOI: 10.1002/biof.1835 PMID: 35294077

Bauer, H., Horowitz, R. E., Levenson, S. M., & Popper, H. (1963). The response of the lymphatic tissue to the microbial flora: Studies on germfree mice. *American Journal of Pathology*, *42*(4), 471–483. PMID: 13966929

Begani, J., Lakhani, J., & Harwani, D. (2018). Current strategies to induce secondary metabolites from microbial biosynthetic cryptic gene clusters. *Annals of Microbiology, 68*(7), 419–432. DOI: 10.1007/s13213-018-1351-1

Belkaid, Y., & Hand, T. W. (2014). Role of the microbiota in immunity and inflammation. *Cell, 157*(1), 121–141. DOI: 10.1016/j.cell.2014.03.011 PMID: 24679531

Bello, M. G. D., et al. (2018). Preserving microbial diversity. *science, 362*(6410), 33-34.

Bemark, M., Pitcher, M. J., Dionisi, C., & Spencer, J. (2024). Gut-associated lymphoid tissue: A microbiota-driven hub of B cell immunity. *Trends in Immunology, 45*(3), 211–223. DOI: 10.1016/j.it.2024.01.006 PMID: 38402045

Bergman, E. N. (1990). Energy contributions of volatile fatty acids from the gastrointestinal tract in various species. *Physiological Reviews, 70*(2), 567–590. DOI: 10.1152/physrev.1990.70.2.567 PMID: 2181501

Berni Canani, R., Sangwan, N., Stefka, A. T., Nocerino, R., Paparo, L., Aitoro, R., Calignano, A., Khan, A. A., Gilbert, J. A., & Nagler, C. R. (2016). *Lactobacillus rhamnosus* GG-supplemented formula expands butyrate-producing bacterial strains in food allergic infants. *The ISME Journal, 10*(3), 742–750. DOI: 10.1038/ismej.2015.151

Berry, S. E., Valdes, A. M., Drew, D. A., Asnicar, F., Mazidi, M., Wolf, J., & Segal, E. (2020). Human postprandial responses to food and potential for precision nutrition. *Nature Medicine, 26*(6), 964–973. DOI: 10.1038/s41591-020-0934-0 PMID: 32528151

Beserra, B. T. S., Fernandes, R., do Rosario, V. A., Mocellin, M. C., Kuntz, M. G. F., & Trindade, E. B. S. M. (2015). A systematic review and meta-analysis of the prebiotics and synbiotics effects on glycaemia, insulin concentrations and lipid parameters in adult patients with overweight or obesity. *Clinical Nutrition (Edinburgh, Lothian), 34*(5), 845–858. DOI: 10.1016/j.clnu.2014.10.004 PMID: 25456608

Bešlo, D., Golubić, N., Rastija, V., Agić, D., Karnaš, M., Šubarić, D., & Lučić, B. (2023). Antioxidant activity, metabolism, and bioavailability of polyphenols in the diet of animals. *Antioxidants, 12*(6), 1141. DOI: 10.3390/antiox12061141 PMID: 37371871

Bharti, S. K., Pathak, V., Alam, T., Arya, A., Basak, G., & Awasthi, M. G. (2020). Materiality of edible film packaging in muscle foods: A worthwhile conception. *Journal of Packaging Technology and Research, 4*(2), 117–132. DOI: 10.1007/s41783-020-00087-9

Bhuiyan, M. N. I., & Nahid, M. (2025). Smart nutrition: AI and 3D printing for personalized diets. *Food and Nutrition, 1*(2), 100032. DOI: 10.1016/j.fnutr.2025.100032

Bhuiyan, M. N. I., Saha, B. K., & Satter, M. A. (2025). Harnessing Artificial Intelligence and Precision Diets for Brain Health and Cognitive Resilience. *The Journal of Nutrition, 155*(10), 3179–3190. Advance online publication. DOI: 10.1016/j.tjnut.2025.08.007 PMID: 40812476

Bhushan, B., Singh, B. P., Saini, K., Kumari, M., Tomar, S. K., & Mishra, V. (2019). Role of microbes, metabolites and effector compounds in host–microbiota interaction: A pharmacological outlook. *Environmental Chemistry Letters, 17*(4), 1801–1820. DOI: 10.1007/s10311-019-00914-9

Biagi, E., Franceschi, C., Rampelli, S., Severgnini, M., Ostan, R., Turroni, S., Consolandi, C., Quercia, S., Scurti, M., Monti, D., Capri, M., Brigidi, P., & Candela, M. (2016). Gut microbiota and extreme longevity. *Current Biology, 26*(11), 1480–1485. DOI: 10.1016/j.cub.2016.04.016 PMID: 27185560

Binns, N., Lee, M. K., & Lee, A. (2015). The relationship between gut microbiota and protein digestion. *Nutrition Research Reviews, 28*(2), 121–135. DOI: 10.1017/S0954422415000100 PMID: 26650242

Birknerova, N., Mancikova, V., Paul, E. D., Matyasovsky, J., Cekan, P., Palicka, V., & Parova, H. (2022). Circulating Cell-Free DNA-Based Methylation Pattern in Saliva for Early Diagnosis of Head and Neck Cancer. *Cancers (Basel), 14*(19), 4882. DOI: 10.3390/cancers14194882 PMID: 36230805

Bisht, V., et al. (2024). Understanding of probiotic origin antimicrobial peptides: a sustainable approach ensuring food safety. *npj Science of Food, 8*(1), 67.

Bjerregård Madsen, J., Kaila, A., Vehviläinen-Julkunen, K., & Miettinen, M. (2016). Time allocation and temporal focus in nursing management: An integrative review. *Journal of Nursing Management, 24*(8), 983–993. DOI: 10.1111/jonm.12411 PMID: 27411357

Blaabjerg, S., Artzi, D. M., & Aabenhus, R. (2017). Probiotics for the prevention of antibiotic-associated diarrhea in outpatients—A systematic review and meta-analysis. *Antibiotics (Basel, Switzerland), 6*(4), 21. DOI: 10.3390/antibiotics6040021 PMID: 29023420

Blevins, S. M., & Bronze, M. S. (2010). Robert Koch and the “golden age” of bacteriology. *International Journal of Infectious Diseases, 14*(9), e744–e751. DOI: 10.1016/j.ijid.2009.12.003 PMID: 20413340

Bloemendaal, A. L., Buchs, N. C., George, B. D., & Guy, R. J. (2016). Intestinal stem cells and intestinal homeostasis in health and in inflammation. *Surgery, 159*(5), 1237–1248. DOI: 10.1016/j.surg.2016.01.014

Borgeraas, H., Johnson, L. K., Skattebu, J., Hertel, J. K., & Hjelmesæth, J. (2018). Effects of probiotics on body weight, body mass index, fat mass and fat percentage in subjects with overweight or obesity: A systematic review and meta-analysis of randomized controlled trials. *Obesity Reviews, 19*(2), 219–232. DOI: 10.1111/obr.12626 PMID: 29047207

Bouchard, C., & Ordovas, J. M. (2012). Fundamentals of nutrigenetics and nutrigenomics. *Progress in Molecular Biology and Translational Science, 108*, 1–15. DOI: 10.1016/B978-0-12-398397-8.00001-0

Bourebaba, Y., Marycz, K., Mularczyk, M., & Bourebaba, L. (2022). Postbiotics as potential new therapeutic agents for metabolic disorders management. *Biomedicine and Pharmacotherapy, 153*, 113138. DOI: 10.1016/j.biopha.2022.113138

Bouziat, R., Hinterleitner, R., Brown, J. J., Stencel-Baerenwald, J. E., Ikizler, M., Mayassi, T., Meisel, M., Kim, S. M., & Jabri, B. (2017). Reovirus infection triggers inflammatory responses to dietary antigens and development of celiac disease. *Science, 356*(6333), 44–50. DOI: 10.1126/science.aah5298

Boyle, R. J., Robins-Browne, R. M., & Tang, M. L. (2006). Probiotic use in clinical practice: What are the risks? *The American Journal of Clinical Nutrition, 83*(6), 1256–1264. DOI: 10.1093/ajcn/83.6.1256 PMID: 16762934

Bradley, E., & Haran, J. (2024). The human gut microbiome and aging. *Gut Microbes, 16*(1), 2359677. DOI: 10.1080/19490976.2024.2359677 PMID: 38831607

Bressa, C., Bailén-Andrino, M., Pérez-Santiago, J., González-Soltero, R., Pérez, M., Montalvo-Lominchar, M. G., Maté-Muñoz, J. L., Domínguez, R., Moreno, D., & Larrosa, M. (2017). Differences in gut microbiota profile between women with active lifestyle and sedentary women. *PLoS One, 12*(2), e0171352. DOI: 10.1371/journal.pone.0171352 PMID: 28187199

Brown, E. M., Clardy, J., & Xavier, R. J. (2023). Gut microbiome lipid metabolism and its impact on host physiology. *Cell Host & Microbe, 31*(2), 173–186. DOI: 10.1016/j.chom.2023.01.009 PMID: 36758518

Bryrup, T., Thomsen, C. W., Kern, T., Allin, K. H., Brandslund, I., Jørgensen, N. R., Vestergaard, H., Hansen, T., Hansen, T. H., Pedersen, O., & Nielsen, T. (2019). Metformin-induced changes of the gut microbiota in healthy young men: Results of a non-blinded, one-armed intervention study. *Diabetologia*, *62*(6), 1024–1035. DOI: 10.1007/s00125-019-4848-7 PMID: 30904939

Bull, M. J., & Plummer, N. T. (2014). Part 1: The human gut microbiome in health and disease. *Integrative Medicine (Encinitas, Calif.)*, *13*(6), 17–22. PMID: 26770121

Bultman, S. J. (2014). Molecular pathways: Gene-environment interactions regulating dietary fiber induction of proliferation and apoptosis via butyrate for cancer prevention. *Clinical Cancer Research*, *20*(4), 799–803. DOI: 10.1158/1078-0432.CCR-13-2483 PMID: 24270685

Bunyavanich, S., Shen, N., Grishin, A., Jones, S. M., Leung, D. Y. M., Sampson, H., Sicherer, S., & Clemente, J. C. (2016). Early-life gut microbiome composition and milk allergy resolution. *The Journal of Allergy and Clinical Immunology*, *138*(4), 1122–1130. DOI: 10.1016/j.jaci.2016.03.041

Camelo-Castillo, A., Rivera-Caravaca, J. M., Orenes-Piñero, E., Ramírez-Macías, I., Roldán, V., Lip, G. Y. H., & Marín, F. (2021). Gut microbiota and the quality of oral anticoagulation in vitamin K antagonists users: A review of potential implications. *Journal of Clinical Medicine*, *10*(4), 715. DOI: 10.3390/jcm10040715 PMID: 33670220

Caminero, A., Guzman, M., Libertucci, J., & Lomax, A. E. (2023). The emerging roles of bacterial proteases in intestinal diseases. *Gut Microbes*, *15*(1), 2181922. DOI: 10.1080/19490976.2023.2181922

Campbell, J. H., Foster, C. M., Vishnivetskaya, T., Campbell, A. G., Yang, Z. K., Wymore, A., Palumbo, A. V., Chesler, E. J., & Podar, M. (2012). Host genetic and environmental effects on mouse intestinal microbiota. *The ISME Journal*, *6*(11), 2033–2044. DOI: 10.1038/ismej.2012.54 PMID: 22695862

Campos-Perez, W., & Martinez-Lopez, E. (2021). Effects of short chain fatty acids on metabolic and inflammatory processes in human health. *Biochimica et Biophysica Acta (BBA)-. Biochimica et Biophysica Acta. Molecular and Cell Biology of Lipids*, *1866*(5), 158900. DOI: 10.1016/j.bbalip.2021.158900 PMID: 33571672

Canfora, E. E., Jocken, J. W., & Blaak, E. E. (2015). Short-chain fatty acids in control of body weight and insulin sensitivity. *Nature Reviews. Endocrinology*, *11*(10), 577–591. DOI: 10.1038/nrendo.2015.128 PMID: 26260141

Cani, P. D., Amar, J., Iglesias, M. A., Poggi, M., Knauf, C., Bastelica, D., Neyrinck, A. M., Fava, F., Tuohy, K. M., Chabo, C., Waget, A., Delmée, E., Cousin, B., Sulpice, T., Chamontin, B., Ferrières, J., Tanti, J. F., Gibson, G. R., Casteilla, L., & Burcelin, R. (2007). Metabolic endotoxemia initiates obesity and insulin resistance. *Diabetes*, *56*(7), 1761–1772. DOI: 10.2337/db06-1491 PMID: 17456850

Cani, P. D., & de Vos, W. M. (2017). Next-generation beneficial microbes: The case of Akkermansia muciniphila. *Frontiers in Microbiology*, *8*, 1765. DOI: 10.3389/fmicb.2017.01765 PMID: 29018410

Cani, P. D., Possemiers, S., Van de Wiele, T., Guiot, Y., Everard, A., Rottier, O., Geurts, L., Naslain, D., Neyrinck, A., Lambert, D. M., Muccioli, G. G., & Delzenne, N. M. (2009). Changes in gut microbiota control inflammation in obese mice through a mechanism involving GLP-2-driven improvement of gut permeability. *Gut*, *58*(8), 1091–1103. DOI: 10.1136/gut.2008.165886 PMID: 19240062

Cani, P. D., Van Hul, M., & Delzenne, N. M. (2019). Microbiome and metabolic health: From mechanisms to therapeutic perspectives. *Nature Reviews. Endocrinology*, *15*(2), 69–85. DOI: 10.1038/s41574-018-0143-9 PMID: 30602737

Cannizzaro, R., Maiero, S., Pelizzo, P., Gulotta, M., Facchin, S., Tessarolo, G., Zucchetto, A., Matrone, F., Realdon, S., & Bortolus, R. (2025). Microencapsulated sodium butyrate in the prevention of acute radiotherapy proctitis: Single-center prospective study. *Journal of Clinical Medicine*, *14*(13), 4783. Advance online publication. DOI: 10.3390/jcm14134783 PMID: 40649157

Cantu-Jungles, T., & Hamaker, B. (2020). New view on dietary fiber selection for predictable shifts in gut microbiota. *mBio*, *11*(1), 02179–02119. DOI: 10.1128/mBio.02179-19 PMID: 32071263

Cao, X., Dong, A., Kang, G., Wang, X., Duan, L., Hou, H., Zhao, T., Wu, S., Liu, X., Huang, H., & Wu, R. (2022). Modeling spatial interaction networks of the gut microbiota. *Gut Microbes*, *14*(1), 2106103. DOI: 10.1080/19490976.2022.2106103 PMID: 35921525

Carbonero, F., Benefiel, A. C., & Gaskins, H. R. (2012). Contributions of the microbial hydrogen economy to colonic homeostasis. *Nature Reviews. Gastroenterology & Hepatology*, *9*(9), 504–518. DOI: 10.1038/nrgastro.2012.85 PMID: 22585131

Cardona, F., Andrés-Lacueva, C., Tulipani, S., Tinahones, F. J., & Queipo-Ortuño, M. I. (2013). Benefits of polyphenols on gut microbiota and implications in human health. *The Journal of Nutritional Biochemistry*, *24*(8), 1415–1422. DOI: 10.1016/j.jnutbio.2013.05.001 PMID: 23849454

Cardon, P., Fleischmann, C., Aritz, J., Logemann, M., & Heidewald, J. (2023). The challenges and opportunities of AI-assisted writing: Developing AI literacy for the AI age. *Business and Professional Communication Quarterly*, *86*(3), 257–295. DOI: 10.1177/23294906231176517

Carlos-Reyes, Á., López-González, J. S., Meneses-Flores, M., Gallardo-Rincón, D., Ruíz-García, E., Marchat, L. A., Astudillo-de la Vega, H., Hernández de la Cruz, O. N., & López-Camarillo, C. (2019). Dietary Compounds as Epigenetic Modulating Agents in Cancer. *Frontiers in Genetics*, *10*, 79. DOI: 10.3389/fgene.2019.00079

Carson, C., & Lawson, H. A. (2018). Epigenetics of metabolic syndrome. *Physiological Genomics*, *50*(11), 947–955. DOI: 10.1152/physiolgenomics.00072.2018 PMID: 30240346

Carvalho, B. M., & Saad, M. J. A. (2013). Influence of gut microbiota on subclinical inflammation and insulin resistance. *Mediators of Inflammation*, *986734*, 1–13. Advance online publication. DOI: 10.1155/2013/986734 PMID: 23840101

Casadevall, G., Duran, C., & Osuna, S. (2023). AlphaFold2 and deep learning for elucidating enzyme conformational flexibility and its application for design. *JACS Au*, *3*(6), 1554–1566. DOI: 10.1021/jacsau.3c00188 PMID: 37388680

Casado, J. M. R. (2017). Centenario de Elie Metchnikoff (1845-1916). *Educación Médica*, *18*(2), 136–143. DOI: 10.1016/j.edumed.2016.11.009

Cazzaniga, M., Cardinali, M., Di Pierro, F., Zonzini, G. B., Palazzi, C. M., Gregoretti, A., Zerbinati, N., Guasti, L., & Bertuccioli, A. (2024). The potential role of probiotics, especially butyrate producers, in the management of gastrointestinal mucositis induced by oncologic chemo-radiotherapy. *International Journal of Molecular Sciences*, *25*(4), 2306. Advance online publication. DOI: 10.3390/ijms25042306 PMID: 38396981

Chassaing, B., Vijay-Kumar, M., & Gewirtz, A. T. (2017). How diet can impact gut microbiota to promote or endanger health. *Current Opinion in Gastroenterology*, *33*(6), 417–421. DOI: 10.1097/MOG.0000000000000401 PMID: 29019865

Chaudhary, D., Guleria, D., Aggarwal, H., Mishra, V., Chauhan, A., Dufossé, L., & Joshi, N. C. (2025). Nutrigenomics and Personalized Diets-Tailoring Nutrition for Optimal Health. *Applied Food Research*, *100980*(1), 100980. Advance online publication. DOI: 10.1016/j.afres.2025.100980

Chelakkot, C., Choi, Y., Kim, D.-K., Park, H. T., Ghim, J., Kwon, Y., Jeon, J., Kim, M.-S., Jee, Y.-K., Gho, Y. S., Park, H.-S., Kim, Y.-K., & Ryu, S. H. (2018). Akkermansia muciniphila-derived extracellular vesicles influence gut permeability through the regulation of tight junctions. *Experimental & Molecular Medicine*, *50*(2), e450. DOI: 10.1038/emm.2017.282 PMID: 29472701

Chelakkot, C., Ghim, J., & Ryu, S. H. (2018). Mechanisms regulating intestinal barrier integrity and its pathological implications. *Experimental & Molecular Medicine*, *50*(8), 1–9. DOI: 10.1038/s12276-018-0126-x PMID: 30115904

Cheng, F. S., Pan, D., Chang, B., Jiang, M., & Sang, L. X. (2020). Probiotic mixture VSL# 3: An overview of basic and clinical studies in chronic diseases. *World Journal of Clinical Cases*, *8*(8), 1361–1384. DOI: 10.12998/wjcc.v8.i8.1361 PMID: 32368530

Cheng, J., Hu, J., Geng, F., & Nie, S. (2022). Bacteroides utilization for dietary polysaccharides and their beneficial effects on gut health. *Food Science and Human Wellness*, *11*(5), 1101–1110. DOI: 10.1016/j.fshw.2022.04.002

Chen, J., Zhao, K.-N., & Vitetta, L. (2019). Effects of intestinal microbial–elaborated butyrate on oncogenic signaling pathways. *Nutrients*, *11*(5), 1026. DOI: 10.3390/nu11051026 PMID: 31067776

Chen, L., Zhernakova, D. V., Kurilshikov, A., Andreu-Sánchez, S., Wang, D., Augustijn, H. E., Vich Vila, A., Weersma, R. K., Medema, M. H., Netea, M. G., Kuipers, F., Wijmenga, C., Zhernakova, A., & Fu, J. (2022). Influence of the microbiome, diet and genetics on inter-individual variation in the human plasma metabolome. *Nature Medicine*, *28*(11), 2333–2343. DOI: 10.1038/s41591-022-02014-8 PMID: 36216932

Chen, S., Zhang, Z., Liu, S., Chen, T., Lu, Z., Zhao, W., Mou, X., & Liu, S. (2024). Consistent signatures in the human gut microbiome of longevous populations. *Gut Microbes*, *16*(1), 2393756. DOI: 10.1080/19490976.2024.2393756 PMID: 39197040

Chen, Y., & Esmaeilzadeh, P. (2024). Generative AI in medical practice: In-depth exploration of privacy and security challenges. *Journal of Medical Internet Research*, *26*, e53008. DOI: 10.2196/53008 PMID: 38457208

Chen, Y., Zhang, S., Zeng, B., Zhao, J., Yang, M., Zhang, M., Li, Y., Ni, Q., Wu, D., & Li, Y. (2020). Transplant of microbiota from long-living people to mice reduces aging-related indices and transfers beneficial bacteria. *Aging (Albany NY)*, *12*(6), 4778–4793. DOI: 10.18632/aging.102872 PMID: 32176868

Chen, Z., Guan, D., Wang, Z., Li, X., Dong, S., Huang, J., & Zhou, W. (2023). Microbiota in cancer: Molecular mechanisms and therapeutic interventions. *MedComm*, *4*(6), e417. DOI: 10.1002/mco2.417 PMID: 37937304

Chetty, A., & Blekhman, R. (2024). Multi-omic approaches for host-microbiome data integration. *Gut Microbes*, *16*(1), 2297860. DOI: 10.1080/19490976.2023.2297860 PMID: 38166610

Chieffi, D., Fanelli, F., & Fusco, V. (2022). Legislation of probiotic foods and supplements. In *Probiotics for human nutrition in health and disease* (pp. 25–44). Academic Press., DOI: 10.1016/B978-0-323-89908-6.00013-3

Chignell, J. F., De Long, S. K., & Reardon, K. F. (2018). Meta-proteomic analysis of protein expression distinctive to electricity-generating biofilm communities in air-cathode microbial fuel cells. *Biotechnology for Biofuels*, *11*(1), 121. DOI: 10.1186/s13068-018-1111-2

Chigurupati, M. (2025). Unraveling the Causal Effects of Risk Factors on Diabetes Mellitus Insights from Mendelian Randomization Studies. *North American Journal of Engineering Research*, *6*(1).

Cho, I., & Blaser, M. J. (2012). The human microbiome at the interface of health and disease. *Nature Reviews. Genetics*, *13*(4), 260–270. DOI: 10.1038/nrg3182 PMID: 22411464

Cho, M. S., Kim, S. Y., Suk, K. T., & Kim, B. Y. (2018). Modulation of gut microbiome in nonalcoholic fatty liver disease: Pro-, pre-, syn-, and antibiotics. *Journal of Microbiology (Seoul, Korea)*, *56*(12), 855–867. DOI: 10.1007/s12275-018-8346-2

Chopra, G., Kaushik, S., & Kain, P. (2022). Nutrient sensing via gut in *Drosophila melanogaster. International Journal of Molecular Sciences*, *23*(5), 2694. Advance online publication. DOI: 10.3390/ijms23052694 PMID: 35269834

Christ, A., Lauterbach, M., & Latz, E. (2019). Western diet and the immune system: An inflammatory connection. *Immunity*, *51*(5), 794–811. DOI: 10.1016/j.immuni.2019.09.020 PMID: 31747581

Chrysostomou, D., Roberts, L. A., Marchesi, J. R., & Kinross, J. M. (2023). Gut microbiota modulation of efficacy and toxicity of cancer chemotherapy and immunotherapy. *Gastroenterology*, *164*(2), 198–213. DOI: 10.1053/j.gastro.2022.10.018 PMID: 36309208

Chu, H., & Mazmanian, S. K. (2013). Innate immune recognition of the microbiota promotes host-microbial symbiosis. *Nature Immunology*, *14*(7), 668–675. DOI: 10.1038/ni.2635 PMID: 23778794

Chung, W. S. F., Meijerink, M., Zeuner, B., Holck, J., Louis, P., Meyer, A. S., Wells, J. M., Flint, H. J., & Duncan, S. H. (2017). Prebiotic potential of pectin and pectic oligosaccharides to promote anti-inflammatory commensal bacteria in the human colon. *FEMS Microbiology Ecology*, *93*(11), fix127. Advance online publication. DOI: 10.1093/femsec/fix127 PMID: 29029078

Church, D. L., Cerutti, L., Gürtler, A., Griener, T., Zelazny, A., & Emler, S. (2020). Performance and application of 16S rRNA gene cycle sequencing for routine identification of bacteria in the clinical microbiology laboratory. *Clinical Microbiology Reviews*, *33*(4), 10–1128. DOI: 10.1128/CMR.00053-19

Cicenia, A., Santangelo, F., Gambardella, L., Pallotta, L., Iebba, V., Scirocco, A., Marignani, M., Tellan, G., Carabotti, M., Corazziari, E. S., Schippa, S., & Severi, C. (2016). Protective role of postbiotic mediators secreted by Lactobacillus rhamnosus GG versus lipopolysaccharide-induced damage in human colonic smooth muscle cells. *Journal of Clinical Gastroenterology*, *50*(Supplement 2), S140–S144. DOI: 10.1097/MCG.0000000000000681

Clemente, A., & Olias, R. (2017). Beneficial effects of legumes in gut health. *Current Opinion in Food Science*, *14*, 32–36. DOI: 10.1016/j.cofs.2017.01.005

Clemente, J. C., Ursell, L. K., Parfrey, L. W., & Knight, R. (2012). The impact of the gut microbiota on human health: An integrative view. *Cell*, *148*(6), 1258–1270. DOI: 10.1016/j.cell.2012.01.035 PMID: 22424233

Clevers, H. (2013). The intestinal crypt, a prototype stem cell compartment. *Cell*, *154*(2), 274–284. DOI: 10.1016/j.cell.2013.07.004

Clevers, H. C., & Bevins, C. L. (2013). Paneth cells: Maestros of the small intestinal crypts. *Annual Review of Physiology*, *75*(1), 289–311. DOI: 10.1146/annurev-physiol-030212-183744

Clooney, A. G., Bernstein, C. N., Leslie, W. D., Vagianos, K., Sargent, M., Laserna-Mendieta, E. J., Claesson, M. J., & Targownik, L. E. (2016). A comparison of the gut microbiome between long-term users and non-users of proton pump inhibitors. *Alimentary Pharmacology & Therapeutics*, *43*(9), 974–984. DOI: 10.1111/apt.13568 PMID: 26923470

Collins, J. T.. (2024). Anatomy, abdomen and pelvis, small intestine. In *StatPearls* [Internet]. StatPearls Publishing.

Collins, S. L., Stine, J. G., Bisanz, J. E., Okafor, C. D., & Patterson, A. D. (2023). Bile acids and the gut microbiota: Metabolic interactions and impacts on disease. *Nature Reviews. Microbiology*, *21*(4), 236–247. DOI: 10.1038/s41579-022-00805-x PMID: 36253479

Collins, S. M., Surette, M., & Bercik, P. (2012). The interplay between the intestinal microbiota and the brain. *Nature Reviews. Microbiology*, *10*(11), 735–742. DOI: 10.1038/nrmicro2876 PMID: 23000955

Cong, X., Henderson, W. A., Graf, J., & McGrath, J. M. (2015). Early life experience and gut microbiome: The brain–gut–microbiota signaling system. *Advances in Neonatal Care*, *15*(5), 314–323. DOI: 10.1097/ANC.0000000000000191 PMID: 26240939

Conrado, R., Gomes, T. C., Roque, G. S. C., & De Souza, A. O. (2022). Overview of bioactive fungal secondary metabolites: Cytotoxic and antimicrobial compounds. *Antibiotics (Basel, Switzerland)*, *11*(11), 1604. DOI: 10.3390/antibiotics11111604 PMID: 36421247

Cotillard, A., Kennedy, S. P., Kong, L. C., Prifti, E., Pons, N., Le Chatelier, E., Almeida, M., Quinquis, B., Levenez, F., Galleron, N., Gougis, S., Rizkalla, S., Batto, J.-M., Renault, P., Doré, J., Zucker, J.-D., Clément, K., Ehrlich, S. D., Blottière, H., & Layec, S. (2013). Dietary intervention impact on gut microbial gene richness. *Nature*, *500*(7464), 585–588. DOI: 10.1038/nature12480 PMID: 23985875

Cresci, G. A., & Bawden, E. (2015). Gut microbiome: What we do and don't know. *Nutrition in Clinical Practice*, *30*(6), 734–746. DOI: 10.1177/0884533615609899 PMID: 26449893

Crespo-Escobar, P., Mearin, M. L., Hervás, D., Auricchio, R., Castillejo, G., Gyimesi, J., Martínez-Ojinaga, E., Werkstetter, K., & Koletzko, S. (2017). The role of gluten consumption at an early age in celiac disease development: A further analysis of the prospective PreventCD cohort study. *The American Journal of Clinical Nutrition*, *105*(4), 890–896. DOI: 10.3945/ajcn.116.144352

Cross, K. L., Campbell, J. H., Balachandran, M., Campbell, A. G., Cooper, C. J., Griffen, A., Heaton, M., Joshi, S., Klingeman, D., Leys, E., Yang, Z., Parks, J. M., & Podar, M. (2019). Targeted isolation and cultivation of uncultivated bacteria by reverse genomics. *Nature Biotechnology*, *37*(11), 1314–1321. DOI: 10.1038/s41587-019-0260-6

Cryan, J. F., & Dinan, T. G. (2012). Mind-altering microorganisms: The impact of the gut microbiota on brain and behaviour. *Nature Reviews. Neuroscience*, *13*(10), 701–712. DOI: 10.1038/nrn3346 PMID: 22968153

Cryan, J. F., O'Riordan, K. J., Cowan, C. S. M., Sandhu, K. V., Bastiaanssen, T. F. S., Boehme, M., Codagnone, M. G., Cussotto, S., Fulling, C., Golubeva, A. V., Guzzetta, K. E., Jaggar, M., Long-Smith, C. M., Lyte, J. M., Martin, J. A., Molinero-Perez, A., Moloney, G., Morelli, E., Morillas, E., & Dinan, T. G. (2019). The microbiota–gut–brain axis. *Physiological Reviews*, *99*(4), 1877–2013. DOI: 10.1152/physrev.00018.2018 PMID: 31460832

Cucick, A. C. C., Bedani, R., Ribeiro, L. S., Franco, B. D. G. D. M., & Saad, S. M. I. (2024). Effect of fruit by-products and orange pectin on folate (vitamin B9) production by selected starter and probiotic strains. *International Journal of Food Science & Technology*, *59*(6), 3929–3938. DOI: 10.1111/ijfs.17141

Cummings, J. H., & Macfarlane, G. T. (1997). Role of intestinal bacteria in nutrient metabolism. *Clinical Nutrition (Edinburgh, Lothian)*, *16*(1), 3–11. DOI: 10.1016/S0261-5614(97)80252-X PMID: 9406136

Cusumano, G., Angeles Flores, G., Venanzoni, R., & Angelini, P. (2025). The impact of antibiotic therapy on intestinal microbiota: Dysbiosis, antibiotic resistance, and restoration strategies. *Antibiotics (Basel, Switzerland)*, *14*(4), 371. Advance online publication. DOI: 10.3390/antibiotics14040371 PMID: 40298495

D'Aimmo, M. R.. (2023). Folate-producing bifidobacteria: Metabolism, genetics, and relevance. *Microbiome Research Reports*, *3*(1), 11. PMID: 38455078

Dabrowska, K., & Witkiewicz, W. (2016). Correlations of host genetics and gut microbiome composition. *Frontiers in Microbiology*, *7*, 1357. DOI: 10.3389/fmicb.2016.01357 PMID: 27625642

Daguet, D., Pinheiro, I., Verhelst, A., Possemiers, S., & Marzorati, M. (2016). Arabinogalactan and fructooligosaccharides improve the gut barrier function in distinct areas of the colon in the Simulator of the Human Intestinal Microbial Ecosystem. *Journal of Functional Foods*, *20*, 369–379. DOI: 10.1016/j.jff.2015.11.005

Das, B., & Nair, G. B. (2019). Homeostasis and dysbiosis of the gut microbiome in health and disease. *Journal of Biosciences*, *44*(5), 117. DOI: 10.1007/s12038-019-9926-y PMID: 31719226

Das, P., Babaei, P., & Nielsen, J. (2019). Metagenomic analysis of microbe-mediated vitamin metabolism in the human gut microbiome. *BMC Genomics*, *20*(1), 208. DOI: 10.1186/s12864-019-5591-7 PMID: 30866812

Das, T. K., Pradhan, S., Chakrabarti, S., Mondal, K. C., & Ghosh, K. (2022). Current status of probiotic and related health benefits. *Applied Food Research*, *2*(2), 100185. DOI: 10.1016/j.afres.2022.100185

David, L. A., Maurice, C. F., Carmody, R. N., Gootenberg, D. B., Button, J. E., Wolfe, B. E., Ling, A. V., Devlin, A. S., Varma, Y., Fischbach, M. A., Biddinger, S. B., Dutton, R. J., & Turnbaugh, P. J. (2014). Diet rapidly and reproducibly alters the human gut microbiome. *Nature*, *505*(7484), 559–563. DOI: 10.1038/nature12820 PMID: 24336217

Davie, J. R. (2003). Inhibition of Histone Deacetylase Activity by Butyrate. *The Journal of Nutrition*, *133*(7), 2485S–2493S. DOI: 10.1093/jn/133.7.2485S PMID: 12840228

de Almada, C. N., Almada, C. N., Martinez, R. C., & Sant'Ana, A. S. (2016). Paraprobiotics: Evidences on their ability to modify biological responses, inactivation methods and perspectives on their application in foods. *Trends in Food Science & Technology*, *58*, 96–114. DOI: 10.1016/j.tifs.2016.09.011

De Filippis, F., Pellegrini, N., Vannini, L., Jeffery, I. B., La Storia, A., Laghi, L., Serrazanetti, D. I., Di Cagno, R., Ferrocino, I., Lazzi, C., Turroni, S., Cocolin, L., Brigidi, P., Neviani, E., Gobbetti, M., O'Toole, P. W., & Ercolini, D. (2016). High-level adherence to a Mediterranean diet beneficially impacts the gut microbiota and associated metabolome. *Gut*, *65*(11), 1812–1821. DOI: 10.1136/gutjnl-2015-309957 PMID: 26416813

De Filippo, C., Cavalieri, D., Di Paola, M., Ramazzotti, M., Poullet, J. B., Massart, S., Collini, S., Pieraccini, G., & Lionetti, P. (2010). Impact of diet in shaping gut microbiota revealed by a comparative study in children from Europe and rural Africa. *Proceedings of the National Academy of Sciences of the United States of America*, *107*(33), 14691–14696. DOI: 10.1073/pnas.1005963107 PMID: 20679230

de Marcellis-Warin, N., Marty, F., Thelisson, E., & Warin, T. (2022). Artificial intelligence and consumer manipulations: From consumer's counter algorithms to firm's self-regulation tools. *AI and Ethics*, *2*(2), 259–268. DOI: 10.1007/s43681-022-00149-5

de Mattos, P. B. G., de Souza Vandenberghe, L. P., Valladares-Diestra, K. K., Neyra, L. C. R., Vieira, S., Letti, L. A. J., & Soccol, C. R. (2024). Recent developments in xylooligosaccharides: Sustainable production, characterization, beneficial properties and applications. *Food Research International*, *197*, 115206. DOI: 10.1016/j.foodres.2024.115206

Dedeyne, L., Deschodt, M., Verschueren, S., Tournoy, J., & Gielen, E. (2017). Effects of multi-domain interventions in (pre)frail elderly on frailty, functional, and cognitive status: A systematic review. *Clinical Interventions in Aging*, *12*, 873–896. DOI: 10.2147/CIA.S130794 PMID: 28579766

Deiuliis, J. A. (2016). MicroRNAs as regulators of metabolic disease: Pathophysiologic significance and emerging role as biomarkers and therapeutics. *International Journal of Obesity, 40*(1), 88–101. DOI: 10.1038/ijo.2015.170 PMID: 26311337

Dekaboruah, E., Suryavanshi, M. V., Chettri, D., & Verma, A. K. (2020). Human microbiome: An academic update on human body site-specific surveillance and its possible role. *Archives of Microbiology, 202*(8), 2147–2167. DOI: 10.1007/s00203-020-01931-x PMID: 32524177

Dekker, J., Rossen, J. W., Büller, H. A., & Einerhand, A. W. (2002). The MUC family: An obituary. *Trends in Biochemical Sciences, 27*(3), 126–131. DOI: 10.1016/S0968-0004(01)02052-7

Delgobo, M., Paludo, K. S., Fernandes, D., Oliveira, J. G., Ortolan, G. L., & Favero, G. M. (2019). Gut: Key element on immune system regulation. *Brazilian Archives of Biology and Technology, 62*, e19180654. DOI: 10.1590/1678-4324-2019180654

den Besten, G., van Eunen, K., Groen, A. K., Venema, K., Reijngoud, D.-J., & Bakker, B. M. (2013). The role of short-chain fatty acids in the interplay between diet, gut microbiota, and host energy metabolism. *Journal of Lipid Research, 54*(9), 2325–2340. DOI: 10.1194/jlr.R036012 PMID: 23821742

Deng, Z., Guo, L., Chen, X., & Wu, W. (2023). Smart Wearable Systems for Health Monitoring. *Sensors (Basel), 23*(5), 2479. DOI: 10.3390/s23052479 PMID: 36904682

Deng, Z., Lu, L., Li, B., Shi, X., Jin, H., & Hu, W. (2023). The roles of inflammasomes in cancer. *Frontiers in Immunology, 14*, 1195572. DOI: 10.3389/fimmu.2023.1195572 PMID: 37497237

Dethlefsen, L., & Relman, D. A. (2011). Incomplete recovery and individualized responses of the human distal gut microbiota to repeated antibiotic perturbation. *Proceedings of the National Academy of Sciences of the United States of America, 108*(Suppl. 1), 4554–4561. DOI: 10.1073/pnas.1000087107 PMID: 20847294

Devkota, S., Wang, Y., Musch, M. W., Leone, V., Fehlner-Peach, H., Nadimpalli, A., Antonopoulos, D. A., Jabri, B., & Chang, E. B. (2012). Dietary-fat-induced taurocholic acid promotes pathobiont expansion and colitis in IL-10−/− mice. *Nature, 487*(7405), 104–108. DOI: 10.1038/nature11225 PMID: 22722865

Dhopatkar, N., Keeler, J. L., Mutwalli, H., Whelan, K., Treasure, J., & Himmerich, H. (2023). Gastrointestinal symptoms, gut microbiome, probiotics and prebiotics in anorexia nervosa: A review of mechanistic rationale and clinical evidence. *Psychoneuroendocrinology, 147*, 105959. DOI: 10.1016/j.psyneuen.2022.105959

Diabetes Technol. Ther. (2024). *Noninvasive real-time glucose monitoring in the near future*. DOI: 10.1089/dia.2024.0005

Diagnostics. (2019). *RF and microwave techniques for non-invasive glucose monitoring*. DOI: 10.3390/diagnostics9010008

Dimidi, E., Cox, S. R., Rossi, M., & Whelan, K. (2019). Fermented Foods: Definitions and Characteristics, Impact on the Gut Microbiota and Effects on Gastrointestinal Health and Disease. *Nutrients*, *11*(8), 1806. DOI: 10.3390/nu11081806 PMID: 31387262

Ding, L., Weger, B. D., Liu, J. Y., Zhou, L., Lim, Y., Wang, D., & Sassone-Corsi, P. (2024). Maternal high fat diet induces circadian clock-independent endocrine alterations impacting the metabolism of the offspring. *iScience*, *27*(5), 110343. Advance online publication. DOI: 10.1016/j.isci.2024.110343 PMID: 39045103

Dixit, Y., Wagle, A., & Vakil, B. (2016). Patents in the field of probiotics, prebiotics, synbiotics: A review. *J Food Microbiol Saf Hyg*, *1*(02), 1–13. DOI: 10.4172/2476-2059.1000111

do Carmo, M. M., Walker, J. C., Novello, D., Caselato, V. M., Sgarbieri, V. C., Ouwehand, A. C., Andreollo, N. A., Hiane, P. A., & Dos Santos, E. F. (2016). Polydextrose: Physiological Function, and Effects on Health. *Nutrients*, *8*(9), 553. DOI: 10.3390/nu8090553

Dogra, S. K., Chung, C., Wang, D., Sakwinska, O., Colombo Mottaz, S., & Sprenger, N. (2021). Nurturing the early life gut microbiome and immune maturation for long term health. *Microorganisms*, *9*(10), 2110. DOI: 10.3390/microorganisms9102110 PMID: 34683431

Donath, M. Y., & Shoelson, S. E. (2011). Type 2 diabetes as an inflammatory disease. *Nature Reviews. Immunology*, *11*(2), 98–107. DOI: 10.1038/nri2925 PMID: 21233852

Dong, Y., Wei, Z., & Xue, C. (2021). Recent advances in carrageenan-based delivery systems for bioactive ingredients: A review. *Trends in Food Science & Technology*, *112*, 348–362. DOI: 10.1016/j.tifs.2021.04.012

Duan, L., Zhao, J., & Wang, X.. (2025). Wearable Electrochemical Biosensors for Advanced Healthcare Monitoring. *Advancement of Science*, *202411433*(2), 2411433. Advance online publication. DOI: 10.1002/advs.202411433 PMID: 39588557

Dubois, N., Muñoz-Garcia, J., Heymann, D., & Renodon-Cornière, A. (2023). High glucose exposure drives intestinal barrier dysfunction by altering its morphological, structural and functional properties. *Biochemical Pharmacology, 216*, 115765. DOI: 10.1016/j.bcp.2023.115765

Dudley, R., Dodgson, G., Sarll, G., Halhead, R., Bolas, H., & McCarthy-Jones, S. (2014). The effect of arousal on auditory threat detection and the relationship to auditory hallucinations. *Journal of Behavior Therapy and Experimental Psychiatry, 45*(3), 311–318. DOI: 10.1016/j.jbtep.2014.02.002 PMID: 24632145

Du, W., Zou, Z.-P., Ye, B.-C., & Zhou, Y. (2025). Gut microbiota and associated metabolites: Key players in high-fat diet-induced chronic diseases. *Gut Microbes, 17*(1), 2494703. DOI: 10.1080/19490976.2025.2494703 PMID: 40260760

Eaton, S. E., Kaczmarek, J., Mahmood, D., McDiarmid, A. M., Norarfan, A. N., Scott, E. G., Then, C. K., Tsui, H. Y., & Kiltie, A. E. (2022). Exploiting dietary fibre and the gut microbiota in pelvic radiotherapy patients. *British Journal of Cancer, 127*(9), 1535–1546. DOI: 10.1038/s41416-022-01980-7 PMID: 36175620

Eckburg, P. B., Bik, E. M., Bernstein, C. N., Purdom, E., Dethlefsen, L., Sargent, M., Gill, S. R., Nelson, K. E., & Relman, D. A. (2005). Diversity of the human intestinal microbial flora. *Science, 308*(5728), 1635–1638. DOI: 10.1126/science.1110591 PMID: 15831718

Eisenstein, M. (2020). The hunt for a healthy microbiome. *Nature, 577*(7792), S6–S8. DOI: 10.1038/d41586-020-00193-3 PMID: 31996823

Eissa, M. (2024). The Gut Microbiome: A Potential Therapeutic Path in Complementary Medicine. *Journal of Research in Complementary Medicine, 1*(2), 55–55. DOI: 10.5455/JRCM.20240509063048

Ejtahed, H.-S., Tito, R. Y., Siadat, S.-D., Hasani-Ranjbar, S., Hoseini-Tavassol, Z., Rymenans, L., Verbeke, K., Soroush, A. R., Raes, J., & Larijani, B. (2019). Metformin induces weight loss associated with gut microbiota alteration in non-diabetic obese women: A randomized double-blind clinical trial. *European Journal of Endocrinology, 180*(3), 165–176. DOI: 10.1530/EJE-18-0826 PMID: 30540558

Elazzazy, A. M., Baeshen, M. N., Alasmi, K. M., Alqurashi, S. I., Desouky, S. E., & Khattab, S. M. R. (2025). Where Biology Meets Engineering: Scaling up microbial nutraceuticals to bridge nutrition, therapeutics, and global impact. *Microorganisms, 13*(3), 566. DOI: 10.3390/microorganisms13030566 PMID: 40142459

Emran, T. B., Islam, F., Mitra, S., Paul, S., Nath, N., Khan, Z., Das, R., Chandran, D., Sharma, R., Lima, C. M. G., Awadh, A. A. A., Almazni, I. A., Alhasaniah, A. H., & Guiné, R. P. F. (2022). Pectin: A Bioactive Food Polysaccharide with Cancer Preventive Potential. *Molecules (Basel, Switzerland)*, *27*(21), 7405. DOI: 10.3390/molecules27217405

Engevik, M. A., Morra, C. N., Röth, D., Engevik, K., Spinler, J. K., Devaraj, S., Crawford, S. E., Estes, M. K., Kalkum, M., & Versalovic, J. (2019). Microbial Metabolic Capacity for Intestinal Folate Production and Modulation of Host Folate Receptors. *Frontiers in Microbiology*, *10*, 2305. DOI: 10.3389/fmicb.2019.02305 PMID: 31649646

Ercolini, D., & Fogliano, V. (2018). Food design to feed the human gut microbiota. *Journal of Agricultural and Food Chemistry*, *66*(15), 3754–3758. DOI: 10.1021/acs.jafc.8b00456 PMID: 29565591

Eriguchi, Y., Takashima, S., Oka, H., Shimoji, S., Nakamura, K., & Teshima, T. (2012). Graft-versus-host disease disrupts intestinal microbial ecology by inhibiting Paneth cell production of α-defensins. *Blood*, *120*(1), 223–231. DOI: 10.1182/blood-2011-12-401166

Escriva, P. P., Bernardino, C. C. T., & Letellier, E. (2025). De-coding the complex role of microbial metabolites in cancer. *Cell Reports*, *44*(3). PMID: 40023841

Eslami, M., Naderian, R., Bahar, A., Babaeizad, A., Rezanavaz Gheshlagh, S., Oksenych, V., & Tahmasebi, H. (2025). Microbiota as diagnostic biomarkers: Advancing early cancer detection and personalized therapeutic approaches through microbiome profiling. *Frontiers in Immunology*, *16*, 1559480. DOI: 10.3389/fimmu.2025.1559480 PMID: 40406094

Esterházy, D., Canesso, M. C. C., Mesin, L., Muller, P. A., de Castro, T. B. R., Lockhart, A., ElJalby, M., Faria, A. M. C., & Mucida, D. (2019). Compartmentalized gut lymph node drainage dictates adaptive immune responses. *Nature*, *569*(7754), 126–130. DOI: 10.1038/s41586-019-1125-3

Estrada, J. A., & Contreras, I. (2019). Nutritional modulation of immune and central nervous system homeostasis: The role of diet in development of neuroinflammation and neurological disease. *Nutrients*, *11*(5), 1076. DOI: 10.3390/nu11051076 PMID: 31096592

Everard, A., Belzer, C., Geurts, L., Ouwerkerk, J. P., Druart, C., Bindels, L. B., Guiot, Y., Derrien, M., Muccioli, G. G., Delzenne, N. M., de Vos, W. M., & Cani, P. D. (2013). Cross-talk between Akkermansia muciniphila and intestinal epithelium controls diet-induced obesity. *Proceedings of the National Academy of Sciences of the United States of America, 110*(22), 9066–9071. DOI: 10.1073/pnas.1219451110 PMID: 23671105

Fang, X., et al. (2025). Precision microbiome: A new era of targeted therapy with core probiotics. *Research, 8*, 0658.

Fan, Y., & Pedersen, O. (2021). Gut microbiota in human metabolic health and disease. *Nature Reviews. Microbiology, 19*(1), 55–71. DOI: 10.1038/s41579-020-0433-9 PMID: 32887946

Farhat, E. K., Sher, E. K., Džidić-Krivić, A., Banjari, I., & Sher, F. (2023). Functional biotransformation of phytoestrogens by gut microbiota with impact on cancer treatment. *The Journal of Nutritional Biochemistry, 118*, 109368. DOI: 10.1016/j.jnutbio.2023.109368 PMID: 37100304

Farin, H. F., Jordens, I., Mosa, M. H., Basak, O., Korving, J., Tauriello, D. V., de Punder, K., Angers, S., Peters, P. J., Maurice, M. M., & Clevers, H. (2016). Visualization of a short-range Wnt gradient in the intestinal stem-cell niche. *Nature, 530*(7590), 340–343. DOI: 10.1038/nature16937

Farré-Maduell, E., & Casals-Pascual, C. (2019). The origins of gut microbiome research in Europe: From Escherich to Nissle. *Human Microbiome Journal, 14*, 100065. Advance online publication. DOI: 10.1016/j.humic.2019.100065

Fekete, E., and Buret, A. G. (2023). The role of mucin O-glycans in microbiota dysbiosis, intestinal homeostasis, and host-pathogen interactions. *American Journal of Physiology-Gastrointestinal and Liver Physiology, 324*(5), G452–G465. DOI: 10.1152/ajpgi.00261.2022

Feng, T., & Wang, J. (2020). Oxidative stress tolerance and antioxidant capacity of lactic acid bacteria as probiotic: A systematic review. *Gut Microbes, 12*(1), 1801944. DOI: 10.1080/19490976.2020.1801944

Feng, Y., Wassie, T., Gan, R., & Wu, X. (2023). Structural characteristics and immunomodulatory effects of sulfated polysaccharides derived from marine algae. *Critical Reviews in Food Science and Nutrition, 63*(24), 7180–7196. DOI: 10.1080/10408398.2022.2043823

Fernandes, A., Oliveira, A., Soares, R., & Barata, P. (2021). The effects of ionizing radiation on gut microbiota: A systematic review. *Nutrients*, *13*(9), 3025. Advance online publication. DOI: 10.3390/nu13093025 PMID: 34578902

Ferrucci, L., & Fabbri, E. (2018). Inflammageing: Chronic inflammation in ageing, cardiovascular disease, and frailty. *Nature Reviews. Cardiology*, *15*(9), 505–522. DOI: 10.1038/s41569-018-0064-2 PMID: 30065258

Flint, H. J. (2020). *Why gut microbes matter*. Springer. DOI: 10.1007/978-3-030-43246-1

Flint, H. J., Scott, K. P., Duncan, S. H., Louis, P., & Forano, E. (2012). Microbial degradation of complex carbohydrates in the gut. *Gut Microbes*, *3*(4), 289–306. DOI: 10.4161/gmic.19897 PMID: 22572875

Foley, M. H., O'Flaherty, S., Barrangou, R., & Theriot, C. M. (2019). Bile salt hydrolases: Gatekeepers of bile acid metabolism and host-microbiome crosstalk in the gastrointestinal tract. *PLoS Pathogens*, *15*(3), e1007581. DOI: 10.1371/journal.ppat.1007581 PMID: 30845232

Food and Drug Administration, HHS. (2007). Current good manufacturing practice in manufacturing, packaging, labeling, or holding operations for dietary supplements. Final rule. *Federal Register*, *72*(121), 34751–34958.

Forslund, K., Hildebrand, F., Nielsen, T., Falony, G., Le Chatelier, E., Sunagawa, S., Prifti, E., Vieira-Silva, S., Gudmundsdottir, V., Pedersen, H. K., Arumugam, M., Kristiansen, K., Voigt, A. Y., Vestergaard, H., Hercog, R., Costea, P. I., Kultima, J. R., Li, J., Jørgensen, T., & Pedersen, O. (2015). Disentangling type 2 diabetes and metformin treatment signatures in the human gut microbiota. *Nature*, *528*(7581), 262–266. DOI: 10.1038/nature15766 PMID: 26633628

Franceschi, C., Bonafè, M., Valensin, S., Olivieri, F., De Luca, M., Ottaviani, E., & De Benedictis, G. (2000). Inflamm-aging: An evolutionary perspective on immunosenescence. *Annals of the New York Academy of Sciences*, *908*(1), 244–254. DOI: 10.1111/j.1749-6632.2000.tb06651.x PMID: 10911963

Franzosa, E. A., Huang, K., Meadow, J. F., Gevers, D., Lemon, K. P., Bohannan, B. J. M., & Huttenhower, C. (2015). Identifying personal microbiomes using metagenomic codes. *Proceedings of the National Academy of Sciences of the United States of America*, *112*(22), E2930–E2938. DOI: 10.1073/pnas.1423854112 PMID: 25964341

Franzosa, E. A., McIver, L. J., Rahnavard, G., Thompson, L. R., Schirmer, M., Weingart, G., Lipson, K. S., Knight, R., Caporaso, J. G., Segata, N., & Huttenhower, C. (2015). Species-level functional profiling of metagenomes and metatranscriptomes. *Nature Methods, 15*(11), 962–968. DOI: 10.1038/s41592-018-0176-y PMID: 30377376

Frioux, C., Ansorge, R., Özkurt, E., Nedjad, C. G., Fritscher, J., Quince, C., Waszak, S. M., & Hildebrand, F. (2023). Enterosignatures define common bacterial guilds in the human gut microbiome. *Cell Host & Microbe, 31*(7), 1111–1125.e6. DOI: 10.1016/j.chom.2023.05.024 PMID: 37339626

Front. Anal. Sci. (2024). *Future directions: What lies ahead for smart biochemical wearables*. DOI: 10.3389/frans.2024.1509815

Front. Physiol. (2024). *Integrated framework of load monitoring: smartphone + wearables + point of care*. [DOI pending]

Frontiers in Bioeng. Biotechnol. (2025). *Wearable sensors–based assistive technologies for patient health monitoring*. DOI: 10.3389/fbioe.2025.1437877

Frontiers in Digital Health. (2025). *Returning individual wearable sensor results to participants*. DOI: 10.3389/fdgth.2025.1569452

Fry, M. (2024). The discovery of archaea: From observed anomaly to consequential restructuring of the phylogenetic tree. *History and Philosophy of the Life Sciences, 46*(2), 16. Advance online publication. DOI: 10.1007/s40656-024-00616-8 PMID: 38530473

Fui-Hoon Nah, F., Zheng, R., Cai, J., Siau, K., & Chen, L. (2023). Generative AI and ChatGPT: Applications, challenges, and AI-human collaboration. *Journal of Information Technology Case and Application Research, 25*(3), 277–304. DOI: 10.1080/15228053.2023.2233814

Fu, J., & Wu, H. (2023). Structural mechanisms of NLRP3 inflammasome assembly and activation. *Annual Review of Immunology, 41*(1), 301–316. DOI: 10.1146/annurev-immunol-081022-021207 PMID: 36750315

Gao, R., Zhu, C., Li, H., Yin, M., Pan, C., Huang, L., Kong, C., Wang, X., Zhang, Y., Qu, S., & Qin, H. (2018). Dysbiosis signatures of gut microbiota along the sequence from healthy, young patients to those with overweight and obesity. *Obesity (Silver Spring, Md.), 26*(2), 351–361. DOI: 10.1002/oby.22088 PMID: 29280312

Gasaly, N., de Vos, P., & Hermoso, M. A. (2021). Impact of bacterial metabolites on gut barrier function and host immunity: A focus on bacterial metabolism and its relevance for intestinal inflammation. *Frontiers in Immunology*, *12*, 658354. DOI: 10.3389/fimmu.2021.658354 PMID: 34122415

Gasaly, N., Hermoso, M. A., & Gotteland, M. (2021). Butyrate and the fine-tuning of colonic homeostasis: Implication for inflammatory bowel diseases. *International Journal of Molecular Sciences*, *22*(6), 3061. DOI: 10.3390/ijms22063061 PMID: 33802759

Gasbarrini, G., Bonvicini, F., & Gramenzi, A. (2016). Probiotics history. *Journal of Clinical Gastroenterology*, *50*(Supplement 2), S116–S119. DOI: 10.1097/MCG.0000000000000697

Gaur, V. K., Gupta, S., Sharma, P., Gupta, P., Varjani, S., Srivastava, J. K., & Rodriguez-Couto, S. (2022). Metabolic cascade for remediation of plastic waste: A case study on microplastic degradation. *Current Pollution Reports*, *8*(1), 30–42. DOI: 10.1007/s40726-021-00210-7

Gayap, H. T., & Akhloufi, M. A. (2024). Deep machine learning for medical diagnosis, application to lung cancer detection: A review. *BioMedInformatics*, *4*(1), 236–257. DOI: 10.3390/biomedinformatics4010015

Geirnaert, A., Calatayud, M., Grootaert, C., Laukens, D., Devriese, S., Smagghe, G., De Vos, M., Boon, N., & Van de Wiele, T. (2017). Butyrate-producing bacteria supplemented in vitro to Crohn's disease patient microbiota increased butyrate production and enhanced intestinal epithelial barrier integrity. *Scientific Reports*, *7*(1), 11450. DOI: 10.1038/s41598-017-11734-8

Gensollen, T., Iyer, S. S., Kasper, D. L., & Blumberg, R. S. (2016). How colonization by microbiota in early life shapes the immune system. *Science*, *352*(6285), 539–544. DOI: 10.1126/science.aad9378 PMID: 27126036

Gerber, G. K. (2014). The dynamic microbiome. *FEBS Letters*, *588*(22), 4131–4139. DOI: 10.1016/j.febslet.2014.02.037 PMID: 24583074

Ghaisas, S., Maher, J., & Kanthasamy, A. (2016). Gut microbiome in health and disease: Linking the microbiome-gut-brain axis and environmental factors in the pathogenesis of systemic and neurodegenerative diseases. *Pharmacology & Therapeutics*, *158*, 52–62. DOI: 10.1016/j.pharmthera.2015.11.012 PMID: 26627987

Ghare, M., Vishwakarma, K., Tripathi, S., Dixit, G. P., & Soren, K. R. (2024). Unveiling the benefits of resistant starch in legumes: Overview of current and future prospective. *Stärke*, *76*(7-8), 2300212. DOI: 10.1002/star.202300212

Ghoshal, U. C., & Srivastava, D. (2014). Irritable bowel syndrome and small intestinal bacterial overgrowth: Meaningful association or unnecessary hype. *World Journal of Gastroenterology*, *20*(10), 2482–2491. DOI: 10.3748/wjg.v20.i10.2482 PMID: 24627585

Ghosh, T. S., Rampelli, S., Jeffery, I. B., Santoro, A., Neto, M. C., Capri, M., & Candela, M. (2020). Mediterranean diet intervention alters the gut microbiome in older people reducing frailty and improving health status. *Gut*, *69*(7), 1218–1228. DOI: 10.1136/gutjnl-2019-319654 PMID: 32066625

Gibson, G. R., Hutkins, R., Sanders, M. E., Prescott, S. L., Reimer, R. A., Salminen, S. J., Scott, K., Stanton, C., Swanson, K. S., Cani, P. D., Verbeke, K., & Reid, G. (2017). Expert consensus document: The International Scientific Association for Probiotics and Prebiotics (ISAPP) consensus statement. *Nature Reviews. Gastroenterology & Hepatology*, *14*(8), 491–502. DOI: 10.1038/nrgastro.2017.75 PMID: 28611480

Gibson, G. R., & Roberfroid, M. B. (1995). Dietary modulation of the human colonic microbiota: Introducing the concept of prebiotics. *The Journal of Nutrition*, *125*(6), 1401–1412. DOI: 10.1093/jn/125.6.1401 PMID: 7782892

Gieryńska, M., Szulc-Dąbrowska, L., Struzik, J., Mielcarska, M. B., & Gregorczyk-Zboroch, K. P. (2022). Integrity of the intestinal barrier: The involvement of epithelial cells and microbiota—A mutual relationship. *Animals (Basel)*, *12*(2), 145. Advance online publication. DOI: 10.3390/ani12020145 PMID: 35049768

Gilbert, J. A., Blaser, M. J., Caporaso, J. G., Jansson, J. K., Lynch, S. V., & Knight, R. (2018). Current understanding of the human microbiome. *Nature Medicine*, *24*(4), 392–400. DOI: 10.1038/nm.4517 PMID: 29634682

Gomez de Agüero, M., Ganal-Vonarburg, S. C., Fuhrer, T., Rupp, S., Uchimura, Y., Li, H., Steinert, A., Heikenwalder, M., Hapfelmeier, S., Sauer, U., McCoy, K. D., & Macpherson, A. J. (2016). The maternal microbiota drives early postnatal innate immune development. *Science*, *351*(6279), 1296–1302. DOI: 10.1126/science.aad2571

González-Hernández, A., Escamilla, A., Pérez-Ruiz, E., Rios, A., Frecha, C., Vaca-Paniagua, F., & Tenorio, J. (2025). From genes to personalized cancer care: A systematic review of toxicity-associated genetic variants in solid tumor treatments. *bioRxiv*. DOI: 10.1101/2025.10.21.25338446

Goodrich, J. K., Waters, J. L., Poole, A. C., Sutter, J. L., Koren, O., Blekhman, R., Beaumont, M., Van Treuren, W., Knight, R., Bell, J. T., Spector, T. D., Clark, A. G., & Ley, R. E. (2014). Human genetics shape the gut microbiome. *Cell*, *159*(4), 789–799. DOI: 10.1016/j.cell.2014.09.053 PMID: 25417156

Górczyńska-Kosiorz, S., Lejawa, M., Goławski, M., Tomaszewska, A., Fronczek, M., Maksym, B., Banach, M., & Osadnik, T. (2024). The Impact of Haplotypes of the FTO Gene, Lifestyle, and Dietary Patterns on BMI and Metabolic Syndrome in Polish Young Adult Men. *Nutrients, 16*(11), 1615. DOI: 10.3390/nu16111615

Gorthy, S., Sargar, P., Hugar, C., Li, J., & Habyarimana, E. (2024). Summary of the potential and exploitation of omics and biotechnological breakthroughs in sorghum. In *Sorghum science and biotechnology* (p. 405). Springer., DOI: 10.1007/978-981-97-4347-6_17

Gou, H. Z., Zhang, Y. L., & Zhang, L. (2022). How do intestinal probiotics restore the intestinal barrier? *Frontiers in Microbiology, 13*, 929346. DOI: 10.3389/fmicb.2022.929346

Goyal, V. K., Rani, D., Arora, R., Mehrotra, S., Deng, C., & Wang, Y. (2023). Unlocking the potential of nano-enabled precision agriculture for efficient and sustainable farming. *Plants, 12*(21), 3744. Advance online publication. DOI: 10.3390/plants12213744 PMID: 37960100

Grandi, F. C., Modi, H., Kampman, L., & Corces, M. R. (2022). Chromatin accessibility profiling by ATAC-seq. *Nature Protocols, 17*(6), 1518–1552. DOI: 10.1038/s41596-022-00692-9 PMID: 35478247

Greer, J. B., & O'Keefe, S. J. (2011). Microbial induction of immunity, inflammation, and cancer. *Frontiers in Physiology, 1*, 168. DOI: 10.3389/fphys.2010.00168 PMID: 21423403

Griffith, R., O'Connell, M., & Smith, K. (2017). The importance of product reformulation versus consumer choice in improving diet quality. *Economica, 84*(333), 34–53. DOI: 10.1111/ecca.12192

Guan, P., Yu, K., Wei, W., Tan, Y., & Wu, J. (2023). Big data analytics on lung cancer diagnosis framework with deep learning. *IEEE/ACM Transactions on Computational Biology and Bioinformatics, 21*(2), 757–770. DOI: 10.1109/TCBB.2023.3281638 PMID: 37256795

Guanzon, D., Ross, J. P., Ma, C., Berry, O., & Liew, Y. J. (2024). Comparing methylation levels assayed in GC-rich regions with current and emerging methods. *BMC Genomics, 25*(1), 741. DOI: 10.1186/s12864-024-10605-7 PMID: 39080541

Gulliver, E. L., Young, R. B., Chonwerawong, M., D'Adamo, G. L., Thomason, T., Widdop, J. T., Rutten, E. L., Rossetto Marcelino, V., Bryant, R. V., Costello, S. P., O'Brien, C. L., Hold, G. L., Giles, E. M., & Forster, S. C. (2022). Review article: The future of microbiome-based therapeutics. *Alimentary Pharmacology & Therapeutics*, *56*(2), 192–208. DOI: 10.1111/apt.17049 PMID: 35611465

Guo, L., Da, F., Gao, Q., Miao, X., Guo, J., Zhang, W., Li, J., Wang, J., & Liu, J. (2023). Irradiation-induced intestinal injury is associated with disorders of bile acids metabolism. *International Journal of Radiation Oncology, Biology, Physics*, *115*(2), 490–500. DOI: 10.1016/j.ijrobp.2022.08.007 PMID: 35948117

Gupta, V. K., Kim, M., Bakshi, U., Cunningham, K. Y., Davis, J. M.III, Lazaridis, K. N., Nelson, H., Chia, N., & Sung, J. (2020). A predictive index for health status using species-level gut microbiome profiling. *Nature Communications*, *11*(1), 4635. DOI: 10.1038/s41467-020-18476-8 PMID: 32934239

Hadrich, D. (2018). Microbiome research is becoming the key to better understanding health and nutrition. *Frontiers in Genetics*, *9*, 212. DOI: 10.3389/fgene.2018.00212 PMID: 29951086

Hall, J. A., Grainger, J. R., Spencer, S. P., & Belkaid, Y. (2011). The role of retinoic acid in tolerance and immunity. *Immunity*, *35*(1), 13–22. DOI: 10.1016/j.immuni.2011.07.002

Hamasalim, H. J. (2016). Synbiotic as feed additives relating to animal health and performance. *Advances in Microbiology*, *6*(04), 288–302. DOI: 10.4236/aim.2016.64028

Haran, J. P., Zeamer, A., Ward, D. V., Dutta, P., Bucci, V., & McCormick, B. A. (2021). The nursing home older adult gut microbiome composition shows time-dependent dysbiosis and is influenced by medication exposures, age, environment, and frailty. *The Journals of Gerontology. Series A, Biological Sciences and Medical Sciences*, *76*(11), 1930–1938. DOI: 10.1093/gerona/glab167 PMID: 34125200

Harindranath, S., & Desai, D. (2025). Wearable technology in inflammatory bowel disease: Current state and future direction. *Expert Review of Medical Devices*, *22*(2), 121–126. DOI: 10.1080/17434440.2025.2453561 PMID: 39798078

Harley, I. T. W., & Karp, C. L. (2012). Obesity and the gut microbiome: Striving for causality. *Molecular Metabolism*, *1*(1-2), 21–31. DOI: 10.1016/j.molmet.2012.07.002 PMID: 24024115

Hashem, Z. S. (2025). Bacterial Metabolites in Defense: A Crucial Aspect of Microbial Interaction and Host Protection. In *Metabolic Dynamics in Host-Microbe Interaction* (pp. 101-120). Springer. DOI: 10.1007/978-981-96-1305-2_5

Hasin, Y., Seldin, M., & Lusis, A. (2017). Multi-omics approaches to disease. *Genome Biology*, *18*(1), 83. DOI: 10.1186/s13059-017-1215-1 PMID: 28476144

Hassan, A., Khan, H., Ali, A., Din, I. U., Sajid, A., Husain, M., & Amin, R. (2024). An enhanced lung cancer identification and classification based on advanced deep learning and convolutional neural network. [BBE]. *Bulletin of Business and Economics*, *13*(1), 136–150. DOI: 10.61506/01.00308

Heidari, M., Maleki Vareki, S., Yaghobi, R., & Karimi, M. H. (2024). Microbiota activation and regulation of adaptive immunity. *Frontiers in Immunology*, *15*, 1429436. DOI: 10.3389/fimmu.2024.1429436 PMID: 39445008

Heinken, A., Basile, A., Hertel, J., Thinnes, C., & Thiele, I. (2021). Genome-scale metabolic modeling of the human microbiome in the era of personalized medicine. *Annual Review of Microbiology*, *75*(1), 199–222. DOI: 10.1146/annurev-micro-060221-012134

Heinken, A., & Thiele, I. (2015). Systems biology of host–microbe metabolomics. *Wiley Interdisciplinary Reviews. Systems Biology and Medicine*, *7*(4), 195–219. DOI: 10.1002/wsbm.1301 PMID: 25929487

He, J., Zhang, P., Shen, L., Niu, L., Tan, Y., Chen, L., Zhao, Y., Bai, L., Hao, X., Li, X., Zhang, S., & Zhu, L. (2020). Short-chain fatty acids and their association with signalling pathways in inflammation, glucose and lipid metabolism. *International Journal of Molecular Sciences*, *21*(17), 6356. DOI: 10.3390/ijms21176356 PMID: 32887215

Hemmati, M. A., Monemi, M., Asli, S., Mohammadi, S., Foroozanmehr, B., Haghmorad, D., Oksenych, V., & Eslami, M. (2024). Using new technologies to analyze gut microbiota and predict cancer risk. *Cells*, *13*(23), 1987. DOI: 10.3390/cells13231987

Henao-Mejia, J., Elinav, E., Jin, C., Hao, L., Mehal, W. Z., Strowig, T., Thaiss, C. A., Kau, A. L., Eisenbarth, S. C., Jurczak, M. J., Camporez, J. P., Shulman, G. I., Gordon, J. I., Hoffman, H. M., & Flavell, R. A. (2012). Inflammasome-mediated dysbiosis regulates progression of NAFLD and obesity. *Nature*, *482*(7384), 179–185. DOI: 10.1038/nature10809 PMID: 22297845

Henke, M. T., Kenny, D. J., Cassilly, C. D., Vlamakis, H., Xavier, R. J., & Clardy, J. (2019). *Ruminococcus gnavus*, a member of the human gut microbiome associated with Crohn's disease, produces an inflammatory polysaccharide. *Proceedings of the National Academy of Sciences of the United States of America*, *116*(26), 12672–12677. DOI: 10.1073/pnas.1904099116 PMID: 31182571

He, R., Qi, P., Shu, L., Ding, Y., Zeng, P., Wen, G., Xiong, Y., & Deng, H. (2025). Dysbiosis and extraintestinal cancers. *Journal of Experimental & Clinical Cancer Research : CR, 44*(1), 44. DOI: 10.1186/s13046-025-03313-x PMID: 39915884

Herran, A. R., Pérez-Andrés, J., Caminero, A., Nistal, E., Vivas, S., Ruiz de Morales, J. M., Casqueiro, J., & Sollid, L. M. (2017). Gluten-degrading bacteria are present in the human small intestine of healthy volunteers and celiac patients. *Research in Microbiology, 168*(7), 673–684. DOI: 10.1016/j.resmic.2017.04.008

Heterogeneity in VEGFR3 levels drives lymphatic vessel hyperplasia through cell-autonomous and non-cell-autonomous mechanisms | Nature Communications. (n.d.). Retrieved October 18, 2025, from https://www.nature.com/articles/s41467-018-03692-0

He, Y., Huang, J., Li, Q., Xia, W., Zhang, C., Liu, Z., Xiao, J., Yi, Z., Deng, H., Xiao, Z., Hu, J., Li, H., Zu, X., Quan, C., & Chen, J. (2022). Gut microbiota and tumor immune escape: A new perspective for improving tumor immunotherapy. *Cancers (Basel), 14*(21), 5317. DOI: 10.3390/cancers14215317 PMID: 36358736

Hill, C., Guarner, F., Reid, G., Gibson, G. R., Merenstein, D. J., Pot, B., Morelli, L., Canani, R. B., Flint, H. J., Salminen, S., Calder, P. C., & Sanders, M. E. (2014). Expert consensus document: The International Scientific Association for Probiotics and Prebiotics consensus statement on the scope and appropriate use of the term probiotic. *Nature Reviews. Gastroenterology & Hepatology, 11*(8), 506–514. DOI: 10.1038/nrgastro.2014.66 PMID: 24912386

Hill, M. J. (2012). Microbial vitamin K and cardiovascular disease. *Microbial Biotechnology, 5*(1), 98–107. DOI: 10.1111/j.1751-7915.2011.00228.x PMID: 21958386

Hodgkinson, K., El Abbar, F., Dobranowski, P., Manoogian, J., Butcher, J., Figeys, D., Mack, D., & Stintzi, A. (2023). Butyrate's role in human health and the current progress towards its clinical application to treat gastrointestinal disease. *Clinical Nutrition (Edinburgh, Lothian), 42*(1), 61–75. DOI: 10.1016/j.clnu.2022.10.024

Hofmann, A. F. (1999). Bile Acids: The Good, the Bad, and the Ugly. *Physiology (Bethesda, MD), 14*(1), 24–29. DOI: 10.1152/physiologyonline.1999.14.1.24 PMID: 11390813

Holzapfel, C., Waldenberger, M., Lorkowski, S., & Daniel, H. (2022). Genetics and epigenetics in personalized nutrition: Evidence, expectations, and experiences. *Molecular Nutrition & Food Research, 66*(17), 2200077. DOI: 10.1002/mnfr.202200077

Honda, K., & Littman, D. R. (2016). The microbiome in infectious disease and inflammation. *Annual Review of Immunology*, *34*, 307–336. DOI: 10.1146/annurev-immunol-041015-055728 PMID: 22224764

Hoofnagle, C. J., Van Der Sloot, B., & Borgesius, F. Z. (2019). The European union general data protection regulation: What it is and what it means. *Information & Communications Technology Law*, *28*(1), 65–98. DOI: 10.1080/13600834.2019.1573501

Hooper, L. V., & Macpherson, A. J. (2010). Immune adaptations that maintain homeostasis with the intestinal microbiota. *Nature Reviews. Immunology*, *10*(3), 159–169. DOI: 10.1038/nri2710 PMID: 20182457

Hossain, K. S., Amarasena, S., & Mayengbam, S. (2022). B vitamins and their roles in gut health. *Microorganisms*, *10*(6), 1168. DOI: 10.3390/microorganisms10061168 PMID: 35744686

Hotamisligil, G. S. (2006). Inflammation and metabolic disorders. *Nature*, *444*(7121), 860–867. DOI: 10.1038/nature05485 PMID: 17167474

Hou, M., Yu, Q. Q., Yang, L., Zhao, H., Jiang, P., Qin, L., & Zhang, Q. (2024). The role of short-chain fatty acid metabolism in the pathogenesis, diagnosis and treatment of cancer. *Frontiers in Oncology*, *14*, 1451045. DOI: 10.3389/fonc.2024.1451045 PMID: 39435279

Hou, Q., Ye, L., Huang, L., & Yu, Q. (2017). The research progress on intestinal stem cells and its relationship with intestinal microbiota. *Frontiers in Immunology*, *8*, 599. DOI: 10.3389/fimmu.2017.00599

Hou, Y., Li, J., & Ying, S. (2023). Tryptophan metabolism and gut microbiota: A novel regulatory axis integrating the microbiome, immunity, and cancer. *Metabolites*, *13*(11), 1166. DOI: 10.3390/metabo13111166 PMID: 37999261

Hrubša, M., Siatka, T., Nejmanová, I., Vopršalová, M., Kujovská Krčmová, L., Matoušová, K., Javorská, L., Macáková, K., Mercolini, L., Remião, F., Máťuš, M., & Mladěnka, P. (2022). Biological properties of vitamins of the B-complex, part 1: Vitamins B1, B2, B3, and B5. *Nutrients*, *14*(3), 484. DOI: 10.3390/nu14030484 PMID: 35276844

Huang, C., Feng, S., Huo, F., & Liu, H. (2022). Effects of four antibiotics on the diversity of the intestinal microbiota. *Microbiology Spectrum*, *10*(2), e01904–e01921. DOI: 10.1128/spectrum.01904-21 PMID: 35311555

Huang, G., Khan, R., Zheng, Y., Lee, P. C., Li, Q., & Khan, I. (2023). Exploring the role of gut microbiota in advancing personalized medicine. *Frontiers in Microbiology*, *14*, 1274925. DOI: 10.3389/fmicb.2023.1274925 PMID: 38098666

Huang, S.-C., He, Y.-F., Chen, P., Liu, K.-L., & Shaukat, A. (2023). Gut microbiota as a target in the bone health of livestock and poultry: Roles of short-chain fatty acids. *Animal Diseases*, *3*(1), 23. DOI: 10.1186/s44149-023-00089-5

Huang, Y., He, S., Li, J. Z., Seo, Y. K., Osborne, T. F., Cohen, J. C., & Hobbs, H. H. (2010). A feed-forward loop amplifies nutritional regulation of PNPLA3. *Proceedings of the National Academy of Sciences of the United States of America*, *107*(17), 7892–7897. DOI: 10.1073/pnas.1003585107

Hubballi, R. B., Selvakumar, P., Seenivasan, R., & Basava Aradhya, S. G., Dinesh, N., & Seelam, P. K. (2025). Overview of Current AI Technologies in Education. In L. Kyei-Blankson & E. Ntuli (Eds.), *Transformative AI Practices for Personalized Learning Strategies* (pp. 1–26). IGI Global. DOI: 10.4018/979-8-3693-8744-3.ch001

Hullar, M. A. J., & Fu, B. C. (2014). Diet, the Gut Microbiome, and Epigenetics. *Cancer Journal (Sudbury, Mass.)*, *20*(3), 170–175. DOI: 10.1097/PPO.0000000000000053 PMID: 24855003

Human Microbiome Project Consortium. (2012). Structure, function and diversity of the healthy human microbiome. *Nature*, *486*(7402), 207–214. DOI: 10.1038/nature11234 PMID: 22699609

Huynh, U., & Zastrow, M. L. (2023). Metallobiology of Lactobacillaceae in the gut microbiome. *Journal of Inorganic Biochemistry*, *238*, 112023. DOI: 10.1016/j.jinorgbio.2022.112023

Hwang, C. H., Lee, N. K., & Paik, H. D. (2022). The anti-cancer potential of heat-killed Lactobacillus brevis KU15176 upon AGS cell lines through intrinsic apoptosis pathway. *International Journal of Molecular Sciences*, *23*(8), 4073. DOI: 10.3390/ijms23084073

Iacomino, G., Rufián-Henares, J. Á., & Lauria, F. (2024). Editorial: Personalized nutrition and gut microbiota: Current and future directions. *Frontiers in Nutrition*, *11*, 1375157. Advance online publication. DOI: 10.3389/fnut.2024.1375157 PMID: 38487630

Iacovacci, J., Serafini, M. S., Avuzzi, B., Badenchini, F., Cicchetti, A., Devecchi, A., Dispinzieri, M., Doldi, V., Giandini, T., Gioscio, E., Mancinelli, E., Noris Chiorda, B., Orlandi, E., Palorini, F., Possenti, L., Reis Ferreira, M., Villa, S., Zaffaroni, N., De Cecco, L., & Rancati, T. (2024). Intestinal microbiota composition is predictive of radiotherapy-induced acute gastrointestinal toxicity in prostate cancer patients. *EBioMedicine*, *106*, 105246. Advance online publication. DOI: 10.1016/j.ebiom.2024.105246 PMID: 39029427

Ianiro, G., Eusebi, L. H., Black, C. J., Gasbarrini, A., Cammarota, G., & Ford, A. C. (2019). Systematic review with meta-analysis: Efficacy of faecal microbiota transplantation for the treatment of irritable bowel syndrome. *Alimentary Pharmacology & Therapeutics, 50*(3), 240–248. DOI: 10.1111/apt.15330 PMID: 31136009

Indira, M., Venkateswarulu, T. C., Prabhakar, K. V., Peele, K. A., & Krupanidhi, S. (2018). Isolation and characterization of bacteriocin producing Enterococcus casseliflavus and its antagonistic effect on Pseudomonas aeruginosa. *Karbala International Journal of Modern Science, 4*(4), 361–368. DOI: 10.1016/j.kijoms.2018.09.002

Influences of diet and the gut microbiome on epigenetic modulation in cancer and other diseases | Clinical Epigenetics. (n.d.). Retrieved October 18, 2025, from https://link.springer.com/article/10.1186/s13148-015-0144-7

Iriart, J. A. B. (2019). Precision medicine/personalized medicine: A critical analysis of movements in the transformation of biomedicine in the early 21st century. *Cadernos de Saude Publica, 35*, e00153118. DOI: 10.1590/0102-311x00153118 PMID: 30916181

ISAPP. (2022). Definition of postbiotics: A panel debate in Amsterdam. International Scientific Association for Probiotics and Prebiotics (ISAPP). Available at: https://isappscience.org/definition-of-postbiotics-a-panel-debate-in-amsterdam/ (Accessed 27 July 2025).

Islam, F., Azmat, F., Imran, A., Zippi, M., Hong, W., Tariq, F., Shehzadi, U., Fatima, A., Safdar, M., Ahmed, H., Ijaz, M., Zeeshan, F., Ali, R., Asif Shah, M., & Suleria, H. A. (2024). Role of postbiotics in food and health: A comprehensive review. *CYTA: Journal of Food, 22*(1), 2386412. DOI: 10.1080/19476337.2024.2386412

Ivanov, S., Soliman, M., Tuomi, A., Alkathiri, N. A., & Al-Alawi, A. N. (2024). Drivers of generative AI adoption in higher education through the lens of the theory of planned behaviour. *Technology in Society, 77*, 102521. DOI: 10.1016/j.techsoc.2024.102521

Ivleva, E. A., & Grivennikov, S. I. (2022). Microbiota-driven mechanisms at different stages of cancer development. *Neoplasia : an International Journal for Oncology Research, 32*, 100829. DOI: 10.1016/j.neo.2022.100829 PMID: 35933824

Jackson, P. P. J., Wijeyesekera, A., & Rastall, R. A. (2022). Inulin-type fructans and short-chain fructooligosaccharides-their role within the food industry as fat and sugar replacers and texture modifiers-what needs to be considered! *Food Science & Nutrition, 11*(1), 17–38. DOI: 10.1002/fsn3.3040

Jackson, S. A., Schoeni, J. L., Vegge, C., Pane, M., Stahl, B., Bradley, M., & Sanders, M. E. (2019). Improving end-user trust in the quality of commercial probiotic products. *Frontiers in Microbiology, 10*, 739. DOI: 10.3389/fmicb.2019.00739

Jagannath, B., Lin, K.-C., Pali, M., Sankhala, D., Muthukumar, S., & Prasad, S. (2024). A sweat-based wearable enabling technology for real-time monitoring of IL-1β and CRP as potential markers for inflammatory bowel disease. *Inflammatory Bowel Diseases*. Advance online publication. DOI: 10.1093/ibd/izaa191 PMID: 32720974

Jain, N. (2020). The early life education of the immune system: Moms, microbes and (missed) opportunities. *Gut Microbes, 12*(1), 1824564. DOI: 10.1080/19490976.2020.1824564 PMID: 33043833

Jameus, A., Dougherty, J., Narendrula, R., Levert, D., Valiquette, M., Pirkkanen, J., Lalonde, C., Bonin, P., Gagnon, J. D., Appanna, V. D., Tharmalingam, S., & Thome, C. (2024). Acute impacts of ionizing radiation exposure on the gastrointestinal tract and gut microbiome in mice. *International Journal of Molecular Sciences, 25*(6), 3339. Advance online publication. DOI: 10.3390/ijms25063339 PMID: 38542312

Janda, J. M., & Abbott, S. L. (2007). 16S rRNA gene sequencing for bacterial identification in the diagnostic laboratory: Pluses, perils, and pitfalls. *Journal of Clinical Microbiology, 45*(9), 2761–2764. DOI: 10.1128/JCM.01228-07 PMID: 17626177

Jang, W., Kim, S., Son, Y., Kim, S., Lee, S., Kim, H. J., Jo, H., Park, J., Lee, K., Lee, H., Rahmati, M., Woo, S., Hwang, J., Kang, J., Smith, L., & Yon, D. K. (2025). Global, regional, and national burden of pharyngeal cancer and projections to 2050 in 185 countries: A population-based systematic analysis of GLOBOCAN 2022. *Journal of Korean Medical Science, 40*(30), e177. DOI: 10.3346/jkms.2025.40.e177 PMID: 40762594

JanssenDuijghuijsen, L., Looijesteijn, E., van den Belt, M., Gerhard, B., Ziegler, M., Ariens, R., Tjoelker, R., & Geurts, J.JanssenDuijghuijsen. (2024). Changes in gut microbiota and lactose intolerance symptoms before and after daily lactose supplementation in individuals with the lactase nonpersistent genotype. *The American Journal of Clinical Nutrition, 119*(3), 702–710. DOI: 10.1016/j.ajcnut.2023.12.016 PMID: 38159728

Javdan, B., Lopez, J. G., Chankhamjon, P., Lee, Y.-C. J., Hull, R., Wu, Q., Wang, X., Chatterjee, S., & Donia, M. S. (2020). Personalized Mapping of Drug Metabolism by the Human Gut Microbiome. *Cell, 181*(7), 1661–1679.e22. DOI: 10.1016/j.cell.2020.05.001 PMID: 32526207

Jeffery, I. B., Lynch, D. B., & O'Toole, P. W. (2016). Composition and temporal stability of the gut microbiota in older persons. *The ISME Journal, 10*(1), 170–182. DOI: 10.1038/ismej.2015.88 PMID: 26090993

Jenkins, E. L., Ilicic, J., Barklamb, A. M., & McCaffrey, T. A. (2020). Assessing the credibility and authenticity of social media content for applications in health communication: Scoping review. *Journal of Medical Internet Research, 22*(7), e17296. DOI: 10.2196/17296 PMID: 32706675

Jennis, M., Cavanaugh, C. R., Leo, G. C., Mabus, J. R., Lenhard, J., & Hornby, P. J. (2017). Microbiota-derived tryptophan indoles increase after gastric bypass surgery and reduce intestinal permeability in vitro and in vivo. *Neurogastroenterology and Motility, 30*(2), e13178. DOI: 10.1111/nmo.13178 PMID: 28782205

Jia, W., Xie, G., & Jia, W. (2018). Bile acid-microbiota crosstalk in gastrointestinal inflammation and carcinogenesis. *Nature Reviews. Gastroenterology & Hepatology, 15*(2), 111–128. DOI: 10.1038/nrgastro.2017.119 PMID: 29018272

Johansson, M. E., Phillipson, M., Petersson, J., Velcich, A., Holm, L., & Hansson, G. C. (2008). The inner of the two Muc2 mucin-dependent mucus layers in colon is devoid of bacteria. *Proceedings of the National Academy of Sciences of the United States of America, 105*(39), 15064–15069. DOI: 10.1073/pnas.0803124105

Johnson, A. J., Vangay, P., Al-Ghalith, G. A., Hillmann, B. M., Ward, T. L., Shields-Cutler, R. R., Kim, A. D., Shmagel, A. K., Syed, A. N., Walter, J., Menon, R., Koecher, K., & Knights, D. (2019). Daily sampling reveals personalized diet-microbiome associations in humans. *Cell Host & Microbe, 25*(6), 789–802. DOI: 10.1016/j.chom.2019.05.005 PMID: 31194939

Johnson, J. S., Spakowicz, D. J., Hong, B. Y., Petersen, L. M., Demkowicz, P., Chen, L., Leopold, S. R., Hanson, B. M., Agresta, H. O., Gerstein, M., Sodergren, E., & Weinstock, G. M. (2019). Evaluation of 16S rRNA gene sequencing for species and strain-level microbiome analysis. *Nature Communications, 10*(1), 5029. DOI: 10.1038/s41467-019-13036-1

Joseph, T. A., & Pe'er, I. (2021). An introduction to whole-metagenome shotgun sequencing studies. *Deep sequencing data analysis*, 107-122.

Jovel, J., Patterson, J., Wang, W., Hotte, N., O'Keefe, S., Mitchel, T., Perry, T., Kao, D., Mason, A. L., Madsen, K. L., & Wong, G. K. (2016). Characterization of the gut microbiome using 16S or shotgun metagenomics. *Frontiers in Microbiology, 7*, 459. DOI: 10.3389/fmicb.2016.00459 PMID: 27148170

Joyner, M. J., Paneth, N., & Ioannidis, J. P. A. (2019). What happens when underpowered studies are pooled? *Nature*, *569*(7758), 447–449. DOI: 10.1038/d41586-019-01409-7

Jump, R. L. P., Crnich, C. J., Mody, L., Bradley, S. F., Nicolle, L. E., & Yoshikawa, T. T. (2018). Infectious diseases in older adults of long-term care facilities: Update on approach to diagnosis and management. *Journal of the American Geriatrics Society*, *66*(4), 789–803. DOI: 10.1111/jgs.15248 PMID: 29667186

Kahn, J., Pregartner, G., & Schemmer, P. (2020). Effects of both Pro- and Synbiotics in Liver Surgery and Transplantation with Special Focus on the Gut-Liver Axis-A Systematic Review and Meta-Analysis. *Nutrients*, *12*(8), 2461. DOI: 10.3390/nu12082461

Kalyanaraman, B., Cheng, G., & Hardy, M. (2024). The role of short-chain fatty acids in cancer prevention and cancer treatment. *Archives of Biochemistry and Biophysics*, *761*, 110172. DOI: 10.1016/j.abb.2024.110172 PMID: 39369836

Kameoka, S., Motooka, D., Watanabe, S., Kubo, R., Jung, N., Midorikawa, Y., Shinozaki, N. O., Sawai, Y., Takeda, A. K., & Nakamura, S. (2021). Benchmark of 16S rRNA gene amplicon sequencing using Japanese gut microbiome data from the V1–V2 and V3–V4 primer sets. *BMC Genomics*, *22*(1), 527. DOI: 10.1186/s12864-021-07746-4

Kandari, A., Odat, M. A., Alzaid, F., & Scott, K. P. (2024). Biotics and bacterial function: Impact on gut and host health. *The ISME Journal*, *18*(1), wrae226. Advance online publication. DOI: 10.1093/ismejo/wrae226

Kandpal, M., Indari, O., Baral, B., Jakhmola, S., Tiwari, D., Bhandari, V., Pandey, R. K., Bala, K., Sonawane, A., & Jha, H. C. (2022). Dysbiosis of gut microbiota from the perspective of the gut–brain axis: Role in the provocation of neurological disorders. *Metabolites*, *12*(11), 1064. DOI: 10.3390/metabo12111064 PMID: 36355147

Kang, J., Cho, Y.-H., & Lee, Y. (2022). Pyocyanin and 1-Hydroxyphenazine promote anaerobic killing of Pseudomonas aeruginosa via single-electron transfer with ferrous iron. *Microbiology Spectrum*, *10*(6), e02312–e02322. DOI: 10.1128/spectrum.02312-22 PMID: 36321913

Karam, F., El Deghel, Y., Iratni, R., Dakroub, A. H., & Eid, A. H. (2025). The gut microbiome and colorectal cancer: An integrative review of the underlying mechanisms. *Cell Biochemistry and Biophysics*, *83*(3), 1–14. DOI: 10.1007/s12013-025-01683-9 PMID: 39946032

Karhus, L. L., Gunnes, N., Størdal, K., & Ludvigsson, J. F. (2018). Influenza and risk of later celiac disease: A cohort study of 2.6 million people. *Scandinavian Journal of Gastroenterology*, *53*(1), 15–23. DOI: 10.1080/00365521.2017.1362464

Karnwal, A., Dohroo, A., & Malik, T. (2023). Unveiling the potential of bioinoculants and nanoparticles in sustainable agriculture for enhanced plant growth and food security. *BioMed Research International*, *2023*(1), 6911851. Advance online publication. DOI: 10.1155/2023/6911851 PMID: 38075309

Kashyap, P. C., Chia, N., Nelson, H., Segal, E., & Elinav, E. (2017, December). Microbiome at the frontier of personalized medicine. In Mayo Clinic Proceedings (Vol. 92, No. 12, pp. 1855-1864). *Elsevier*. https://doi.org/DOI: 10.1016/j.mayocp.2017.10.004

Kassem, N. M., Abdelmegid, Y. A., El-Sayed, M. K., Sayed, R. S., Abdel-Aalla, M. H., & Kassem, H. A. (2023). Nutrigenomics and microbiome shaping the future of personalized medicine: A review article. *Journal of Genetic Engineering and Biotechnology*, *21*(1), 134. DOI: 10.1186/s43141-023-00599-2

Kau, A. L., Ahern, P. P., Griffin, N. W., Goodman, A. L., & Gordon, J. I. (2011). Human nutrition, the gut microbiome and the immune system. *Nature*, *474*(7351), 327–336. DOI: 10.1038/nature10213 PMID: 21677749

Kaur, N., Pandey, S., & Bhushan, K. (2025). Recent Developments in Extraction, Molecular Characterization, Bioactivity, and Application of Brewers Spent Grain Arabinoxylans. *Journal of Food Science*, *90*(5), e70239. DOI: 10.1111/1750-3841.70239

Kawamoto, S., Maruya, M., Kato, L. M., Suda, W., Atarashi, K., Doi, Y., Tsutsui, Y., Qin, H., Honda, K., Okada, T., Hattori, M., & Fagarasan, S. (2014). Foxp3^{+} T cells regulate immunoglobulin A selection and facilitate diversification of bacterial species responsible for immune homeostasis. *Immunity*, *41*(1), 152–165. DOI: 10.1016/j.immuni.2014.05.016 PMID: 25017466

Kawasaki, T., & Kawai, T. (2014). Toll-like receptor signaling pathways. *Frontiers in Immunology*, *5*, 461. DOI: 10.3389/fimmu.2014.00461 PMID: 25309543

Kayama, H., Okumura, R., & Takeda, K. (2020). Interaction between the microbiota, epithelia, and immune cells in the intestine. *Annual Review of Immunology*, *38*(1), 23–48. DOI: 10.1146/annurev-immunol-070119-115104

Kemppainen, K. M., Lynch, K. F., Liu, E., Lönnrot, M., Simell, V., Briese, T., Koletzko, S., Hagopian, W., Rewers, M., She, J.-X., Simell, O., Toppari, J., Ziegler, A.-G., Akolkar, B., Krischer, J. P., Lernmark, Å., Hyöty, H., Triplett, E. W., & Agardh, D. (2017). Factors that increase risk of celiac disease autoimmunity after a gastrointestinal infection in early life. *Clinical Gastroenterology and Hepatology, 15*(5), 694–702. DOI: 10.1016/j.cgh.2016.10.033

Keyhani, G., Hosseini, H. M., & Salimi, A. (2022). Effect of extracellular vesicles of Lactobacillus rhamnosus GG on the expression of CEA gene and protein released by colorectal cancer cells. *Iranian Journal of Microbiology, 14*(1), 90. DOI: 10.18502/ijm.v14i1.8809

Khan, R. H., Miah, J., Nipun, S. A. A., Islam, M., Amin, M. S., & Taluckder, M. S. (2023). Enhancing lung cancer diagnosis with machine learning methods and systematic review synthesis. In 2021 7th International Conference on Electrical, Electronics and Information Engineering (ICEEIE) (p. 1). IEEE. DOI: 10.1109/ICEEIE59078.2023.10334739

Khan, I., Bai, Y., Ullah, N., Liu, G., Rajoka, M. S. R., & Zhang, C. (2022). Differential susceptibility of the gut microbiota to DSS treatment interferes in the conserved microbiome association in mouse models of colitis and is related to the initial gut microbiota difference. *Advanced Gut & Microbiome Research, 2022*, 7813278. Advance online publication. DOI: 10.1155/2022/7813278

Khodoun, M. V., Tomar, S., Tocker, J. E., Wang, Y. H., & Finkelman, F. D. (2018). Prevention of food allergy development and suppression of established food allergy by neutralization of thymic stromal lymphopoietin, IL-25, and IL-33. *The Journal of Allergy and Clinical Immunology, 141*(1), 171–179. DOI: 10.1016/j.jaci.2017.02.046

Kim, B.-S., Choi, C. W., Shin, H., Jin, S.-P., Bae, J.-S., Han, M., Seo, E. Y., Chun, J., & Chung, J. H. (2019). Comparison of the gut microbiota of centenarians in longevity villages of South Korea with those of other age groups. *Journal of Microbiology and Biotechnology, 29*(3), 429–440. DOI: 10.4014/jmb.1811.11023 PMID: 30661321

Kim, B., Song, A., Son, A., & Shin, Y. (2024). Gut microbiota and epigenetic choreography: Implications for human health. *Revista de Medicina (São Paulo), 103*(29), e39051. DOI: 10.1097/MD.0000000000039051 PMID: 39029010

Kim, C. H. (2018). Immune regulation by microbiome metabolites. *Immunology, 154*(2), 220–229. DOI: 10.1111/imm.12930 PMID: 29569377

Kim, H., Caulfield, L. E., Garcia-Larsen, V., Steffen, L. M., Coresh, J., & Rebholz, C. M. (2019a). Plant-based diets are associated with a lower risk of incident cardiovascular disease, cardiovascular disease mortality, and all-cause mortality in a general population of middle-aged adults. *Journal of the American Heart Association*, *8*(16), e012865. DOI: 10.1161/JAHA.119.012865 PMID: 31387433

Kim, H., Caulfield, L. E., Garcia-Larsen, V., Steffen, L. M., Grams, M. E., Coresh, J., & Rebholz, C. M. (2019b). Plant-based diets and incident CKD and kidney function. *Clinical Journal of the American Society of Nephrology; CJASN*, *14*(5), 682–691. DOI: 10.2215/CJN.12391018 PMID: 31023928

Kim, J., & Lee, H. K. (2022). Potential role of the gut microbiome in colorectal cancer progression. *Frontiers in Immunology*, *12*, 807648. DOI: 10.3389/fimmu.2021.807648 PMID: 35069592

Kim, N., Ma, J., Kim, W., Kim, J., Belenky, P., & Lee, I. (2024). Genome-resolved metagenomics: A game changer for microbiome medicine. *Experimental & Molecular Medicine*, *56*(7), 1501–1512. DOI: 10.1038/s12276-024-01262-7

Kim, S. A., & Shin, J. (2018). Role of the gut microbiome in obesity and metabolic syndrome. *Experimental & Molecular Medicine*, *50*(11), 1–9. DOI: 10.1038/s12276-018-0178-y PMID: 30429461

Kim, S. K., Guevarra, R. B., Kim, Y. T., Kwon, J., Kim, H., Cho, J. H., Kim, H. B., & Lee, J. H. (2019). Role of probiotics in human gut microbiome-associated diseases. *Journal of Microbiology and Biotechnology*, *29*(9), 1335–1340. DOI: 10.4014/jmb.1906.06064 PMID: 31434172

Kim, Y. C.. (2020). An integrated wearable microneedle array for the continuous monitoring of multiple biomarkers in interstitial fluid. *Nature Biomedical Engineering*, *6*(11), 1214–1222. DOI: 10.1038/s41551-022-00887-1 PMID: 35534575

Kiousi, D. E., Kouroutzidou, A. Z., Neanidis, K., Karavanis, E., Matthaios, D., Pappa, A., & Galanis, A. (2023). The role of the gut microbiome in cancer immunotherapy: Current knowledge and future directions. *Cancers (Basel)*, *15*(7), 2101. DOI: 10.3390/cancers15072101 PMID: 37046762

Knight, R., Vrbanac, A., Taylor, B. C., Aksenov, A., Callewaert, C., Debelius, J., Gonzalez, A., Kosciolek, T., McCall, L.-I., McDonald, D., Melnik, A. V., Morton, J. T., Navas, J., Quinn, R. A., Sanders, J. G., Swafford, A. D., Thompson, L. R., Tripathi, A., Xu, Z. Z., & Dorrestein, P. C. (2018). Best practices for analysing microbiomes. *Nature Reviews. Microbiology*, *16*(7), 410–422. DOI: 10.1038/s41579-018-0029-9 PMID: 29795328

Koh, A., De Vadder, F., Kovatcheva-Datchary, P., & Bäckhed, F. (2016). From dietary fiber to host physiology: Short-chain fatty acids as key bacterial metabolites. *Cell, 165*(6), 1332–1345. DOI: 10.1016/j.cell.2016.05.041 PMID: 27259147

Koh, A., Molinaro, A., Ståhlman, M., Khan, M. T., Schmidt, C., Mannerås-Holm, L., Wu, H., Carreras, A., Jeong, H., Olofsson, L. E., Bergh, P. O., Gerdes, V., Hartstra, A., de Brauw, M., Perkins, R., Nieuwdorp, M., Bergström, G., & Bäckhed, F. (2018). Microbially produced imidazole propionate impairs insulin signaling through mTORC1. *Cell, 175*(4), 947–961.e17. DOI: 10.1016/j.cell.2018.09.055 PMID: 30401435

Kolodziejczyk, A. A., Zheng, D., & Elinav, E. (2019). Diet–microbiota interactions and personalized nutrition. *Nature Reviews. Microbiology, 17*(12), 742–753. DOI: 10.1038/s41579-019-0256-8 PMID: 31541197

Kong, F., Hua, Y., Zeng, B., Ning, R., Li, Y., & Zhao, J. (2016). Gut microbiota signatures of longevity. *Current Biology, 26*(18), R832–R833. DOI: 10.1016/j.cub.2016.08.015 PMID: 27676296

Konopelski, P., & Mogilnicka, I. (2022). Biological effects of indole-3-propionic acid, a gut microbiota-derived metabolite, and its precursor tryptophan in mammals' health and disease. *International Journal of Molecular Sciences, 23*(3), 1222. DOI: 10.3390/ijms23031222 PMID: 35163143

Koo, B.-K., Spit, M., Jordens, I., Low, T. Y., Stange, D. E., van de Wetering, M., van Es, J. H., & Clevers, H. (2012). Tumour suppressor RNF43 is a stem-cell E3 ligase that induces endocytosis of Wnt receptors. *Nature, 488*(7413), 665–669. DOI: 10.1038/nature11308

Kootte, R. S., Levin, E., Salojärvi, J., Smits, L. P., Hartstra, A. V., Udayappan, S. D., Hermes, G., Bouter, K. E., Koopen, A. M., Holst, J. J., Knop, F. K., Blaak, E. E., Zhao, J., Smidt, H., Harms, A. C., Hankemeijer, T., Bergström, G., & Nieuwdorp, M. (2017). Improvement of Insulin Sensitivity after Lean Donor Feces in Metabolic Syndrome Is Driven by Baseline Intestinal Microbiota Composition. *Cell Metabolism, 26*(4), 611–619.e6. DOI: 10.1016/j.cmet.2017.09.008 PMID: 28978426

Koponen, K. K., Salosensaari, A., Ruuskanen, M. O., Havulinna, A. S., Männistö, S., Jousilahti, P., Palmu, J., Salido, R., Sanders, K., Brennan, C., Humphrey, G. C., Sanders, J. G., Meric, G., Cheng, S., Inouye, M., Jain, M., Niiranen, T. J., Valsta, L. M., Knight, R., & Salomaa, V. V. (2021). Associations of healthy food choices with gut microbiota profiles. *The American Journal of Clinical Nutrition, 114*(2), 605–616. DOI: 10.1093/ajcn/nqab077 PMID: 34020448

Koppel, N., Maini Rekdal, V., & Balskus, E. P. (2017). Chemical transformation of xenobiotics by the human gut microbiota. *Science*, *356*(6344), eaag2770. Advance online publication. DOI: 10.1126/science.aag2770

Korčok, D. J., Tršić-Milanović, N. A., Ivanović, N. D., & Đorđević, B. I. (2018). Development of probiotic formulation for the treatment of iron deficiency anemia. *Chemical & Pharmaceutical Bulletin*, *66*(4), 347–352. DOI: 10.1248/cpb.c17-00634

Korpela, K. (2018). Diet, microbiota, and metabolic health: Trade-off between saccharolytic and proteolytic fermentation. *Annual Review of Food Science and Technology*, *9*(1), 65–84. DOI: 10.1146/annurev-food-030117-012830 PMID: 29298101

Korpela, K. (2021). Impact of delivery mode on infant gut microbiota. *Annals of Nutrition & Metabolism*, *77*(Suppl. 3), 11–19. DOI: 10.1159/000518498 PMID: 34515049

Kotte, K. R., Attaluri, V., & Selvakumar, P. (2025). Revolutionising Retail Banking with AI and Virtual Technologies AI-Driven Financial Training. In Nair, A. J., Manohar, S., Limbu, Y. B., & Huhmann, B. A. (Eds.), *Intersecting Natural Language Processing and FinTech Innovations in Service Marketing* (pp. 421–440). IGI Global., DOI: 10.4018/979-8-3693-9944-6.ch020

Kovatcheva-Datchary, P., Nilsson, A., Akrami, R., Lee, Y. S., De Vadder, F., Arora, T., Hallen, A., Martens, E., Björck, I., & Bäckhed, F. (2015). Dietary fiber-induced improvement in glucose metabolism is associated with increased abundance of *Prevotella*. *Cell Metabolism*, *22*(6), 971–982. DOI: 10.1016/j.cmet.2015.10.001 PMID: 26552345

Krautkramer, K. A., Dhillon, R. S., Denu, J. M., & Carey, H. V. (2017). Metabolic programming of the epigenome: Host and gut microbial metabolite interactions with host chromatin. *Translational Research; the Journal of Laboratory and Clinical Medicine*, *189*, 30–50. DOI: 10.1016/j.trsl.2017.08.005 PMID: 28919341

Krautkramer, K. A., Fan, J., & Bäckhed, F. (2021). Gut microbial metabolites as multi-kingdom intermediates. *Nature Reviews. Microbiology*, *19*(2), 77–94. DOI: 10.1038/s41579-020-0438-4 PMID: 32968241

Krautkramer, K. A., Kreznar, J. H., Romano, K. A., Vivas, E. I., Barrett-Wilt, G. A., Rabaglia, M. E., Keller, M. P., Attie, A. D., Rey, F. E., & Denu, J. M. (2016). Diet-Microbiota Interactions Mediate Global Epigenetic Programming in Multiple Host Tissues. *Molecular Cell*, *64*(5), 982–992. DOI: 10.1016/j.molcel.2016.10.025 PMID: 27889451

Kubelkova, K., Benuchova, M., Kozakova, H., Sinkora, M., Krocova, Z., Pejchal, J., & Macela, A. (2016). Gnotobiotic mouse model's contribution to understanding host–pathogen interactions. *Cellular and Molecular Life Sciences : CMLS*, *73*(20), 3961–3969. DOI: 10.1007/s00018-016-2341-8 PMID: 27544211

Kuczynski, J., Stombaugh, J., Walters, W. A., González, A., Caporaso, J. G., & Knight, R. (2012). Using QIIME to analyze 16S rRNA gene sequences from microbial communities. *Current Protocols in Bioinformatics*, Chapter 10, Unit 10.7. DOI: 10.1002/0471250953.bi1007s36

Kuhnle, G. G. C., Story, G. W., Reda, T., Mani, A. R., Moore, K. P., Lunn, J. C., & Bingham, S. A. (2007). Diet-induced endogenous formation of nitroso compounds in the GI tract. *Free Radical Biology & Medicine*, *43*(7), 1040–1047. DOI: 10.1016/j.freeradbiomed.2007.03.011 PMID: 17761300

Kuipers, F., Bloks, V. W., & Groen, A. K. (2014). Beyond intestinal soap–bile acids in metabolic control. *Nature Reviews. Endocrinology*, *10*(8), 488–498. DOI: 10.1038/nrendo.2014.60 PMID: 24821328

Kumar, A. (2019). Ethical considerations in microbiome research. *Frontiers in Microbiology*, *10*, 1801. DOI: 10.3389/fmicb.2019.01801

Kundra, P., Rachmühl, C., Lacroix, C., & Geirnaert, A. (2021). Role of dietary micronutrients on gut microbial dysbiosis and modulation in inflammatory bowel disease. *Molecular Nutrition & Food Research*, *65*(5), 1901271. DOI: 10.1002/mnfr.201901271

Kunst, C., Schmid, S., Michalski, M., Tümen, D., Buttenschön, J., Müller, M., Gülow, K., & Falk-Paulsen, M. (2023). The influence of gut microbiota on oxidative stress and the immune system. *Biomedicines*, *11*(5), 1388. DOI: 10.3390/biomedicines11051388

Kussmann, M., & van Bladeren, P. J. (2011). The extended nutrigenomics – understanding the interplay between the genomes of food, gut microbes, and human host. *Frontiers in Genetics*, *2*, 21. DOI: 10.3389/fgene.2011.00021

Lagier, J.-C., Hugon, P., Khelaifia, S., Fournier, P.-E., La Scola, B., & Raoult, D. (2015). The rebirth of culture in microbiology through the example of culturomics to study human gut microbiota. *Clinical Microbiology Reviews*, *28*(1), 237–264. DOI: 10.1128/CMR.00014-14 PMID: 25567229

Lagier, J.-C., Khelaifia, S., Alou, M. T., Ndongo, S., Dione, N., Hugon, P., Caputo, A., Cadoret, F., Traore, S. I., Seck, E. H., Dubourg, G., Durand, G., Mourembou, G., Guilhot, E., Togo, A., Bellali, S., Bachar, D., Cassir, N., Bittar, F., & Raoult, D. (2016). Culture of previously uncultured members of the human gut microbiota by culturomics. *Nature Microbiology*, *1*(12), 16203. DOI: 10.1038/nmicrobiol.2016.203 PMID: 27819657

Lagier, J.-C., & Raoult, D. (2016). Greffe de microbiote fécal et infections. *Medecine Sciences*, *32*(11), 1015–1020. DOI: 10.1051/medsci/20163211015 PMID: 28008840

Lagoumintzis, G., & Patrinos, G. P. (2023). Triangulating nutrigenomics, metabolomics and microbiomics toward personalized nutrition and healthy living. *Human Genomics*, *17*(1), 109. DOI: 10.1186/s40246-023-00561-w

Lagoumintzis, G., & Patrinos, G. P. (2024). Nutrigenomics and personalized nutrition: Advancing basic, clinical, and translational research. *Frontiers in Nutrition*, *11*, 1435475. DOI: 10.3389/fnut.2024.1435475

Lakshminarayanan, B., Stanton, C., O'Toole, P. W., & Ross, R. P. (2014). Compositional dynamics of the human intestinal microbiota with aging: Implications for health. *The Journal of Nutrition, Health & Aging*, *18*(9), 773–786. DOI: 10.1007/s12603-014-0549-6 PMID: 25389954

Lante, A., Canazza, E., & Tessari, P. (2023). Beta-glucans of cereals: Functional and technological properties. *Nutrients*, *15*(9), 2124. DOI: 10.3390/nu15092124

Lanzaro, F., Barlabà, A., De Nigris, D., Di Domenico, F., Verde, V. L., Del Giudice, E. M., & Staiano, A. (2023). Pediatric diabetic nephropathy: Novel insights from microRNAs. *Journal of Clinical Medicine*, *12*(4), 1447. Advance online publication. DOI: 10.3390/jcm12041447 PMID: 36835983

Larson, P. J., Zhou, W., Santiago, A., Driscoll, S., Fleming, E., Voigt, A. Y., Chun, O. K., Grady, J. J., Kuchel, G. A., Robison, J. T., & Oh, J. (2022). Associations of the skin, oral and gut microbiome with aging, frailty and infection risk reservoirs in older adults. *Nature Aging*, *2*(10), 941–955. DOI: 10.1038/s43587-022-00287-9 PMID: 36398033

Le Chatelier, E., Nielsen, T., Qin, J., Prifti, E., Hildebrand, F., Falony, G., Almeida, M., Arumugam, M., Batto, J.-M., Kennedy, S., Leonard, P., Li, J., Burgdorf, K., Grarup, N., Jørgensen, T., Brandslund, I., Nielsen, H. B., Juncker, A. S., Bertalan, M., & Pedersen, O. (2013). Richness of human gut microbiome correlates with metabolic markers. *Nature*, *500*(7464), 541–546. DOI: 10.1038/nature12506 PMID: 23985870

Lee, J.-Y., et al. (2022). The microbiome and gut homeostasis. *science, 377*(6601), eabp9960.

Lee, J., d'Aigle, J., Atadja, L., Quaicoe, V., Honarpisheh, P., Ganesh, B. P., Hassan, A., Graf, J., Petrosino, J., Putluri, N., Zhu, L., Durgan, D. J., Bryan, R. M.Jr, McCullough, L. D., & Venna, V. R. (2020). Gut microbiota–derived short-chain fatty acids promote poststroke recovery in aged mice. *Circulation Research, 127*(4), 453–465. DOI: 10.1161/CIRCRESAHA.119.316448 PMID: 32354259

Lee, J., Park, S., Oh, N., Park, J., Kwon, M., Seo, J., & Roh, S. (2021). Oral intake of Lactobacillus plantarum L-14 extract alleviates TLR2-and AMPK-mediated obesity-associated disorders in high-fat-diet-induced obese C57BL/6J mice. *Cell Proliferation, 54*(6), e13039. DOI: 10.1111/cpr.13039

Lee, K. S., Palatinszky, M., Pereira, F. C., Nguyen, J., Fernandez, V. I., Mueller, A. J., Menolascina, F., Daims, H., Berry, D., Wagner, M., & Stocker, R. (2019). An automated Raman-based platform for the sorting of live cells by functional properties. *Nature Microbiology, 4*(6), 1035–1048. DOI: 10.1038/s41564-019-0394-9

Lee, S. H., You, H. S., Kang, H. G., Kang, S. S., & Hyun, S. H. (2020). Association between altered blood parameters and gut microbiota after synbiotic intake in healthy, elderly Korean women. *Nutrients, 12*(10), 3112. DOI: 10.3390/nu12103112 PMID: 33053824

Lee, Y. S., Kim, T. Y., Kim, Y., Lee, S. H., Kim, S., Kang, S. W., Yang, J.-Y., Baek, I.-J., Sung, Y. H., Park, Y.-Y., & Kweon, M.-N. (2018). Microbiota-derived lactate accelerates intestinal stem-cell-mediated epithelial development. *Cell Host & Microbe, 24*(6), 833–846.e6. DOI: 10.1016/j.chom.2018.11.002

Le, H. D., Wolinska, J. M., Baertschiger, R. M., & Himidan, S. A. (2023). Complication is inevitable, but suffering is optional—Psychological aspects of dealing with complications in surgery. *European Journal of Pediatric Surgery, 33*(03), 181–190. DOI: 10.1055/s-0043-1767830 PMID: 36948212

León, E. D., & Francino, M. P. (2022). Roles of secretory immunoglobulin A in host–microbiota interactions in the gut ecosystem. *Frontiers in Microbiology, 13*, 880484. Advance online publication. DOI: 10.3389/fmicb.2022.880484 PMID: 35722300

Leviatan, S., & Segal, E. (2020). Identifying gut microbes that affect human health. *Nature, 587*(7834), 373–374. DOI: 10.1038/d41586-020-03069-8

Levy, M., Kolodziejczyk, A. A., Thaiss, C. A., & Elinav, E. (2017). Dysbiosis and the immune system. *Nature Reviews. Immunology*, *17*(4), 219–232. DOI: 10.1038/nri.2017.7 PMID: 28260787

Lewandowska-Pietruszka, Z., Figlerowicz, M., & Mazur-Melewska, K. (2022). The history of the intestinal microbiota and the gut–brain axis. *Pathogens (Basel, Switzerland)*, *11*(12), 1540. Advance online publication. DOI: 10.3390/pathogens11121540 PMID: 36558874

Ley, R. E., Turnbaugh, P. J., Klein, S., & Gordon, J. I. (2006). Microbial ecology: Human gut microbes associated with obesity. *Nature*, *444*(7122), 1022–1023. DOI: 10.1038/4441022a PMID: 17183309

Li, C. (2023). Understanding interactions among diet, host and gut microbiota for personalized nutrition. *Life Sciences*, *312*, 121265. DOI: 10.1016/j.lfs.2022.121265 PMID: 36473543

Li, D., Li, Y., Yang, S., Lu, J., Jin, X., & Wu, M. (2022). Diet-gut microbiota-epigenetics in metabolic diseases: From mechanisms to therapeutics. *Biomedicine and Pharmacotherapy*, *153*, 113290. DOI: 10.1016/j.biopha.2022.113290 PMID: 35724509

Li, H. Y., Zhou, D. D., Gan, R. Y., Huang, S. Y., Zhao, C. N., Shang, A., Xu, X. Y., & Li, H. B. (2021). Effects and Mechanisms of Probiotics, Prebiotics, Synbiotics, and Postbiotics on Metabolic Diseases Targeting Gut Microbiota: A Narrative Review. *Nutrients*, *13*(9), 3211. DOI: 10.3390/nu13093211

Li, J. (2023). Information avoidance in the age of COVID-19: A meta-analysis. *Information Processing & Management*, *60*(1), 103163. DOI: 10.1016/j.ipm.2022.103163 PMID: 36405670

Li, J., Wu, T., Li, N., Wang, X., Chen, G., & Lyu, X. (2019). Bilberry anthocyanin extract promotes intestinal barrier function and inhibits digestive enzyme activity by regulating the gut microbiota in aging rats. *Food & Function*, *10*(1), 333–343. DOI: 10.1039/C8FO01962B PMID: 30575836

Li, K., Epperly, M. W., Acosta Barreto, G., Greenberger, J. S., & Methé, B. A. (2021). Longitudinal fecal microbiome study of total body irradiated mice treated with radiation mitigators identifies bacterial associations with survival. *Frontiers in Cellular and Infection Microbiology*, *11*, 715396. Advance online publication. DOI: 10.3389/fcimb.2021.715396 PMID: 34621689

Li, L., Abou-Samra, E., Ning, Z., Zhang, X., Mayne, J., Wang, J., Cheng, K., Walker, K., Stintzi, A., & Figeys, D. (2019). An in vitro model maintaining taxon-specific functional activities of the gut microbiome. *Nature Communications*, *10*(1), 4146. DOI: 10.1038/s41467-019-12087-8 PMID: 31515476

Li, L., Yang, C., Jia, M., Wang, Y., Zhao, Y., Li, Q., Gong, J., He, Y., Xu, K., Liu, X., Chen, X., Hu, J., & Liu, Z. (2024). Synbiotic therapy with Clostridium sporogenes and xylan promotes gut-derived indole-3-propionic acid and improves cognitive impairments in an Alzheimer's disease mouse model. *Food & Function*, *15*(15), 7865–7882. DOI: 10.1039/D4FO00886C PMID: 38967039

Li, M., van Esch, B. C. A. M., Henricks, P. A. J., Folkerts, G., & Garssen, J. (2018). The anti-inflammatory effects of short chain fatty acids on lipopolysaccharide-or tumor necrosis factor α-stimulated endothelial cells via activation of GPR41/43 and inhibition of HDACs. *Frontiers in Pharmacology*, *9*, 533. DOI: 10.3389/fphar.2018.00533 PMID: 29875665

Ling, L. L., Schneider, T., Peoples, A. J., Spoering, A. L., Engels, I., Conlon, B. P., Mueller, A., Schäberle, T. F., Hughes, D. E., Epstein, S., Jones, M., Lazarides, L., Steadman, V. A., Cohen, D. R., Felix, C. R., Fetterman, K. A., Millett, W. P., Nitti, A. G., Zullo, A. M., & Lewis, K. (2015). A new antibiotic kills pathogens without detectable resistance. *Nature*, *517*(7535), 455–459. DOI: 10.1038/nature14098

Liong, M. T. (2008). Roles of probiotics and prebiotics in colon cancer prevention: Postulated mechanisms and in-vivo evidence. *International Journal of Molecular Sciences*, *9*(5), 854–863. DOI: 10.3390/ijms9050854 PMID: 19325789

Li, S. (2023). Modulation of immunity by tryptophan microbial metabolites. *Frontiers in Nutrition*, *10*, 1209613. DOI: 10.3389/fnut.2023.1209613 PMID: 37521424

Li, S., Heng, X., Guo, L., Lessing, D. J., & Chu, W. (2022). SCFAs improve disease resistance via modulate gut microbiota, enhance immune response and increase antioxidative capacity in the host. *Fish & Shellfish Immunology*, *120*, 560–568. DOI: 10.1016/j.fsi.2021.12.035 PMID: 34958920

Liu, H. (2024). Integrative Approaches in Computational Genomics: Combining Omics Data to Study Gene Evolution. Computational Molecular Biology, 14(0). https://bioscipublisher.com/index.php/cmb/article/view/3990

Liu, B., Zhou, H., Tan, L., Siu, K. T. H., & Guan, X. (2024). Exploring treatment options in cancer: Tumor treatment strategies. *Signal Transduction and Targeted Therapy*, *9*(1), 175. Advance online publication. DOI: 10.1038/s41392-024-01856-7 PMID: 39013849

Liu, Q., Yu, Z., Tian, F., Zhao, J., Zhang, H., Zhai, Q., & Chen, W. (2020). Surface components and metabolites of probiotics for regulation of intestinal epithelial barrier. *Microbial Cell Factories*, *19*(1), 23. DOI: 10.1186/s12934-020-1289-4 PMID: 32024520

Liu, R., Zhang, X., Cai, Y., Xu, S., Xu, Q., Ling, C., Li, X., Li, W., Liu, P., & Liu, W. (2024). Research progress on medicinal components and pharmacological activities of polygonatum sibiricum. *Journal of Ethnopharmacology*, *328*, 118024. DOI: 10.1016/j.jep.2024.118024

Liu, W., Yu, L., Chen, Q., Zhang, C., Wang, L., Yu, N., Peng, D., Ou, J., Chen, W., Zhang, Y., & Wang, Y. (2025). Poria cocos polysaccharides alleviate obesity-related adipose tissue insulin resistance via gut microbiota-derived short-chain fatty acids activation of FGF21/PI3K/AKT signaling. *Food Research International*, *215*, 116671. DOI: 10.1016/j.foodres.2025.116671

Liu, X., Shao, J., Liao, Y.-T., Wang, L.-N., Jia, Y., Dong, P., Liu, Z., He, D., Li, C., & Zhang, X. (2023). Regulation of short-chain fatty acids in the immune system. *Frontiers in Immunology*, *14*, 1186892. DOI: 10.3389/fimmu.2023.1186892 PMID: 37215145

Liu, Y., Tang, Y., Cheng, Y., Huang, W., & Xiang, L. (2022). Electrochemical Biosensors Based on Saliva Electrolytes for Rapid Detection and Diagnosis. *Journal of Materials Chemistry. B*, *11*(1), 33–45. DOI: 10.1039/D2TB02031A PMID: 36484271

Liu, Y., Tran, D. Q., & Rhoads, J. M. (2018). Probiotics in disease prevention and treatment. *Journal of Clinical Pharmacology*, *58*(S10), S164–S179. DOI: 10.1002/jcph.1121

Li, Y., Wang, D. D., Satija, A., Ivey, K. L., Li, J., Wilkinson, J. E., Wu, Y., Ding, E. L., Rimm, E. B., Hu, F. B., & Sun, Q. (2021). Plant-based diet index and metabolic risk in men: Exploring the role of the gut microbiome. *The Journal of Nutrition*, *151*(9), 2780–2789. DOI: 10.1093/jn/nxab175 PMID: 34114015

Li, Z., Ke, X., Zuo, D., Wang, Z., Fang, F., & Li, B. (2022). New insights into the relationship between gut microbiota and radiotherapy for cancer. *Nutrients*, *15*(1), 48. DOI: 10.3390/nu15010048 PMID: 36615706

Li, Z., Xiong, W., Liang, Z., Wang, J., Zeng, Z., Kołat, D., Li, X., Zhou, D., Xu, X., & Zhao, L. (2024). Critical role of the gut microbiota in immune responses and cancer immunotherapy. *Journal of Hematology & Oncology*, *17*(1), 33. DOI: 10.1186/s13045-024-01541-w PMID: 38745196

Lockis, V. R., Cruz, A. G., Walter, E. H., Faria, J. A., Granato, D., & Sant'Ana, A. S. (2011). Prerequisite programs at schools: Diagnosis and economic evaluation. *Foodborne Pathogens and Disease*, *8*(2), 213–220. DOI: 10.1089/fpd.2010.0645

Longo, S., Rizza, S., & Federici, M. (2023). Microbiota-gut-brain axis: Relationships among the vagus nerve, gut microbiota, obesity, and diabetes. *Acta Diabetologica*, *60*(8), 1007–1017. DOI: 10.1007/s00592-023-02088-x PMID: 37058160

Longo, V. D., & Panda, S. (2016). Fasting, circadian rhythms, and time-restricted feeding in healthy lifespan. *Cell Metabolism*, *23*(6), 1048–1059. DOI: 10.1016/j.cmet.2016.06.001 PMID: 27304506

Lopomo, A., Burgio, E., & Migliore, L. (2016). Chapter Six—Epigenetics of Obesity. In Tao, Y.-X. (Ed.), *Progress in Molecular Biology and Translational Science* (Vol. 140, pp. 151–184). Academic Press., DOI: 10.1016/bs.pmbts.2016.02.002

Louis, P., & Flint, H. J. (2017). Formation of propionate and butyrate by the human colonic microbiota. *Environmental Microbiology*, *19*(1), 29–41. DOI: 10.1111/1462-2920.13589 PMID: 27928878

Louis, S., Tappu, R. M., Damms-Machado, A., Huson, D. H., & Bischoff, S. C. (2016). Characterization of the gut microbial community of obese patients following a weight-loss intervention using whole metagenome shotgun sequencing. *PLoS One*, *11*(2), e0149564. DOI: 10.1371/journal.pone.0149564 PMID: 26919743

Lozenov, S., Krastev, B., Nikolaev, G., Peshevska-Sekulovska, M., Peruhova, M., & Velikova, T. (2023). Gut microbiome composition and its metabolites are a key regulating factor for malignant transformation, metastasis and antitumor immunity. *International Journal of Molecular Sciences*, *24*(6), 5978. DOI: 10.3390/ijms24065978 PMID: 36983053

Luczynski, P., Neufeld, K. A. M. V., Oriach, C. S., Clarke, G., Dinan, T. G., & Cryan, J. F. (2016). Growing up in a bubble: Using germ-free animals to assess the influence of the gut microbiota on brain and behavior. *The International Journal of Neuropsychopharmacology*, *19*(8), pyw020. Advance online publication. DOI: 10.1093/ijnp/pyw020 PMID: 26912607

Luda, K. M., Joeris, T., Persson, E. K., Rivollier, A., Demiri, M., Sitnik, K. M., Pool, L., Holm, J. B., Melo-Gonzalez, F., & Agace, W. W. (2016). IRF8 transcription-factor-dependent classical dendritic cells are essential for intestinal T cell homeostasis. *Immunity*, *44*(4), 860–874. DOI: 10.1016/j.immuni.2016.02.008

Lumeng, C. N., & Saltiel, A. R. (2011). Inflammatory links between obesity and metabolic disease. *The Journal of Clinical Investigation*, *121*(6), 2111–2117. DOI: 10.1172/JCI57132 PMID: 21633179

Luo, C., Xu, X., Wei, X., Feng, W., Huang, H., Liu, H., Xu, R., Lin, J., Han, L., & Zhang, D. (2019). Natural medicines for the treatment of fatigue: Bioactive components, pharmacology, and mechanisms. *Pharmacological Research*, *148*, 104409. DOI: 10.1016/j.phrs.2019.104409

Luu, M., Riester, Z., Baldrich, A., Reichardt, N., Yuille, S., Busetti, A., Klein, M., Wempe, A., Leister, H., Raifer, H., Picard, F., Muhammad, K., Ohl, K., Romero, R., Fischer, F., Bauer, C. A., Huber, M., Gress, T. M., Lauth, M., & Visekruna, A. (2021). Microbial short-chain fatty acids modulate CD8+ T cell responses and improve adoptive immunotherapy for cancer. *Nature Communications*, *12*(1), 4077. DOI: 10.1038/s41467-021-24331-1 PMID: 34210970

Lv, J., Hao, P., Zhou, Y., Liu, T., Wang, L., Song, C., Wang, Z., Liu, Z., & Liu, Y. (2025). Role of the intestinal flora-immunity axis in the pathogenesis of rheumatoid arthritis-mechanisms regulating short-chain fatty acids and Th17/Treg homeostasis. *Molecular Biology Reports*, *52*(1), 1–11. DOI: 10.1007/s11033-025-10714-w PMID: 40544212

Lynch, S. V., & Pedersen, O. (2016). The human intestinal microbiome in health and disease. *The New England Journal of Medicine*, *375*(24), 2369–2379. DOI: 10.1056/NEJMra1600266 PMID: 27974040

Mabsor-Zgandaoui, S., Moussaif, A., El Hessni, A., Mesfioui, A., El Mzibri, M., Iddar, A., & Moutaouakkil, A. (2025). Ionising and ultraviolet radiation induce the secretion of melanin in *Tetrahymena pyriformis. The International Journal of Environmental Studies*, *82*(1), 1–14. DOI: 10.1080/00207233.2024.2412455

Mabsor-Zgandaoui, S., Rachmoune, K., El Hessni, A., El Mzibri, M., Iddar, A., & Moutaouakkil, A. (2025). Effect of hydrogen peroxide pre-treatment on enhancing the cellular resistance of *Tetrahymena pyriformis* exposed to ionizing radiation. *Toxicological and Environmental Chemistry*, *107*(2), 294–309. DOI: 10.1080/02772248.2025.2460804

Macpherson, A. J., & Uhr, T. (2004). Induction of protective IgA by intestinal dendritic cells carrying commensal bacteria. *Science*, *303*(5664), 1662–1665. DOI: 10.1126/science.1091334 PMID: 15016999

Mafe, A. N., & Büsselberg, D. (2025). The Effect of Microbiome-Derived Metabolites in Inflammation-Related Cancer Prevention and Treatment. *Biomolecules*, *15*(5), 688. DOI: 10.3390/biom15050688 PMID: 40427581

Maheswaran, K., Selvakumar, P., Shaikh, M., Shashank, G., Gupta, S., & Manjunath, T. C. (2025). The Evolution of Smart Urban Mobility With Emerging Technologies. In Ponnusamy, S., Assaf, M., Youssef, B., Jeon, G., & Kalyanaraman, S. (Eds.), *Leveraging VANETs and Blockchain Technology for Urban Mobility* (pp. 1–28). IGI Global., DOI: 10.4018/979-8-3373-0265-2.ch001

Mahmoud, A. M. (2022). An Overview of Epigenetics in Obesity: The Role of Lifestyle and Therapeutic Interventions. *International Journal of Molecular Sciences*, *23*(3), 1341. DOI: 10.3390/ijms23031341 PMID: 35163268

Maia, J. M., Solon, I. G., Soriano, R. N., & Branco, L. G. S. (2024). Exploring the links between pro-inflammatory diets, gut dysbiosis, serotonin, and their implications for psychiatric and neurodegenerative disorders. *Brain Behavior and Immunity Integrative*, *8*, 100097. DOI: 10.1016/j.bbii.2024.100097

Maier, L., Pruteanu, M., Kuhn, M., Zeller, G., Telzerow, A., Anderson, E. E., & Typas, A. (2018). Extensive impact of non-antibiotic drugs on human gut bacteria. *Nature*, *555*(7698), 623–628. DOI: 10.1038/nature25979 PMID: 29555994

Mak, J. W. Y., Chan, F. K. L., & Ng, S. C. (2020). Probiotics and COVID-19: One size does not fit all. *The Lancet. Gastroenterology & Hepatology*, *5*(7), 644–645. DOI: 10.1016/S2468-1253(20)30122-9

Maldonado Galdeano, C., et al. (2015). Role of probiotics and functional foods in health: gut immune stimulation by two probiotic strains and a potential probiotic yoghurt. *Endocrine, Metabolic & Immune Disorders-Drug Targets (Formerly Current Drug Targets-Immune, Endocrine & Metabolic Disorders), 15*(1), 37-45.

Ma, N., & Ma, X. (2019). Dietary amino acids and the gut-microbiome-immune axis: Physiological metabolism and therapeutic prospects. *Comprehensive Reviews in Food Science and Food Safety*, *18*(1), 221–242. DOI: 10.1111/1541-4337.12401 PMID: 33337014

Manjunath, M., Ogwu, M. C., Udayakumar, S., Kuchipudi, J. D., Rengarajan, C., Selvakumar, P., & Manjunath, T. C. (2026). Chromatography in Food Contaminant Analysis: Principles, Advances, and Applications for Food Safety. In Ogwu, M., & Izah, S. (Eds.), *Detection, Identification, and Monitoring of Food Contaminants* (pp. 207–238). IGI Global Scientific Publishing., DOI: 10.4018/979-8-3373-3982-5.ch007

Manshouri, S., Seif, F., Kamali, M., Bahar, M. A., Mashayekh, A., & Molatefi, R. (2024). The interaction of inflammasomes and gut microbiota: Novel therapeutic insights. *Cell Communication and Signaling : CCS*, *22*(1), 209. DOI: 10.1186/s12964-024-01504-1 PMID: 38566180

Marcobal, A., Kashyap, P. C., Nelson, T. A., Aronov, P. A., Donia, M. S., Spormann, A., Fischbach, M. A., & Sonnenburg, J. L. (2013). A metabolomic view of how the human gut microbiota impacts the host metabolome using humanized and gnotobiotic mice. *The ISME Journal*, *7*(10), 1933–1943. DOI: 10.1038/ismej.2013.89 PMID: 23739052

Marcum, J. A. (2020). Nutrigenetics/nutrigenomics, personalized nutrition, and precision healthcare. *Current Nutrition Reports*, *9*(4), 338–345. DOI: 10.1007/s13668-020-00327-z

Marim, A. V. C., & Gabardo, S. (2021). Xylooligosaccharides: Prebiotic potential from agro-industrial residue, production strategies and prospects. *Biocatalysis and Agricultural Biotechnology*, *37*, 102190. DOI: 10.1016/j.bcab.2021.102190

Markowiak, P., & Śliżewska, K. (2017). Effects of probiotics, prebiotics, and synbiotics on human health. *Nutrients*, *9*(9), 1021. DOI: 10.3390/nu9091021 PMID: 28914794

Markowiak, P., & Śliżewska, K. (2018). The role of probiotics, prebiotics and synbiotics in animal nutrition. *Gut Pathogens*, *10*(1), 21. DOI: 10.1186/s13099-018-0250-0 PMID: 29930711

Maron, D. J., Fazio, S., & Linton, M. F. (2000). Current perspectives on statins. *Circulation*, *101*(2), 207–213. DOI: 10.1161/01.CIR.101.2.207 PMID: 10637210

Martinez, F. D. (2014). The human microbiome. Early life determinant of health outcomes. *Annals of the American Thoracic Society*, *11*(Supplement 1), S7–S12. DOI: 10.1513/AnnalsATS.201306-186MG PMID: 24437411

Martinez, K. B., Mackert, J. D., & McIntosh, M. K. (2017). Polyphenols and intestinal health. In Watson, R. R. (Ed.), *Nutrition and Functional Foods for Healthy Aging* (pp. 191–210). Elsevier., DOI: 10.1016/B978-0-12-805376-8.00018-6

Maurel, S. (2024). *Rôle de l'implantation du microbiote intestinal sur la susceptibilité au syndrome de l'intestin irritable à l'âge adulte* (Doctoral dissertation). Université Paris-Saclay.

MDPI. (2024). Recent advances in wearable healthcare devices: From material to application. *Biosensors (Basel)*, *11*(4), 358. DOI: 10.3390/bios11040358 PMID: 38671780

Meena, K., Visarada, K., & Meena, D. K. (2022). *Sorghum bicolor* (L.) Moench a multifarious crop—Fodder to therapeutic potential and biotechnological applications: A future food for the millennium. *Future Foods : a Dedicated Journal for Sustainability in Food Science, 6*, 100188. Advance online publication. DOI: 10.1016/j.fufo.2022.100188

Mehtab, W., Agarwal, A., Singh, N., Malhotra, A., & Makharia, G. (2019). All that a physician should know about FODMAPs. *Indian Journal of Gastroenterology, 38*(5), 378–390. DOI: 10.1007/s12664-019-01002-0 PMID: 31802437

Meijer, K., de Vos, P., & Priebe, M. G. (2010). Butyrate and other short-chain fatty acids as modulators of immunity: What relevance for health? *Current Opinion in Clinical Nutrition and Metabolic Care, 13*(6), 715–721. DOI: 10.1097/MCO.0b013e32833eebe5 PMID: 20823773

Meissner, A., Gnirke, A., Bell, G. W., Ramsahoye, B., Lander, E. S., & Jaenisch, R. (2005). Reduced representation bisulfite sequencing for comparative high-resolution DNA methylation analysis. *Nucleic Acids Research, 33*(18), 5868–5877. DOI: 10.1093/nar/gki901 PMID: 16224102

Melin, P. (2004). Proteomics as a tool to study microbial interactions. *Current Proteomics, 1*(1), 27–34. DOI: 10.2174/1570164043488261

Meng, N., Zhou, Y., Zhang, Q., Yu, X., Li, H., Liu, Y., Liu, M., & Li, Q. (2023). Using inflammatory biological age to evaluate the preventing aging effect of a polyphenol-probiotic-enhanced dietary pattern in adults aged 50 years and older. *Journal of Agricultural and Food Chemistry, 71*(16), 6314–6325. DOI: 10.1021/acs.jafc.2c07241 PMID: 37057839

Meral, G., Aslan, E. S., Tunaligil, V., Burkay, N., Alper Acar, E. G., & Alp, M. Y. (2024). The importance of nutrigenetics and microbiota in personalized medicine: From phenotype to genotype. *Cureus, 16*(5), 61256. DOI: 10.7759/cureus.61256

Metchnikoff, É. (1907). *The prolongation of life: Optimistic studies*. Heinemann. https://archive.org/details/prolongationofli00metc

Metchnikoff, I. I. (2004). *The prolongation of life: Optimistic studies (Reprint of* (1907 ed.). Springer.

Metwaly, A., Kriaa, A., Hassani, Z., Carraturo, F., Druart, C., Arnauts, K., & de Vos, W. M. (2025). A consensus statement on establishing causality, therapeutic applications and the use of preclinical models in microbiome research. *Nature Reviews. Gastroenterology & Hepatology, 22*(5), 343–357. DOI: 10.1038/s41575-025-01041-3 PMID: 40033063

Microbiota in health and diseases | Signal Transduction and Targeted Therapy. (n.d.-a). Retrieved October 18, 2025, from https://www.nature.com/articles/s41392-022-00974-4

Microbiota in health and diseases | Signal Transduction and Targeted Therapy. (n.d.-b). Retrieved October 18, 2025, from https://www.nature.com/articles/s41392-022-00974-4

Micromachines. (2022). Flexible wearable sensors for sports: kinematics to physiologies. DOI: 10.3390/mi13010058

MicroRNAs as regulators of metabolic disease: Pathophysiologic significance and emerging role as biomarkers and therapeutics | International Journal of Obesity. (n.d.). Retrieved October 18, 2025, from https://www.nature.com/articles/ijo2015170

Mikkelsen, K., & Apostolopoulos, V. (2019). B vitamins and ageing. *Biochemistry and cell biology of ageing: Part I biomedical science*, 451-470.

Miller, M. B., & Bassler, B. L. (2001). Quorum sensing in bacteria. *Annual Review of Microbiology, 55*(1), 165–199. DOI: 10.1146/annurev.micro.55.1.165 PMID: 11544353

Missiego-Beltrán, J., & Beltrán-Velasco, A. I. (2024). The Role of Microbial Metabolites in the Progression of Neurodegenerative Diseases—Therapeutic Approaches: A Comprehensive Review. *International Journal of Molecular Sciences, 25*(18), 10041. DOI: 10.3390/ijms251810041 PMID: 39337526

Modulation of the Gut Microbiota by Nutrition and Its Relationship to Epigenetics. (n.d.). Retrieved October 18, 2025, from https://www.mdpi.com/1422-0067/25/2/1228

Monteagudo-Mera, A., Rastall, R. A., Gibson, G. R., Charalampopoulos, D., & Chatzifragkou, A. (2019). Adhesion mechanisms mediated by probiotics and prebiotics and their potential impact on human health. *Applied Microbiology and Biotechnology, 103*(16), 6463–6472. DOI: 10.1007/s00253-019-09978-7 PMID: 31267231

Moore, J. W., Millard, S., Babidge, W., Rowland, R., & Roediger, W. E. (1997). Hydrogen sulphide produces diminished fatty acid oxidation in the rat colon in vivo: Implications for ulcerative colitis. *ANZ Journal of Surgery, 67*(4), 245–249. DOI: 10.1111/j.1445-2197.1997.tb01961.x PMID: 9152152

Moradi, M., Molaei, R., & Guimarães, J. T. (2021). A review on preparation and chemical analysis of postbiotics from lactic acid bacteria. *Enzyme and Microbial Technology, 143*, 109722. DOI: 10.1016/j.enzmictec.2020.109722

Morais, L. H., Schreiber, H. L.IV, & Mazmanian, S. K. (2021). The gut microbiota–brain axis in behaviour and brain disorders. *Nature Reviews. Microbiology*, *19*(4), 241–255. DOI: 10.1038/s41579-020-00460-0 PMID: 33093662

Moretto, M. M., Harrow, D. I., Hawley, T. S., & Khan, I. A. (2015). Interleukin-12-producing CD103+CD11b−CD8+ dendritic cells are responsible for eliciting gut intraepithelial lymphocyte response against *Encephalitozoon cuniculi*. *Infection and Immunity*, *83*(12), 4719–4730. DOI: 10.1128/IAI.00820-15

Mostafavi Abdolmaleky, H., & Zhou, J. R. (2024). Gut microbiota dysbiosis, oxidative stress, inflammation, and epigenetic alterations in metabolic diseases. *Antioxidants*, *13*(8), 985. DOI: 10.3390/antiox13080985 PMID: 39199231

Mowat, A. M. (2018). To respond or not to respond: A personal perspective of intestinal tolerance. *Nature Reviews. Immunology*, *18*(6), 405–415. DOI: 10.1038/s41577-018-0002-x PMID: 29491358

Mudannayake, D. C., Jayasena, D. D., Wimalasiri, K. M., Ranadheera, C. S., & Ajlouni, S. (2022). Inulin fructans–food applications and alternative plant sources: A review. *International Journal of Food Science & Technology*, *57*(9), 5764–5780. DOI: 10.1111/ijfs.15947

Muhammad, A. Y., Amonov, M., Baig, A. A., & Alvi, F. J. (2024). Gut Microbiome: An Intersection between Human Genome, Diet, and Epigenetics. *Advanced Gut & Microbiome Research*, *2024*(1), 6707728. DOI: 10.1155/2024/6707728

Mukherjee, A., Breselge, S., Dimidi, E., Marco, M. L., & Cotter, P. D. (2024). Fermented foods and gastrointestinal health: Underlying mechanisms. *Nature Reviews. Gastroenterology & Hepatology*, *21*(4), 248–266. DOI: 10.1038/s41575-023-00869-x PMID: 38081933

Mullins, V. A., Bresette, W., Johnstone, L., Hallmark, B., & Chilton, F. H. (2020). Genomics in Personalized Nutrition: Can You "Eat for Your Genes"? *Nutrients*, *12*(10), 3118. DOI: 10.3390/nu12103118

Murph, A., Marston, C., Bramley, D., Trevelyan, C., & Allington, G. (2024). Dynamic token contextualization for adaptive knowledge synthesis in large language models. *OSF Preprints*. DOI: 10.31219/osf.io/8dsa7

Muthukumar, J., Selvasekaran, P., Lokanadham, M., and Chidambaram, R. (2020). Food and food products associated with food allergy and food intolerance—An overview. *Food Research International, 138*(Part B), 109780. DOI: 10.1016/j.foodres.2020.109780

Myhrstad, M. C., Tunsjø, H., Charnock, C., & Telle-Hansen, V. H. (2020). Dietary fiber, gut microbiota, and metabolic regulation—Current status in human randomized trials. *Nutrients*, *12*(3), 859. DOI: 10.3390/nu12030859 PMID: 32210176

Nadeem, M. A., Nawaz, M. A., Shahid, M. Q., Doğan, Y., Cömertpay, G., Yıldız, M., & Baloch, F. S. (2017). DNA molecular markers in plant breeding: Current status and recent advancements in genomic selection and genome editing. *Biotechnology, Biotechnological Equipment*, *32*(2), 261–285. DOI: 10.1080/13102818.2017.1400401

Nagao-Kitamoto, H., & Kamada, N. (2017). Host-microbial cross-talk in inflammatory bowel disease. *Immune Network*, *17*(1), 1–12. DOI: 10.4110/in.2017.17.1.1 PMID: 28261015

Nakato, R., & Sakata, T. (2021). Methods for ChIP-seq analysis: A practical workflow and advanced applications. *Methods (San Diego, Calif.)*, *187*, 44–53. DOI: 10.1016/j.ymeth.2020.03.005 PMID: 32240773

Nakkarach, A., Foo, H. L., Song, A. A.-L., Mutalib, N. E. A., Nitisinprasert, S., & Withayagiat, U. (2021). Anti-cancer and anti-inflammatory effects elicited by short chain fatty acids produced by Escherichia coli isolated from healthy human gut microbiota. *Microbial Cell Factories*, *20*(1), 36. DOI: 10.1186/s12934-020-01477-z PMID: 33546705

Nascimento, C. E. O., Simões, L. C. O., Pereira, J. C., da Silva, R. R., de Lima, E. A., de Almeida, G. C., Penna, A. L. B., Boscolo, M., Gomes, E., & da Silva, R. (2022). Application of a recombinant GH10 endoxylanase from Thermoascus aurantiacus for xylooligosaccharide production from sugarcane bagasse and probiotic bacterial growth. *Journal of Biotechnology*, *347*, 1–8. DOI: 10.1016/j.jbiotec.2022.02.003

Nat. Electron. (2021). Wearable devices for COVID-19 detection. DOI: 10.1038/s41928-020-00505-5

Nature Biomedical Engineering. (2022). Integrated wearable microneedle array for biomarker monitoring. DOI: 10.1038/s41551-022-00916-z

Nature Electronics. (2021). Smart lens COVID-19 detection. DOI: 10.1038/s41928-020-00504-6

Nature Reviews Materials. (2022). End-to-end design of wearable sensors. DOI: 10.1038/s41578-022-00460-x

Nazir, A., Hussain, F. H. N., & Raza, A. (2024). Advancing microbiota therapeutics: The role of synthetic biology in engineering microbial communities for precision medicine. *Frontiers in Bioengineering and Biotechnology*, *12*, 1511149. Advance online publication. DOI: 10.3389/fbioe.2024.1511149 PMID: 39698189

Neurath, M. F., Artis, D., & Becker, C. (2025). The intestinal barrier: A pivotal role in health, inflammation, and cancer. *The Lancet. Gastroenterology & Hepatology*, *10*(6), 573–592. Advance online publication. DOI: 10.1016/S2468-1253(24)00390-X PMID: 40086468

Newgard, C. B., An, J., Bain, J. R., Muehlbauer, M. J., Stevens, R. D., Lien, L. F., Haqq, A. M., Shah, S. H., Arlotto, M., Slentz, C. A., Rochon, J., Gallup, D., Ilkayeva, O., Wenner, B. R., Yancy, W. S.Jr, Eisenson, H., Musante, G., Surwit, R. S., Millington, D. S., & Svetkey, L. P. (2009). A branched-chain amino acid-related metabolic signature that differentiates obese and lean humans and contributes to insulin resistance. *Cell Metabolism*, *9*(4), 311–326. DOI: 10.1016/j.cmet.2009.02.002 PMID: 19356713

Ngandu, T., Lehtisalo, J., Solomon, A., Levälahti, E., Ahtiluoto, S., Antikainen, R., Bäckman, L., Hänninen, T., Jula, A., Laatikainen, T., Lindström, J., Mangialasche, F., Paajanen, T., Pajala, S., Peltonen, M., Rauramaa, R., Stigsdotter-Neely, A., Strandberg, T., Tuomilehto, J., & Kivipelto, M. (2015). A 2-year multidomain intervention of diet, exercise, cognitive training, and vascular risk monitoring versus control to prevent cognitive decline in at-risk elderly people (FINGER): A randomised controlled trial. *Lancet*, *385*(9984), 2255–2263. DOI: 10.1016/S0140-6736(15)60461-5 PMID: 25771249

Ng, S. C., Kamm, M. A., Yeoh, Y. K., Chan, P. K., Zuo, T., Tang, W., Sood, A., Andoh, A., Ohmiya, N., Zhou, Y., Ooi, C. J., Mahachai, V., Wu, C.-Y., Zhang, F., Sugano, K., & Chan, F. K. L. (2020). Scientific frontiers in faecal microbiota transplantation: Joint document of Asia-Pacific Association of Gastroenterology (APAGE) and Asia-Pacific Society for Digestive Endoscopy (APSDE). *Gut*, *69*(1), 83–91. DOI: 10.1136/gutjnl-2019-319407 PMID: 31611298

Niamah, A. K., Abdulmuttaleb, A. M., & Hussain, N. A. (2020). Antibacterial spectrum of produced reuterin from new isolates of Lactobacillus reuteri. *Journal of Microbiology, Biotechnology and Food Sciences*, *10*(1), 134–139. DOI: 10.15414/jmbfs.2020.10.1.134-139

Nicholson, J. K., Holmes, E., Kinross, J., Burcelin, R., Gibson, G., Jia, W., & Pettersson, S. (2012). Host-gut microbiota metabolic interactions. *Science*, *336*(6086), 1262–1267. DOI: 10.1126/science.1223813 PMID: 22674330

Nistal, E., Caminero, A., Herran, A. R., Arias, L., Vivas, S., de Morales, J. M. R., Calleja, S., de Miera, L. E. S., Arroyo, P., & Casqueiro, J. (2016). Study of duodenal bacterial communities by 16s rRNA gene analysis in adults with active celiac disease versus non celiac disease controls. *Journal of Applied Microbiology*, *120*(6), 1691–1700. DOI: 10.1111/jam.13111

Nogacka, A. M., Salazar, N., Arboleya, S., Suárez, M., Fernández, N., Solís, G., de los Reyes-Gavilán, C. G., & Gueimonde, M. (2018). Early microbiota, antibiotics and health. *Cellular and Molecular Life Sciences : CMLS*, *75*(1), 83–91. DOI: 10.1007/s00018-017-2670-2 PMID: 28988290

Noronha, A., Modamio, J., Jarosz, Y., Guerard, E., Sompairac, N., Preciat, G., Daníelsdóttir, A. D., Krecke, M., Merten, D., Haraldsdóttir, H. S., Heinken, A., Heirendt, L., Magnúsdóttir, S., Ravcheev, D. A., Sahoo, S., Gawron, P., Friscioni, L., Garcia, B., Prendergast, M., & Thiele, I. (2019). The Virtual Metabolic Human database: Integrating human and gut microbiome metabolism with nutrition and disease. *Nucleic Acids Research*, *47*(D1), D614–D624. DOI: 10.1093/nar/gky992 PMID: 30371894

NPJ Digital Medicine. (2020). Wireless monitoring of CSF shunts. DOI: 10.1038/s41746-020-00408-x

O'Connor, P. M., Kuniyoshi, T. M., Oliveira, R. P. S., Hill, C., Ross, R. P., & Cotter, P. D. (2020). Antimicrobials for food and feed; a bacteriocin perspective. *Current Opinion in Biotechnology*, *61*, 160–167. DOI: 10.1016/j.copbio.2019.12.023 PMID: 31968296

O'Toole, P. W., & Jeffery, I. B. (2015). Gut microbiota and aging. *Science*, *350*(6265), 1214–1215. DOI: 10.1126/science.aac8469 PMID: 26785481

O'Toole, P. W., Marchesi, J. R., & Hill, C. (2017). Next-generation probiotics: The spectrum from probiotics to live biotherapeutics. *Nature Microbiology*, *2*(5), 1–6. DOI: 10.1038/nmicrobiol.2017.57

Obayya, M., Arasi, M. A., Alruwais, N., Alsini, R., Mohamed, A., & Yaseen, I. (2023). Biomedical image analysis for colon and lung cancer detection using tuna swarm algorithm with deep learning model. *IEEE Access : Practical Innovations, Open Solutions*, *11*, 94705–94720. DOI: 10.1109/ACCESS.2023.3309711

Ocvirk, S., Wilson, A. S., Appolonia, C. N., Thomas, T. K., & O'Keefe, S. J. D. (2019). Fiber, fat, and colorectal cancer: New insight into modifiable dietary risk factors. *Current Gastroenterology Reports*, *21*(11), 62. DOI: 10.1007/s11894-019-0725-2 PMID: 31792624

Odamaki, T., Bottacini, F., Kato, K., Mitsuyama, E., Yoshida, K., Horigome, A., Xiao, J., & van Sinderen, D. (2018). Genomic diversity and distribution of *Bifidobacterium longum* subsp. *longum* across the human lifespan. *Scientific Reports*, *8*(1), 85. DOI: 10.1038/s41598-017-18391-x PMID: 29311585

Odamaki, T., Kato, K., Sugahara, H., Hashikura, N., Takahashi, S., Xiao, J., Abe, F., & Osawa, R. (2016). Age-related changes in gut microbiota composition from newborn to centenarian: A cross-sectional study. *BMC Microbiology*, *16*(1), 90. DOI: 10.1186/s12866-016-0708-5 PMID: 27220822

Oh, S., Lee, J., Chun, S., Choi, J. E., Kim, M. N., Chon, Y. E., Ha, Y., Hwang, S. G., Choi, S. W., & Hong, K. W. (2023). Interaction between the PNPLA3 Gene and Nutritional Factors on NAFLD Development: The Korean Genome and Epidemiology Study. *Nutrients*, *15*(1), 152. DOI: 10.3390/nu15010152

Okumura, R., & Takeda, K. (2018). Maintenance of intestinal homeostasis by mucosal barriers. *Inflammation and Regeneration*, *38*(1), 5. DOI: 10.1186/s41232-018-0063-z PMID: 29619131

Oliphant, K., & Allen-Vercoe, E. (2019). Macronutrient metabolism by the human gut microbiome: Major fermentation by-products and their impact on host health. *Microbiome*, *7*(1), 91. DOI: 10.1186/s40168-019-0704-8 PMID: 31196177

Oliver, A., Chase, A. B., Weihe, C., Orchanian, S. B., Riedel, S. F., Hendrickson, C. L., Lay, M., Sewall, J. M., Martiny, J. B. H., & Whiteson, K. (2021). High-fiber, whole-food dietary intervention alters the human gut microbiome but not fecal short-chain fatty acids. *mSystems*, *6*(2), 00115–00121. DOI: 10.1128/msystems.00115-21 PMID: 33727392

Olofsson, L. E., & Bäckhed, F. (2022). The metabolic role and therapeutic potential of the microbiome. *Endocrine Reviews*, *43*(5), 907–926. DOI: 10.1210/endrev/bnac004 PMID: 35094076

Otto-Dobos, L. D., Strehle, L. D., Loman, B. R., Seng, M. M., Sardesai, S. D., Williams, N. O., Gatti-Mays, M. E., Stover, D. G., Sudheendra, P. K., Wesolowski, R., Andridge, R. R., Bailey, M. T., & Pyter, L. M. (2024). Baseline gut microbiome alpha diversity predicts chemotherapy-induced gastrointestinal symptoms in patients with breast cancer. *NPJ Breast Cancer*, *10*(1), 99. DOI: 10.1038/s41523-024-00707-6 PMID: 39548124

Owaga, E., Hsieh, R. H., Mugendi, B., Masuku, S., Shih, C. K., & Chang, J. S. (2015). Th17 cells as potential probiotic therapeutic targets in inflammatory bowel diseases. *International Journal of Molecular Sciences*, *16*(9), 20841–20858. DOI: 10.3390/ijms160920841 PMID: 26340622

Owens, J. A., Saeedi, B. J., Naudin, C. R., Hunter-Chang, S., Barbian, M. E., Eboka, R. U., Askew, L., Darby, T. M., Robinson, B. S., & Jones, R. M. (2021). Lactobacillus rhamnosus GG orchestrates an antitumor immune response. *Cellular and Molecular Gastroenterology and Hepatology*, *12*(4), 1311–1327. DOI: 10.1016/j.jcmgh.2021.06.001 PMID: 34111601

Owusu-Apenten, R. K., & Vieira, E. R. (2023). *Elementary food science (No. 303022)*. Springer., DOI: 10.1007/978-3-030-65433-7

Palm, N. W., de Zoete, M. R., Cullen, T. W., Barry, N. A., Stefanowski, J., Hao, L., Degnan, P. H., Hu, J., Peter, I., Zhang, W., Ruggiero, E., Cho, J. H., Goodman, A. L., & Flavell, R. A. (2014). Immunoglobulin A coating identifies colitogenic bacteria in inflammatory bowel disease. *Cell*, *158*(5), 1000–1010. DOI: 10.1016/j.cell.2014.08.006 PMID: 25171403

Paone, P., & Cani, P. D. (2020). Mucus barrier, mucins and gut microbiota: The expected slimy partners? *Gut*, *69*(12), 2232–2243. DOI: 10.1136/gutjnl-2020-322260

Parada Venegas, D., De la Fuente, M. K., Landskron, G., González, M. J., Quera, R., Dijkstra, G., Harmsen, H. J. M., Faber, K. N., & Hermoso, M. A. (2019). Short chain fatty acids (SCFAs)-mediated gut epithelial and immune regulation and its relevance for inflammatory bowel diseases. *Frontiers in Immunology*, *10*, 277. DOI: 10.3389/fimmu.2019.00277 PMID: 30915065

Parker, A., Romano, S., Ansorge, R., Aboelnour, A., Le Gall, G., Savva, G. M., Pontifex, M. G., Telatin, A., Baker, D., Jones, E., Vauzour, D., Rudder, S., Blackshaw, L. A., Jeffery, G., & Carding, S. R. (2022). Fecal microbiota transfer between young and aged mice reverses hallmarks of the aging gut, eye, and brain. *Microbiome*, *10*(1), 1–25. DOI: 10.1186/s40168-022-01243-w PMID: 35501923

Pasini, E., Corsetti, G., Assanelli, D., Testa, C., Romano, C., Dioguardi, F. S., & Aquilani, R. (2019). Effects of chronic exercise on gut microbiota and intestinal barrier in human with type 2 diabetes. *Minerva Medica*, *110*(1), 3–11. DOI: 10.23736/S0026-4806.18.05589-1 PMID: 30667205

Patil, S., & Mehdi, S. F. S. (2025). The Gut-Brain Axis and Mental Health: How Diet Shapes Our Cognitive and Emotional Well-Being. *Cureus*, *17*(7). Advance online publication. DOI: 10.7759/cureus.88420 PMID: 40842787

Patra, D. (2024). Synthetic biology-enabled engineering of probiotics for precision and targeted therapeutic delivery applications. *Exon*, *1*(2), 54–66. DOI: 10.69936/en11y0024

Patti, G. J., Yanes, O., & Siuzdak, G. (2012). Innovation: Metabolomics: the apogee of the omics trilogy. *Nature Reviews. Molecular Cell Biology*, *13*(4), 263–269. DOI: 10.1038/nrm3314 PMID: 22436749

Pattnaik, S., Imchen, M., Kumavath, R., Prasad, R., & Busi, S. (2022). Bioactive microbial metabolites in cancer therapeutics: Mining, repurposing, and their molecular targets. *Current Microbiology*, *79*(10), 300. DOI: 10.1007/s00284-022-02990-7 PMID: 36002695

Pawar, P., Anute, N., Tripathi, S., Ahluwalia, G. K., Kalshetti, P., & Selvakumar, P. (2026). AI and Its Importance in the Development of Luxury Consumption. In Vale, V. (Ed.), *Multidisciplinary Approach to Luxury Consumption and AI* (pp. 1–34). IGI Global Scientific Publishing., DOI: 10.4018/979-8-3693-8422-0.ch001

Pedersen, H. K., Gudmundsdottir, V., Nielsen, H. B., Hyotylainen, T., Nielsen, T., Jensen, B. A., Forslund, K., Hildebrand, F., Prifti, E., Falony, G., Le Chatelier, E., Levenez, F., Doré, J., Mattila, I., Plichta, D. R., Pöhö, P., Hellgren, L. I., Arumugam, M., Sunagawa, S., & Pedersen, O. (2016). Human gut microbes impact host serum metabolome and insulin sensitivity. *Nature*, *535*(7612), 376–381. DOI: 10.1038/nature18646 PMID: 27409811

Pedroza Matute, S., & Iyavoo, S. (2023). Exploring the gut microbiota: Lifestyle choices, disease associations, and personal genomics. *Frontiers in Nutrition*, *10*, 1225120. DOI: 10.3389/fnut.2023.1225120

Penders, J., Thijs, C., Vink, C., Stelma, F. F., Snijders, B., Kummeling, I., & Stobberingh, E. E. (2006). Factors influencing the composition of the intestinal microbiota in early infancy. *Pediatrics*, *118*(2), 511–521. DOI: 10.1542/peds.2005-2824 PMID: 16882802

Peng, X., Hao, M., Zhao, Y., Cai, Y., Chen, X., Chen, H., Zhang, Y., Dong, L., Liu, X., Ding, C., Liu, W., Yang, M., & Luo, Y. (2021). Red ginseng has stronger anti-aging effects compared to ginseng possibly due to its regulation of oxidative stress and the gut microbiota. *Phytomedicine*, *93*, 153772. DOI: 10.1016/j.phymed.2021.153772 PMID: 34753028

Pereira-Marques, J., Ferreira, R. M., & Figueiredo, C. (2024). A metatranscriptomics strategy for efficient characterization of the microbiome in human tissues with low microbial biomass. *Gut Microbes*, *16*(1), 2323235. DOI: 10.1080/19490976.2024.2323235

Perrier, C., & Corthésy, B. (2011). Gut permeability and food allergies. *Clinical and Experimental Allergy*, *41*(1), 20–28. DOI: 10.1111/j.1365-2222.2010.03639.x

Perry, R. J., Peng, L., Barry, N. A., Cline, G. W., Zhang, D., Cardone, R. L., Petersen, K. F., Kibbey, R. G., Goodman, A. L., & Shulman, G. I. (2016). Acetate mediates a microbiome-brain-β-cell axis to promote metabolic syndrome. *Nature*, *534*(7606), 213–217. DOI: 10.1038/nature18309 PMID: 27279214

Peters, D. L., Wang, W., Zhang, X., Ning, Z., Mayne, J., & Figeys, D. (2019). Metaproteomic and metabolomic approaches for characterizing the gut microbiome. *Proteomics*, *19*(16), 1800363. DOI: 10.1002/pmic.201800363

Philippot, L., Griffiths, B. S., & Langenheder, S. (2021). Microbial community resilience across ecosystems and multiple disturbances. *Microbiology and Molecular Biology Reviews : MMBR*, *85*(2), 00026–00020. DOI: 10.1128/MMBR.00026-20 PMID: 33789927

Picó, C., Serra, F., Rodríguez, A. M., Keijer, J., & Palou, A. (2019). Biomarkers of Nutrition and Health: New Tools for New Approaches. *Nutrients*, *11*(5), 1092. DOI: 10.3390/nu11051092 PMID: 31100942

Pimentel, M., Kong, Y., & Park, S. (2004). IBS subjects with methane on lactulose breath test have lower postprandial serotonin levels than subjects with hydrogen. *Digestive Diseases and Sciences*, *49*(1), 84–47. DOI: 10.1023/B:DDAS.0000011607.24171.c0 PMID: 14992440

Pires, L., Gonzalez-Paramás, A. M., Heleno, S. A., & Calhelha, R. C. (2024). Gut microbiota as an endocrine organ: Unveiling its role in human physiology and health. *Applied Sciences (Basel, Switzerland)*, *14*(20), 9383. DOI: 10.3390/app14209383

Plasmonic Sensor for Hydrogen Sulfide in Saliva: Multisensor Platform and Bag Format. *Talanta*, 245, 123449. DOI: 10.1016/j.talanta.2022.123449

Plaza-Diaz, J., Ruiz-Ojeda, F. J., Gil-Campos, M., & Gil, A. (2019). Mechanisms of action of probiotics. *Advances in Nutrition*, *10*(S1), S49–S66. DOI: 10.1093/advances/nmy063 PMID: 30721959

Plummer, E. L., Lozinsky, A. C., Axelrad, C., Garland, S. M., Jacobs, S. E., & Tang, M. L. K. (2020). Postnatal probiotics and allergic disease in very preterm infants: Sub-study to the ProPrems randomized trial. *Allergy*, *75*(1), 83–88. DOI: 10.1111/all.14088

Pluznick, J. L., Protzko, R. J., Gevorgyan, H., Peterlin, Z., Sipos, A., Han, J., Brunet, I., Wan, L. X., Rey, F., Wang, T., Firestein, S. J., Yanagisawa, M., Gordon, J. I., Eichmann, A., Peti-Peterdi, J., & Caplan, M. J. (2013). Olfactory receptor responding to gut microbiota-derived signals plays a role in renin secretion and blood pressure regulation. *Proceedings of the National Academy of Sciences of the United States of America, 110*(11), 4410–4415. DOI: 10.1073/pnas.1215927110 PMID: 23401498

Pollock, J., Glendinning, L., Wisedchanwet, T., & Watson, M. (2018). The madness of microbiome: Attempting to find consensus "best practice" for 16S microbiome studies. *Applied and Environmental Microbiology, 84*(7), e02627–e17. DOI: 10.1128/AEM.02627-17 PMID: 29427429

Pols, T. W., Noriega, L. G., Nomura, M., Auwerx, J., & Schoonjans, K. (2011). The bile acid membrane receptor TGR5 as an emerging target in metabolism and inflammation. *Journal of Hepatology, 54*(6), 1263–1272. DOI: 10.1016/j.jhep.2010.12.004 PMID: 21145931

Pompei, A.. (2007). Genome sequence and characterization of Bifidobacterium breve strain UCC2003. *Journal of Bacteriology, 189*(19), 6878–6884. DOI: 10.1128/JB.00719-07

Porcari, S., Mullish, B. H., Asnicar, F., Ng, S. C., Zhao, L., Hansen, R., & Segal, E. (2024). International consensus statement on microbiome testing in clinical practice. *The Lancet. Gastroenterology & Hepatology, 10*(2), 154–163. DOI: 10.1016/S2468-1253(24)00311-X PMID: 39647502

Portik, D. M., Brown, C. T., & Pierce-Ward, N. T. (2022). Evaluation of taxonomic classification and profiling methods for long-read shotgun metagenomic sequencing datasets. *BMC Bioinformatics, 23*(1), 541. DOI: 10.1186/s12859-022-05103-0

Pradhan, S., Karve, S. S., Weiss, A. A., Hawkins, J., Poling, H. M., Helmrath, M. A., Wells, J. M., & McCauley, H. A. (2020). Tissue responses to Shiga toxin in human intestinal organoids. *Cellular and Molecular Gastroenterology and Hepatology, 10*(1), 171–190. DOI: 10.1016/j.jcmgh.2020.02.006

Preshaw, P. M. (2018). Host modulation therapy with anti-inflammatory agents. *Periodontology 2000, 76*(1), 131–149. DOI: 10.1111/prd.12148 PMID: 29193331

Qin, J., Li, R., Raes, J., Arumugam, M., Burgdorf, K. S., Manichanh, C., Nielsen, T., Pons, N., Levenez, F., Yamada, T., Mende, D. R., Li, J., Xu, J., Li, S., Li, D., Cao, J., Wang, B., Liang, H., Zheng, H., & Wang, J. (2010). A human gut microbial gene catalogue established by metagenomic sequencing. *Nature, 464*(7285), 59–65. DOI: 10.1038/nature08821 PMID: 20203603

Qin, J., Li, Y., Cai, Z., Li, S., Zhu, J., Zhang, F., Liang, S., Zhang, W., Guan, Y., Shen, D., Peng, Y., Zhang, D., Jie, Z., Wu, W., Qin, Y., Xue, W., Li, J., Han, L., Lu, D., & Wang, J. (2012). A metagenome-wide association study of gut microbiota in type 2 diabetes. *Nature*, *490*(7418), 55–60. DOI: 10.1038/nature11450 PMID: 23023125

Qin, Y. Q., Wang, L. Y., Yang, X. Y., Xu, Y. J., Fan, G., Fan, Y. G., Ren, J. N., An, Q., & Li, X. (2023). Inulin: Properties and health benefits. *Food & Function*, *14*(7), 2948–2968. DOI: 10.1039/D2FO01096H

Qiu, X., Zou, Z., Lin, T., Guo, C., & Lin, D. (2025). Engineered Lactobacillus rhamnosus Producing 3-Hydroxybutyrate: A Dual-Action Therapeutic Strategy for Colon Cancer Cachexia. *Biotechnology and Bioengineering*, *122*(6), 1574–1589. DOI: 10.1002/bit.28972 PMID: 40055977

Qi, X., Zhang, Y., Zhang, Y., Luo, F., Song, K., Wang, G., & Ling, F. (2023). Vitamin B12 produced by Cetobacterium somerae improves host resistance against pathogen infection through strengthening the interactions within gut microbiota. *Microbiome*, *11*(1), 135. DOI: 10.1186/s40168-023-01574-2 PMID: 37322528

Quagebeur, R., Dalile, B., Raes, J., Van Oudenhove, L., Verbeke, K., & Vrieze, E. (2023). The role of short-chain fatty acids (SCFAs) in regulating stress responses, eating behavior, and nutritional state in anorexia nervosa: Protocol for a randomized controlled trial. *Journal of Eating Disorders*, *11*(1), 191. DOI: 10.1186/s40337-023-00917-6 PMID: 37884972

Qu, D., Wang, G., Yu, L., Tian, F., Chen, W., & Zhai, Q. (2021). The effects of diet and gut microbiota on the regulation of intestinal mucin glycosylation. *Carbohydrate Polymers*, *258*, 117651. DOI: 10.1016/j.carbpol.2021.117651

Quince, C., Walker, A. W., Simpson, J. T., Loman, N. J., & Segata, N. (2017). Shotgun metagenomics, from sampling to analysis. *Nature Biotechnology*, *35*(9), 833–844. DOI: 10.1038/nbt.3935 PMID: 28898207

Quinn, A. M., Bottery, M. J., Thompson, H., & Friman, V.-P. (2022). Resistance evolution can disrupt antibiotic exposure protection through competitive exclusion of the protective species. *The ISME Journal*, *16*(10), 2433–2447. DOI: 10.1038/s41396-022-01285-w PMID: 35859161

Rahman, M. S., Lee, Y., Park, D. S., & Kim, Y. S. (2022). Bifidobacterium bifidum DS0908 and Bifidobacterium longum DS0950 culture-supernatants ameliorate obesity-related characteristics in mice with high-fat diet-induced obesity. *Journal of Microbiology and Biotechnology*, *33*(1), 96–105. DOI: 10.4014/jmb.2210.10046

Rahman, S.. (2023). Gut microbial metabolites and its impact on human health. *Annals of Gastroenterology*, *36*(4), 360. DOI: 10.20524/aog.2023.0809 PMID: 37396009

Rajpoot, A., & Tiwari, S. (2025). Predictive modeling of structural performance using machine learning: A comprehensive review. *Deleted Journal*, *3*(1), 25–40. DOI: 10.47392/IRJAEH.2025.0005

Raj, R., Bhope, A., Kodmalwar, P. A., Sudindra, V. R., Sharma, A., Selvakumar, P., & Manjunath, T. C. (2026). Exchange Rates and Trade Dynamics. In Canguende-Valentim, C., Madaleno, M., Victorino, S., & Jungo, J. (Eds.), *Monetary Dynamics and Socio-Economic Development in Emerging Economies* (pp. 195–220). IGI Global Scientific Publishing., DOI: 10.4018/979-8-3693-9765-7.ch007

Raj, R., Lavanya, K., Chavan, S., Gokila, S., Hubballi, R. B., Selvakumar, P., & Manjunath, T. (2026). Econometric Models to Explain the Economic Growth of a Country or Region. In Reyes Ruiz, G. (Ed.), *Impacts of Military Spending on Economic Growth* (pp. 43–72). IGI Global Scientific Publishing., DOI: 10.4018/979-8-3373-3456-1.ch002

Rakyan, V. K., Down, T. A., Balding, D. J., & Beck, S. (2011). Epigenome-wide association studies for common human diseases. *Nature Reviews. Genetics*, *12*(8), 529–541. DOI: 10.1038/nrg3000 PMID: 21747404

Ramezani, A., & Raj, D. S. (2014). The gut microbiome, kidney disease, and targeted interventions. *Journal of the American Society of Nephrology*, *25*(4), 657–670. DOI: 10.1681/ASN.2013080905

Ramírez-Pérez, O.. (2018). The role of the gut microbiota in bile acid metabolism. *Annals of Hepatology*, *16*(1), 21–26.

Ramos-Lopez, O. (2023). Epigenetic Biomarkers of Metabolic Responses to Lifestyle Interventions. *Nutrients*, *15*(19), 4251. DOI: 10.3390/nu15194251 PMID: 37836535

Ramos-Lopez, O., Martinez, J. A., & Milagro, F. I. (2022). Holistic Integration of Omics Tools for Precision Nutrition in Health and Disease. *Nutrients*, *14*(19), 4074. DOI: 10.3390/nu14194074 PMID: 36235725

Rampelli, S., Candela, M., Turroni, S., Biagi, E., Collino, S., Franceschi, C., O'Toole, P. W., & Brigidi, P. (2013). Functional metagenomic profiling of intestinal microbiome in extreme ageing. *Aging (Albany NY)*, *5*(12), 902–912. DOI: 10.18632/aging.100623 PMID: 24334635

Rampelli, S., Soverini, M., D'Amico, F., Barone, M., Tavella, T., Monti, D., Capri, M., Astolfi, A., Brigidi, P., Biagi, E., Franceschi, C., Turroni, S., & Candela, M. (2020). Shotgun metagenomics of gut microbiota in humans with up to extreme longevity and the increasing role of xenobiotic degradation. *mSystems*, *5*(2), e00124–e20. DOI: 10.1128/mSystems.00124-20 PMID: 32209716

Rao, B., & Arshad, M. Y. (2023). Early detection of lung cancer using machine learning technique. In *2022 International Conference on Computer Communication and Informatics (ICCCI)* (p. 1). IEEE. DOI: 10.1109/ICCCI56745.2023.10128389

Rastall, R. A., Gibson, G. R., Gill, H. S., Guarner, F., Klaenhammer, T. R., Pot, B., Reid, G., Rowland, I. R., & Sanders, M. E. (2005). Modulation of the microbial ecology of the human colon by probiotics, prebiotics and synbiotics to enhance human health: An overview of enabling science and potential applications. *FEMS Microbiology Ecology*, *52*(2), 145–152. DOI: 10.1016/j.femsec.2005.01.003 PMID: 16329901

Ratajczak, W., Rył, A., Mizerski, A., Walczakiewicz, K., Sipak, O., & Laszczyńska, M. (2019). Immunomodulatory potential of gut microbiome-derived short-chain fatty acids (SCFAs). *Acta Biochimica Polonica*, *66*(1), 1–12. DOI: 10.18388/abp.2018_2648 PMID: 30831575

Ratiner, K., Ciocan, D., Abdeen, S. K., & Elinav, E. (2023). Utilization of the microbiome in personalized medicine. *Nature Reviews. Microbiology*, *22*(4), 291–305. DOI: 10.1038/s41579-023-00998-9 PMID: 38110694

Rawat, D., Sharma, S., & Bhadula, S. (2023). Deep learning techniques in digital clinical diagnostic system for lung cancer. In 2022 8th International Conference on Advanced Computing and Communication Systems (ICACCS) (p. 1232). IEEE. DOI: 10.1109/ICACCS57279.2023.10113055

Reijnders, D., Goossens, G. H., Hermes, G. D., Neis, E. P., van der Beek, C. M., Most, J., Holst, J. J., Lenaerts, K., Kootte, R. S., Nieuwdorp, M., Groen, A. K., Olde Damink, S. W., Boekschoten, M. V., Smidt, H., Zoetendal, E. G., Dejong, C. H. C., & Blaak, E. E. (2016). Effects of gut microbiota manipulation by antibiotics on host metabolism in obese humans: A randomized double-blind placebo-controlled trial. *Cell Metabolism*, *24*(1), 63–74. DOI: 10.1016/j.cmet.2016.06.016 PMID: 27411009

Reinke, H., & Asher, G. (2019). Crosstalk between metabolism and circadian clocks. *Nature Reviews. Molecular Cell Biology*, *20*(4), 227–241. DOI: 10.1038/s41580-018-0096-9 PMID: 30635659

Ridlon, J. M., Harris, S. C., Bhowmik, S., Kang, D. J., & Hylemon, P. B. (2016). Consequences of bile salt biotransformations by intestinal bacteria. *Gut Microbes*, *7*(1), 22–39. DOI: 10.1080/19490976.2015.1127483 PMID: 26939849

Ridlon, J. M., Kang, D. J., & Hylemon, P. B. (2006). Bile salt biotransformations by human intestinal bacteria. *Journal of Lipid Research*, *47*(2), 241–259. DOI: 10.1194/jlr.R500013-JLR200 PMID: 16299351

Ridlon, J. M., Kang, D. J., Hylemon, P. B., & Bajaj, J. S. (2014). Bile acids and the gut microbiome. *Current Opinion in Gastroenterology*, *30*(3), 332–338. DOI: 10.1097/MOG.0000000000000057 PMID: 24625896

Rinninella, E., Cintoni, M., Raoul, P., Lopetuso, L. R., Scaldaferri, F., Pulcini, G., Miggiano, G. A. D., Gasbarrini, A., & Mele, M. C. (2019). Food components and dietary habits: Keys for a healthy gut microbiota composition. *Nutrients*, *11*(10), 2393. DOI: 10.3390/nu11102393 PMID: 31591348

Ríos-Covián, D., Ruas-Madiedo, P., Margolles, A., Gueimonde, M., de los Reyes-Gavilán, C. G., & Salazar, N. (2016). Intestinal short chain fatty acids and their link with diet and human health. *Frontiers in Microbiology*, *7*, 185. DOI: 10.3389/fmicb.2016.00185 PMID: 26925050

Risdian, C., Mozef, T., & Wink, J. (2019). Biosynthesis of polyketides in Streptomyces. *Microorganisms*, *7*(5), 124. DOI: 10.3390/microorganisms7050124 PMID: 31064143

Roberto, C. A., Ng, S. W., Ganderats-Fuentes, M., Hammond, D., Barquera, S., Jauregui, A., & Taillie, L. S. (2021). The influence of front-of-package nutrition labeling on consumer behavior and product reformulation. *Annual Review of Nutrition*, *41*(1), 529–550. DOI: 10.1146/annurev-nutr-111120-094932

Rodriguez-Arrastia, M., Martinez-Ortigosa, A., Rueda-Ruzafa, L., Folch Ayora, A., & Ropero-Padilla, C. (2021). Probiotic supplements on oncology patients' treatment-related side effects: A systematic review of randomized controlled trials. *International Journal of Environmental Research and Public Health*, *18*(8), 4265. DOI: 10.3390/ijerph18084265 PMID: 33920572

Rodriguez-Castaño, G. P., Caro-Quintero, A., Reyes, A., & Lizcano, F. (2017). Advances in Gut Microbiome Research, Opening New Strategies to Cope with a Western Lifestyle. *Frontiers in Genetics*, *7*, 224. DOI: 10.3389/fgene.2016.00224 PMID: 28119734

Rodríguez-Colman, M. J., Schewe, M., Meerlo, M., Pras-Raves, M., Sacchetti, A., & Burgering, B. M. (2017). Interplay between metabolic identities in the intestinal crypt supports stem cell function. *Nature*, *543*(7645), 424–427. DOI: 10.1038/nature21673

Ross, J. P., van Dijk, S., Phang, M., Skilton, M. R., Molloy, P. L., & Oytam, Y. (2022). Batch-effect detection, correction and characterisation in Illumina HumanMethylation450 and MethylationEPIC BeadChip array data. *Clinical Epigenetics*, *14*(1), 58. DOI: 10.1186/s13148-022-01277-9 PMID: 35488315

Rothschild, D., Weissbrod, O., Barkan, E., Kurilshikov, A., Korem, T., Zeevi, D., Costea, P. I., Godneva, A., Kalka, I. N., Bar, N., Shilo, S., Lador, D., Vila, A. V., Zmora, N., Pevsner-Fischer, M., Israeli, D., Kosower, N., Malka, G., Wolf, B. C., & Segal, E. (2018). Environment dominates over host genetics in shaping human gut microbiota. *Nature*, *555*(7695), 210–215. DOI: 10.1038/nature25973 PMID: 29489753

Rouskas, K., Guela, M., Pantoura, M., Pagkalos, I., Hassapidou, M., Lalama, E., Pfeiffer, A. F. H., Decorte, E., Cornelissen, V., Wilson-Barnes, S., Hart, K., Mantovani, E., Dias, S. B., Hadjileontiadis, L., Gymnopoulos, L. P., Dimitropoulos, K., & Argiriou, A. (2025). The Influence of an AI-Driven Personalized Nutrition Program on the Human Gut Microbiome and Its Health Implications. *Nutrients*, *17*(7), 1260. DOI: 10.3390/nu17071260 PMID: 40219016

Rowland, I., Gibson, G., Heinken, A., Scott, K., Swann, J., Thiele, I., & Tuohy, K. (2018). Gut microbiota functions: Metabolism of nutrients and other food components. *European Journal of Nutrition*, *57*(1), 1–24. DOI: 10.1007/s00394-017-1445-8 PMID: 28393285

Roy, S., & Dhaneshwar, S. (2023). Role of prebiotics, probiotics, and synbiotics in management of inflammatory bowel disease: Current perspectives. *World Journal of Gastroenterology*, *29*(14), 2078–2100. DOI: 10.3748/wjg.v29.i14.2078

Rueda, G. H., Causada-Calo, N., Borojevic, R., Nardelli, A., Pinto-Sanchez, M. I., Constante, M., Libertucci, J., Mohan, V., Langella, P., Loonen, L. M. P., Wells, J. M., Collins, S. M., Sokol, H., Verdu, E. F., & Bercik, P. (2024). Oral tryptophan activates duodenal aryl hydrocarbon receptor in healthy subjects: A crossover randomized controlled trial. *American Journal of Physiology. Gastrointestinal and Liver Physiology*, *326*(6), G687–G696. DOI: 10.1152/ajpgi.00306.2023 PMID: 38591144

Rui, S., Fengrui, G., Yining, Z., Hong, S., Xuewen, Y., Changping, W., & Chunjia, Y. (2025). Biological activity of secondary metabolites of actinomycetes and their potential sources as antineoplastic drugs: A review. *Frontiers in Microbiology, 16*, 1550516. DOI: 10.3389/fmicb.2025.1550516 PMID: 40406345

Ruszkowski, J., & Witkowski, J. M. (2019). Lactulose: Patient- and dose-dependent prebiotic properties in humans. *Anaerobe, 59*, 100–106. DOI: 10.1016/j.anaerobe.2019.06.002

Saad, N., Delattre, C., Urdaci, M., Schmitter, J. M., & Bressollier, P. (2013). An overview of the last advances in probiotic and prebiotic field. *Lebensmittel-Wissenschaft + Technologie, 50*(1), 1–16. DOI: 10.1016/j.lwt.2012.05.014

Saak, C. C., Pierce, E. C., Dinh, C. B., Portik, D., Hall, R., Ashby, M., & Dutton, R. J. (2023). Longitudinal, multi-platform metagenomics yields a high-quality genomic catalog and guides an in vitro model for cheese communities. *mSystems, 8*(1), e00701–e00722. DOI: 10.1128/msystems.00701-22 PMID: 36622155

Saberi, M., Woods, N. B., de Luca, C., Schenk, S., Lu, J. C., Bandyopadhyay, G., Verma, I. M., & Olefsky, J. M. (2009). Hematopoietic cell-specific deletion of toll-like receptor 4 ameliorates hepatic and adipose tissue insulin resistance in high-fat-fed mice. *Cell Metabolism, 10*(5), 419–429. DOI: 10.1016/j.cmet.2009.09.006 PMID: 19883619

Sadeghi, A., Ebrahimi, M., Kharazmi, M. S., & Jafari, S. M. (2023). Effects of microbial-derived biotics (meta/pharma/post-biotics) on the modulation of gut microbiome and metabolome; general aspects and emerging trends. *Food Chemistry, 411*, 135478. DOI: 10.1016/j.foodchem.2023.135478

Saha, T.. (2022). Non-invasive monitoring of interstitial fluid lactate through an epidermal iontophoretic device. *Talanta, 254*, 124122. DOI: 10.1016/j.talanta.2022.124122 PMID: 36459870

Sakthivel, M., Jaganathan, A., Mohanraj, M., & Selvakumar, P. Mohit, & Manjunath, T. (2025). Brand Loyalty through AI and Personalisation: AI-Generated Content for Financial Marketing. In A. J. Nair, S. Manohar, Y. B. Limbu, & B. A. Huhmann (Eds.), *Intersecting Natural Language Processing and FinTech Innovations in Service Marketing* (pp. 77–96). IGI Global. DOI: 10.4018/979-8-3693-9944-6.ch006

Salem, A. E., Singh, R., Ayoub, Y. K., Khairy, A. M., & Mullin, G. E. (2018). The gut microbiome and irritable bowel syndrome: State of art review. *Arab Journal of Gastroenterology, 19*(3), 136–141. DOI: 10.1016/j.ajg.2018.02.008 PMID: 29935865

Salminen, S., Collado, M. C., Endo, A., Hill, C., Lebeer, S., Quigley, E. M., & von Wright, A. (2021). The International Scientific Association of Probiotics and Prebiotics (ISAPP) consensus statement on the definition and scope of postbiotics. *Nature Reviews. Gastroenterology & Hepatology*, *18*(9), 649–667. DOI: 10.1038/s41575-021-00440-6 PMID: 33948025

Salsinha, A. S., Pimentel, L. L., Fontes, A. L., Gomes, A. M., & Rodríguez-Alcalá, L. M. (2018). Microbial production of conjugated linoleic acid and conjugated linolenic acid relies on a multienzymatic system. *Microbiology and Molecular Biology Reviews : MMBR*, *82*(4), 00019–00018. DOI: 10.1128/MMBR.00019-18 PMID: 30158254

Salva, S., Kolling, Y., Ivir, M., Gutiérrez, F., & Alvarez, S. (2021). The role of immunobiotics and postbiotics in the recovery of immune cell populations from respiratory mucosa of malnourished hosts: Effect on the resistance against respiratory infections. *Frontiers in Nutrition*, *8*, 704868. DOI: 10.3389/fnut.2021.704868

Salvi, P. S., & Cowles, R. A. (2021). Butyrate and the intestinal epithelium: Modulation of proliferation and inflammation in homeostasis and disease. *Cells*, *10*(7), 1775. DOI: 10.3390/cells10071775 PMID: 34359944

Salvo-Romero, E., Stokes, P., & Gareau, M. G. (2020). Microbiota–immune interactions: From gut to brain. *LymphoSign Journal*, *7*(1), 1–23. DOI: 10.14785/lymphosign-2019-0018

Sanders, M. E., Heimbach, J. T., Pot, B., Tancredi, D. J., Lenoir-Wijnkoop, I., Lähteenmäki-Uutela, A., Gueimonde, M., & Bañares, S. (2011). Health claims substantiation for probiotic and prebiotic products. *Gut Microbes*, *2*(3), 127–133. DOI: 10.4161/gmic.2.3.16174 PMID: 21646865

Sanders, M. E., Merenstein, D. J., Reid, G., Gibson, G. R., & Rastall, R. A. (2019). Probiotics and prebiotics in intestinal health and disease: From biology to the clinic. *Nature Reviews. Gastroenterology & Hepatology*, *16*(10), 605–616. DOI: 10.1038/s41575-019-0173-3 PMID: 31296969

Santaló, J., & Berdasco, M. (2022). Ethical implications of epigenetics in the era of personalized medicine. *Clinical Epigenetics*, *14*(1), 44. DOI: 10.1186/s13148-022-01263-1 PMID: 35337378

Sardans, J., Lambers, H., Preece, C., Alrefaei, A. F., & Penuelas, J. (2023). Role of mycorrhizas and root exudates in plant uptake of soil nutrients (calcium, iron, magnesium, and potassium): Has the puzzle been completely solved? *The Plant Journal*, *114*(6), 1227–1242. DOI: 10.1111/tpj.16184 PMID: 36917083

Sato, T., van Es, J. H., Snippert, H. J., Stange, D. E., Barker, N., Shroyer, N. F., & Clevers, H. (2011). Paneth cells constitute the niche for Lgr5 stem cells in intestinal crypts. *Nature*, *469*(7330), 415–418. DOI: 10.1038/nature09637

Sato, T., Vries, R. G., Snippert, H. J., van de Wetering, M., Barker, N., Stange, D. E., van Es, J. H., Abo, A., Kujala, P., Peters, P. J., & Clevers, H. (2009). Single Lgr5 stem cells build crypt-villus structures in vitro without a mesenchymal niche. *Nature*, *459*(7244), 262–265. DOI: 10.1038/nature07935 PMID: 19329995

Saulnier, D. M. A., Gibson, G. R., & Kolida, S. (2008). In vitro effects of selected synbiotics on the human faecal microbiota composition. *FEMS Microbiology Ecology*, *66*(3), 516–527. DOI: 10.1111/j.1574-6941.2008.00561.x PMID: 18673391

Sayin, S. I., Wahlström, A., Felin, J., Jäntti, S., Marschall, H. U., Bamberg, K., Angelin, B., Hyötyläinen, T., Orešič, M., & Bäckhed, F. (2013). Gut microbiota regulates bile acid metabolism by reducing the levels of tauro-beta-muricholic acid, a naturally occurring FXR antagonist. *Cell Metabolism*, *17*(2), 225–235. DOI: 10.1016/j.cmet.2013.01.003 PMID: 23395169

Scepanovic, P., Hodel, F., Mondot, S., Partula, V., Byrd, A., Hammer, C., Alanio, C., Bergstedt, J., Patin, E., Touvier, M., Lantz, O., Albert, M. L., Duffy, D., Quintana-Murci, L., & Fellay, J. (2019). A comprehensive assessment of demographic, environmental, and host genetic associations with gut microbiome diversity in healthy individuals. *Microbiome*, *7*(1), 130. DOI: 10.1186/s40168-019-0747-x PMID: 31519223

Scheithauer, T. P., Rampanelli, E., Nieuwdorp, M., Vallance, B. A., Verchere, C. B., van Raalte, D. H., & Herrema, H. (2020). Gut microbiota as a trigger for metabolic inflammation in obesity and type 2 diabetes. *Frontiers in Immunology*, *11*, 571731. DOI: 10.3389/fimmu.2020.571731 PMID: 33178196

Schroeder, B. O. (2019). Fight them or feed them: How the intestinal mucus layer manages the gut microbiota. *Gastroenterology Report*, *7*(1), 3–12. DOI: 10.1093/gastro/goy052

Schwarzer, M., Hermanova, P., Srutkova, D., Hudcovic, T., Akgün, J., Wiedermann, U., & Kozakova, H. (2017). Diet matters: Endotoxin in the diet impacts the level of allergic sensitization in germ-free mice. *PLoS One*, *12*(1), e0167786. DOI: 10.1371/journal.pone.0167786

Science Translational Medicine. (2018). Epidermal electronics for shunt monitoring. DOI: 10.1126/scitranslmed.aau2423

Scientific Reports. (2022). Reshaping healthcare with wearable biosensors. DOI: 10.1038/s41598-022-26951-z

Seganfredo, F. B., Blume, C. A., Moehlecke, M., Giongo, A., Casagrande, D. S., Spolidoro, J. V. N., Padoin, A. V., Schaan, B. D., & Mottin, C. C. (2017). Weight-loss interventions and gut microbiota changes in overweight and obese patients: A systematic review. *Obesity Reviews*, *18*(8), 832–851. DOI: 10.1111/obr.12541 PMID: 28524627

Sekirov, I., Russell, S. L., Antunes, L. C. M., & Finlay, B. B. (2010). Gut microbiota in health and disease. *Physiological Reviews*, *90*(3), 859–904. DOI: 10.1152/physrev.00045.2009 PMID: 20664075

Selma, M. V., Espín, J. C., & Tomás-Barberán, F. A. (2009). Interaction between phenolics and gut microbiota: Role in human health. *Journal of Agricultural and Food Chemistry*, *57*(15), 6485–6501. DOI: 10.1021/jf902107d PMID: 19580283

Selvakumar, P., & Haashni, S. SudhaAnanthi, G., & Manjunath, T. C. (2026). Cybernetic Systems Thinking: Foundations for Organizational Adaptability. In L. Tsvasman (Ed.), Cybernetic Leadership for Sustainable Innovation (pp. 99-124). IGI Global Scientific Publishing. DOI: 10.4018/979-8-3373-2484-5.ch004

Sempionatto, J. R., Lin, M., & Yin, L.. (2019). Pacifier Biosensor: Toward Noninvasive Saliva Biomarker Monitoring. *Analytical Chemistry*, *91*(23), 13883–13891. DOI: 10.1021/acs.analchem.9b03379 PMID: 31573188

Sender, R., Fuchs, S., & Milo, R. (2016). Are we really vastly outnumbered? Revisiting the ratio of bacterial to host cells in humans. *Cell*, *164*(3), 337–340. DOI: 10.1016/j.cell.2016.01.013 PMID: 26824647

Seo, S.-K., & Kwon, B. (2023). Immune regulation through tryptophan metabolism. *Experimental & Molecular Medicine*, *55*(7), 1371–1379. DOI: 10.1038/s12276-023-01028-7 PMID: 37394584

Sepp, E., Smidt, I., Rööp, T., Tšepetova, J., Kõljalg, S., Mikelsaar, M., Soidla, I., Ainsaar, M., Kolk, H., Vallas, M., Jaagura, M., & Mändar, R. (2022). Comparative analysis of gut microbiota in centenarians and young people: Impact of eating habits and childhood living environment. *Frontiers in Cellular and Infection Microbiology*, *12*, 851404. DOI: 10.3389/fcimb.2022.851404 PMID: 35372105

Seshanna, S. V., Gopalakrishnan, G., Anute, N., Deepthi Reddy, K., Sharma, M., Selvakumar, P., & Manjunath, T. C. (2026). Digital Transformation and Cybersecurity. In Saeed, S., & Tahir, S. (Eds.), *User-Centric Cybersecurity Implications for Sustainable Digital Transformation* (pp. 1–30). IGI Global Scientific Publishing., DOI: 10.4018/979-8-3373-3171-3.ch001

Shabbir, K., Noureldin, M., & Sim, S. (2024). Data-driven model for seismic assessment, design, and retrofit of structures using explainable artificial intelligence. *Computer-Aided Civil and Infrastructure Engineering*. Advance online publication. DOI: 10.1111/mice.13338

Shadab, A., Mahjoor, M., Abbasi-Kolli, M., Afkhami, H., Moeinian, P., & Safdarian, A. R. (2023). Divergent functions of NLRP3 inflammasomes in cancer: A review. *Cell Communication and Signaling : CCS*, *21*(1), 232. DOI: 10.1186/s12964-023-01235-9 PMID: 37715239

Shafique, B., Ranjha, M. M. A. N., Murtaza, M. A., Walayat, N., Nawaz, A., Khalid, W., Mahmood, S., Nadeem, M., Manzoor, M. F., Ameer, K., Aadil, R. M., & Ibrahim, S. A. (2022). Recent trends and applications of nanoencapsulated bacteriocins against microbes in food quality and safety. *Microorganisms*, *11*(1), 85. DOI: 10.3390/microorganisms11010085 PMID: 36677377

Shah, S. C., Day, L. W., Somsouk, M., & Sewell, J. L. (2013). Meta-analysis: Antibiotic therapy for small intestinal bacterial overgrowth. *Alimentary Pharmacology & Therapeutics*, *38*(8), 925–934. DOI: 10.1111/apt.12479 PMID: 24004101

Shajari, S., Kuruvinashetti, K., Komeili, A., & Sundararaj, U.MDPI. (2023). The emergence of AI-based wearable sensors for digital health. *Sensors (Basel)*, *23*(23), 9498. DOI: 10.3390/s23239498 PMID: 38067871

Shanahan, E. R., McMaster, J. J., & Staudacher, H. M. (2021). Conducting research on diet–microbiome interactions: A review of current challenges, essential methodological principles, and recommendations for best practice in study design. *Journal of Human Nutrition and Dietetics*, *34*(4), 631–644. DOI: 10.1111/jhn.12868 PMID: 33639033

Shang, Z., Pai, L., & Patil, S. (2024). Unveiling the dynamics of gut microbial interactions: A review of dietary impact and precision nutrition in gastrointestinal health. *Frontiers in Nutrition*, *11*, 1395664. Advance online publication. DOI: 10.3389/fnut.2024.1395664 PMID: 38873568

Shapira, S. N., & Christofk, H. R. (2020). Metabolic regulation of tissue stem cells. *Trends in Cell Biology*, *30*(7), 566–576. DOI: 10.1016/j.tcb.2020.04.004 PMID: 32359707

Sharafi, H., Divsalar, E., Rezaei, Z., Liu, S. Q., & Moradi, M. (2024). The potential of postbiotics as a novel approach in food packaging and biopreservation: A systematic review of the latest developments. *Critical Reviews in Food Science and Nutrition*, *64*(33), 12524–12554. DOI: 10.1080/10408398.2023.2253909

Sharpton, T. J. (2014). An introduction to the analysis of shotgun metagenomic data. *Frontiers in Plant Science*, *5*, 209. DOI: 10.3389/fpls.2014.00209

Shen, H., Zhang, C., Li, S., Liang, Y., Lee, L. T., Aggarwal, N., & Lu, T. K. (2024). Prodrug-conjugated tumor-seeking commensals for targeted cancer therapy. *Nature Communications*, *15*(1), 4343. Advance online publication. DOI: 10.1038/s41467-024-48661-y PMID: 38773197

Shen, X., Tilves, C., Kim, H., Tanaka, T., Spira, A. P., Chia, C. W., Talegawkar, S. A., Ferrucci, L., & Mueller, N. T. (2024). Plant-based diets and the gut microbiome: Findings from the Baltimore Longitudinal Study of Aging. *The American Journal of Clinical Nutrition*, *119*(4), 628–638. DOI: 10.1016/j.ajcnut.2024.01.006 PMID: 38218318

Shi, M., Zhang, Y.-Z., & Holmes, E. C. (2018). Meta-transcriptomics and the evolutionary biology of RNA viruses. *Virus Research*, *243*, 83–90. DOI: 10.1016/j.virusres.2017.10.016 PMID: 29111455

Shimizu, H.. (2019). Regulation of host energy metabolism by gut microbiota-derived short-chain fatty acids. *Glycative Stress Research*, *6*(3), 181–191.

Shin, N. R., Whon, T. W., & Bae, J. W. (2015). Proteobacteria: Microbial signature of dysbiosis in gut microbiota. *Trends in Biotechnology*, *33*(9), 496–503. DOI: 10.1016/j.tibtech.2015.06.011 PMID: 26210164

Shi, X., Ma, T., Sakandar, H. A., Menghe, B., & Sun, Z. (2022). Gut microbiome and aging nexus and underlying mechanism. *Applied Microbiology and Biotechnology*, *106*(17), 5349–5358. DOI: 10.1007/s00253-022-12089-5 PMID: 35882675

Shock, T., Badang, L., Ferguson, B., & Martinez-Guryn, K. (2021a). The interplay between diet, gut microbes, and host epigenetics in health and disease. *The Journal of Nutritional Biochemistry*, *95*, 108631. DOI: 10.1016/j.jnutbio.2021.108631 PMID: 33789148

Shoelson, S. E., Lee, J., & Goldfine, A. B. (2006). Inflammation and insulin resistance. *The Journal of Clinical Investigation*, *116*(7), 1793–1801. DOI: 10.1172/JCI29069 PMID: 16823477

Shroyer, N. F., Helmrath, M. A., Wang, V. Y.-C., Antalffy, B., Henning, S. J., & Zoghbi, H. Y. (2007). Intestine-specific ablation of mouse atonal homolog 1 (Math1) reveals a role in cellular homeostasis. *Gastroenterology, 132*(7), 2478–2488. DOI: 10.1053/j.gastro.2007.03.047

Shukla, P. K., Gangwar, R., Manda, B., Meena, A. S., Yadav, N., Szabo, E., Balogh, A., Lee, S. C., Tigyi, G., & Rao, R. K. (2016). Rapid disruption of intestinal epithelial tight junction and barrier dysfunction by ionizing radiation in mouse colon in vivo: Protection by N-acetyl-L-cysteine. *American Journal of Physiology. Gastrointestinal and Liver Physiology, 310*(9), G705–G715. DOI: 10.1152/ajpgi.00314.2015 PMID: 26822914

Silvester, J. A., & Leffler, D. A. (2017). The effect of gastrointestinal viral infections and vaccination on risk of celiac disease autoimmunity. *Clinical Gastroenterology and Hepatology, 15*(5), 703–705. DOI: 10.1016/j.cgh.2016.12.014

Singh, A., Rajput, V. D., Rawat, S., Sharma, R., Singh, A. K., Kumar, P., & Minkina, T. (2022). Geoinformatics and nanotechnological approaches for coping up abiotic and biotic stress in crop plants. In *Nanotechnology in plant growth promotion and protection* (p. 337). Wiley., DOI: 10.1002/9781119808565.ch17

Singh, P., Arora, A., Strand, T. A., Leffler, D. A., Catassi, C., Green, P. H., Kelly, C. P., Ahuja, V., & Makharia, G. K. (2018). Global prevalence of celiac disease: Systematic review and meta-analysis. *Clinical Gastroenterology and Hepatology, 16*(6), 823–836. DOI: 10.1016/j.cgh.2017.06.037

Singh, R. K., Chang, H. W., Yan, D., Lee, K. M., Ucmak, D., Wong, K., Abrouk, M., Farahnik, B., Nakamura, M., Zhu, T. H., Bhutani, T., & Liao, W. (2017). Influence of diet on the gut microbiome and implications for human health. *Journal of Translational Medicine, 15*(1), 73. DOI: 10.1186/s12967-017-1175-y PMID: 28388917

Singh, R., Zogg, H., Wei, L., Bartlett, A., Ghoshal, U. C., Rajender, S., & Ro, S. (2021). Gut microbial dysbiosis in the pathogenesis of gastrointestinal dysmotility and metabolic disorders. *Journal of Neurogastroenterology and Motility, 27*(1), 19–34. DOI: 10.5056/jnm20149 PMID: 33166939

Singh, V. (2023). Current challenges and future implications of exploiting the omics data into nutrigenetics and nutrigenomics for personalized diagnosis and nutrition-based care. *Nutrition (Burbank, Los Angeles County, Calif.), 110*, 112002. DOI: 10.1016/j.nut.2023.112002 PMID: 36940623

Singh, V., Shirbhate, E., Kore, R., Vishwakarma, S., Parveen, S., Veerasamy, R., Tiwari, A. K., & Rajak, H. (2025). Microbial metabolites-induced epigenetic modifications for inhibition of colorectal cancer: Current status and future perspectives. *Mini-Reviews in Medicinal Chemistry*, *25*(1), 76–93. DOI: 10.2174/0113895575320344240625080555 PMID: 38982701

Sinrod, A. J. G., Shah, I. M., Surek, E., & Barile, D. (2023). Uncovering the promising role of grape pomace as a modulator of the gut microbiome: An in-depth review. *Heliyon*, *9*(10), e20499. DOI: 10.1016/j.heliyon.2023.e20499

Sirisinha, S. (2016). The potential impact of gut microbiota on your health: Current status and future challenges. *Asian Pacific Journal of Allergy and Immunology*, *34*(4), 249–264. DOI: 10.12932/AP0803 PMID: 28042926

Skinner, M. K. (2024). Epigenetic biomarkers for disease susceptibility and preventative medicine. *Cell Metabolism*, *36*(2), 263–277. DOI: 10.1016/j.cmet.2023.11.015 PMID: 38176413

Slifer, Z. M., & Blikslager, A. T. (2020). The integral role of tight junction proteins in the repair of injured intestinal epithelium. *International Journal of Molecular Sciences*, *21*(3), 972. DOI: 10.3390/ijms21030972

Smits, S. A.. (2019). Public health interventions targeting the microbiome: A new frontier in disease prevention. *Nature Reviews. Microbiology*, *17*(9), 654–668. DOI: 10.1038/s41579-019-0236-9

Smits, S. A., Leach, J., Sonnenburg, E. D., Gonzalez, C. G., Lichtman, J. S., Reid, G., Knight, R., Manjurano, A., Changalucha, J., Elias, J. E., Dominguez-Bello, M. G., & Sonnenburg, J. L. (2017). Seasonal cycling in the gut microbiome of the Hadza hunter-gatherers of Tanzania. *Science*, *357*(6353), 802–806. DOI: 10.1126/science.aan4834 PMID: 28839072

Smolinska, S., Popescu, F. D., & Zemelka-Wiacek, M. (2025). A Review of the Influence of Prebiotics, Probiotics, Synbiotics, and Postbiotics on the Human Gut Microbiome and Intestinal Integrity. *Journal of Clinical Medicine*, *14*(11), 3673. DOI: 10.3390/jcm14113673

Sniffen, J. C., McFarland, L. V., Evans, C. T., & Goldstein, E. J. (2018). Choosing an appropriate probiotic product for your patient: An evidence-based practical guide. *PLoS One*, *13*(12), e0209205. DOI: 10.1371/journal.pone.0209205

Sokol, H., Pigneur, B., Watterlot, L., Lakhdari, O., Bermúdez-Humarán, L. G., Gratadoux, J. J., Blugeon, S., Bridonneau, C., Furet, J. P., Corthier, G., Grangette, C., Vasquez, N., Pochart, P., Trugnan, G., Thomas, G., Blottière, H. M., Doré, J., Marteau, P., Seksik, P., & Langella, P. (2008). *Faecalibacterium prausnitzii* is an anti-inflammatory commensal bacterium identified by gut microbiota analysis of Crohn disease patients. *Proceedings of the National Academy of Sciences of the United States of America, 105*(43), 16731–16736. DOI: 10.1073/pnas.0804812105 PMID: 18936492

Soldado-Gordillo, A., & Álvarez-Mercado, A. I. (2024). Epigenetics, Microbiota, and Breast Cancer: A Systematic Review. *Life (Chicago, Ill.), 14*(6), 705. DOI: 10.3390/life14060705 PMID: 38929688

Soldán, M., Argalášová, Ľ., Hadvinová, L., Galileo, B., & Babjaková, J. (2024). The effect of dietary types on gut microbiota composition and development of non-communicable diseases: A narrative review. *Nutrients, 16*(18), 3134. DOI: 10.3390/nu16183134 PMID: 39339734

Soletsky, B., & Feig, D. I. (2012). Uric Acid Reduction Rectifies Prehypertension in Obese Adolescents. *Hypertension, 60*(5), 1148–1156. DOI: 10.1161/HYPERTENSIONAHA.112.196980 PMID: 23006736

Sollid, L. M., & Jabri, B. (2013). Triggers and drivers of autoimmunity: Lessons from coeliac disease. *Nature Reviews. Immunology, 13*(4), 294–302. DOI: 10.1038/nri3407

Solopova, A., Bottacini, F., Venturi degli Esposti, E., Amaretti, A., Raimondi, S., Rossi, M., & van Sinderen, D. (2020). Riboflavin biosynthesis and overproduction by a derivative of the human gut commensal Bifidobacterium longum subsp. infantis ATCC 15697. *Frontiers in Microbiology, 11*, 573335. DOI: 10.3389/fmicb.2020.573335 PMID: 33042083

Sommer, F., Anderson, J. M., Bharti, R., Raes, J., & Rosenstiel, P. (2017). The resilience of the intestinal microbiota influences health and disease. *Nature Reviews. Microbiology, 15*(10), 630–638. DOI: 10.1038/nrmicro.2017.58 PMID: 28626231

Son, J. W., Shoaie, S., & Lee, S. (2020). Systems biology: A multi-omics integration approach to metabolism and the microbiome. *Endocrinology and Metabolism (Seoul, Korea), 35*(3), 507–514. DOI: 10.3803/EnM.2020.303 PMID: 32981293

Sonnenburg, E. D., & Sonnenburg, J. L. (2019). The ancestral and industrialized gut microbiota and implications for human health. *Nature Reviews. Microbiology, 17*(6), 383–390. DOI: 10.1038/s41579-019-0191-8 PMID: 31089293

Sonnenburg, E. D., & Sonnenburg, J. L. (2019). *The good gut: Taking control of your weight, your mood, and your long-term health.* Penguin Press.

Sonnenburg, J. L., & Bäckhed, F. (2016). Diet–microbiota interactions as moderators of human metabolism. *Nature, 535*(7610), 56–64. DOI: 10.1038/nature18846

Spencer, M. D., Hamp, T. J., Reid, R. W., Fischer, L. M., Zeisel, S. H., & Fodor, A. A. (2011). Association between composition of the human gastrointestinal microbiome and development of fatty liver with choline deficiency. *Gastroenterology, 140*(3), 976–986. DOI: 10.1053/j.gastro.2010.11.049 PMID: 21129376

Speybroeck, L. V., De Waele, D., & Van de Vijver, G. (2002). Theories in early embryology: Close connections between epigenesis, preformationism, and self-organization. *Annals of the New York Academy of Sciences, 981*(1), 7–49. DOI: 10.1111/j.1749-6632.2002.tb04910.x PMID: 12547672

St Germain, M. M., Mortazavi, A., & Bakovic, M. (2025). Advancing Personalized Nutrition Through Genetic Nutritional Insights. *Nutrients, 17*(13), 2166. DOI: 10.3390/nu17132166

Stolfi, C., Maresca, C., Monteleone, G., & Laudisi, F. (2022). Implication of intestinal barrier dysfunction in gut dysbiosis and diseases. *Biomedicines, 10*(2), 289. DOI: 10.3390/biomedicines10020289 PMID: 35203499

Sturm, G., Mojarrad, M., & Kaster, A. K. (2023). Targeted cell labeling and sorting of prokaryotes for cultivation and omics approaches. *Microbial Physiology, 33*(1), 63–84. DOI: 10.1159/000532088

Subhan, F. B., & Chan, C. B. (2016). Review of Dietary Practices of the 21st Century: Facts and Fallacies. *Canadian Journal of Diabetes, 40*(4), 348–354. DOI: 10.1016/j.jcjd.2016.05.005 PMID: 27497150

Su, C., Hsu, Y., Thangudu, S., Chen, W., Huang, Y., Yu, C., & Wu, M. (2021). Application of multiparametric MR imaging to predict the diversification of renal function in miR29a-mediated diabetic nephropathy. *Scientific Reports, 11*(1), 81519. Advance online publication. DOI: 10.1038/s41598-021-81519-7 PMID: 33479331

Suez, J., Zmora, N., Zilberman-Schapira, G., Mor, U., & Elinav, E. (2019). Personalized microbiome-based approaches to prophylaxis against food allergy and other non-communicable diseases. *Trends in Immunology, 40*(8), 682–700. DOI: 10.1016/j.it.2019.06.008

Sunaga, S., Tsunoda, J., Teratani, T., Mikami, Y., & Kanai, T. (2022). Heterogeneity of ILC2s in the intestine; homeostasis and pathology. *Frontiers in Immunology, 13*, 867351. DOI: 10.3389/fimmu.2022.867351

Sun, J., Chen, F., & Wu, G. (2023). Potential effects of gut microbiota on host cancers: Focus on immunity, DNA damage, cellular pathways, and anticancer therapy. *The ISME Journal*, *17*(10), 1535–1551. DOI: 10.1038/s41396-023-01483-0 PMID: 37553473

Sun, J., Chen, S., Zang, D., Sun, H., Sun, Y., & Chen, J. (2024). Butyrate as a promising therapeutic target in cancer: From pathogenesis to clinic [Review]. *International Journal of Oncology*, *64*(4), 44. Advance online publication. DOI: 10.3892/ijo.2024.5632 PMID: 38426581

Sun, M.-F., & Shen, Y.-Q. (2018). Dysbiosis of gut microbiota and microbial metabolites in Parkinson's Disease. *Ageing Research Reviews*, *45*, 53–61. DOI: 10.1016/j.arr.2018.04.004 PMID: 29705121

Swallah, M. S., Fan, H., Wang, S., Yu, H., & Piao, C. (2021). Prebiotic Impacts of Soybean Residue (Okara) on Eubiosis/Dysbiosis Condition of the Gut and the Possible Effects on Liver and Kidney Functions. *Molecules (Basel, Switzerland)*, *26*(2), 326. DOI: 10.3390/molecules26020326

Świątkiewicz, I., Woźniak, A., & Taub, P. R. (2021). Time-restricted eating and metabolic syndrome: Current status and future perspectives. *Nutrients*, *13*(1), 221. Advance online publication. DOI: 10.3390/nu13010221 PMID: 33466692

Synergistic Interplay of Diet, Gut Microbiota, and Insulin Resistance: Unraveling the Molecular Nexus—Gopal—2024—Molecular Nutrition & Food Research—Wiley Online Library. (n.d.). Retrieved October 18, 2025, from https://onlinelibrary.wiley.com/doi/abs/10.1002/mnfr.202400677

Tahara, Y., & Shibata, S. (2013). Chronobiology and nutrition. *Neuroscience*, *253*, 78–88. DOI: 10.1016/j.neuroscience.2013.08.049 PMID: 24007937

Tang, J. (2011). Microbial metabolomics. *Current Genomics*, *12*(6), 391–403. DOI: 10.2174/138920211797248619 PMID: 22379393

Tang, W. H., Wang, Z., Levison, B. S., Koeth, R. A., Britt, E. B., Fu, X., Wu, Y., & Hazen, S. L. (2013). Intestinal microbial metabolism of phosphatidylcholine and cardiovascular risk. *The New England Journal of Medicine*, *368*(17), 1575–1584. DOI: 10.1056/NEJMoa1109400 PMID: 23614584

Tanwar, R., Panghal, A., Chaudhary, G., Kumari, A., & Chhikara, N. (2023). Nutritional, phytochemical and functional potential of sorghum: A review. *Food Chemistry Advances*, *3*, 100501. Advance online publication. DOI: 10.1016/j.focha.2023.100501

Tap, J., Derrien, M., Törnblom, H., Brazier, L., Cools-Portier, S., Doré, J., Störsrud, S., le Nevé, B., Öhman, L., & Simrén, M. (2017). Identification of an intestinal microbiota signature associated with severity of irritable bowel syndrome. *Gastroenterology, 152*(1), 111–123.e8. DOI: 10.1053/j.gastro.2016.09.049 PMID: 27725146

Tedeschi, L. O. (2019). ASN-ASAS SYMPOSIUM: FUTURE OF DATA ANALYTICS IN NUTRITION: Mathematical modeling in ruminant nutrition: approaches and paradigms, extant models, and thoughts for upcoming predictive analytics. *Journal of Animal Science, 97*(5), 1921–1944. DOI: 10.1093/jas/skz092 PMID: 30882142

Thaiss, C. A., Levy, M., Grosheva, I., Zheng, D., Soffer, E., Blacher, E., Braverman, S., Tengeler, A. C., Serradas, P., & Elinav, E. (2018). Hyperglycemia drives intestinal barrier dysfunction and risk for enteric infection. *Science, 359*(6382), 1376–1383. DOI: 10.1126/science.aar3318

Thanoon, M. A., Zulkifley, M. A., Zainuri, M. A. A. M., & Abdani, S. R. (2023). A review of deep learning techniques for lung cancer screening and diagnosis based on CT images. *Diagnostics (Basel), 13*(16), 2617. Advance online publication. DOI: 10.3390/diagnostics13162617 PMID: 37627876

The interplay between diet and the gut microbiome: Implications for health and disease | Nature Reviews Microbiology. (n.d.). Retrieved October 18, 2025, from https://www.nature.com/articles/s41579-024-01068-4

The role of the gut microbiota in the onset and progression of heart failure: Insights into epigenetic mechanisms and aging | Clinical Epigenetics. (n.d.). Retrieved October 18, 2025, from https://link.springer.com/article/10.1186/s13148-024-01786-9

Thevaranjan, N., Puchta, A., Schulz, C., Naidoo, A., Szamosi, J. C., Verschoor, C. P., Loukov, D., Schenck, L. P., Jury, J., Foley, K. P., Schertzer, J. D., Larche, M. J., Davidson, D. J., Verdu, E. F., Surette, M. G., & Bowdish, D. M. E. (2017). Age-associated microbial dysbiosis promotes intestinal permeability, systemic inflammation, and macrophage dysfunction. *Cell Host & Microbe, 21*(4), 455–466.e4. DOI: 10.1016/j.chom.2017.03.002 PMID: 28407483

Thirumurugan, D., et al. (2018). An introductory chapter: secondary metabolites. *Secondary metabolites-sources and applications, 1*, 13.

Thomas, C., Gioiello, A., Noriega, L., Strehle, A., Oury, J., Rizzo, G., Macchiarulo, A., Yamamoto, H., Mataki, C., Pruzanski, M., Pellicciari, R., Auwerx, J., & Schoonjans, K. (2009). TGR5-mediated bile acid sensing controls glucose homeostasis. *Cell Metabolism, 10*(3), 167–177. DOI: 10.1016/j.cmet.2009.08.001 PMID: 19723493

Thorakkattu, P., Khanashyam, A. C., Shah, K., Babu, K. S., Mundanat, A. S., Deliephan, A., Deokar, G. S., Santivarangkna, C., & Nirmal, N. P. (2022). Postbiotics: Current trends in food and pharmaceutical industry. *Foods*, *11*(19), 3094. DOI: 10.3390/foods11193094

Thursby, E., & Juge, N. (2017). Introduction to the human gut microbiota. *The Biochemical Journal*, *474*(11), 1823–1836. DOI: 10.1042/BCJ20160510 PMID: 28512250

Tiangpook, S., Nhim, S., Prangthip, P., Pason, P., Tachaapaikoon, C., Ratanakhanokchai, K., & Waeonukul, R. (2023). Production of a Series of Long-Chain Isomaltooligosaccharides from Maltose by *Bacillus subtilis* AP-1 and Associated Prebiotic Properties. *Foods*, *12*(7), 1499. DOI: 10.3390/foods12071499

Tiderencel, K. A., Hutcheon, D. A., & Ziegler, J. (2020). Probiotics for the treatment of type 2 diabetes: A review of randomized controlled trials. *Diabetes/Metabolism Research and Reviews*, *36*(1), e3213. DOI: 10.1002/dmrr.3213

Tiffon, C. (2018). The impact of nutrition and environmental epigenetics on human health and disease. *International Journal of Molecular Sciences*, *19*(11), 3425. DOI: 10.3390/ijms19113425

Tilg, H., Zmora, N., Adolph, T. E., & Elinav, E. (2020). The intestinal microbiota fuelling metabolic inflammation. *Nature Reviews. Immunology*, *20*(1), 40–54. DOI: 10.1038/s41577-019-0198-4 PMID: 31388093

Tiwari, S., Yadav, S. K., Sahu, V. K., & Tripathi, M. K. (2018). Current status and future prospects of marker assisted breeding for genetic improvement of minor millets. *International Journal of Current Microbiology and Applied Sciences*, *7*(12), 2587–2601. DOI: 10.20546/ijcmas.2018.712.293

Tomlinson, C., Khoury, J., & Dainty, K. N. (2019). Cultural competence in personalized nutrition: Integrating microbiome data. *Nutrients*, *11*(10), 2410. DOI: 10.3390/nu11102410 PMID: 31600938

Topolska, K., Florkiewicz, A., & Filipiak-Florkiewicz, A. (2021). Functional food—Consumer motivations and expectations. *International Journal of Environmental Research and Public Health*, *18*(10), 5327. DOI: 10.3390/ijerph18105327

Torres-Fuentes, C., Schellekens, H., Dinan, T. G., & Cryan, J. F. (2017). The microbiota-gut-brain axis in obesity. *The Lancet. Gastroenterology & Hepatology*, *2*(10), 747–756. DOI: 10.1016/S2468-1253(17)30147-4 PMID: 28844808

Tremaroli, V., & Bäckhed, F. (2012). Functional interactions between the gut microbiota and host metabolism. *Nature*, *489*(7415), 242–249. DOI: 10.1038/nature11552 PMID: 22972297

Tremaroli, V., Karlsson, F. H., Werling, M., Ståhlman, M., Kovatcheva-Datchary, P., Olbers, T., Fändriks, L., Le Roux, C. W., Nielsen, J., & Bäckhed, F. (2015). Roux-en-Y Gastric Bypass and Vertical Banded Gastroplasty Induce Long-Term Changes on the Human Gut Microbiome Contributing to Fat Mass Regulation. *Cell Metabolism*, *22*(2), 228–238. DOI: 10.1016/j.cmet.2015.07.009 PMID: 26244932

Tripathi, A., Pandey, V. K., Panesar, P. S., Taufeeq, A., Mishra, H., Rustagi, S., Malik, S., Kovács, B., Suthar, T., & Shaikh, A. M. (2024). Fermentative production of vitamin B12 by Propionibacterium shermanii and Pseudomonas denitrificans and its promising health benefits: A review. *Food Science & Nutrition*, *12*(11), 8675–8691. DOI: 10.1002/fsn3.4428 PMID: 39619983

Tsasis, P., & Bains, J. (2008). Management of complex chronic disease: Facing the challenges in the Canadian health-care system. *Health Services Management Research*, *21*(4), 228–235. DOI: 10.1258/hsmr.2008.008001 PMID: 18957400

Tuikhar, N., Keisam, S., Labala, R. K., Ramakrishnan, P., Arunkumar, M. C., Ahmed, G., Biagi, E., & Jeyaram, K. (2019). Comparative analysis of the gut microbiota in centenarians and young adults shows a common signature across genotypically non-related populations. *Mechanisms of Ageing and Development*, *179*, 23–35. DOI: 10.1016/j.mad.2019.02.001 PMID: 30738080

Tun, M. H., Tun, H. M., Mahoney, J. J., Konya, T. B., Guttman, D. S., Becker, A. B., Mandhane, P. J., Turvey, S. E., Subbarao, P., Sears, M. R., Brook, J. R., Lou, W., Takarao, T. K., Scott, J. A., & Kozyrskyj, A. L. (2018). Postnatal exposure to household disinfectants, infant gut microbiota and subsequent risk of overweight in children. *Canadian Medical Association Journal*, *190*(37), E1097–E1107. DOI: 10.1503/cmaj.170809 PMID: 30224442

Turnbaugh, P. J., & Gordon, J. I. (2009). The core gut microbiome, energy balance and obesity. *The Journal of Physiology*, *587*(17), 4153–4158. DOI: 10.1113/jphysiol.2009.174136 PMID: 19491241

Turnbaugh, P. J., Hamady, M., Yatsunenko, T., Cantarel, B. L., Duncan, A., Ley, R. E., Sogin, M. L., Jones, W. J., Roe, B. A., Affourtit, J. P., Egholm, M., Henrissat, B., Heath, A. C., Knight, R., & Gordon, J. I. (2009). A core gut microbiome in obese and lean twins. *Nature*, *457*(7228), 480–484. DOI: 10.1038/nature07540 PMID: 19043404

Turnbaugh, P. J., Ley, R. E., Hamady, M., Fraser-Liggett, C. M., Knight, R., & Gordon, J. I. (2007). The human microbiome project. *Nature*, *449*(7164), 804–810. DOI: 10.1038/nature06244 PMID: 17943116

Turnbaugh, P. J., Ley, R. E., Mahowald, M. A., Magrini, V., Mardis, E. R., & Gordon, J. I. (2006). An obesity-associated gut microbiome with increased capacity for energy harvest. *Nature*, *444*(7122), 1027–1031. DOI: 10.1038/nature05414 PMID: 17183312

Turner, J. R. (2009). Intestinal mucosal barrier function in health and disease. *Nature Reviews. Immunology*, *9*(11), 799–809. DOI: 10.1038/nri2653

Ubeda, C., Taur, Y., Jenq, R. R., Equinda, M. J., Son, T., Samstein, M., Viale, A., Socci, N. D., van den Brink, M. R. M., Kamboj, M., & Pamer, E. G. (2010). Vancomycin-resistant *Enterococcus* domination of intestinal microbiota is enabled by antibiotic treatment in mice and precedes bloodstream invasion in humans. *The Journal of Clinical Investigation*, *120*(12), 4332–4341. DOI: 10.1172/JCI43918 PMID: 21099116

Ulita, N., Kartanegara, A. T., Salsabila, J., Saleh, A., & Queen, Z. (2024). Empathy map gen z towards healthy food: A foodpreneur design strategy. [ATT]. *Aptisi Transactions on Technopreneurship*, *6*(2), 242–253. DOI: 10.34306/att.v6i2.404

Ülker, I., & Yildiran, H. (2018). The effects of bariatric surgery on gut microbiota in patients with obesity: A review of the literature. *Bioscience of Microbiota, Food and Health*, *38*(1), 3–9. DOI: 10.12938/bmfh.18-018 PMID: 30705797

Ullah, H., Arbab, S., Tian, Y., Liu, C. Q., Chen, Y., Qijie, L., Khan, M. I. U., Hassan, I. U., & Li, K. (2023). The gut microbiota–brain axis in neurological disorder. *Frontiers in Neuroscience*, *17*, 1225875. Advance online publication. DOI: 10.3389/fnins.2023.1225875 PMID: 37600019

Utreja, S. (2023). *Unlocking the Power of Next Generation Sequencing for Microbiome Analysis*. State University of New York at Buffalo.

Valdes, A. M., Walter, J., Segal, E., & Spector, T. D. (2018). Role of the gut microbiota in nutrition and health. *BMJ (Clinical Research Ed.)*, *361*, k2179. DOI: 10.1136/bmj.k2179 PMID: 29899036

Valero-Cases, E., Cerdá-Bernad, D., Pastor, J.-J., & Frutos, M.-J. (2020). Non-dairy fermented beverages as potential carriers to ensure probiotics, prebiotics, and bioactive compounds arrival to the gut and their health benefits. *Nutrients*, *12*(6), 1666. DOI: 10.3390/nu12061666 PMID: 32503276

Valitutti, F., Cucchiara, S., & Fasano, A. (2019). Celiac disease and the microbiome. *Nutrients, 11*(10), 2403. DOI: 10.3390/nu11102403 PMID: 31597349

Valladares-Diestra, K. K., de Souza Vandenberghe, L. P., Vieira, S., Goyzueta-Mamani, L. D., de Mattos, P. B. G., Manzoki, M. C., Soccol, V. T., & Soccol, C. R. (2023). The Potential of Xylooligosaccharides as Prebiotics and Their Sustainable Production from Agro-Industrial by-Products. *Foods, 12*(14), 2681. DOI: 10.3390/foods12142681

Vallianou, N., Stratigou, T., Christodoulatos, G. S., & Dalamaga, M. (2019). Understanding the role of the gut microbiome and microbial metabolites in obesity and obesity-associated metabolic disorders: Current evidence and perspectives. *Current Obesity Reports, 8*(3), 317–332. DOI: 10.1007/s13679-019-00352-2 PMID: 31175629

Van den Elsen, L. W., Garssen, J., Burcelin, R., & Verhasselt, V. (2019). Shaping the gut microbiota by breastfeeding: The gateway to allergy prevention? *Frontiers in Pediatrics, 7*, 47. DOI: 10.3389/fped.2019.00047 PMID: 30873394

van der Post, S., Jabbar, K. S., & Hansson, G. C. (2019). Structural weakening of the colonic mucus barrier is an early event in ulcerative colitis pathogenesis. *Gut, 68*(12), 2142–2151. DOI: 10.1136/gutjnl-2018-317571

van Zanten, A. R. (2023). Personalized nutrition therapy in critical illness and convalescence: Moving beyond one-size-fits-all to phenotyping and endotyping. *Current Opinion in Critical Care, 29*(4), 281–285. DOI: 10.1097/MCC.0000000000001060 PMID: 37431268

Vancamelbeke, M., & Vermeire, S. (2017). The intestinal barrier: A fundamental role in health and disease. *Expert Review of Gastroenterology & Hepatology, 11*(9), 821–834. DOI: 10.1080/17474124.2017.1343143 PMID: 28650209

Vangay, P., Johnson, A. J., Ward, T. L., Al-Ghalith, G. A., Shields-Cutler, R. R., Hillmann, B. M., Lucas, S. K., Beura, L. K., Thompson, E. A., Till, L. M., Batres, R., Paw, B., Pergament, S. L., Saenyakul, P., Xiong, M., Kim, A. D., Kim, G., Masopust, D., Martens, E. C., & Knights, D. (2018). US immigration westernizes the human gut microbiome. *Cell, 175*(4), 962–972. DOI: 10.1016/j.cell.2018.10.029 PMID: 30388453

Vanuytsel, T., Tack, J., & Farre, R. (2021). The role of intestinal permeability in gastrointestinal disorders and current methods of evaluation. *Frontiers in Nutrition, 8*, 717925. DOI: 10.3389/fnut.2021.717925

Varshney, N.. (2024). Significance of microbial biomolecules, secondary metabolites, and their impact on the diverse aspects of human health. In *Industrial microbiology and biotechnology: an insight into current trends* (pp. 99–127). Springer. DOI: 10.1007/978-981-97-1912-9_6

Veiga, P., Suez, J., Derrien, M., & Elinav, E. (2020). Moving from probiotics to precision probiotics. *Nature Microbiology*, *5*(7), 878–880. DOI: 10.1038/s41564-020-0721-1

Vera-Santander, V. E., Hernández-Figueroa, R. H., Jiménez-Munguía, M. T., Mani-López, E., & López-Malo, A. (2023). Health benefits of consuming foods with bacterial probiotics, postbiotics, and their metabolites: A review. *Molecules (Basel, Switzerland)*, *28*(3), 1230. DOI: 10.3390/molecules28031230

Verbeke, K. (2018). Nonceliac gluten sensitivity: What is the culprit? *Gastroenterology*, *154*(3), 471–473. DOI: 10.1053/j.gastro.2018.01.013

Verdi, S., Jackson, M. A., Beaumont, M., Bowyer, R. C. E., Bell, J. T., Spector, T. D., & Steves, C. J. (2018). An investigation into physical frailty as a link between the gut microbiome and cognitive health. *Frontiers in Aging Neuroscience*, *10*, 398. DOI: 10.3389/fnagi.2018.00398 PMID: 30564113

Verma, M., ... (2018). Challenges in personalized nutrition and health. In (Vol. 5, pp. 117): Frontiers Media SA. DOI: 10.3389/fnut.2018.00117

Verma, A., Inslicht, S. S., & Bhargava, A. (2024). Gut-brain axis: Role of microbiome, metabolomics, hormones, and stress in mental health disorders. *Cells*, *13*(17), 1436. DOI: 10.3390/cells13171436 PMID: 39273008

Vernocchi, P., Del Chierico, F., & Putignani, L. (2016). Gut microbiota profiling: Metabolomics based approach to unravel compounds affecting human health. *Frontiers in Microbiology*, *7*, 1144. DOI: 10.3389/fmicb.2016.01144

Vernocchi, P., Del Chierico, F., & Putignani, L. (2020). Gut microbiota metabolism and interaction with food components. *International Journal of Molecular Sciences*, *21*(10), 3688. DOI: 10.3390/ijms21103688 PMID: 32456257

Vieira-Silva, S., Falony, G., Belda, E., Nielsen, T., Aron-Wisnewsky, J., Chakaroun, R., Forslund, S. K., Assmann, K., Valles-Colomer, M., Nguyen, T. T. D., Proost, S., Prifti, E., Tremaroli, V., Pons, N., Le Chatelier, E., Andreelli, F., Bastard, J.-P., Coelho, L. P., Galleron, N., & Raes, J. (2020). Statin therapy is associated with lower prevalence of gut microbiota dysbiosis. *Nature*, *581*(7808), 310–315. DOI: 10.1038/s41586-020-2269-x PMID: 32433607

Vijay, J., ... (2025). Precision Nutrition Through Nutritional Informatics: Futuristic Technologies for Health Advancement. In *Exploration of Transformative Technologies in Healthcare 6.0* (pp. 329-360). IGI Global Scientific Publishing.

Vila, A. V., Collij, V., Sanna, S., Sinha, T., Imhann, F., Bourgonje, A. R., Mujagic, Z., Jonkers, D. M. A. E., Masclee, A. A. M., Fu, J., Kurilshikov, A., Gacesa, R., & Weersma, R. K. (2020). Impact of commonly used drugs on the composition and metabolic function of the gut microbiota. *Nature Communications*, *11*(1), 362. DOI: 10.1038/s41467-019-14177-z PMID: 31953381

Vinayamohan, P., Joseph, D., Viju, L. S., Baskaran, S. A., & Venkitanarayanan, K. (2024). Efficacy of probiotics in reducing pathogenic potential of infectious agents. *Fermentation (Basel, Switzerland)*, *10*(12), 599. Advance online publication. DOI: 10.3390/fermentation10120599

Vogtmann, E., Hua, X., Zeller, G., Sunagawa, S., Voigt, A. Y., Hercog, R., Goedert, J. J., Shi, J., Bork, P., & Sinha, R. (2016). Colorectal cancer and the human gut microbiome: Reproducibility with whole-genome shotgun sequencing. *PLoS One*, *11*(5), e0155362. DOI: 10.1371/journal.pone.0155362

Vrieze, A., Van Nood, E., Holleman, F., Salojärvi, J., Kootte, R. S., Bartelsman, J. F., Dallinga-Thie, G. M., Ackermans, M. T., Serlie, M. J., Oozeer, R., Derrien, M., Druesne, A., Van Hylckama Vlieg, J. E., Bloks, V. W., Groen, A. K., Heilig, H. G., Zoetendal, E. G., Stroes, E. S., de Vos, W. M., & Nieuwdorp, M. (2012). Transfer of intestinal microbiota from lean donors increases insulin sensitivity in individuals with metabolic syndrome. *Gastroenterology*, *143*(4), 913–916.e7. DOI: 10.1053/j.gastro.2012.06.031 PMID: 22728514

Waclawiková, B., & El Aidy, S. (2018). Role of microbiota and tryptophan metabolites in the remote effect of intestinal inflammation on brain and depression. *Pharmaceuticals (Basel, Switzerland)*, *11*(3), 63. DOI: 10.3390/ph11030063 PMID: 29941795

Wahlström, A., Sayin, S. I., Marschall, H. U., & Bäckhed, F. (2016). Intestinal Crosstalk between Bile Acids and Microbiota and Its Impact on Host Metabolism. *Cell Metabolism*, *24*(1), 41–50. DOI: 10.1016/j.cmet.2016.05.005 PMID: 27320064

Walker, A. W., Ince, J., Duncan, S. H., Webster, L. M., Holtrop, G., Ze, X., Brown, D., Stares, M. D., Scott, P., Bergerat, A., Louis, P., McIntosh, F., Johnstone, A. M., Lobley, G. E., Parkhill, J., & Flint, H. J. (2011). Dominant and diet-responsive groups of bacteria within the human colonic microbiota. *The ISME Journal*, *5*(2), 220–230. DOI: 10.1038/ismej.2010.118 PMID: 20686513

Walker, W. A. (2017). The importance of appropriate initial bacterial colonization of the intestine in newborn, child, and adult health. *Pediatric Research, 82*(3), 387–395. DOI: 10.1038/pr.2017.111 PMID: 28426649

Wall, R., et al. (2014). Bacterial neuroactive compounds produced by psychobiotics. *Microbial endocrinology: The microbiota-gut-brain axis in health and disease*, 221-239.

Walsh, L. H., Coakley, M., Walsh, A. M., O'Toole, P. W., & Cotter, P. D. (2023). Bioinformatic approaches for studying the microbiome of fermented food. *Critical Reviews in Microbiology, 49*(6), 693–725. DOI: 10.1080/1040841X.2022.2132850 PMID: 36287644

Wang, B. X., Wu, C. M., & Ribbeck, K. (2021). Home, sweet home: How mucus accommodates our microbiota. *The FEBS Journal, 288*(6), 1789–1799. DOI: 10.1111/febs.15504

Wang, C., Wang, H., & Li, Y.. (2024). Factors influencing university students' behavioral intention to use generative artificial intelligence: Integrating the theory of planned behavior and AI literacy. *International Journal of Human-Computer Interaction*, •••, 1–23. DOI: 10.1080/10447318.2024.2383033

Wang, F., Baden, M. Y., Guasch-Ferré, M., Wittenbecher, C., Li, J., Li, Y., Sun, Q., Rimm, E. B., Manson, J. E., Willett, W. C., Hu, F. B., & Qi, L. (2022a). Plasma metabolite profiles related to plant-based diets and the risk of type 2 diabetes. *Diabetologia, 65*(7), 1119–1132. DOI: 10.1007/s00125-022-05692-8 PMID: 35391539

Wang, F., Ugai, T., Haruki, K., Wan, Y., Akimoto, N., Arima, K., Zhong, R., Twombly, T. S., Wu, K., Yin, K., Zhang, X., Giovannucci, E. L., Willett, W. C., & Ogino, S. (2022b). Healthy and unhealthy plant-based diets in relation to the incidence of colorectal cancer overall and by molecular subtypes. *Clinical and Translational Medicine, 12*(8), e893. DOI: 10.1002/ctm2.893 PMID: 35998061

Wang, J., Haq, A. U., Afzal, N., Khan, S., Alsolai, H., Alanazi, S. M., & Alshammari, W. M. (2025). Developing an innovative lung cancer detection model for accurate diagnosis in AI healthcare systems. *Scientific Reports, 15*(1), 22945. Advance online publication. DOI: 10.1038/s41598-025-03960-2 PMID: 40592932

Wang, J., Qie, J., Zhu, D., Zhang, X., Zhang, Q., Xu, Y., Wang, Y., Mi, K., Pei, Y., Liu, Y., Jia, G., & Liu, X. (2022). The landscape in the gut microbiome of long-lived families reveals new insights on longevity and aging – relevant neural and immune function. *Gut Microbes, 14*(1), e2107288. DOI: 10.1080/19490976.2022.2107288 PMID: 35939616

Wang, J., Zhu, N., Su, X., Gao, Y., & Yang, R. (2023). Gut-microbiota-derived metabolites maintain gut and systemic immune homeostasis. *Cells*, *12*(5), 793. DOI: 10.3390/cells12050793 PMID: 36899929

Wang, L., Wang, X., Zhang, G., Ma, Y., Zhang, Q., Li, Z., Ran, J., Hou, X., Geng, Y., Yang, Z., Feng, S., Li, C., & Zhao, X. (2021). The impact of pelvic radiotherapy on the gut microbiome and its role in radiation-induced diarrhoea: A systematic review. *Radiation Oncology (London, England)*, *16*(1), 187. Advance online publication. DOI: 10.1186/s13014-021-01899-y PMID: 34563216

Wang, L., Zhang, W., Wu, X., Liang, X., Cao, L., Zhai, J., Yang, Y., Chen, Q., Liu, H., Zhang, J., Ding, Y., Zhu, F., & Tang, J. (2022). MIAOME: Human microbiome affect the host epigenome. *Computational and Structural Biotechnology Journal*, *20*, 2455–2463. DOI: 10.1016/j.csbj.2022.05.024 PMID: 35664224

Wang, Q., Wang, K., Wu, W., Giannoulatou, E., Ho, J. W. K., & Li, L. (2019). Host and microbiome multi-omics integration: Applications and methodologies. *Biophysical Reviews*, *11*(1), 55–65. DOI: 10.1007/s12551-018-0491-7 PMID: 30627872

Wang, Q., Xu, G., Yan, O., Wang, S., & Wang, X. (2025). Radiation-induced injury and the gut microbiota: Insights from a microbial perspective. *Therapeutic Advances in Gastroenterology*, *18*, 17562848251347347. Advance online publication. DOI: 10.1177/17562848251347347 PMID: 40535532

Wang, S. P., Rubio, L. A., Duncan, S. H., Donachie, G. E., Holtrop, G., Lo, G., Farquharson, F. M., Wagner, J., Parkhill, J., Louis, P., Walker, A. W., & Flint, H. J. (2020). Pivotal roles for pH, lactate, and lactate-utilizing bacteria in the stability of a human colonic microbial ecosystem. *mSystems*, *5*(5), 00645–00620. DOI: 10.1128/mSystems.00645-20 PMID: 32900872

Wang, S., Walton, K. D., & Gumucio, D. L. (2019). Signals and forces shaping organogenesis of the small intestine. In *Current Topics in Developmental Biology* (Vol. 132, pp. 31–65). Academic Press., DOI: 10.1016/bs.ctdb.2018.12.001

Wang, X., Zeng, H., Li, L., Fang, Z., Xu, L., Shi, W., Li, J., Qian, J., Tan, X., Li, J., Qian, Y., & Xie, L. (2022). Personalized nutrition intervention improves nutritional status and quality of life of colorectal cancer survivors in the community: A randomized controlled trial. *Nutrition (Burbank, Los Angeles County, Calif.)*, *103-104*, 11. DOI: 10.1016/j.nut.2022.111835

Wang, Y., Dilidaxi, D., Wu, Y., Sailike, J., Sun, X., & Nabi, X. (2020). Composite probiotics alleviate type 2 diabetes by regulating intestinal microbiota and inducing GLP-1 secretion in db/db mice. *Biomedicine and Pharmacotherapy*, *125*, 109914. DOI: 10.1016/j.biopha.2020.109914 PMID: 32035395

Wang, Y., Liu, L., Jin, Z., & Zhang, D. (2021). Microbial cell factories for green production of vitamins. *Frontiers in Bioengineering and Biotechnology*, *9*, 661562. DOI: 10.3389/fbioe.2021.661562 PMID: 34222212

Wang, Y., Nie, Y., Wang, P., Li, Y., Ma, Q., & Yu, D. (2022). A novel bacterial imprinted polymers-electrochemiluminescent sensor for Lactobacillus salivarius detection. *Sensors and Actuators. B, Chemical*, *358*, 131467. DOI: 10.1016/j.snb.2022.131467

Wang, Y., Wu, Y., Wang, Y., Xu, H., Mei, X., Yu, D., & Li, W. (2017). Antioxidant properties of probiotic bacteria. *Nutrients*, *9*(5), 521. DOI: 10.3390/nu9050521

Wang, Z., Klipfell, E., Bennett, B. J., Koeth, R., Levison, B. S., Dugar, B., Feldstein, A. E., Britt, E. B., Fu, X., Chung, Y. M., Wu, Y., Schauer, P., Smith, J. D., Allayee, H., Tang, W. H., DiDonato, J. A., Lusis, A. J., & Hazen, S. L. (2011). Gut flora metabolism of phosphatidylcholine promotes cardiovascular disease. *Nature*, *472*(7341), 57–63. DOI: 10.1038/nature09922 PMID: 21475195

Wani, S. H., Choudhary, M., Barmukh, R., Bagaria, P. K., Samantara, K., Razzaq, A., & Kumar, A. (2022). Molecular mechanisms, genetic mapping, and genome editing for insect pest resistance in field crops. *Theoretical and Applied Genetics*, *135*(12), 3875–3901. DOI: 10.1007/s00122-022-04060-9 PMID: 35267056

Wan, Z., Zheng, J., Zhu, Z., Sang, L., Zhu, J., Luo, S., Zhao, Y., Wang, R., Zhang, Y., Hao, K., Chen, L., Du, J., Kan, J., & He, H. (2022). Intermediate role of gut microbiota in vitamin B nutrition and its influences on human health. *Frontiers in Nutrition*, *9*, 1031502. DOI: 10.3389/fnut.2022.1031502 PMID: 36583209

Wardman, J. F., Bains, R. K., Rahfeld, P., & Withers, S. G. (2022). Carbohydrate-active enzymes (CAZymes) in the gut microbiome. *Nature Reviews. Microbiology*, *20*(9), 542–556. DOI: 10.1038/s41579-022-00712-1 PMID: 35347288

Warren, C. M., Jiang, J., & Gupta, R. S. (2020). Epidemiology and burden of food allergy. *Current Allergy and Asthma Reports*, *20*(2), 6. DOI: 10.1007/s11882-020-0898-7

Watson, H., Mitra, S., Croden, F. C., Taylor, M., Wood, H. M., Perry, S. L., & Hold, G. L. (2018). A randomised trial of the effect of omega-3 polyunsaturated fatty acid supplements on the human intestinal microbiota. *Gut*, *67*(11), 1974–1983. DOI: 10.1136/gutjnl-2017-314968 PMID: 28951525

Watts, G., Youens-Clark, K., Slepian, M. J., Wolk, D. M., Oshiro, M. M., Metzger, G. S., Dhingra, D., Cranmer, L. D., & Hurwitz, B. L. (2017). 16S rRNA gene sequencing on a benchtop sequencer: Accuracy for identification of clinically important bacteria. *Journal of Applied Microbiology*, *123*(6), 1584–1596. DOI: 10.1111/jam.13590 PMID: 28940494

Weersma, R. K., Zhernakova, A., & Fu, J. (2020). Interaction between drugs and the gut microbiome. *Gut*, *69*(8), 1510–1519. DOI: 10.1136/gutjnl-2019-320204 PMID: 32409589

Wei, C., Nawi, H. M., & Naeem, S. B. (2024). The uses and gratifications (U&G) model for understanding fake news sharing behavior on social media. *Journal of Academic Librarianship*, *50*(5), 102938. DOI: 10.1016/j.acalib.2024.102938

Wei, L. Q., Cheong, I. H., Yang, G. H., Li, X. G., Kozlakidis, Z., Ding, L., Liu, N. N., & Wang, H. (2021). The application of high-throughput technologies for the study of microbiome and cancer. *Frontiers in Genetics*, *12*, 699793. DOI: 10.3389/fgene.2021.699793 PMID: 34394190

Weir, T. L. (2023). Grand challenges: Actualizing the potential of the gut microbiome to address global nutrition challenges. *Frontiers in Microbiomes*, *2*, 1146827. Advance online publication. DOI: 10.3389/frmbi.2023.1146827

Wei, Y., Shen, F., Song, H., Zhao, R., Feng, W., Pan, Y., Li, X., Yu, H., Familiari, G., Relucenti, M., Aschner, M., Shi, H., Chen, R., Nie, G., & Chen, H. (2024). The challenge and opportunity of gut microbiota-targeted nanomedicine for colorectal cancer therapy. *iMeta*, *3*(4), e213. DOI: 10.1002/imt2.213 PMID: 39135695

Whelan, K., Alexander, M., Gaïani, C., Lunken, G., Holmes, A., Staudacher, H. M., & Whelan, K. (2024). Design and reporting of prebiotic and probiotic clinical trials in the context of diet and the gut microbiome. *Nature Microbiology*, *9*(11), 2785–2796. DOI: 10.1038/s41564-024-01831-6 PMID: 39478082

Whitman, J. A., Doherty, L. A., Pantoja-Feliciano de Goodfellow, I. G., Racicot, K., Anderson, D. J., Kensil, K., Karl, J. P., Gibson, G. R., & Soares, J. W. (2024). In vitro fermentation shows polyphenol and fiber blends have an additive beneficial effect on gut microbiota states. *Nutrients*, *16*(8), 1159. DOI: 10.3390/nu16081159 PMID: 38674850

Wiersinga, W. J., Rhodes, A., Cheng, A. C., Peacock, S. J., & Prescott, H. C. (2020). Pathophysiology, transmission, diagnosis, and treatment of coronavirus disease 2019 (COVID-19): A review. *Journal of the American Medical Association*, *324*(8), 782–793. DOI: 10.1001/jama.2020.12839

Wikoff, W. R., Anfora, A. T., Liu, J., Schultz, P. G., Lesley, S. A., Peters, E. C., & Siuzdak, G. (2009). Metabolomics analysis reveals large effects of gut microflora on mammalian blood metabolites. *Proceedings of the National Academy of Sciences of the United States of America, 106(10)*, 3698–3703. DOI: 10.1073/pnas.0812874106

Wilkinson, J. E., Franzosa, E. A., Everett, C., Li, C., Bae, S., Berzansky, I., Bhosle, A., Bjørnevik, K., Brennan, C. A., Cao, Y. G., Chun, E., Clay, S. L., Fenn, K., Hall, A. B., Lennon, D., Lobel, L., Ma, S., Ma, W., Maharjan, S., & Huttenhower, C. (2021). A framework for microbiome science in public health. *Nature Medicine, 27*(5), 766–774. DOI: 10.1038/s41591-021-01258-0 PMID: 33820996

Williamson, G., & Clifford, M. N. (2017). Colonic metabolites of berry polyphenols: The missing link to biological activity? *British Journal of Nutrition, 118*(4), 317–328. DOI: 10.1017/S0007114517001864 PMID: 20955650

Wilmanski, T., Rappaport, N., Diener, C., Gibbons, S. M., & Price, N. D. (2021). From taxonomy to metabolic output: What factors define gut microbiome health? *Gut Microbes, 13*(1), 1907270. DOI: 10.1080/19490976.2021.1907270

Windey, K., De Preter, V., & Verbeke, K. (2012). Relevance of protein fermentation to gut health. *Molecular Nutrition & Food Research, 56*(1), 184–196. DOI: 10.1002/mnfr.201100542 PMID: 22121108

Wong, C. C., & Yu, J. (2023). Gut microbiota in colorectal cancer development and therapy. *Nature Reviews. Clinical Oncology, 20*(7), 429–452. DOI: 10.1038/s41571-023-00766-x PMID: 37169888

Wong, G. W.-K. (2024). Food allergies around the world. *Frontiers in Nutrition, 11*, 1391631. DOI: 10.3389/fnut.2024.1373110

Wu, L., Xie, X., Li, Y., Liang, T., Zhong, H., Yang, L., Li, Y., & Liu, S. (2022). Gut microbiota as an antioxidant system in centenarians associated with high antioxidant activities of gut-resident *Lactobacillus. NPJ Biofilms and Microbiomes, 8*(1), 102. DOI: 10.1038/s41522-022-00366-0

Wu, L., Zeng, T., Zinellu, A., Rubino, S., Kelvin, D. J., & Carru, C. (2019). A cross-sectional study of compositional and functional profiles of gut microbiota in Sardinian centenarians. *mSystems, 4*(4), e00325–e19. DOI: 10.1128/mSystems.00325-19 PMID: 31289141

Wysocki, O., Davies, J. K., Vigo, M., Armstrong, A. C., Landers, D., Lee, R., & Freitas, A. (2023). Assessing the communication gap between AI models and healthcare professionals: Explainability, utility and trust in AI-driven clinical decision-making. *Artificial Intelligence, 316*, 103839. DOI: 10.1016/j.artint.2022.103839

Xavier-Santos, D., Padilha, M., Fabiano, G. A., Vinderola, G., Gomes Cruz, A., Sivieri, K., & Costa Antunes, A. E. (2022). Evidences and perspectives of the use of probiotics, prebiotics, synbiotics, and postbiotics as adjuvants for prevention and treatment of COVID-19: A bibliometric analysis and systematic review. *Trends in Food Science & Technology*, *120*, 174–192. DOI: 10.1016/j.tifs.2021.12.033

Xiaoli, L., Figler, H. M., Banerjee, K. G., Hayes, C. S., Dudley, E. G., & Moxley, R. A. (2018). Non-pathogenic *Escherichia coli* enhance Stx2a production of *E. coli* O157:H7 through both bamA-dependent and independent mechanisms. *Frontiers in Microbiology*, *9*, 1325. DOI: 10.3389/fmicb.2018.01325

Xiao, Y., Dong, J., Yin, Z., Wu, Q., Zhou, Y., & Zhou, X. (2018). Procyanidin B2 protects against d-galactose-induced mimetic aging in mice: Metabolites and microbiome analysis. *Food and Chemical Toxicology*, *119*, 141–149. DOI: 10.1016/j.fct.2018.05.017 PMID: 29751077

Xia, T., Teng, K., Liu, Y., Guo, Y., Huang, F., Tahir, M., Wang, T., & Zhong, J. (2023). A novel two-component bacteriocin, acidicin P, and its key residues for inhibiting Listeria monocytogenes by targeting the cell membrane. *Microbiology Spectrum*, *11*(4), e05210–e05222. DOI: 10.1128/spectrum.05210-22

Xie, L. W., Cai, S., Lu, H. Y., Tang, F. L., Zhu, R. Q., Tian, Y., & Li, M. (2024). Microbiota-derived I3A protects the intestine against radiation injury by activating AhR/IL-10/Wnt signaling and enhancing the abundance of probiotics. *Gut Microbes*, *16*(1), 2347722. Advance online publication. DOI: 10.1080/19490976.2024.2347722 PMID: 38706205

Xu, H. Y., Li, Q. C., Zhou, W. J., Zhang, H. B., Chen, Z. X., Peng, N., Gong, S. Y., Liu, B., & Zeng, F. (2023). Anti-oxidative and anti-aging effects of probiotic fermented ginseng by modulating gut microbiota and metabolites in Caenorhabditis elegans. *Plant Foods for Human Nutrition (Dordrecht, Netherlands)*, *78*(2), 320–328. DOI: 10.1007/s11130-023-01055-9 PMID: 36947370

Xu, J., & Zhao, F. (2018). Single-cell metagenomics: Challenges and applications. *Protein & Cell*, *9*(5), 501–510. DOI: 10.1007/s13238-018-0544-5

Xu, Y., Wang, M., Bao, L., Cheng, Z., & Li, X. (2024). A cross-sectional study based on the comprehensive model of information seeking: Which factors influence health information-seeking behavior in patients with periodontitis. *BMC Oral Health*, *24*(1), 1307. DOI: 10.1186/s12903-024-05068-x PMID: 39468496

Yang, D., Wang, Z., Chen, Y., Guo, Q., & Dong, Y. (2023). Interactions between gut microbes and NLRP3 inflammasome in the gut-brain axis. *Computational and Structural Biotechnology Journal, 21*, 2215–2227. DOI: 10.1016/j.csbj.2023.03.017 PMID: 37035548

Yang, J., & Yu, J. (2018). The association of diet, gut microbiota and colorectal cancer: What we eat may imply what we get. *Protein & Cell, 9*(5), 474–487. DOI: 10.1007/s13238-018-0543-6 PMID: 29713943

Yang, K., Li, G., Li, Q., Wang, W., Zhao, X., Shao, N., Qiu, H., Liu, J., Xu, L., & Zhao, J. (2025). Distribution of gut microbiota across intestinal segments and their impact on human physiological and pathological processes. *Cell & Bioscience, 15*(1), 47. Advance online publication. DOI: 10.1186/s13578-025-01385-y PMID: 40241220

Yang, S., Liu, H., & Liu, Y. (2025). Advances in intestinal epithelium and gut microbiota interaction. *Frontiers in Microbiology, 16*, 1499202. Advance online publication. DOI: 10.3389/fmicb.2025.1499202 PMID: 40104591

Yan, K. S., Janda, C. Y., Chang, J., Zheng, G. X. Y., Larkin, K. A., Luca, V. C., Chia, L. A., Mah, A. T., Han, A., Terry, J. M., Ootani, A., Roelf, K., Lee, M., Yuan, J., Li, X., Bolen, C. R., Wilhelmy, J., Davies, P. S., Ueno, H., & Kuo, C. J. (2017). Non-equivalence of Wnt and R-spondin ligands during Lgr5+ intestinal stem-cell self-renewal. *Nature, 545*(7653), 238–242. DOI: 10.1038/nature22313

Yao, S., Zhou, C., Li, S., Li, Y., Shen, C., Tao, Y., & Li, X. (2024). Microbial diversity across tea varieties and ecological niches: Correlating tea polyphenol contents with stress resistance. *Frontiers in Microbiology, 15*, 1439630. DOI: 10.3389/fmicb.2024.1439630 PMID: 39252833

Yassine, F., Najm, A., & Bilen, M. (2025). The role of probiotics, prebiotics, and synbiotics in the treatment of inflammatory bowel diseases: An overview of recent clinical trials. *Frontiers in Systems Biology, 5*, 1561047. DOI: 10.3389/fsysb.2025.1561047

Yatsunenko, T., Rey, F. E., Manary, M. J., Trehan, I., Dominguez-Bello, M. G., Contreras, M., Magris, M., Hidalgo, G., Baldassano, R. N., Anokhin, A. P., Heath, A. C., Warner, B., Reeder, J., Kuczynski, J., Caporaso, J. G., Lozupone, C. A., Lauber, C., Clemente, J. C., Knights, D., & Gordon, J. I. (2012). Human gut microbiome viewed across age and geography. *Nature, 486*(7402), 222–227. DOI: 10.1038/nature11053 PMID: 22699611

Ye, D., He, J., & He, X. (2024). The role of bile acid receptor TGR5 in regulating inflammatory signalling. *Scandinavian Journal of Immunology*, *99*(4), e13361. DOI: 10.1111/sji.13361 PMID: 38307496

Yeşilyurt, N., Yılmaz, B., Ağagündüz, D., & Capasso, R. (2021). Involvement of probiotics and postbiotics in the immune system modulation. *Biologics (Basel, Switzerland)*, *1*(2), 89–110. DOI: 10.3390/biologics1020006

Ye, X., Li, H., Anjum, K., Zhong, X., Miao, S., Zheng, G., Liu, W., & Li, L. (2022). Dual role of indoles derived from intestinal microbiota on human health. *Frontiers in Immunology*, *13*, 903526. DOI: 10.3389/fimmu.2022.903526 PMID: 35784338

Yim, D., Khuntia, J., Parameswaran, V., & Meyers, A. (2024). Preliminary evidence of the use of generative AI in health care clinical services: Systematic narrative review. *JMIR Medical Informatics*, *12*(1), e52073. DOI: 10.2196/52073 PMID: 38506918

Yin, Y.-N., Yu, Q.-F., Fu, N., Liu, X.-W., & Lu, F.-G. (2010). Effects of four bifidobacteria on obesity in high-fat diet induced rats. *World Journal of Gastroenterology*, *16*(27), 3394–3401. DOI: 10.3748/wjg.v16.i27.3394 PMID: 20632441

Yoha, K. S., Nida, S., Dutta, S., Moses, J. A., & Anandharamakrishnan, C. (2022). Targeted delivery of probiotics: Perspectives on research and commercialization. *Probiotics and Antimicrobial Proteins*, *14*(1), 15–48. DOI: 10.1007/s12602-021-09791-7

Yoo, S., Jung, S. C., Kwak, K., & Kim, J. S. (2024). The role of prebiotics in modulating gut microbiota: Implications for human health. *International Journal of Molecular Sciences*, *25*(9), 4834. DOI: 10.3390/ijms25094834 PMID: 38732060

Yuan, K.-H., Bentler, P. M., & Zhang, W. (2005). The effect of skewness and kurtosis on mean and covariance structure analysis: The univariate case and its multivariate implication. *Sociological Methods & Research*, *34*(2), 240–258. DOI: 10.1177/0049124105280200

Yuan, P.. (2020). Microbial production of vitamins. In *Systems and synthetic biotechnology for production of nutraceuticals* (pp. 159–187). Springer.

Yu, C., Liu, S., Chen, L., Shen, J., Niu, Y., Wang, T., Zhang, W., & Fu, L. (2019). Effect of exercise and butyrate supplementation on microbiota composition and lipid metabolism. *The Journal of Endocrinology*, *243*(2), 125–135. DOI: 10.1530/JOE-19-0122 PMID: 31454784

Yunes, R. A., Poluektova, E. U., Vasileva, E. V., Odorskaya, M. V., Marsova, M. V., Kovalev, G. I., & Danilenko, V. N. (2020). A multi-strain potential probiotic formulation of GABA-producing Lactobacillus plantarum 90sk and Bifidobacterium adolescentis 150 with antidepressant effects. *Probiotics and Antimicrobial Proteins*, *12*(3), 973–979. DOI: 10.1007/s12602-019-09601-1

Yu, X., Wu, X., Qiu, L., Wang, D., Gan, M., Chen, X., Wei, H., & Xu, F. (2015). Analysis of the intestinal microbial community structure of healthy and long-living elderly residents in Gaotian Village of Liuyang City. *Applied Microbiology and Biotechnology*, *99*(19), 9085–9095. DOI: 10.1007/s00253-015-6888-3 PMID: 26298698

Yu, Y., Zhang, J., Wang, J., & Sun, B. (2021). MicroRNAs: The novel mediators for nutrient-modulating biological functions. *Trends in Food Science & Technology*, *114*, 167–175. DOI: 10.1016/j.tifs.2021.05.028

Zalila-Kolsi, I., Dhieb, D., Osman, H. A., & Mekideche, H. (2025). The Gut microbiota and colorectal cancer: Understanding the link and exploring therapeutic interventions. *Biology (Basel)*, *14*(3), 251. DOI: 10.3390/biology14030251 PMID: 40136508

Zang, T., Han, L., Lu, Z., Tan, L., Liang, D., Shen, X., Liao, X., Liu, Y., Ren, H., & Sun, J. (2024). The History and Prediction of Prebiotics and Postbiotics: A Patent Analysis. *Nutrients*, *16*(3), 380. DOI: 10.3390/nu16030380

Zawistowska-Rojek, A., & Zaręba, D. (2020). Food and supplement sources of probiotics and prebiotics. *Critical Reviews in Food Science and Nutrition*, *60*(1), 1–18. DOI: 10.1080/10408398.2019.1572683 PMID: 30277800

Zeb, F., Osaili, T., Obaid, R. S., Naja, F., Radwan, H., Cheikh Ismail, L., Hasan, H., Hashim, M., Alam, I., Sehar, B., & Faris, M. E. (2023). Gut Microbiota and Time-Restricted Feeding/Eating: A Targeted Biomarker and Approach in Precision Nutrition. *Nutrients*, *15*(2), 259. DOI: 10.3390/nu15020259 PMID: 36678130

Zechner, E. L., & Kienesberger, S. (2024). Microbiota-derived small molecule genotoxins: Host interactions and ecological impact in the gut ecosystem. *Gut Microbes*, *16*(1), 2430423. DOI: 10.1080/19490976.2024.2430423 PMID: 39558480

Zeevi, D., Korem, T., Zmora, N., Israeli, D., Rothschild, D., Weinberger, A., Ben-Yacov, O., Lador, D., Avnit-Sagi, T., Lotan-Pompan, M., Suez, J., Mahdi, J. A., Matot, E., Malka, G., Kosower, N., Rein, M., Zilberman-Schapira, G., Dohnalová, L., Pevsner-Fischer, M., & Segal, E. (2015). Personalized nutrition by prediction of glycemic responses. *Cell*, *163*(5), 1079–1094. DOI: 10.1016/j.cell.2015.11.001 PMID: 26590418

Zempleni, J., Chew, Y. C., Hassan, Y. I., & Wijeratne, S. S. (2008). Epigenetic regulation of chromatin structure and gene function by biotin. *Nutrition Reviews*, *66*(Suppl 1), S46–S48. DOI: 10.1111/j.1753-4887.2008.00073.x PMID: 18673490

Zepeda-Rivera, M., Minot, S. S., Bouzek, H., Wu, H., Blanco-Míguez, A., Manghi, P., Jones, D. S., LaCourse, K. D., Wu, Y., McMahon, E. F., Park, S.-N., Lim, Y. K., Kempchinsky, A. G., Willis, A. D., Cotton, S. L., Yost, S. C., Sicinska, E., Kook, J.-K., Dewhirst, F. E., & Johnston, C. D. (2024). A distinct Fusobacterium nucleatum clade dominates the colorectal cancer niche. *Nature*, *628*(8007), 424–432. DOI: 10.1038/s41586-024-07182-w PMID: 38509359

Zevallos, V. F., Raker, V., Tenzer, S., Jimenez-Calvente, C., Ashfaq-Khan, M., Rüssel, N., Pickert, G., Schild, H., Steinbrink, K., & Schuppan, D. (2017). Nutritional wheat amylase-trypsin inhibitors promote intestinal inflammation via activation of myeloid cells. *Gastroenterology*, *152*(5), 1100–1113. DOI: 10.1053/j.gastro.2016.12.006

Zhang, N., Xu, Y., Lu, Q., Zhu, L., An, R., Zhou, X., Wang, Y., Ma, Y., Deng, H., Guo, H., Wang, L., Sun, J., Bo, H., & Wang, X. (2024). Exploring the behavioral intentions of PICC-related thrombosis prevention in breast cancer patients undergoing chemotherapy: A qualitative study based on theory of planned behavior. *Supportive Care in Cancer*, *32*(10), 1–13. DOI: 10.1007/s00520-024-08827-2 PMID: 39235516

Zhang, P. (2022). Influence of Foods and Nutrition on the Gut Microbiome and Implications for Intestinal Health. *International Journal of Molecular Sciences*, *23*(17), 9588. DOI: 10.3390/ijms23179588 PMID: 36076980

Zhang, P.. (2022). Influence of foods and nutrition on the gut microbiome and implications for intestinal health. *Frontiers in Nutrition*, *9*, 833968. DOI: 10.3389/fnut.2022.833968 PMID: 36076980

Zhang, S. (2023). Artificial intelligence and applications in structural and material engineering. Highlights in Science. *Engineering and Technology*, *75*, 240–248. DOI: 10.54097/9qknfc57

Zhang, S.-M., & Huang, S.-L. (2023). The commensal anaerobe Veillonella dispar reprograms its lactate metabolism and short-chain fatty acid production during the stationary phase. *Microbiology Spectrum*, *11*(2), e03558–e03522. DOI: 10.1128/spectrum.03558-22 PMID: 36975840

Zhang, W., Sadeghi, A., Karaca, A. C., Zhang, J., & Jafari, S. M. (2024). Carbohydrate polymer-based carriers for colon targeted delivery of probiotics. *Critical Reviews in Food Science and Nutrition*, *64*(33), 12759–12779. DOI: 10.1080/10408398.2023.2257321

Zhang, Y., Thompson, K. N., Branck, T., Yan Yan, , Nguyen, L. H., Franzosa, E. A., & Huttenhower, C. (2021). Metatranscriptomics for the human microbiome and microbial community functional profiling. *Annual Review of Biomedical Data Science*, *4*(1), 279–311. DOI: 10.1146/annurev-biodatasci-031121-103035 PMID: 34465175

Zhao, L., Zhang, F., Ding, X., Wu, G., Lam, Y. Y., Wang, X., & Zhao, Y. (2018). Gut bacteria selectively promoted by dietary fibers alleviate type 2 diabetes. *Science*, *359*(6380), 1151–1156. DOI: 10.1126/science.aao5774 PMID: 29590046

Zhao, Y., Wang, C., & Goel, A. (2021). Role of gut microbiota in epigenetic regulation of colorectal Cancer. *Biochimica et Biophysica Acta (BBA)-. Revisiones en Cáncer*, *1875*(1), 188490. PMID: 33321173

Zheng, P., Zhang, F., Wang, K., Zhang, W., Li, Y., Sun, Y., Sun, X., Li, C., Dong, B., Wang, L., & Xu, L. (2021). Smart Biosensors and Intelligent Devices for Salivary Biomarker Detection. *Trends in Analytical Chemistry*, *140*, 116281. DOI: 10.1016/j.trac.2021.116281

Zhen, J., Zhou, Z., He, M., Han, H.-X., Lv, E.-H., Wen, P.-B., Liu, X., Wang, Y.-T., Cai, X.-C., Tian, J.-Q., Zhang, M.-Y., Xiao, L., & Kang, X.-X. (2023). The gut microbial metabolite trimethylamine N-oxide and cardiovascular diseases. *Frontiers in Endocrinology*, *14*, 1085041. DOI: 10.3389/fendo.2023.1085041 PMID: 36824355

Zhernakova, A., Elbers, C. C., Ferwerda, B., & Oosting, M. (2010). Evolutionary and functional analysis of celiac risk loci reveals SH2B3 as a protective factor against bacterial infection. *American Journal of Human Genetics*, *86*(6), 970–977. DOI: 10.1016/j.ajhg.2010.05.004

Zhernakova, A., Kurilshikov, A., Bonder, M. J., Tigchelaar, E. F., Schirmer, M., Vatanen, T., Mujagic, Z., Vila, A. V., Falony, G., Vieira-Silva, S., Wang, J., Imhann, F., Brandsma, E., Jankipersadsing, S. A., Joossens, M., Cenit, M. C., Deelen, P., Swertz, M. A., Weersma, R. K., & Fu, J. (2016). Population-based metagenomics analysis reveals markers for gut microbiome composition and diversity. *Science*, *352*(6285), 565–569. DOI: 10.1126/science.aad3369 PMID: 27126040

Zhong, C., Qu, C., Wang, B., Liang, S., & Zeng, B. (2017). Probiotics for preventing and treating small intestinal bacterial overgrowth: A meta-analysis and systematic review of current evidence. *Journal of Clinical Gastroenterology*, *51*(4), 300–311. DOI: 10.1097/MCG.0000000000000814 PMID: 28267052

Zhong, J.-G., Lan, W.-T., Feng, Y.-Q., Li, Y.-H., Shen, Y.-Y., Gong, J.-H., Zou, Z., & Hou, X. (2023). Associations between dysbiosis gut microbiota and changes of neurotransmitters and short-chain fatty acids in valproic acid model rats. *Frontiers in Physiology*, *14*, 1077821. DOI: 10.3389/fphys.2023.1077821 PMID: 37035670

Zhou, X., et al. (2019). Early-life food nutrition, microbiota maturation and immune development shape life-long health. *Critical reviews in food science and nutrition, 59*(sup1), S30-S38.

Zhou, H., Yuan, Y., Wang, H., Xiang, W., Li, S., Zheng, H., Wen, Y., Ming, Y., Chen, L., & Zhou, J. (2021). Gut microbiota: A potential target for cancer interventions. *Cancer Management and Research, 13*, 8281–8296. DOI: 10.2147/CMAR.S328249 PMID: 34764691

Zhou, L., Hörmann, S., & Schuppan, D. (2017). Abrogation of immunogenic properties of gliadin peptides through transamination by microbial transglutaminase is acyl-acceptor dependent. *Journal of Agricultural and Food Chemistry*, *65*(34), 7542–7552. DOI: 10.1021/acs.jafc.7b02557

Zhou, M., Fan, Y., Xu, L., Yu, Z., Wang, S., Xu, H., Zhang, J., Zhang, L., Liu, W., Wu, L., Yu, J., Yao, H., Wang, J., & Gao, R. (2023). Microbiome and tryptophan metabolomics analysis in adolescent depression: Roles of the gut microbiota in the regulation of tryptophan-derived neurotransmitters and behaviors in human and mice. *Microbiome*, *11*(1), 145. DOI: 10.1186/s40168-023-01589-9 PMID: 37386523

Zhou, M., Huang, Z., Ma, Z., Chen, J., Lin, S., Yang, X., & Xu, X. (2025). The next frontier in antibody-drug conjugates: Challenges and opportunities in cancer and autoimmune therapy. *Cancer Drug Resistance (Alhambra, Calif.)*, *8*(1), 34–52. DOI: 10.20517/cdr.2025.49 PMID: 40843358

Zimmermann, M. B., Chassard, C., Rohner, F., N'Goran, E. K., Nindjin, C., Dostal, A., Utzinger, J., Ghattas, H., Lacroix, C., & Hurrell, R. F. (2010). The effects of iron fortification on the gut microbiota in African children: A randomized controlled trial. *The American Journal of Clinical Nutrition*, *92*(6), 1406–1415. DOI: 10.3945/ajcn.110.004564 PMID: 20962160

Zimmermann, P. (2023). The immunological interplay between vaccination and the intestinal microbiota. *NPJ Vaccines*, *8*(1), 24. DOI: 10.1038/s41541-023-00627-9

Zinöcker, M. K., & Lindseth, I. A. (2018). The western diet–microbiome-host interaction and its role in metabolic disease. *Nutrients*, *10*(3), 365. DOI: 10.3390/nu10030365 PMID: 29562591

Zmora, N. (2019). *Microbiome-based personalized interventions*. The Weizmann Institute of Science.

Zmora, N., Suez, J., & Elinav, E. (2019). You are what you eat: Diet, health and the gut microbiota. *Nature Reviews. Gastroenterology & Hepatology*, *16*(1), 35–56. DOI: 10.1038/s41575-018-0061-2 PMID: 30262901

Zmora, N., Zeevi, D., Korem, T., Segal, E., & Elinav, E. (2016). Taking it Personally: Personalized Utilization of the Human Microbiome in Health and Disease. *Cell Host & Microbe*, *19*(1), 12–20. DOI: 10.1016/j.chom.2015.12.016 PMID: 26764593

Zmora, N., Zeevi, D., Korem, T., Segal, E., & Elinav, E. (2019). Personalized gut mucosal colonization resistance to empiric probiotics is associated with unique host and microbiome features. *Cell*, *174*(6), 1388–1405.e21. DOI: 10.1016/j.cell.2018.08.041 PMID: 30193112

Zmora, N., Zeevi, D., Korem, T., Segal, E., & Elinav, E. (2019). Taking it personally: Personalized utilization of the human microbiome in health and disease. *Cell Host & Microbe*, *25*(2), 324–330. DOI: 10.1016/j.chom.2019.01.017 PMID: 30763539

Żółkiewicz, J., Marzec, A., Ruszczyński, M., & Feleszko, W. (2020). Postbiotics—A step beyond pre-and probiotics. *Nutrients*, *12*(8), 2189. DOI: 10.3390/nu12082189

Zommiti, M., Feuilloley, M. G. J., & Connil, N. (2020). Update of Probiotics in Human World: A Nonstop Source of Benefactions till the End of Time. *Microorganisms*, *8*(12), 1907. DOI: 10.3390/microorganisms8121907

Zuo, T., Zhang, F., Lui, G. C. Y., & Ng, S. C. (2021). Alterations in gut microbiota of patients with COVID-19 during time of hospitalization. *Gastroenterology*, *159*(3), 944–955. DOI: 10.1053/j.gastro.2020.05.048

About the Contributors

Neethu Asokan is a distinguished microbiologist, researcher, and educator with expertise in industrial microbiology, gut microbiome, microbial biotechnology, bioenergy, natural products and environmental microbiology. Currently serving as an Assistant Professor of Life Sciences at Sri Satya Sai University for Human Excellence (SSSUHE), India, she specializes in several areas of life sciences like biobutanol production from sago spent waste, focusing on fermentation optimization, pretreatment strategies, and economic feasibility. Her research extends into microbial and nano-biotechnology, bioremediation, algal biotechnology, and medical microbiology, including antibiotic resistance and psychomicrobiology. With a strong background in teaching and mentoring, she has guided multiple graduate students, supervised research projects, and contributed significantly to the scientific community through publications, book chapters, and patents. She is also an active member of various professional societies and has been recognized with multiple awards for her contributions. Passionate about sustainability and innovation, Dr. Neethu's work integrates scientific research with real-world applications to advance bioenergy, environmental sustainability, and microbial-based solutions for healthcare and agriculture.

Abdel Rahman Mohammad Said Al-Tawaha is a distinguished professor of plant ecophysiology at Al-Hussein Bin Talal University, Jordan. He earned his Ph.D. in Plant Science from McGill University, Canada. His research spans plant physiology, crop productivity, sustainable agriculture, and the use of natural elicitors for enhancing plant growth. He has published over 500 scholarly articles and books, with more than 7,000 citations. Dr. Al-Tawaha also serves as Editor-in-Chief of Advances in Environmental Biology and contributes extensively to international research collaborations and academic leadership. His work significantly advances the understanding of Mediterranean plant ecology and agricultural sustainability.

Santosh Kumar Singh is an Associate Professor and Head of the Department of Life Sciences at Sri Sathya Sai University for Human Excellence (SSSUHE) in Kalaburagi, Karnataka. He also serves as the university's IQAC Coordinator. Holding an M.Sc. and D.Phil in Life Sciences, Dr. Singh specializes in plant tissue culture, phytochemistry, molecular markers (RAPD, ISSR, AFLP), and antioxidant studies. His research prominently features medicinal plants, including species like Ocimum and Acmella oleracea. With over 40 publications and more than 550 citations, he actively mentors Ph.D. scholars and contributes to interdisciplinary research in plant biotechnology and conservation.

Rajeshwari Ullagaddi is an Assistant Professor in the Department of Life Sciences at Sri Sathya Sai University for Human Excellence (SSSUHE) in Kalaburagi, Karnataka. She specializes in phytochemistry, nutraceuticals, and functional foods, focusing on their roles in combating oxidative stress and promoting health. Her research includes studies on the antioxidant properties of medicinal plants like coriander, aniseed, and mulberry leaves. Dr. Ullagaddi has authored over 20 publications, with more than 700 citations, and has an h-index of 14. She actively contributes to interdisciplinary research in plant-based therapeutics and nutrition education.

***

Banzeer Ahsan Abbasi received her graduate degree in Botany from Quaid-i-Azam University, Islamabad, Pakistan. Dr. Banzeer is currently working as an Assistant Professor at Department of Botany, Rawalpindi Women University, Rawalpindi, Pakistan. She has published more than 60 research articles in various international journals and 10 chapters in reputed publishers (ELSIEVER, RSC and SPRINGER). Currently, she is supervising 2 Ph.D, 6 MPhil and 6 BS students. She has expertise in the synthesis of novel nanomaterials from medicinal plants and their multiple biological and envirnemental applications. Her research is also focusing on phytochemistry, natural products of medicinal plants and Phylogenetics. She has a very decent research background with research published in well-reputed journals with H-index 28, i-10 index 44 and overall citations 3317.

Renu Agarwal is currently serving as Assistant Professor and has been the Vice Principal and Director of the SDNB Centre for Skill Development from June 2023 - March 2025. She previously held the positions of Dean of Management Studies (2022–2023), Dean of New Age Sciences (2017–2022), and Head of Department (2013–2022) at SDNB Vaishnav College for Women, Chromepet, Chennai, Tamil Nadu. With a total of 17.5 years of teaching and research experience, including 12.5

years at SDNB, she has published over 50 research papers and articles in nationally and internationally reputed journals. Dr. Agarwal has supervised 34 postgraduate research projects, including 14 projects funded by SDNB Vaishnav College and 2 funded by TANSCST. She holds two patents and serves as a member of the Board of Studies for undergraduate and postgraduate syllabus revision at the University of Madras (academic years 2021–2024) and TNPSC. In addition to a distinguished academic and research career, she has demonstrated strong leadership qualities and received numerous awards and grants recognizing her exceptional performance. She also secured 5th place in the Tamil Nadu State Level Women's Chess Tournament in 2015.

Sameel Hassan is a researcher in the Department of Agriculture and Forest Sciences at the University of Tuscia, Italy, where he specializes in microbiome analysis, sustainable agriculture, and plant–microbe interactions. His work emphasizes the role of microbial metabolites in influencing plant nutrition, crop resilience, and human health, alongside studies on soil health, stress adaptation, and eco-friendly agricultural practices.

Radhika Kande is a results-driven Senior Cloud and DevOps Engineer with over 9 years of experience designing, automating, and optimizing cloud and infrastructure ecosystems across AWS, Azure, and hybrid enterprise environments. She specializes in building secure, scalable, and highly available architectures using Infrastructure as Code, Kubernetes, and CI/CD automation. Known for driving DevOps transformation, Radhika helps organizations enhance reliability, reduce operational risk, and accelerate software delivery. She excels at cross-functional collaboration, mentoring engineering teams, and implementing cost-efficient cloud solutions. Passionate about automation and innovation, she continuously leverages emerging cloud technologies to deliver impactful business outcomes.

Sumit Kushwaha is an Associate Professor in the Department of the Centre for Research and AI Development Learning Ecosystem (CRADLE) Cell at Chandigarh University Uttar Pradesh, Unnao, India. He is engaged in teaching, research, and academic leadership, with a focus on fostering innovation and research-oriented learning in the areas of artificial intelligence and emerging technologies. His professional contributions include mentoring researchers, promoting interdisciplinary collaboration, and supporting the development of a robust research culture aligned with the university's academic and innovation goals.

Saloua Mabsor-Zgandaoui holds a PhD in Cell Biology, Biotechnology, and Health from the Faculty of Sciences at Ibn Tofail University, Kenitra. Her doctoral research was conducted in collaboration with the National Centre for Nuclear Energy,

Science, and Technology (CNESTEN), where she investigated the enzymatic and molecular mechanisms of cellular response to ionizing radiation, contributing to advances in radiobiology and antioxidant defense strategies. She has authored several peer-reviewed publications and book chapters in internationally indexed platforms. Dr. Mabsor-Zgandaoui is currently an associate member of the Biology and Health Laboratory, Department of Biology, Faculty of Sciences, Ibn Tofail University, where she continues to develop research at the interface of molecular biology, biotechnology, and cellular stress responses.

T.C. Manjunath was born on 6th February 1967. He did his B.E. from RV College of Engg. in 1989 (B'lore Univ), M.E. in Robotics & Automation from Govt.'s LD College of Engg., (Gujarat Univ., Ahmedabad) in 1992 with FCD-First Rank & PhD in Systems & Control Engg. from IIT Bombay in the year 2007, got best research scholar award for the entire IITB. He is currently working as the Dean Research (R & D) and as Professor in Dept. of Computer Science & Engg. with specialization in IoT, Cyber Security, Blockchain Technology in Rajarajeswari College of Engineering, Bengaluru, Karnataka. He has got a teaching (academic), research & administrative experience of more than 35+ years (10 years as Principal & 8 years as HoD, 1 year as Dean Research & rest as faculty) and has published more than 1500+ research papers in various national & international journals & conferences, with 175+ patents, 100+ book-chapters, 25 awards, 100s of Keynote talks and also published 25 text books in various field of science, engineering & technology, completed projects worth Rs. 9 Crores till date & guided 10 PhD scholars in VTU. He is a member of 30 Professional Society Chapters and is a fellow of IE, IETE, AMIEE, Sr. Member of IEEE and a chartered engineer.

Anupama Mohabansi is an Assistant Professor in the Department of Electronics and Telecommunication Engineering at G. H. Raisoni College of Engineering and Management, Nagpur, Maharashtra (Postal Code: 440032). She has been serving at GHRCEMN for the past four years and brings a total teaching experience of 9.4 years. With her extensive academic exposure, she is actively involved in teaching, mentoring students, and contributing to the academic growth of the ETC department.

SaranrajP. holds a Ph.D. in Microbiology from Annamalai University, Chidambaram, India, and is NET (ASRB–ICAR) qualified in Microbiology. He is currently serving as Assistant Professor and Head, Department of Microbiology, at Sacred Heart College (Autonomous), Tirupattur, Tamil Nadu, India. Dr. Saranraj has over 15 years of research experience and 10 years of teaching experience in the fields of Environmental Microbiology, Agricultural Microbiology, Industrial Microbiology, Bioremediation, Microbial Biotechnology, and Sustainable

Ecosystem Management. His research work has focused on Microbial degradation of pollutants, Effluent treatment, Soil health improvement, Plant–microbe interactions, and Applied environmental sustainability. He has an extensive publication record, with more than 240 international research articles, over 90 books (international and national), and 70+ book chapters published with reputed academic publishers.

SelvakumarP. currently serves as an Associate Professor in the Department of Science and Humanities at Nehru Institute of Technology, Coimbatore, Tamil Nadu, India. With a teaching career spanning over a decade, he previously held positions as an Assistant Professor in the Department of Science and Humanities at various engineering colleges in Coimbatore from 2011 to 2023. Dr. P. Selvakumar's primary area of academic and research interest is phytochemistry, where he has made substantial contributions. His research credentials include 30 journal publications, 14 patents, and 25 conference papers. He has actively promoted faculty and student development by organizing 5 Faculty Development Programs (FDPs) and completing 3 NPTEL courses along with 60 Coursera certifications. His dedication to student success is evident in his role as a committed mentor, consistently guiding and supporting his students academically and personally. Recognized for his excellence in teaching, Dr. P. Selvakumar has received numerous accolades, including Best Teacher Awards. He is also an active member of MISTE (The Indian Society for Technical Education) and continues to play a vital role in both acade

P. Parthiban is an accomplished researcher in Biochemistry, Environmental Biotechnology, and Microbial Technology, with over ten years of experience in interdisciplinary research, innovation management, and analytical instrumentation. His work spans bioprocess development, wastewater and sludge valorization, microbial degradation pathways, nano-bioformulations, and phytochemical-based therapeutics. He has contributed to major DST and DRDO-funded projects exceeding 10 crore and has published 30+ peer-reviewed SCI/Scopus articles, reflecting a strong commitment to high-impact research. Dr. Parthiban is also an active innovator, holding 4 utility patents and 7 design patents, and his additional role as a Patent Analyst has strengthened his expertise in prior art search, patent drafting, and technology evaluation. His research aims to develop sustainable, scalable bioprocesses while bridging scientific discovery with societal and industrial applications.

LokeshS. is an academic professional serving as an Assistant Professor in the Department of Electronics and Communication Engineering at SRM Institute of Science and Technology. In his role, he is actively involved in teaching, mentoring students, and contributing to academic and institutional development. His academic engagement reflects a commitment to excellence in engineering education and the advancement of knowledge in the field of electronics and communication engineering.

T. Saminathan is an Assistant Professor in the Department of Electronics and Communication Engineering at SRM Institute of Science and Technology. He is actively involved in teaching, research, and academic development in the field of electronics and communication engineering. With a strong commitment to technical education and innovation, Dr. Saminathan contributes to mentoring students and advancing knowledge through his academic and research activities.

Sirikonda Shwetha is an Assistant Professor in the Department of Computer Science and Engineering at Sumathi Reddy Institute of Technology for Women, with more than 12 years of experience in academia. Her teaching and research interests include machine learning, deep learning, medical image analysis, and optimization techniques. She is actively engaged in developing intelligent systems with practical relevance.

Naresh Kumar S. is a Professor in the Department of Computer Science and Engineering at SR University, with over 21 years of academic experience. His expertise includes deep learning, machine learning, medical image analysis, and optimization techniques, and his research focuses on developing efficient intelligent systems for real-world applications

Rakesh Kumar Yadav is affiliated with KU Leuven, Belgium. His research integrates molecular biology, metagenomics, microbiome analysis, and translational biomedical sciences, with a focus on understanding microbial community dynamics across environmental and host-associated systems. His scholarly work spans environmental microbiomes, gut microbiota studies, genomic surveillance, microbial enzyme discovery, and bioinformatic analysis, reflecting a translational approach that links basic molecular research with applications in health, ecology, and biotechnology.

Tabassum Yaseen obtained his M.Sc. and M.Phil and Ph.D degree in Botany from Department of Botany University of Peshawar, Pakistan. Dr. Yaseen is currently working as an Assistant Professor and Chairperson of the Department at Bacha Khan University, Charsadda, Pakistan. Her research group is involved in vesicular arbuscular mycorrhizal fungi, synthesis of nanoparticles from medicinal plants for biomedical and environmental applications. She has published more than 83 research articles in various journals of international repute, and is a co-author of several book chapters

Wajeeha Zarwa holds an M.Phil. in Plant Sciences from Quaid-i-Azam University, Islamabad, with research focused on plant biochemistry, microbial interactions, and biofuel development. She has co-authored multiple publications and contributed to international research on sustainable environmental solutions.

Index

A

B

D

E

F

G

H

I

L

M

T

V

W

www.ingramcontent.com/pod-product-compliance
Lightning Source LLC
LaVergne TN
LVHW061532290926
849162LV00004B/764